Cataract Surgery in Complicated Cases

Lucio Buratto, MD
Centro Ambrosiano Oftalmico
Milan, Italy

Stephen F. Brint, MD, FACS
Associate Clinical Professor of Ophthalmology
Tulane University School of Medicine
New Orleans, Louisiana

Luigi Caretti, MD
Chief Consultant
UOC (Complex Operative Unit)
Eye Department of ULSS 16 Health Trust
Padua, Italy

CRC Press
Taylor & Francis Group
Boca Raton London New York

CRC Press is an imprint of the
Taylor & Francis Group, an **informa** business

Illustrations courtesy of Massimiliano Crespi and Lucio Burrato.

First published 2013 by SLACK Incorporated

Published 2024 by CRC Press
2385 NW Executive Center Drive, Suite 320, Boca Raton FL 33431

and by CRC Press
4 Park Square, Milton Park, Abingdon, Oxon, OX14 4RN

CRC Press is an imprint of Taylor & Francis Group, LLC

Library of Congress Cataloging-in-Publication Data

Buratto, Lucio.
Cataract surgery in complicated cases / Lucio Buratto, Stephen Brint, Luigi Caretti.
; cm.
Rev. ed. of: Cataract surgery in complicated cases, c2000.
Includes bibliographical references and index.

ISBN 978-1-61711-607-0 (hardback : alk. paper)
I. Brint, Stephen F., 1946- II. Caretti, Luigi. III. Cataract surgery in complicated cases. IV. Title.
[DNLM: 1. Cataract Extraction. WW 260]

617.7'42059--dc23
2012039642

ISBN: 9781617116070 (hbk)
ISBN: 9781003522904 (ebk)

DOI: 10.1201/9781003522904

Dedication

To my little grandchildren, Bianca, Achille, and Kaito.

Lucio Buratto, MD

To Mark and those who have taught me cataract surgery through the years.

Stephen F. Brint, MD, FACS

To my father and my mother.

Luigi Caretti, MD

Contents

Dedication ... *iii*
Acknowledgments ... *v*
About the Authors ... *vi*
Introduction ... *vii*

Chapter 1 Pediatric Cataract ... 1
Chapter 2 Congenital Subluxation of the Crystalline Lens ... 11
Chapter 3 Cataract and Glaucoma ... 27
Chapter 4 Pseudoexfoliation Syndrome ... 59
Chapter 5 Phacoemulsification With a Small Pupil ... 77
Chapter 6 Cataract Surgery in Age-Related Macular Degeneration ... 93
Chapter 7 Brunescent Cataract ... 99
Chapter 8 Cataract in High Myopia ... 105
Chapter 9 Cataract in Severe Hyperopia ... 111
Chapter 10 Cataract in Retinitis Pigmentosa ... 117
Chapter 11 Cataract Surgery in Patients With Uveitis ... 121
Chapter 12 Floppy Iris Syndrome ... 131
Chapter 13 Management of Cataract in Diabetic Patients ... 141
Chapter 14 Role of Vitreoretinal Surgery in Cataract Surgery ... 149
Chapter 15 Traumatic Cataract ... 155
Chapter 16 Cataract in Aniridic Eyes and Other Iris Defects ... 169
Chapter 17 Cataract and Corneal Pathology ... 177
Chapter 18 Cataract Surgery Following Implantation of a Phakic Intraocular Lens ... 203
Chapter 19 Secondary Intraocular Lens Implants in Eyes With or Without Capsular Support ... 213
Chapter 20 Intraocular Lens Explantation and Replacement ... 231

Index ... *247*

Acknowledgments

Publishing a book is a very exhausting task. There is an incredible amount of work involved. All this would not have been possible without the smooth-running organization and help of a number of people who I would now like to thank personally: Luigi Caretti, with his surgical knowledge and his clinical background, contributed to the highly scientific content of this book. My sincere appreciation to Steve Brint for his invaluable contribution, his scientific skill, and for supervision of the English translation. My sincere thanks goes to Massimiliano Crespi, the artist who realized all the magnificent drawings and particularly for his ability to transfer the author's thoughts onto paper; also Salvatore Ferrandes, who was responsible for the clinical iconographic portions. I also would like to thank the staff of Medicongress Camo, in particular Monica Gingardi, for the organizational and operational support provided. My translator, Fiona Johnston for her precise and accurate translation of the Italian texts. Many thanks also to Vittorio Picardo, a warm friend, for supervision of the final text in Italian and AISO (Accademia Italiana di Scienze Oftalmologiche) for the scientific support and grant for the publication of this work. Finally I would like to thank SLACK Incorporated, my publisher, for asking me to produce a new book on cataract surgery.

Lucio Buratto, MD

About the Authors

Lucio Buratto, MD, is a leading international expert in cataract and myopia surgery and a pioneer in ocular techniques, intraocular lens (IOL) implantation, in the phacoemulsification procedure for the cataract, and in laser techniques for myopia, astigmatism, and hyperopia. In 1978, he began using the Kelman phacoemulsification technique and in 1979, started using posterior chamber IOLs. Since 1980, he has organized and presided over 48 updating congresses on the cataract and glaucoma surgeries and on laser therapy, has taken part as spokesman and teacher for more than 400 courses and congresses, and has organized 54 practical courses for the teaching of eye surgery. In 1989, he presented the excimer laser intrastromal keratomileusis, and was the first surgeon in the world to use it, while concurrently he started to treat low myopia using PRK techniques. In 1995, he was appointed Monitor of the US Food and Drug Administration (FDA). In 1996, he was the first surgeon in the world to use the Down-Up LASIK technique that improved the previous LASIK procedure for the correction of myopia and for which he holds a USA patent. For teaching purposes, he has performed surgical operations during live surgery sessions for more than 200 international and Italian congresses and has performed surgery during satellite broadcasts to 54 countries on 4 different continents. He has designed and produced 143 instruments for ocular surgery. In 2004, he was a speaker at the Binkhorst Medal Lecture during the XXII Annual Meeting of the European Society of Cataract and Refractive Surgeons (ESCRS; Paris, France) and was the first European surgeon to use the new Intralase laser for refractive surgery. In 2011, he was the first western European surgeon to use the Femtosecond laser for cataract surgery.

Dr. Buratto has been published in more than 125 scientific publications and 59 monographs (of which 24 are on cataract surgery, 5 are on glaucoma surgery, and 11 are on myopia). Recent works include *Phakic IOLs: State of the Art*, *LASIK: The Evolution of Refractive Surgery*, and *PPRK: The Past, Present, and Future of Surface Ablation.*

Stephen F. Brint, MD, FACS, was the first physician in the United States to perform the LASIK procedure in June 1991, after working with Dr. Lucio Buratto in Milan to perfect the technique. He was the Medical Monitor of the first US FDA LASIK study and has been a lead investigator for both the Alcon Custom Cornea LASIK procedure as well as the Medical Monitor for all of the US FDA Wavelight Allegretto Wavefront Optimized and Custom studies. He graduated from Tulane University School of Medicine, New Orleans, Louisiana, and completed his residency there as well in 1977, and continues to serve as Associate Clinical Professor of Ophthalmology. In addition to his vast LASIK experience of over 30,000 LASIK procedures, many with the Intralase All Laser LASIK technique, he is a renowned cataract/lens surgeon, having participated in the US FDA clinical trials of the new IOLs including the ReSTOR, ReZoom, and toric IOLs.

Dr. Brint is Board Certified by the American Board of Ophthalmology and a Fellow of the American College of Surgeons. He has been recognized as "The Best Doctor in New Orleans" by *New Orleans Magazine* for the last 10 years and has been selected by his peers for the 2000 to 2012 editions of *The Best Doctors in America.* He is a leading cataract surgeon and instructor and the author of the 3 definitive textbooks on LASIK and cataract surgery including the most recent *Custom LASIK.*

Dr. Brint performs surgery and lectures around the world, including Europe, Russia, China, Japan, Australia, Singapore, Africa, and South America.

Dr. Brint has a passion for education and research, and, most recently, has been involved with the refinement of the intraoperative aberrometer for selecting IOL power and femtosecond laser-assisted cataract surgery.

Luigi Caretti, MD, is the Chief Consultant at UOC (Complex Operative Unit) in the Eye Department of ULSS 16 Health Trust in Padua, Italy.

He has considerable experience in surgery of the anterior and posterior segments and associated ocular structures; as primary surgeon, he has performed more than 5000 surgical procedures. He manages the Vitreo-Retinal Surgery Department of UOC (Complex Operative Unit) in the Eye Department in Padua. He has published 12 scientific articles in national and international journals. He has been appointed Director of Vitreo Retinal Surgery in the UOS of ULSS 16 of Padua.

Introduction

During my professional life, I have published many books on cataract surgery; taking into account the foreign language editions, there are 24.

Atlas of Intraocular Lenses, published in 1984, was the first Italian work to introduce the world of modern intraocular lenses to Italian ophthalmologists. The last, *Phacoemulsification: Principles and Techniques,* published with Stephen Brint by my American publisher SLACK Incorporated in 2003, was an internationally acclaimed work that has provided important information covering the entire operative procedure; this work is still being used today.

Now, almost 10 years later, I am publishing 5 new works on cataract surgery with the help of 5 promising, young ophthalmologists.

The first of this series to be published with Mario Romano is *Cataract Surgery Complications*, about the difficult subject of intra- and postoperative complications, their prevention, and treatment.

The next volume is *Cataract Surgery in Complicated Cases*, with Luigi Caretti, on the surgery of complicated cases—another topic of great interest.

Finally, a three-part series titled *Cataract Surgery*, with each part addressing a different topic. Part 1, with Laura Sacchi, deals with patient preparation and the initial part of the operation. Part 2, with Rosalia Sorce, addresses phacoemulsification. Part 3, with Domenico Boccuzzi, addresses intraocular lenses.

With all those books there is the invaluable contribution of Stephen Brint, a renowned cataract surgeon and a very good friend of mine.

I hope that these books will be useful and will constitute a source for teaching and consultation for all eye surgeons lasting many years, resulting in continuous improvement.

Lucio Buratto, MD

1

Pediatric Cataract

The congenital cataract can be described as an opacity of the lens, present at birth in one or both eyes. Due to its potential inhibitory effect on sight development, it is considered the world's greatest cause of pediatric blindness, affecting Third World countries in particular.[1]

There are a number of factors that contribute to the management difficulties of the congenital cataract, even though surgery used to correct this defect has improved considerably over the past 30 years. In these cases, the most important factor is the young patient's age; the operation should be performed very early in the first months of life. This will avoid the onset of amblyopia from sight deprivation even though the literature reports statistically significant increase in complications with surgery performed earlier than 2 months of life. Consequently, it is recommended to wait until the patient is at least 3 months old. Management of the pediatric cataract is completely different from an adult for a number of different reasons. Surgery in very young patients is challenging to say the least; the tissues of a child's eye react in a completely different way from adult tissue. This means that the anterior segment surgeon has to use a number of unique maneuvers.

A good outcome requires absolute precision in every step of surgery; having said that, late complications may develop with even the most successful surgery, and these may lead to a poor anatomical and functional result. Also these eyes may be affected by ocular anomalies that could jeopardize the outcome of the operation (eg, miosis, capsular, zonular, iris, and angle anomalies) and greatly increase the degree of difficulty.

In several scientific studies, even when the sample group has not been randomized,[2-5] a good clinical outcome has been achieved when the treatment is performed within the first 2 months of life (even though there is a much higher risk of complications), without the implantation of an intraocular lens (IOL), and accompanied by a prolonged and optimal optical correction, intensive occlusive therapy, and good compliance of the family. It has been demonstrated that if surgery can be postponed until the patient has reached his or her first birthday, the postoperative results will be better because of greater ease and a lower incidence of postoperative complications. It is also important that the young patient be supervised long-term by a pediatric ophthalmologist with considerable experience in this area. Contact lenses can be used if necessary, if an IOL has not been implanted. However, in the majority of cases, the intermediate option of operating when the child is between the ages of 3 and 7 months is usually the most appropriate.

The Preoperative Examination

Given that congenital cataract is sometimes associated with genetic syndromes, metabolic disorders, intrauterine infections, and ocular conditions with associated anomalies of the iris and the angle, it is advisable that the preoperative examination by the pediatric ophthalmologist follows that of the pediatrician. Through genetic tests, the pediatrician will be able to classify whether the specific case is a syndrome that affects other organs or systems of the newborn; a negative work-up will confirm the diagnosis of an isolated congenital cataract (ie, a child who is clinically healthy and an absence of infections affecting the mother and fetus during pregnancy). In this case, the family history can indicate whether there have been other cases in the same family and provide an opportunity to construct a model of hereditary transmission (through a dominant, or more infrequently, a recessive gene). If the condition is hereditary, the ophthalmologist and the pediatrician will inform the child's parents of the risks that may affect other pregnancies, depending on the mode of gene transmission

Buratto L, Brint SF, Caretti L.
Cataract Surgery in Complicated Cases (pp 1-10).

and the consequent likelihood of the congenital cataract being expressed in successive pregnancies.

Compared to bilateral cataracts, the unilateral congenital cataract affects vision to a lesser degree because it is not as common; however, it is more frequently associated with other ocular anomalies and the management of the resulting amblyopia is much more difficult.[6,7]

When the doctor examines a child with a congenital cataract, he or she will have to take the age of the patient into consideration. The newborn or young child will not be able to cooperate and this will prevent complete diagnosis; it is much easier to fully examine and evaluate the visual acuity of an older child. When examining a young patient suspected of having a cataract, the first step is to check the presence of the red reflex of the fundus with direct ophthalmoscopy; the cataract will often have greater density at the center and appear to be less significant following pupillary dilatation. If the cataract affects the whole lens, the diagnosis will be facilitated by the characteristic white color seen in the pupil (leucocoria).

Ideally the child should be sedated or under narcosis (indicated for newborns); this will allow detailed observation of the morphology of the cataract and may be indicative of the visual acuity. The complete examination of the globe in children, particularly very young ones, almost always necessitates sedation or general anesthesia. Both eyes should be examined under mydriasis to identify associated malformations.

An important prognostic sign is nystagmus, which appears in the first 2 to 3 months of life. The postoperative visual result may be affected by the persistence of fetal blood vessels or other anomalies of the posterior segment that can be identified by indirect ophthalmoscopy, as long as the transparency of the ocular tissues permits. Strabismus is often present in patients with unilateral cataracts. This may not be obvious until there is irreversible amblyopia. The corneal diameter and the intraocular pressure are also very important measurements and can be performed using the ICare device (ICare Finland, Oy, Finland).

The surgeon must also check the patient's ability to fixate on an immobile object or follow a moving object; the parents will often be asked to assist in these tests. If possible, visual function should be evaluated using the Teller acuity card (Stereo Optical Co, Inc, Chicago, IL). In patients with a unilateral cataract, visual function may not be compromised; in these cases, it may appear much later than in cases with bilateral cataracts. By its very nature, as this type of evaluation necessitates the cooperation of the young patients, an appropriate age must be reached before the examination can be performed.

Finally, the surgeon must calculate the power of the IOL he or she wishes to implant. The axial length and the corneal curvature are essential measurements in this calculation. It should be remembered that in the eyes of children with pathological congenital cataract, the axial length and the corneal diameter are usually shorter than in healthy controls.

The Timing of Surgery

One highly debated issue is the optimal timing of the cataract extraction.[8] The prognosis is impacted by the functional condition of the eye prior to surgery, the timing of the operation, and subsequent visual rehabilitation. The timing is determined largely by the density of the cataract and whether the cataract is uni- or bilateral.

In the event that the opacity of the crystalline lens is zonular, and particularly when the condition is bilateral, the surgeon should postpone the operation. Under those specific conditions, the patient will have a certain amount of sight as the clouded vision caused by the cataract is symmetrical and of moderate severity. Consequently, it is advisable to postpone surgery until the patient reaches an age suitable for the implantation of an IOL. The patient must be closely monitored by a pediatric ophthalmologist. If the evaluation of the patient's sight indicates the ability to fixate on a fixed object, the doctor must keep the patient under close observation and record any changes.

However, in the case of total bilateral cataracts, if visual function is reduced significantly in both eyes, even when the reduction is symmetrical, the development of the patient's vision may be impaired in both eyes and the surgeon should intervene early. Both eyes should be operated during the same surgical session, using different instrument sets (even though this will not provide information on the clinical outcome of the refractive result on the first eye operated). Prior to 3 months of age, implantation of an IOL should be avoided (spectacles or contact lenses are safer options); the implantation can be performed at a later stage when the child is older and his or her ocular development is complete. In the event of a total unilateral cataract, which induces severe amblyopia, early surgical intervention is one of the most important factors that influences good functional outcome.

The timing of the operation is greatly affected by the patient's age. In infants younger than 2 months there may be problems with anesthesia, the operation is more difficult, and implantation of an IOL is impossible. Between 2 and 6 months is the optimal timing for operating bilateral congenital cataracts. Between 6 months and 2 years, the operation is easier and the calculation of the IOL power will be more accurate (Table 1-1).

The Operation

Cataract surgery on a child differs from that on an adult primarily because it must be performed under general anesthesia.

Table 1-1.

Age at Surgery

• Below 2 months: There are problems with anesthesia, problems with the operation, insertion of an intraocular lens is impossible
• 2 to 6 months: The optimal period for operating bilateral congenital cataracts
• 6 months to 2 years: Everything, including the calculation of the IOL power, is easier

Mydriasis can be achieved with an association of diclofenac, tropicamide, and phenylephrine. Phenylephrine can have systemic effects, and for this reason it is avoided (or used sparingly in cases of insufficient mydriasis).

Surgical Technique

The majority of surgeons believe that a posterior capsulotomy and an anterior vitrectomy are essential to achieve a transparent visual axis. Two approaches have been described: anterior with corneal or sclerocorneal access and posterior via pars plana.

Anterior Approach

The surgeon creates a corneal or sclerocorneal tunnel in a superior or temporal position, depending on the surgeon's personal preference. If the pupil is small, prior to the capsulorrhexis, Grieshaber flexible iris retractors (Alcon Laboratories Inc, Forth Worth, TX) should be used or the surgeon may consider pupil stretching or the insertion of dilation rings.

Staining the anterior capsule with vital dyes (0.1% trypan blue) is always useful. The undiluted dye is injected into the anterior chamber, ensuring that it stains the anterior surface of the crystalline lens.

Any excess is removed by irrigation to provide better visualization of the capsule and allow a safer, more controlled manipulation of the edge of the flap (also refer to Chapter 15).

The anterior chamber, often shallow, is expanded by filling with a dispersive viscoelastic substance (VES; DuoVisc [Alcon Laboratories Inc]) or a high molecular weight pseudoadaptive VES (Healon 5 [Abbott Laboratories, Abbott Park, IL]). This will push the anterior capsule backwards and flatten it; there will be less tendency for escape during the creation of the rhexis.

The intact capsular bag is punctured with a 26-gauge cystotome at the beginning of the continuous anterior capsulorrhexis to effectively open the anterior capsule, a very resistant, thick, elastic structure in children (Figure 1-1). The rhexis must be gently guided with capsulorrhexis forceps. This instrument has been designed requiring small successive grasps of the capsule to achieve a progressive extension of the capsulotomy with limited possibilities of escape peripherally. It is extremely important that the capsulorrhexis is kept small because it will expand spontaneously due to the intrinsic elasticity of the tissue. If there is excessive expansion or there is an escape toward the zonules, the surgeon can inject additional VES into the anterior chamber to push the lens backwards and permit better control of the capsulorrhexis.

If the cataract is intumescent, once the capsular bag has been punctured with the cystotome, a white fluid may appear in the anterior chamber. This cortical milk can be aspirated (ideally using a fine cannula mounted on a syringe to remove the milky liquid without aspirating any of the VES, and avoiding an uncontrolled opening of the capsular bag); alternately, pseudoadaptive VES (Healon 5) can be used to plug the continuous capsulotomy prior to completing the rhexis.

Hydrodissection must always be performed with maximum caution and only when the surgeon is certain that the capsulotomy is continuous. This procedure should be the first one-half followed by the other because with posterior polar cataracts, these maneuvers could create posterior capsular rupture (in the event of total cataract, the evaluation of posterior opacity is difficult) with loss of lens material into the vitreous.

Hydrodissection is strongly recommended because it is the key step for the complete removal of the equatorial epithelial cells. Nevertheless, some authors believe that hydrodissection is unnecessary.

Depending on the density of the cataract, the lens material can be removed with the ultrasound phaco tip or the irrigation/aspiration (I/A) tip, given that the cataract is always soft.

We would recommend the use of moderate phaco levels even though the use of the ultrasound is rarely necessary; normally, the surgeon will reduce the power levels of the ultrasound, leaving the values of aspiration and vacuum unchanged.

The bimanual I/A technique is particularly useful in this type of surgery. If the nucleus is soft, the surgeon can avoid the use of an ultrasound tip and aspirate using a 0.5-mm cannula to remove the nucleus (with vacuum levels between 100 and 150 and a flow rate of between 20 and 28). For the removal of the cortex, a 0.3-mm cannula should be used (with vacuum levels between 200 and 300 and a flow rate of between 20 and 28).

Complete removal of the nucleus is essential to avoid postoperative inflammation. Another important step is the accurate removal of the anterior subcapsular epithelium, which reduces the risk of visual axis opacification (VAO) postoperatively.

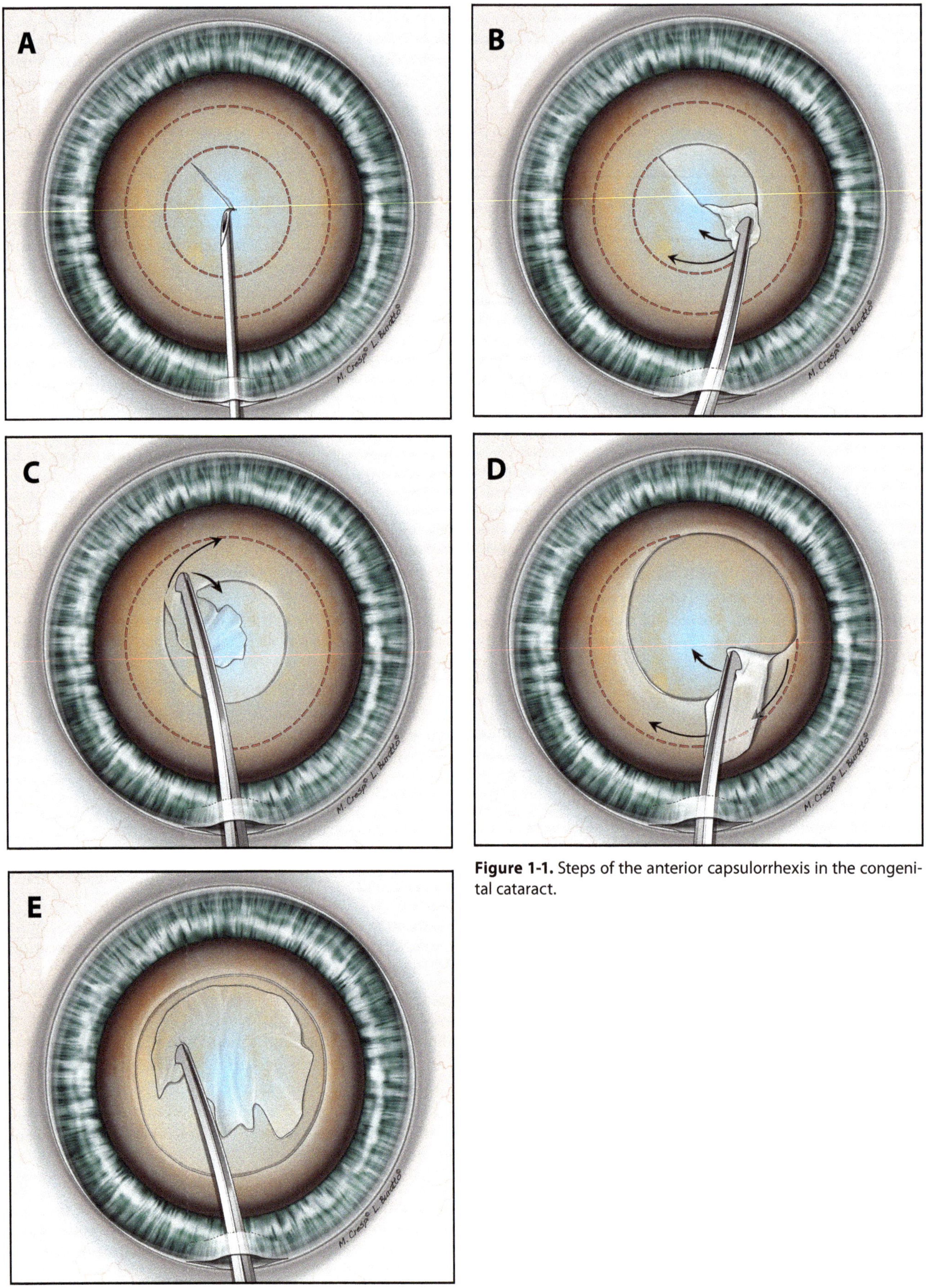

Figure 1-1. Steps of the anterior capsulorrhexis in the congenital cataract.

The surgeon then proceeds with a posterior capsulorrhexis, which is essential in all cases. It must be circular, continuous, and concentric to the anterior one. It allows access to the anterior vitreous and obviously avoids secondary opacification of the posterior capsule.

A small quantity of high viscosity VES is injected into the anterior chamber and into the capsular bag to flatten the posterior capsule or at the point that it is slightly concave. The posterior capsule is perforated with a needle mounted on a syringe of the adhesive viscoelastic, and a bubble of VES is injected between the posterior capsule and the hyaloid membrane to push back the vitreous. At this point, forceps are used to perform the posterior capsulorrhexis, which must be circular, continuous, and concentric to the anterior one and approximately 4 mm in diameter. At the end of the I/A procedure and prior to the injection of VES, the surgeon may decide to inject a small quantity of trypan blue onto the posterior capsule, washing off the excess before injecting the VES; this increases the levels of safety and control of the posterior rhexis. However, it should be remembered that it is easier to determine the diameter of the posterior rhexis without using VES inside the posterior capsule. During this maneuver, the surgeon must pay maximum attention to avoid rupturing the posterior capsule as this could jeopardize the integrity of the capsular bag. Following the correct completion of a posterior capsulotomy, the surgeon must check for and remove any persistent fetal vessels or adhesions to the posterior capsule and the retina.

At this point, the surgeon should perform an anterior vitrectomy, which is automated dry for the most part and small in size to avoid tertiary opacification (Figure 1-2). A dry coaxial vitrectomy is preferable; the infusion line is clamped by the fingers and can be released temporarily if it is necessary to re-expand the anterior chamber. In the event the surgeon uses new 20-gauge vitrectomy probes, the parameters used are normally 5000 cuts, 200 aspiration, and infusion 30 to 35 mm HG.

Recent literature[8,9] has demonstrated that anterior vitrectomy and capture of the IOL optic in the posterior capsulotomy reduce the frequency of VAO. Some surgeons suggest an anterior vitrectomy and a posterior capsulotomy following the implantation of the IOL. This may facilitate the implantation of the IOL in the bag; however, the posterior capsulotomy is more difficult due to the obstruction caused by the optic and the fact that the haptics increase the tension on the posterior capsule, increasing the possibility of escape.

Three articles[10-12] compare different primary surgical procedures to prevent VAO in cataract surgery with implantation of an IOL. Posterior capsulotomy alone is an adequate technique to prevent VAO, except when it is used in slightly older children. Anterior vitrectomy and posterior capsulotomy are considered to be necessary until the child is 5 years of age. Vitrectomy is optional between 5 and 8 years, as shown in recent literature.[10-13]

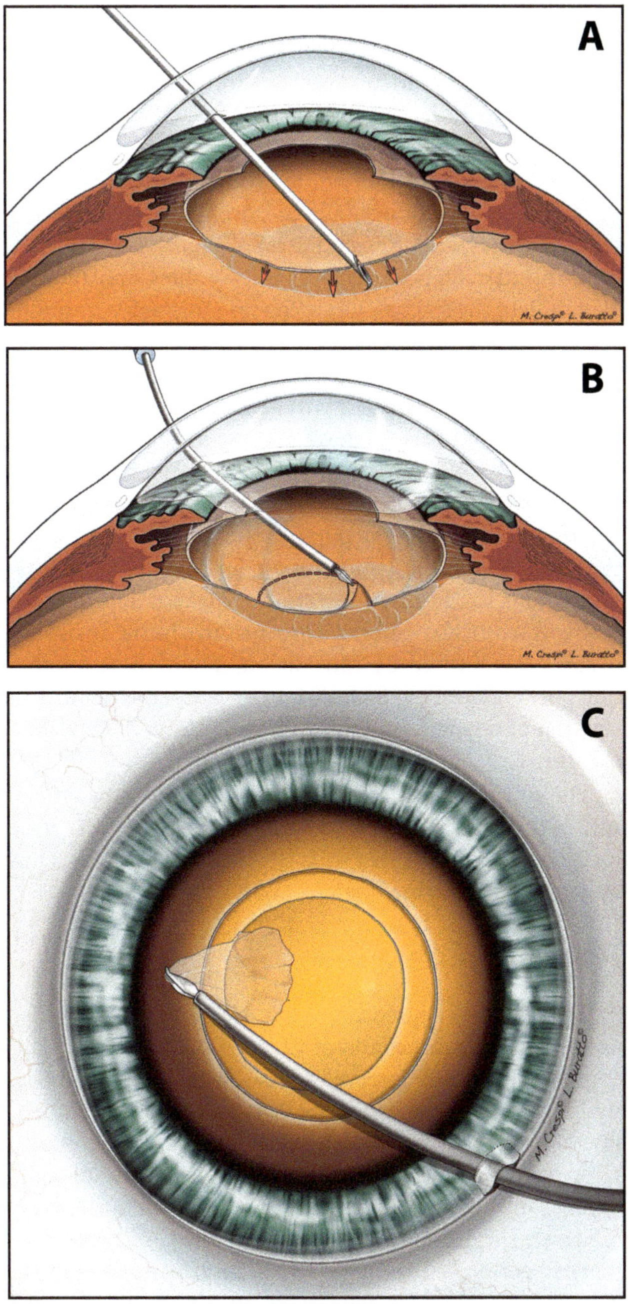

Figure 1-2. Posterior capsulorrhexis. (A) Injection of VES between the posterior capsule and the anterior hyaloid. (B) Initial phase of the posterior capsulorrhexis. (C) Completion of the posterior capsulorrhexis.

With an intact anterior and posterior rhexis, an IOL should be implanted when the corneal diameter is greater than 10 mm and the axial length greater than 17 mm—dimensions seen in children approximately 1 year of age (implantation is difficult below these values).

Regarding the type of IOL to be implanted, the 3-piece IOL, hydrophobic acrylic with an optic diameter 6.0 mm and overall length 13 mm, is most appropriate due to the particular position of the implant itself. It should be injected to minimize the size of the incision.

Implantation of an IOL inside the capsular bag (the technique used in adult patients) leads to a rapid and virtually inevitable VAO. Consequently, the prevention of posterior capsular opacity has an enormous effect on the results of congenital cataract surgery.

If the surgeon decides not to proceed with insertion of the IOL, the operation should prepare the eye for safe secondary implantation (posterior capsulotomy, leaving sufficient capsular support that will at least allow implantation of an IOL in the sulcus). The secondary implant is normally performed when the child is older. Surgical trauma and risk of VAO are lower if the patient is left aphakic. However, with aphakia, posterior synechiae form systematically, which increase difficulties with the secondary implant.

Regardless of whether the surgeon decides to implant an IOL or not, acetylcholine is injected into the anterior chamber to constrict the pupil. If the pupil constricts and the pupil is round, the surgeon can be certain that there is no vitreous in the anterior chamber. Moreover, if vitreous is suspected in the anterior chamber and in the incisions, it can be identified by introducing a spatula through a side port and moving it along the surface of the pupil. Any traction or changes in the pupil will indicate the presence of vitreous.

The softness and elasticity of the sclera induce poor closure of the surgical wounds; consequently, all of the corneal incisions must be sutured with 10-0 nylon. These block any leakage from even the smallest wounds.

Posterior Approach

The posterior approach is rarely used today, and avoided unless there is a concomitant vitreoretinal pathology. This approach is usually reserved for cases of a cataract that is subluxated (with rupture of more than half of the zonular fibers) or luxated (as can happen in rare cases of congenital syndromes such as Marfan's, Weill-Marchesani, and Ehler-Danlos, or in sporadic cases). This technique induces moderate surgical trauma. A pars plana/pars plicata vitrectomy is performed through 2 to 3 20-gauge sclerotomies, positioned 3 mm from the limbus. In the event 2 sclerotomies are used, the one at 2 o'clock is used for the cannula that introduces balanced salt solution (BSS), and the one positioned at 10 o'clock is used for the insertion of the vitrectomy probe, following a 4- to 5-mm opening of the Tenons conjunctiva complex. The 20-gauge needle used for the sclerotomy penetrates the crystalline lens to create an access route for the vitrectomy probe. The posterior capsule and the cataractous material are completely removed; a central anterior capsulotomy is performed without removing the instruments from the eye. If the surgeon decides to implant an IOL during the primary surgery, he or she must create a scleral tunnel. The IOL is inserted in the ciliary sulcus with the residual anterior capsule acting as the support. In the event support is insufficient, as in the cases of luxated or subluxated cataracts, the surgeon proceeds with lens implantation using scleral or iris fixation techniques.

At the end of surgery, it is essential that the surgeon verify the total absence of vitreous from the anterior chamber and the incision. At the end of surgery, the sclerotomies are sutured with 8-0 Vicryl (Ethicon Inc, Cornelia, GA). A conjunctival suture is not needed.

The Intraocular Lens

An IOL should always be implanted because it provides constant optical correction and can limit the onset of amblyopia. It should always be routinely implanted in patients surgically treated for congenital cataract, as a primary or secondary implant. However, there is not agreement on the best types, position, material, and in particular, the exact dioptric power of the IOL. Implantation of an IOL should be obligatory, and the lens should be inserted in infants 2 to 3 months of age if the dimensions of the globe are suitable. There are problems with an implant in very small infants if the globe is small, with a corneal diameter of between 9.5 and 10 mm and an axial length of less than 17 mm.

How and Where to Position the Intraocular Lens

There are a number of different options[8]:

- Haptic in the bag and the optic behind the posterior rhexis (Gimbel's technique)
- Haptic in the bag and optic in the bag
- Haptic in the bag and optic in front of the anterior rhexis
- Haptic in the sulcus and optic behind the anterior rhexis
- Haptic in the sulcus and the optic in front of the noncontinuous anterior capsulotomy

The insertion of an IOL is an extremely critical surgical step because the position of the lens must be stable. Gimbel and DeBroff[14] suggested an implantation technique with the haptics in the capsular bag and the optic behind the posterior rhexis, which should have a diameter of approximately 4 mm, smaller than the diameter of the optic to prevent it moving forward in the bag (Figure 1-3). Apart from stability of the implant, this technique has several advantages: reduction of inflammatory phenomena caused by the absence of contact between vitreous and aqueous and further blockage of secondary membranes that may be responsible for amblyopia. The contact between the anterior and posterior capsules will seal the capsular bag with formation of Sommering's ring and will keep the visual axis clear. If the anterior capsulotomy is not complete,

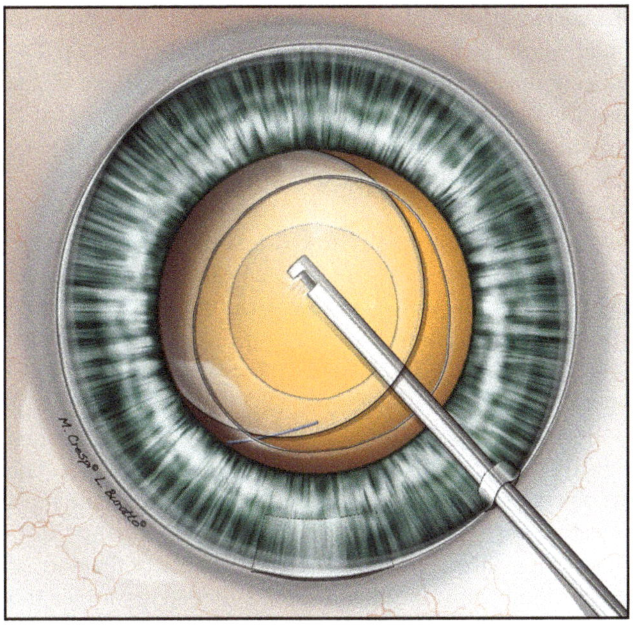

Figure 1-3. Dry vitrectomy behind the IOL optic with high viscosity VES in the anterior chamber.

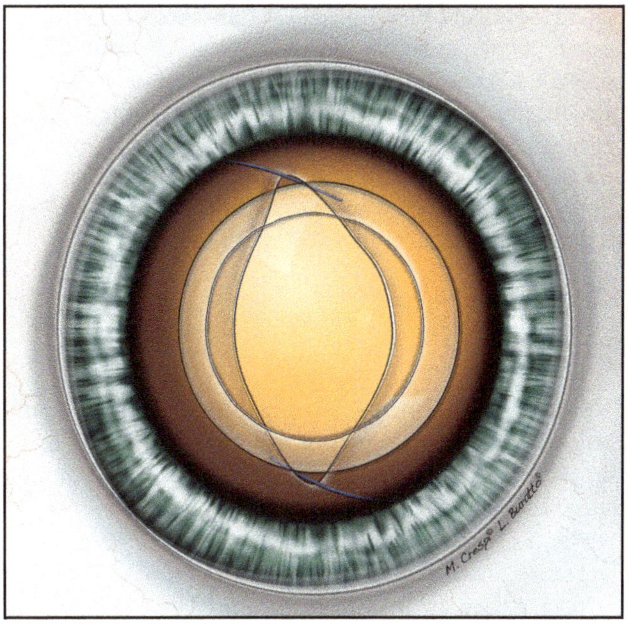

Figure 1-4. Posterior capsulorrhexis with capture of the IOL optic.

the surgeon should place the optic of the IOL behind the posterior capsulorrhexis to reduce the risk of postoperative decentration.

Between the haptics and the optic of the 3-piece acrylic IOL, there is a small spot that, compared to the one-piece IOL, will create greater adhesion of the capsule around the loops. Moreover, a posterior capsulorrhexis that is just slightly smaller than the optic may make it possible to capture the optic but will not prevent the migration of lenticular epithelial cells and the formation of Elschnig pearls (Figure 1-4).

Following implantation, VES in front of the IOL must be completely removed to avoid any increase in the postoperative intraocular pressure.

Surgery performed after 1 year of age produces better results; an IOL implant is recommended, and treatment of complications is easier. However, in patients of this age, prevention of amblyopia is less successful. As mentioned before, the IOL is easier to implant when the corneal diameter is greater than 10 mm and the axial length is greater than 17 mm (below these values, implantation is difficult); these dimensions are usually seen when the child approaches 1 year of age.

Given that amblyopia from sight deprivation is the main problem associated with unilateral cataract, the surgeon should aim for emmetropia. As refraction changes considerably during the early years of life (in particular, the axial length increases significantly until the child is 2 years old, then slows down and stabilizes when the child is between 8 and 10 years; the corneal curvature decreases with age and stabilizes at around 1 year of age), the eye becomes myopic. There are a number of surgical options that can be significantly in the management of this. To compensate for the myopia, which inevitably appears with age, the surgeon would be advised to aim for hyperopia during surgery (when the patient is below 8 years of age), which will vary depending on the patient's age at the time of surgery. The final outcome will be emmetropia or mild myopia. Even with bilateral cataracts, the optimal solution is to reach emmetropia in adulthood. It stands to reason that with emmetropia, as the child develops, the ophthalmologist will prescribe spectacles for near vision or bifocals if the patient has other forms of ametropia. The choice of power of the IOL is still a subject of debate and it is necessary to take a number of factors into consideration: axial length, family refractive history (myopic or hyperopic), and the age of the child. Dahan and Drusedau[15] proposed a series of guidelines that are useful for determining the power of the IOL, but which do not guarantee absolute precision. Numerous formulas to calculate the power of pediatric IOLs have been suggested; however, there is no consensus of opinion in the literature as to which is the most accurate, due to the individual child's growth curve and the consequent refractive variations in the tiny eye.[8] In a recent study,[16] it was demonstrated that the accuracy of the Sanders-Retzlaff-Kraff formula (SRK-II) is superimposable on that of the Pediatric IOL Calculator (ie, a modification of the SRK-II according to the Holladay algorithm, evaluated 3 months after cataract surgery with a primary IOL implant). In another recent article,[17] the 4 formulas (SRK-II, SRK-T, Holladay 1, and Hoffer Q) compared in pediatric eyes basically showed the same degree of reliability (though slightly better for the Hoffer Q).

IOLs that are implanted in children older than 1 year are the same as the IOLs used in adults. Considering the significant postoperative inflammatory reaction seen in pediatric patients, heparinized IOLs are theoretically more appropriate. Hydrophobic acrylic IOLs are the most popular, while silicone IOLs are not indicated because of the high incidence of opacification and contraction of the anterior capsule, as reported in 2001 in *Pediatric Cataract Surgery*[19] and the IOL Survey of the American Society of Cataract and Refractive Surgery and the American Association for Pediatric Ophthalmology and Strabismus.

Postoperative Period

Prophylaxis against endophthalmitis is highly recommended due to the severity of this complication. Prior to surgery, the surgeon should prescribe topical fluoroquinolone antibiotics.

The European Society of Cataract and Refractive Surgeons[20] developed an intraoperative protocol that also includes advice on how to prevent infection in pediatric cases. Postoperatively, treatment is a combination of topical cortisone-antibiotic used 5 to 6 times a day; the dose is tapered over 1 month in cases that are not complicated (1% prednisolone or 0.1% betamethazone or dexamethazone). The patient may not cooperate for obvious reasons and can damage delicate ocular tissues; due to the high reactivity of the tissues, there may also be some severe inflammation, which can compromise the positive outcome of surgery. Highly pigmented eyes are more prone to these problems. Maximum attention must be paid to postoperative therapy to avoid incorrect positioning of the iris, posterior synechiae, and dislocation of the IOL. (The use of mydriatics such as 1% tropicamide or 1% cyclopentolate, 1 to 3 times per day for a week, will reduce ciliary spasm and stabilize the blood-aqueous barrier.) In the event of particularly severe inflammation, the surgeon may decide to prescribe oral prednisolone for 1 week.

Bandages are not necessary after surgery (a plastic shell with a hole in the center is sufficient). This has an enormous psychological impact on the child's family; it also allows the child to have immediate visual function and allows topical therapy to be started immediately.

Postoperative Re-Education and Prevention of Amblyopia

The functional outcome depends on the type of cataract, the timing of the surgery, the quality of the operation, the appearance of complications, the presence of associated pathologies, and particularly the management of amblyopia.[8] Perfect surgery is only the first step; a long period of highly complex visual rehabilitation follows and continues throughout infancy. Postoperatively, the patient must be repeatedly examined by the pediatric ophthalmologist for the correct prescription and possible anti-amblyopic treatment, more difficult to treat in unilateral cataracts. The parents must be trained in the various procedures of the maintenance and use of spectacles and contact lenses that may be prescribed to the young patient. They must also be involved in the strict regime of orthoptic occlusive treatment in patients with a unilateral congenital cataract; this involves covering the healthy eye to stimulate the operated eye. Postoperative visits are frequent and may necessitate light general anesthesia to sedate the more restless child and allow an accurate examination. The initial occlusive treatment must be intensive to force the child to use the operated eye.

Special attention must be paid to the possibility of stabismus that is often present in cases of unilateral cataract. The amblyopic eye cannot fix objects with the fovea (the most sensitive part of the retina and responsible for this function); this is largely due to the predominance of the normal eye. Consequently, the operated eye will tend to wander and follow the pull on tissues surrounding the eye (in particular, the extraocular muscles).

Following surgery, the function must be restored by stimulating fixation capability in the operated eye, and this is achieved by covering the healthy eye. The schedule for occluding the eye will be decided and modified during each examination. During postoperative treatment, the surgeon will decide whether to correct strabismus and when would be the ideal time to operate. The examinations should continue until the patient is at least 7 years old, at intervals of 3 months until the patient is 1 year old and then every 3 to 6 months. This will allow correct prescription of lenses and the identification of possible complications such as VAO, secondary glaucoma, fibrinoid reactions, posterior synechiae, retinal detachment, and pupil decentration. VAO is the most serious postoperative complication and can appear as classical opacification of the posterior capsule or reticular fibrosis of the anterior surface of the vitreous.

Given that the lens is the ocular component with greatest refractive power, following its removal the resulting refractive error should be corrected during surgery (or as soon as possible after the operation) with insertion of an artificial lens to restore a normal visual stimulus as soon as possible. Aphakia for distance and near vision can be corrected with spectacles, contact lenses, IOLs, or a combination of these.

Intraocular Lens

Implanting an IOL is the best way to correct severe hyperopia that results following the removal of a cataract. In this case, the correct lens is inserted into the eye in the same position as the original natural lens. It will not induce the problems of magnification and aberrations induced by spectacles or the risks associated with poor maintenance of contact lenses. The implant results in a sight mechanism very close to the physiological situation.

Clearly, implantation of an IOL reduces the power of correction of the residual refractive error with spectacles and particularly contact lenses, being modified at any time throughout the patient's life.

IOLs and contact lenses have obvious advantages over spectacles. One nonrandomized study[20] published findings on the retrospective evaluation of visual results in children with unilateral cataracts; the study compared the visual results of children with a primary IOL implant and children corrected with aphakic contact lenses. Visual outcome was similar for both groups. The authors also concluded that IOLs encourage better development of the visual capacity when there is poor compliance to contact lenses or when surgery is performed after the patient has reached 1 year of age.

If implantation of an IOL is impossible (or if this option does not produce a satisfactory refractive result), contact lenses will provide the best correction for unilateral aphakia and has 44% compliance. Contact lenses provide better optical correction than spectacles; the visual field is ample and aniseikonia is greatly reduced. In the majority of cases, aphakia is corrected with contact lenses for near-vision correction or spectacles with intolerance to contact lenses in bilateral aphakia. Aphakic spectacles are used to provide satisfactory correction only in cases of bilateral aphakia not affected by anisometropia.

Spectacles

These are now considered to be a primitive optical system; they are esthetically unpleasant and heavy and can deform the delicate structures of the young child's face. They can be easily lost, and this can reduce or alter the visual function. They also greatly magnify the images and induce other functional modifications, such reduced visual field and imperfect image quality. However, spectacles are the elective choice of correction in the immediate postoperative period when an IOL has not been implanted, particularly if surgery was bilateral, or if it was unilateral and it is too early to insert a contact lens into the operated eye. In this case, because of the enormous difference in the size of the images, the sight in the 2 eyes will not be coordinated and simultaneous. It is essential to occlude the healthy eye to force the child to use the operated eye.

Contact Lenses

Compared to spectacles, contact lenses do not cause major problems of aniseikonia even following a unilateral operation. The fact that the lens is almost totally in contact with the eye (with just a layer of tears lying between the 2 systems) will eliminate the irritating problems of image magnification caused by any converging optical system.

Contact lenses are associated with other problems: intolerance, poor maintenance, or, given the young age of the patients, refusal to have them inserted or loss of the lenses. They are still not fully acceptable despite many technological advances.

These can have serious consequences; if the patient refuses to wear the contact lenses, without correction, visual rehabilitation will be impossible. The contact lens can be started in bilateral cataracts several weeks after surgery (spectacles are used in the interim). With unilateral cataract, contact lenses should be used as soon as possible as the insertion of a powerful converging lens (spectacles) in front of the operated eye causes magnification of the images in this eye compared to the healthy eye. The result is that a different image of the same object will be created in the 2 eyes (aniseikonia), and it is unlikely that the brain will "fuse" these into a single image.

Conclusion

The congenital cataract is a severe visual problem that can be treated with appropriate surgery thanks to improvements in surgical techniques and technology used in the production of IOLs or contact lenses. The possibilities of restoring sight to newborns, sufficient for their life requirements, is associated with good surgical results, artificial lens tolerance, general conditions of the eye, and the timing of surgery. It stands to reason that the best results are achieved with early operations in unilateral cataracts, thanks to the uncertain visual behavior of the young patients.

Careful observation by both parents and the pediatrician to identify initial signs of the problem (eg, the white reflex of the pupil, strabismus) is fundamental for the functional prognosis; this will allow the pathology to be diagnosed and treated early. However, good vision cannot be guaranteed by these actions alone. The patient must also undergo adequate postoperative re-education, and the parents' role in all of this is essential.

This type of surgery is extremely difficult, particularly in infants aged 2 to 3 months. Problems arise from the elasticity of the tissue, the dimensions of the cornea and the depth of the anterior chamber, and more generally, hypothalamia and the dimensions of the eye.

There are intraoperative difficulties and an even greater number of postoperative complications, particularly where newborns are concerned. They are frequently difficult to treat.

Implantation of an IOL should be mandatory, even in young infants (aged 2 to 3 months), if the eye has the appropriate dimensions. Once the child has reached 1 year of age, the results of surgery will improve; IOL implantation is almost a routine procedure and the treatment of the complications is easier, however, prevention of amblyopia becomes more difficult.

Amblyopia is one of the main problems associated with pediatric patients with cataract. Consequently, surgery and the optical correction (with IOLs, spectacles, or contact lenses) must aim to overcome this problem.

References

1. Taylor D. In: Cotlier E, Lambert SR, Taylor D, eds. *Congenital Cataracts*. Boca Raton, FL: RG Landes/CRC Press, 1994.
2. Lundvall A, Kugelberg U. Outcome after treatment of congenital unilateral cataract. *Acta Ophthalmol Scand*. 2002;80(6):588-592.
3. Casaer P, Casteels I, Foets B. Surgical treatment outcomes of congenital and juvenile cataracts. *Bull Soc Belge Ophtalmol*. 2005;(297):45-57.
4. Lambert SR, Lynn MJ, Reeves R, Plager DA, Buckley EG, Wilson ME. Is there a latent period for the surgical treatment of children with dense bilateral congenital cataracts? *J AAPOS*. 2006;10(1):30-36.
5. Vishwanath M, Cheong-Leen R, Taylor D, Russell-Eggitt I, Rahi J. Is early surgery for congenital cataract a risk factor for glaucoma? *Br J Ophthalmol*. 2004;88(7):905-910.
6. Rahi JS, Dezateux C. Congenital and infantile cataract in the United Kingdom: underlying or associated factors. British Congenital Cataract Interest Group. *Invest Ophthalmol Vis Sci*. 2000;41(8):2108-2114.
7. Neumann D, Weissman BA, Isenberg SJ, Rosenbaum AL, Bateman JB. The effectiveness of daily wear contact lenses for the correction of infantile aphakia. *Arch Ophthalmol*. 1993;111(7):927-930.
8. Long V, Chen S, Hatt S. Surgical interventions for bilateral congenital cataract. *Cochrane Database Syst Rev*. 2006;3:CD003171.
9. Vasavada AR, Trivedi RH, Nath VC. Visual axis opacification after AcrySof intraocular lens implantation in children. *J Cataract Refract Surg*. 2004;30(5):1073-1081.
10. Müllner-Eidenböck A, Amon M, Moser E, et al. Morphological and functional results of AcrySof intraocular lens implantation in children: prospective randomized study of age-related surgical management. *J Cataract Refract Surg*. 2003;29(2):285-293.
11. Raina UK, Gupta V, Arora R, Mehta DK. Posterior continuous curvilinear capsulorhexis with and without optic capture of the posterior chamber intraocular lens in the absence of vitrectomy. *J Pediatr Ophthalmol Strabismus*. 2002;39(5):278-287.
12. Vasavada AR, Trivedi RH, Singh R. Necessity of vitrectomy when optic capture is performed in children older than 5 years. *J Cataract Refract Surg*. 2001;27(8):1185-1193.
13. Eckstein M, Vijayalakshmi P, Gilbert C, Foster A. Randomised clinical trial of lensectomy versus lens aspiration and primary capsulotomy for children with bilateral cataract in south India. *Br J Ophthalmol*. 1999;83(5):524-529.
14. Gimbel HV, DeBroff BM. Posterior capsulorhexis with optic capture: maintaining a clear visual axis after pediatric cataract surgery. *J Cataract Refract Surg*. 1994;20(6):658-664.
15. Dahan E, Drusedau MU. Choice of lens and dioptric power in pediatric pseudophakia. *J Cataract Refract Surg*. 1997;23 (suppl 1):618-623.
16. Jasman AA, Shaharuddin B, Noor RA, Ismail S, Ghani ZA, Embong Z. Prediction error and accuracy of intraocular lens power calculation in pediatric patient comparing SRK II and Pediatric IOL Calculator. *BMC Ophthalmol*. 2010;10:20.
17. Nihalani BR, VanderVeen DK. Comparison of intraocular lens power calculation formulae in pediatric eyes. *Ophthalmology*. 2010;117(8):1493-1499.
18. Wilson E, Trivedi R, Pandey S. *Pediatric Cataract Surgery, Techniques, Complications and Managements*. Lippincott Williams and Wilkins; 2001.
19. Barry P, Behrens-Baumann W, Pleyer U, Seal D. *ESCRS Guidelines on Prevention, Investigation and Management of Post-Operative Endophthalmitis*. v. 2. http://www.escrs.org/vienna2011/programme/handouts/IC-100/IC-100_Barry_Handout.pdf. Published August 2007. Accessed October 2012.
20. Birch EE, Cheng C, Stager DR Jr, Felius J. Visual acuity development after the implantation of unilateral intraocular lenses in infants and young children. *J AAPOS*. 2005;9(6):527-532.

2

Congenital Subluxation of the Crystalline Lens

Hereditary:

- Marfan's syndrome (bilateral subluxation)
- Homocystinuria (bilateral subluxation)
- Weill-Marchesani syndrome
- Hyperlysinemia
- Deficit of sulfite oxydase
- Essential idiopathic familial ectopia

Acquired:

- Traumatic
- Congenital syphilis
- Hypermature cataract
- Buphthalmos

Subluxation of the lens may be the ocular expression of a number of hereditary diseases (and may also be associated with other systemic abnormalities) such as Marfan's syndrome, homocystinuria, Weill-Marchesani syndrome, hyperlysinemia, a deficit of sulfite oxydase, essential idiopathic familial ectopia, congenital syphilis, or trauma (Figure 2-1).

Progressive subluxation of the lens normally induces significant refractive errors and anisometropia. Moreover, movements of the dislocated lens can create an intermittently phakic or aphakic visual axis resulting in obvious visual disturbances. These problems in the developing vision system of a child frequently cause amblyopia.

With regard to timing of surgery, it is essential to evaluate the degree of lenticular subluxation. In children with significant subluxation, the surgeon should intervene early to prevent amblyopia, or when amblyopia is already present, to initiate therapy to treat it.

Vice versa, surgery can be postponed when a nonprogressive subluxation is present, as this is compatible with development and maintenance of normal vision.

Clinical Evaluation

In these patients, the surgeon should initially determine the best-corrected visual acuity for near and distance vision. The patient may have better vision with phakic or aphakic correction and this should be determined.

If there is little risk of backward or forward dislocation, and it is possible to refract, postponing surgery is justified and treatment of amblyopia should begin.

Surgery should be considered when subluxation of the lens is progressive, splitting the pupil in retroillumination or complete dislocation appears to be imminent. Moreover, if amblyopia cannot be treated adequately by traditional means, such as spectacles, contact lenses, and/or occlusion, the best option may be to remove the lens and implant an intraocular lens (IOL). With older children and adults, poor visual acuity attributed to the subluxated lens is a good reason to consider surgery. The surgeon should consider removing any lens that dislocates forwards or backwards, particularly if unsuccessful nonsurgical attempts have already been attempted to restore vision, with spectacles or aphakic contact lenses.

In the past, surgical removal of the congenital subluxated lens was approached cautiously due to complications and poor visual outcomes.[1-3] In the past, surgery included iridectomy, laser iridotomy, discission, and intracapsular extraction.[4] Following intracapsular surgery, these aphakic patients required spectacles or contact lenses, and rarely epikevatophakia. In more elderly patients, anterior

Buratto L, Brint SF, Caretti L.
Cataract Surgery in Complicated Cases (pp 11-25).

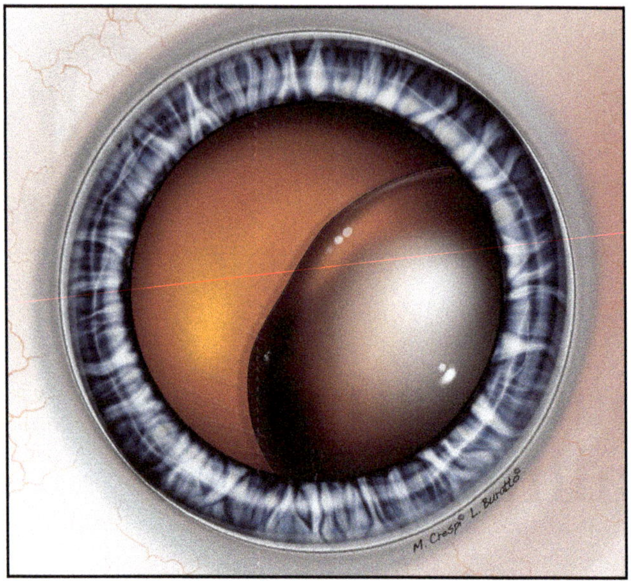

Figure 2-1. Subluxated lens in a young patient with Marfan's syndrome.

chamber IOLs (AC-IOLs) were used. Postoperative complications caused by surgery, such as glaucoma, uveitis, iris retraction, retinal detachment, vitreous loss, and poor visual acuity, were frequently seen in the these patients.

There has been improvement in both surgical and functional results with introduction of new techniques of coaxial microincision lens surgery and new vitrectomy probes with high-frequency cutting rate.

Pars plana vitrectomy and lensectomy, combined with an aphakic contact lens, or in more elderly patients, AC-IOLs, are good surgical options. The problems with these fairly straightforward, effective implants are iritis, pigment dispersion, correctopia, glaucoma, and endothelial cell loss. Another surgical option is a posterior chamber IOL (PC-IOL) sutured in the sulcus or to the iris. Some surgeons favor suturing PC-IOLs in children[5] (refer to Chapter 19).

Presently, capsular tension rings (CTRs) provide surgeons the opportunity to perform phacoemulsification through a small incision with bag PC-IOL implantation.[6]

In any case, zonules that are weak or completely absent present a serious challenge even for highly experienced cataract surgeons and are among the most difficult cases to manage.

Preoperative Evaluation

An extensive preoperative examination will increase the potential of successful cataract surgery. The surgeon must evaluate and describe the area of zonular weakness in terms of the loss (photos/drawings), localize the weak zonules, and evaluate the presence or absence of phacodonesis.

It should be remembered that evaluation of phacodonesis is more obvious in miosis as it is more dramatic prior to dilatation, as dilatation frequently stabilizes the ciliary body and iris, decreasing iris/lens movement.

The surgeon should take extra care when the lens is subluxated inferiorly, as subluxation is often an indication of 360 degrees of zonular weakness combined with effects of gravity. These patients should be reclined and observed with a portable slit lamp to evaluate whether the lens dislocates backwards and confirm that zonular integrity is significantly affected. If the lens does fall backwards, it is unlikely that the surgeon will be able to remove the lens and preserve the bag to support a PC-IOL. A pars plana lensectomy should be considered. This is difficult surgery that should be planned on a case-by-case basis depending on the gravity of the clinical picture. Ideally, the surgeon should use an anterior approach only in cases in which the absence of zonular support is 120 degrees or less (though some have suggested that it is possible to manage these eyes with a lack of support of up to 200 degrees; this will be discussed in more detail later in this chapter). The surgeon should always be prepared to rapidly convert.[6-8]

Elderly patients should also have gonioscopy to check for the presence of synechiae or angle recession, which may prevent AC-IOL implantation. When the surgeon considers a PC-IOL, the patient must be informed that the implantation of a PC-IOL is a possibility or that a CTR may be used. The surgeon should also check for other ocular pathologies that may interfere with visual results and inform the patient.

As many patients with Marfan's syndrome have serious systemic problems that can increase the risk of death or morbidity, they should undergo a full medical examination prior to surgery. Patients on Coumadin (warfarin) for cardiovascular or other problems must be fully informed about the problems associated with discontinuation (or replacement with heparin).

Surgical Treatment

Even though there are a number of different surgical approaches for the subluxated cataract, this section focuses on extraction of the lens using small incision phacoemulsification and PC-IOLs.

With this difficult operation, the surgeon should place the incision away from the area of zonular weakness to reduce stress during phacoemulsification; however, there is often generalized weakness of the zonules in these patients. The surgeon should attempt to place the incision in the quadrant away from the subluxation, given that the zonules on the opposite side are obviously weaker. In any case, the surgeon should not compromise his or her surgical ability by operating in an uncomfortable area.

The surgeon should work with the smallest incision possible without compromising the ability to perform necessary maneuvers. Thus, the amount of liquid escaping from the incision is reduced, and collapse of the chamber is minimized.

We prefer to create an initial entrance into the AC only large enough to insert the viscoelastic (VES) cannula. A generous quantity of high-retention (dispersive or pseudoadaptive) VES is placed above the area of zonular dialysis to tamponade the vitreous, maintain AC depth, and prevent collapse.

A number of different devices have been designed to help stabilize the weakened bag during phacoemulsification: CTRs, capsular tension segments (CTSs), and capsular retractors.

These surgical devices, combined with modern phacoemulsification techniques, allow preservation of the capsular bag even when it is severely weakened.

Capsulorrhexis and Hydrodissection

Capsulorrhexis is difficult and should be started in an area away from the dialysis. This exploits the counterforces of the remaining healthy zonules. A second blunt instrument, such as the Osher nuclear manipulator (Duckworth & Kent, St. Louis, MO), can be used to posteriorly support the lens, where it will be visible if it is significantly decentered. To avoid traction on the zonules, it is frequently necessary to use a technique with traction tangential to the circular shape of the capsulotomy; the surgeon should avoid centrifugal traction that may increase the dialysis. The maneuver is performed more delicately by grasping the flap at its changing insertion point on the capsule and tearing small segments with tangential traction.

When there is loss of or extensive weakness of the zonules, the surgeon may start the opening by cutting the anterior capsule with a cystotome, a sharp 15-degree blade, or a diamond cutter. Once the initial puncture has been created, the surgeon often encounters difficulty with the progression of the capsulorrhexis because of the lack of resistance provided by the zonular fibers.

A large capsulorrhexis (eg, 5.5 to 6.0 mm) is recommended; this will facilitate manipulation of the nucleus. This size is ideal to prevent capsular phimosis; thus, an IOL with an optic diameter less than 6 mm should not be used.

The use of a dispersive or pseudoadaptive VES is recommended; in addition to facilitating the capsulorrhexis, it will reduce mechanical stress on the iris, stabilize the structures, and lasts longer inside the AC. Finally, it reduces the chance of vitreous prolapse.

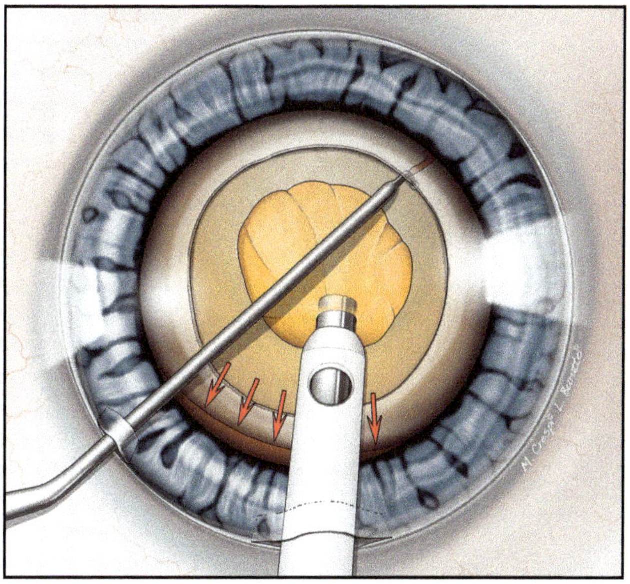

Figure 2-2. "Chopping" technique with traction toward the area of zonular dialysis.

If the rhexis created does not have adequate diameter, the surgeon has the opportunity of enlarging it after having completed the remaining steps of the operation (phaco, aspiration of the cortex, implantation of the IOL, and a CTR, if necessary). Prior to removing the VES, the surgeon may perform an oblique cut at the margin of the rhexis with Vannas scissors (Katena Eye Instruments, Denville, NJ) or with curved vitreous scissors. Starting from the cut, the rhexis can then be enlarged using capsulorrhexis forceps, if possible, for the entire 360 degrees. The maneuver is now much safer and more secure than at the beginning of the operation, thanks to capsular stabilization from the haptics of the IOL and insertion of a CTR.

Hydrodissection must be performed slowly and with extreme care to completely free the nucleus and reduce zonular stress during manipulation of the nucleus. If the nucleus is soft (and it almost always is), complete hydrodissection of the nucleus and its subluxation in the AC will simplify removal and virtually eliminate zonular stress during phacoemulsification.[9]

The surgeon should also attempt hydrodelineation. Rotation of the nucleus prior to phacoemulsification should proceed cautiously and delicately; the nucleus should be rotated slightly or not at all to avoid pulling on the residual zonular fibers (Figure 2-2).

Phacoemulsification and Removal of the Cortex

During phacoemulsification, settings of vacuum and aspiration should be reduced to allow the bottle of BSS to be positioned at a minimal height. A technique developed

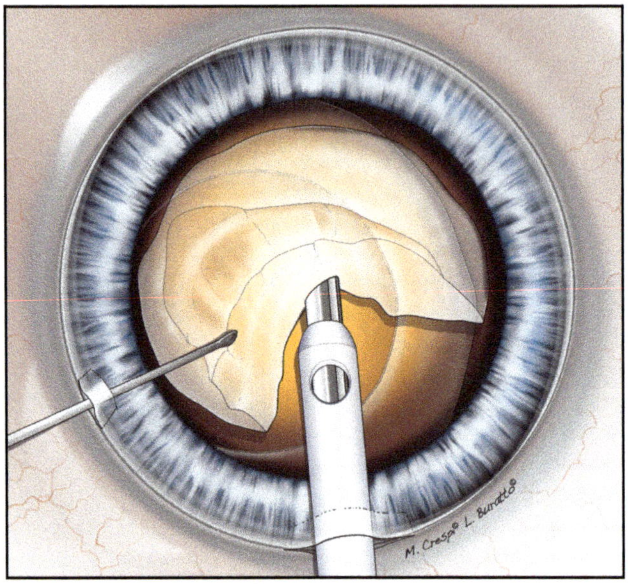

Figure 2-3. Phacoemulsification in the anterior chamber once the nucleus has been visco-expressed outside of the bag.

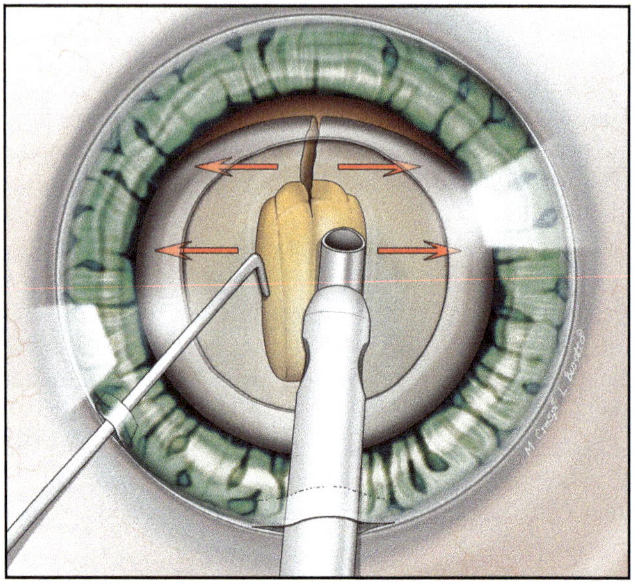

Figure 2-4. "Divide and conquer" technique with traction perpendicular to the area of zonular dialysis.

by Robert Osher, Slow Motion Phaco, may prove useful in these cases.[10] Compared to standard techniques, these alterations lead to reduced pressure in the AC with reduced stress on the fragile and partially absent zonular fibers, a decreased chance of vitreous in the AC, stabilization of the subluxated lens, and finally, generation of less turbulence with less mechanical stimulus on the iris and induced miosis.

Initially, the entrance of the ultrasound tip must occur with the bottle low to avoid fluid entering the eye, excessively deepening the anterior segment, which has already been filled with VES. As soon as some of the VES has been removed, the bottle may be raised slightly.

By contrast, a higher position of the infusion bottle will lead to more infusion and greater intraocular pressure with possibility of fluid passing through areas of zonular weakness and hydration of the vitreous. This may lead to positive vitreous pressure, shallowing of the chamber, and vitreous prolapse.

The bottle should also not be placed too low, creating a situation where anterior and posterior pressures are not balanced.

The "divide and conquer" and particularly the "chopping" techniques are recommended in eyes with zonular weakness. These techniques are ideal for harder nuclei as they minimize zonular stress during phacoemulsification as long as the surgeon applies equal but opposite forces. The phaco tip should never push the nucleus to avoid tearing opposing zonular fibers. Rather than rotating the nucleus, the surgeon should rotate his or her wrist, to limit stress applied to the residual zonular fibers. Another useful maneuver is to rotate the bevel of the phaco tip, directing it (if the surgeon operates at the 12 o'clock position) into the nasal or the temporal segments without rotating the nucleus, to create a greater contact surface when the nuclear mass is engaged, inducing lower levels of zonular stress.

Some surgeons feel the technique is determined by the position of the weak area (as long as this is not widespread); traction forces should be applied toward the strong area and not toward the opposite side to avoid extending the dialysis. Consequently, some surgeons believe that when dealing with zonular lesions near the main incision, the best technique is the "chop": the lens is grasped with the phaco probe, pulled toward the incision, and consequently toward the dialysis, and then fractured with the chopper (Figure 2-3). For zonular lesions positioned opposite the main incision, the "divide and conquer" technique is preferable, pushing toward the weakened area (Figure 2-4).[11,12]

One useful procedure is viscodissection using dispersive or pseudoadaptive VES; this separates the quadrants or halves of the free nucleus from the cortex in the area of zonular weakness. VES is injected between the nuclear quadrants and the peripheral capsular bag, separating the nuclear fragments as well as expanding and stabilizing the bag.

Moreover, cortical viscodissection will limit stress on the remaining zonules during cortical aspiration. Here, the surgeon faces difficulty with aspiration of the cortex due to lack of zonular resistance. This may cause further zonular rupture or dialysis. The use of a standard automated coaxial irrigation/aspiration instrument to remove cortex may lead to hydration of the vitreous, positive pressure, and vitreous prolapse. Buratto bimanual cannulas (Ophthalmic Surgical Instruments, Como, Italy) should be used to stabilize the capsular bag during the maneuvers. The bimanual approach allows the surgeon to maintain a fixed position in the center of the AC; one cannula supplies infusion while the other is used for aspiration, engaging residual pieces of cortex and removing them with extreme care. A tangential forward and backward movement is performed, followed by a movement toward the center of the pupil and successive aspiration. The constant use of positive pressure maintains distention of the bag and prevents the instruments touching and rupturing it.

Occasionally, the surgeon may prefer manual aspiration of the cortex with a 24- to 27-gauge cannula. The cortex is detached tangentially as opposed to radially to limit stress on the zonules; the subincisional cortex may be removed with a J-cannula.

To facilitate phacoemulsification, the surgeon may insert capsular support hooks anchored to the anterior rhexis; this has different benefits, such as support of the lens during removal and distending the capsular diaphragm to prevent vitreous loss.

The problems with phaco with a subluxated lens are extension of the dialysis, vitreous loss, aspiration of the cortex, and the impossibility of implanting an IOL in the bag.

Many recent studies using a CTR have produced encouraging results in the management of zonular dialysis.[6-8] The implantation of a CTR stabilizes the bag and allows the surgeon to complete the phaco and IOL implantation.

If vitreous presents, it should be carefully and completely removed from the anterior segment. If the quantity of vitreous is small, it can be removed using a dry vitrectomy technique with an automated vitrectomy device and the AC filled with VES. On the other hand, for major vitreous presentation, bimanual vitrectomy is required. A lateral side-port incision is used for irrigation with a 25- to 27-gauge cannula, while the vitrectomy handpiece can be inserted either through the primary corneal incision or through the pars plana.

Implantation of the Intraocular Lens

When the lens has been completely removed, the surgeon must decide whether or not to implant an IOL. There is little point implanting a lens in the sulcus if a solid zonular diaphragm is lacking; the same applies to implantation in the bag if it is excessively loose. Prior to surgery, a range of lenses (ie, different powers and models) should be readily available for use as required (for implantation in the bag, sulcus, or AC).

If the surgeon decides to implant an AC-IOL, the residual capsule should be removed. If a PC-IOL is implanted, the surgeon can suture or glue, as promoted by Agarwal, the lens to the sclera or to the iris or implant it in the capsular bag. One should not implant a lens in the sulcus without additional fixation.

Different techniques have been developed and will be discussed for suturing the PC-IOL (see Chapter 19). We will first discuss placement of the IOL in the capsular bag.

An IOL with an optic diameter of 6.0 mm can be easily inserted into the bag, through a corneal microincision in "near clear" cornea, allowing rapid healing of the wound in young patients with extremely elastic sclera.

For these young patients, some surgeons prefer a hydrophobic acrylic IOL, such as the AcrySof MA60 (Alcon Laboratories, Fort Worth, TX), as this has a low inflammatory response and reduced opacification of the PC, as opposed to silicone or hydrophilic acrylic IOLs.[13,14] In particular, plate haptic silicone IOLs should be avoided because they also have a strong tendency to induce fibrosis and anterior capsule contraction with a tendency to IOL decentration. The potential of contraction and fibrosis of the bag is so common that prophylactic cuts along the edge of the capsulorrhexis should be made with the yttrium-aluminum-garnet (YAG) laser if signs appear in the first month after surgery should be considered. The surgeon should always be concerned that placing a PC-IOL in the bag can be a risk when zonular weakness is significant. It is essential to achieve good centration of the IOL and maximize its long-term stability. The use of 3-piece IOLs with a thick edge and loops of stiff polymethylmethacrylate (PMMA) to give greater stability to the bag is recommended. There is a lower incidence of capsular contraction associated with a CTR.[15]

Implantation of an IOL with an optic diameter of 6.0 mm or more can reduce the risk of undesired symptoms, such as edge glare, associated with postoperative decentration. Even though insertion may prove more difficult, an IOL with haptics designed to permit large contact with the equatorial bag increases centration long-term.

For dialysis opposite the incision, the lower haptic is inserted into the bag; the surgeon uses a one-handed or bimanual technique to position the upper haptic in the bag. If the dialysis is located near the incision, positioning the lens will be more difficult. One option is to place the entire lens in the AC, and using a bimanual technique, the upper haptic is inserted into the bag, followed by a similar maneuver for the lower haptic. Alternately, using a foldable lens with an injector greatly simplifies the positioning of the IOL in the PC.

Some surgeons position the haptics along an axis parallel to the dialysis to utilize the remaining strong, intact zonules. This may produce optimal zonular support but may result in ovalization of the bag with greater risk of postoperative decentration.

Positioning the haptics in the bag perpendicular to the zonular dialysis will expand the capsule to a more natural condition with a reduction in ovalization. In some cases, one haptic provides adjacent zonular support alone.

We suggest positioning the haptics along any axis that produces better intraoperative centration of the IOL. This can be achieved through rotation of the IOL, when the initial insertion of the IOL is not well centered.

Also, a CTR can be used to expand the capsular bag and create better stability.

Capsular Tension Rings, Capsule Retractors, and Capsular Tension Segments

Legler and Witschel[16] have been credited with the introduction of the CTR. They demonstrated that a CTR allows both intraoperative and postoperative stabilization of the capsular bag and IOL in patients with zonular dialysis.

Phacoemulsification with implantation of a CTR has been reported as successful in patients with subluxation extending from 90 to 200 degrees,[6-8] even though many are opposed to implantation of a CTR with subluxation greater than 90 degrees.

The CTR is an incomplete ring consisting of a single piece of PMMA, processed to provide good resistance and an excellent degree of flexibility.

A number of sizes are available, from 11 to 13 mm in diameter, depending on the size of the eye. These have been designed specifically for implantation in the capsular bag and are manufactured by a number of companies (eg, Morcher GmbH, Stuttgart, Germany; Ophtec BV, Groningen, Netherlands). There are a number of models with positioning holes at the distal tips; others have 3 positioning holes (2 at the distal tips and 1 at the center of the convexity). They have all been designed to ensure circular expansion of the capsular bag and peripheral stability. The CTR is circular, and because the circle is interrupted, it can adapt to the equatorial circular shape of the bag. They can be inserted into the bag during any step after completion of the capsulorrhexis. The surgeon should attempt to induce the least trauma possible on the residual intact zonular fibers.[17]

Crucial factors using the CTR are creation of the primary incision along the meridian with intact zonules; careful phacoemulsification avoiding zonular damage with the tip; and use (if required) of slow-motion phacoemulsification with low flow rate, low vacuum, and a high infusion bottle height (as described in Chapters 8 and 15).

Prior to inserting the CTR, the surgeon should inject cohesive VES just below the rim of the residual AC to create a space for insertion of the CTR. The cohesive VES can also be used to dissect the cortex from the peripheral capsule, as this will reduce CTR trapping of the cortex.

The CTR can be inserted through an incision in clear cornea using blunt forceps (McPherson [Katena Eye Instruments]), or better still, using an injector such as the Geuder or Ophtec BV shooters through a microincision. The first system is the oldest and is a bimanual technique involving forceps and an IOL hook. One end of the ring is introduced through the corneal incision and successively through the rhexis (Figure 2-5). The surgeon's dominant hand pushes the ring into the capsular bag using blunt forceps; using the nondominant hand, the ring is directed circularly using the hook that is engaged to the positioning hole on the tip that was inserted first (see Figure 2-5). This technique is now obsolete because it is highly traumatic, particularly when the lens is still present.

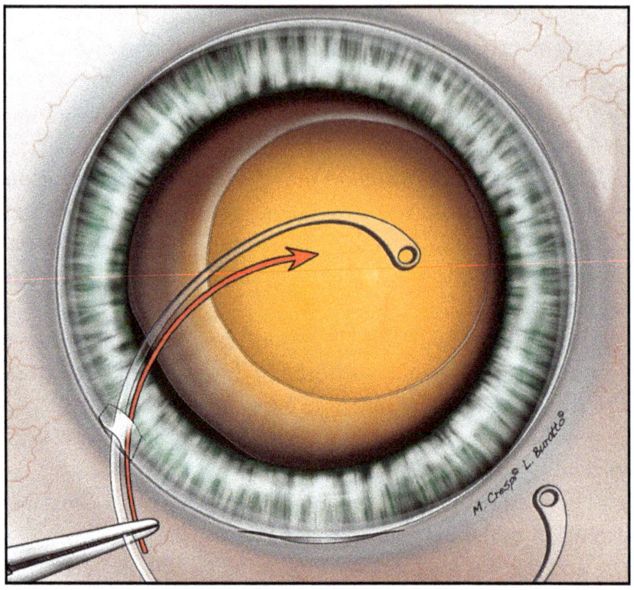

Figure 2-5. PMMA CTR prior to insertion.

The second technique involves an injector similar to those used for IOL implantation. It is less traumatic than the previously described approach (Figure 2-6).

The use of a CTR is contraindicated if there is not a continuous and complete capsulorrhexis, if the posterior capsule has ruptured, or if the zonules are highly compromised (ie, with a loss of more than 90 degrees, even though some authors believe it is possible to implant a CTR with luxations of between 90 to 200 degrees).[6-8]

Positioning a PC-IOL with the aid of a CTR is usually a straightforward procedure, given that the bag is well expanded and supported.

It should be emphasized that a CTR is more useful in patients who have zonular support that is slightly, moderately, or focally compromised, meaning 90 degrees or less (where it is possible to achieve redistribution of capsular forces onto an area of stronger zonular support). With more compromised zonules, adequate stability or centration despite a CTR may not be achieved.

Moreover, long-term stability of the bag and IOL is uncertain in eyes with progressive loss of zonular support, as is the case with Marfan's syndrome. In these cases, capsular retractors are more effective.

The most appropriate timing for CTR insertion is controversial. Some surgeons believe that it should be inserted as soon as any laxity is detected (ie, prior to phacoemulsification)[15]; others believe that it should be prior to irrigation/aspiration or not until implantation of the IOL, which is best if possible.[8] In an experimental study on cadaver eyes,

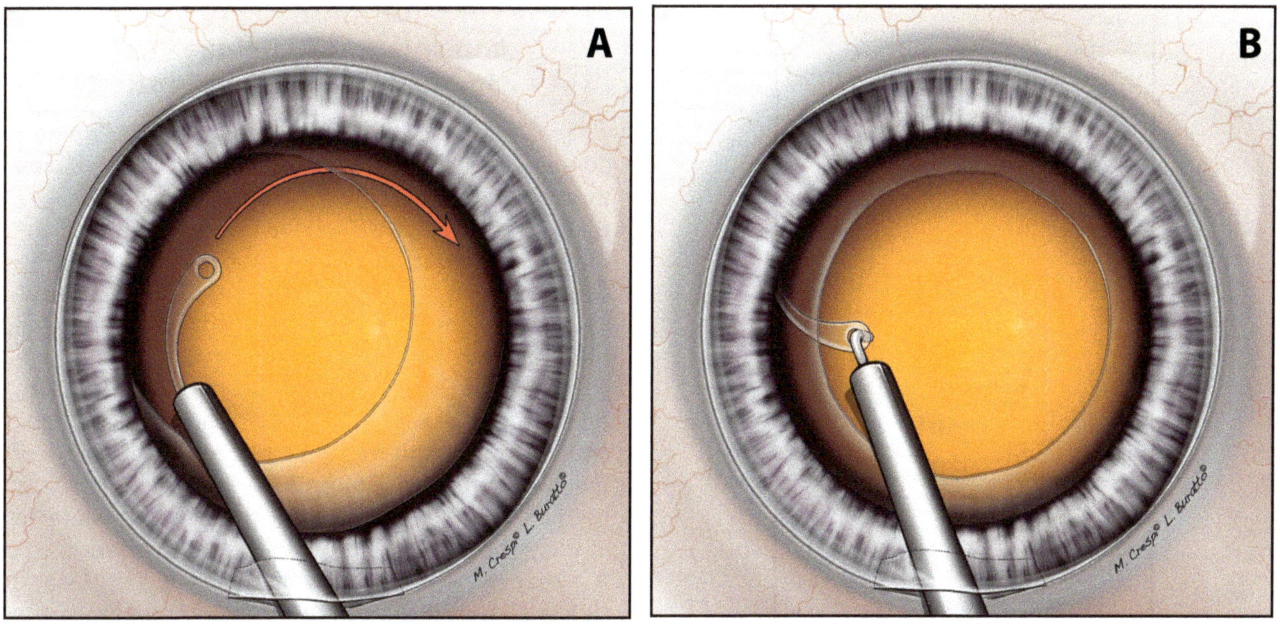

Figure 2-6. Positioning of the Morcher CTR (model 14-A) using the shooter produced by Geuder. (A) Initial phase. (B) Final phase.

Ahmed et al suggested that the ideal timing for the implantation of the CTR should be after the complete removal of the lens.[18]

Insertion of a CTR prior to phaco induces significant torsional stress on the capsular bag and can lead to further dialysis; this does not happen when the CTR is inserted after removal of the cortex. Also, removal of the cortex is more difficult when the CTR is in position, despite the use of a tangential removal technique.

Delayed insertion of the CTR (prior to implanting the IOL) is less traumatic and is not associated with the above problems. However, this does not afford support of the capsule during phaco, and there is potential risk of the bag collapsing and/or complete luxation of the lens, a good reason why hooks or capsular retractors are useful.

Some surgeons avoid CTRs because they believe that a greatly weakened bag over time allows luxation into the vitreous of the IOL-CTR-capsular bag complex.

Some surgeons have presented techniques for suturing the CTR to the sclera for support and better centration when the capsular bag remains dislocated following the insertion of the CTR. Robert Osher[19] demonstrated a technique for suturing the CTR to the sclera; he engaged the CTR with 10-0 Prolene sutures using double-reinforced CIF-4 needles. This technique may work well, but requires the needles to pass through the peripheral capsular bag with the risk of rupturing the bag given that it is under pressure from the CTR.

Pfeifer and Morela[20] suggested the creation of a small peripheral capsulorrhexis to allow passage of the suture. Both techniques offer a solution for bags that are still dislocated after insertion of the CTR. In any case, both of them violate the integrity of the peripheral capsular bag, and there is a risk of capsular rupture following the implantation of the CTR.

Robert Cionni designed a modified CTR (MCTR [FCI Ophthalmics, Pembroke, MA]) that incorporated a hook for unique fixation to achieve scleral fixation without violating the integrity of the capsule[21]; this helps to avoid decentration.

The MCTR is produced by Morcher GmbH based in Stuttgart, Germany. Like the original CTR, it consists of an open, flexible PMMA filament, with the addition of an elevated fixation hole. The hook wraps around the edge of the capsulorrhexis and rests on the residual anterior capsular rim. At the free end of the hook, there is an eyelet for a suture for scleral fixation. This is indicated in patients with greater than 180 degrees zonular dialysis or progressive zonular weakness, as in the case of Marfan's syndrome.

Currently, there are 3 models of MCTR (Morcher) available (Figure 2-7). Model 1-L has a single fixation eyelet that is distant from the insertion tip of the ring. Model 2-C has a single fixation ring close to the insertion extremity of the ring, allowing it to be implanted with the Geuder shooter. Model 2-L has 2 fixation rings. This model is useful for patients with severe zonular weakness. It may also be the elective ring in patients with progressive loss of zonular support, such as with Marfan's syndrome.

The MCTR can be inserted at any time following a successful capsulorrhexis.

However, due to its rigidity and fixed dimension, the MCTR may not be able to fit a deformed or colobomatous lens, increasing the risk of accidental rupture of the capsule during surgery. A useful alternative in these cases could be the use of a CTS of varying dimensions, complete with a fixation eyelet that will induce less mechanical stress on

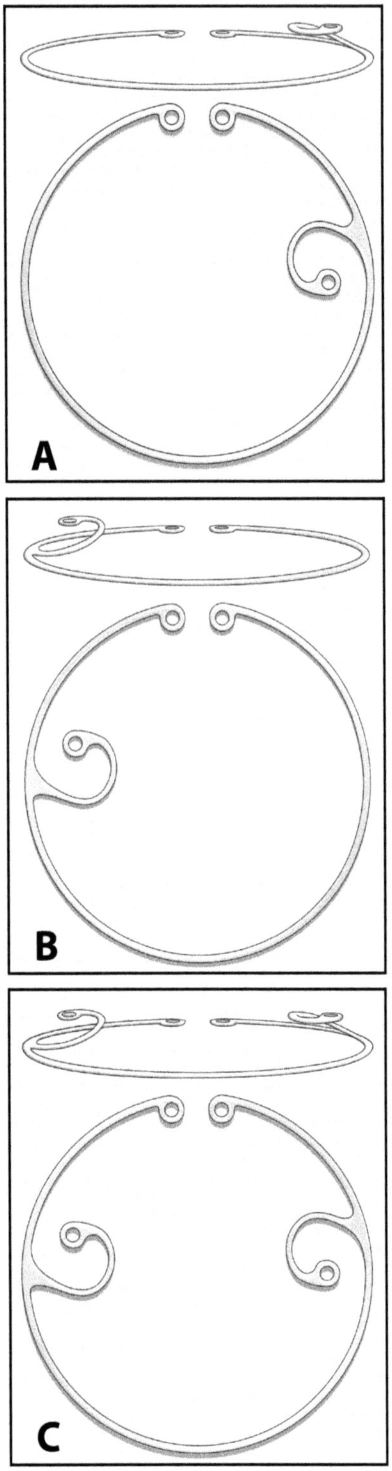

Figure 2-7. Cionni MCTRs. (A) Model 1-L. (B) Model 2-C. (C) Model 2-L.

Implantation Technique for the Modified Capsular Tension Ring

The insertion of the ring begins by prepositioning a double-armed 10-0 Prolene suture using CIF-4 needles, through the eyelet in the ring (Figure 2-8). Alternatively, the suture can be single and the free end of the prolene thread attached to the eyelet of the ring. Following viscodissection to create a space below the residual anterior capsular rim, the MCTR is inserted into the bag. The ring will often "capture" the anterior edge of the capsulorrhexis. If this does not occur, the ring's hook can be easily manipulated anteriorly with an Osher Y-hook and a second blunt instrument to retract the edge of the capsulorrhexis (Figure 2-9). The fixation hook is used to move the MCTR until the eyelet is centered at the dehiscence or in the area of zonular weakness. A Y-shaped hook (Duckworth and Kent, Ltd, Aldock, UK) can be used to push the fixation ring against the sclera wall to ensure that the chosen position results in a centered capsule (Figure 2-10). VES is injected to create a space between the iris and the anterior capsule to prepare for the needle pass. The needles are introduced into the pupil and below the iris through the incision (Figure 2-11). It is essential to always pass the needle and suture in front of the anterior capsule. The needle pass continues with penetration of the sclera wall close to the fixation ring. The needles should exit the sclera approximately 1.5 mm behind the corneal-scleral junction. The ring should be in a fairly posterior position to prevent postoperative iris chaffing. The sutures are tightened until the lens is centered in the capsular bag. A temporary knot is tied.

If a single suture is used, the needle is passed halfway through the scleral thickness, underneath the scleral flap, and the suture is tightened. Following the position of the MCTR, the rest of the procedure is easier. Positioning a MCTR is more difficult when the nucleus is large and hard.

Another excellent technique is to secure the lens with 3 or 4 iris hooks during phacoemulsification. The hooks will stabilize the edge of the complete continuous capsulorrhexis. The MCTR can then be inserted safely.

the bag and the weakened zonules, as suggested by Hasanee and Ahmed.[22]

In otherwise normal eyes with subluxated lenses, the capsulorrhexis must be performed outside the pupil center to ensure that the bag will be centered afterward; thus, the capsulorrhexis will be well centered (Figure 2-12). However, it may require part of the capsulorrhexis to be performed behind the iris without good visualization.

We found that, in these cases, it is easy to inject a foldable acrylic PC-IOL into the capsular bag. Once the PC-IOL is positioned, the temporary knot is released and a permanent knot is created with just enough tension to center the IOL. The knot can then be rotated to lie underneath the sclera

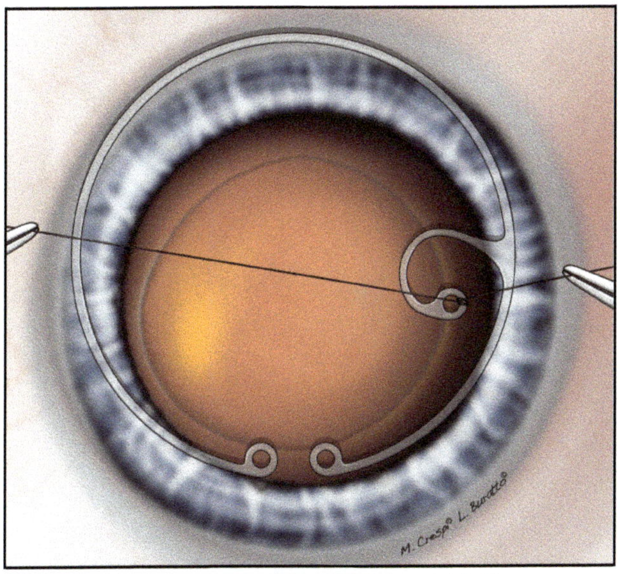

Figure 2-8. Safety suture of the MCTR (model 2-C).

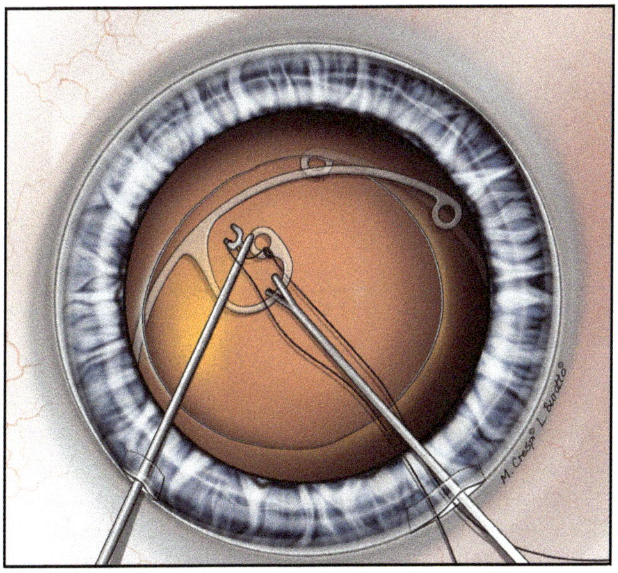

Figure 2-9. Manipulation of the hook on Cionni MCTR.

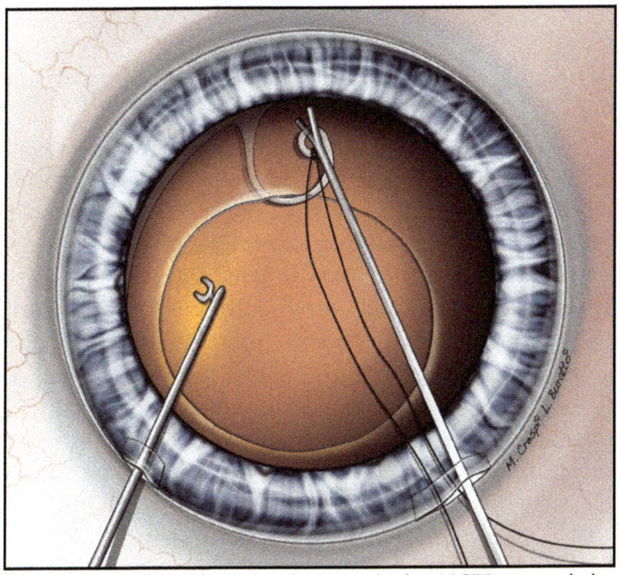

Figure 2-10. Use of a Y-hook to push the MCTR toward the scleral wall. This maneuver will also center the bag.

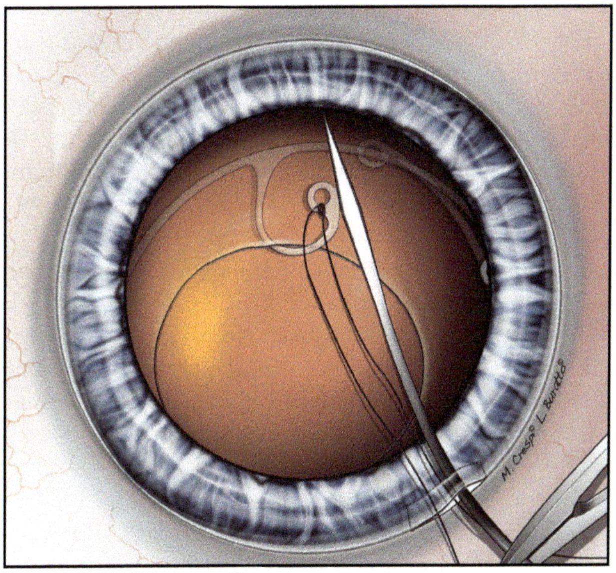

Figure 2-11. CIF-4 needle pass.

or under a scleral flap (having been prepared in advance). If the 2-L hook is used, the fixation site for each hook must be determined by moving each hook toward the scleral wall prior to placing the suture.

Limitations associated with the Cionni MCTR include difficult implantation of the ring with a small rhexis, lenses that are extensively subluxated, large size of the Cionni MCTR compared to the bag of patients with Marfan's syndrome and small bags.

Surgeons feel the MCTR requires a suture inducing tension, which over years may lead to breakage.

There are advantages associated with implantation of a CTR: better centration of the IOL, less IOL tilting, less capsular contraction, and a decreased incidence of anterior and posterior opacity (theoretical). Severe phimosis is often the result of a lack of countertraction in eyes with zonular weakness; over time, this may be responsible for IOL decentration and further zonular weakening.[23] There is no consensus on whether CTRs decrease epithelial cell migration.

Some surgeons feel that a CTR should be positioned in all eyes if zonular laxity occurs during surgery.

Complications may arise during implantation of a CTR (eg, increase in pre-existing zonular dehiscence and tears in the margin of the capsulorrhexis).

Jacob et al[7] reported intraoperative extension of dialysis in 9.52% of eyes, and in one case, conversion to pars plana vitrectomy to remove nuclear fragments luxated in the vitreous. Regarding tears in the margin of the capsulorrhexis,

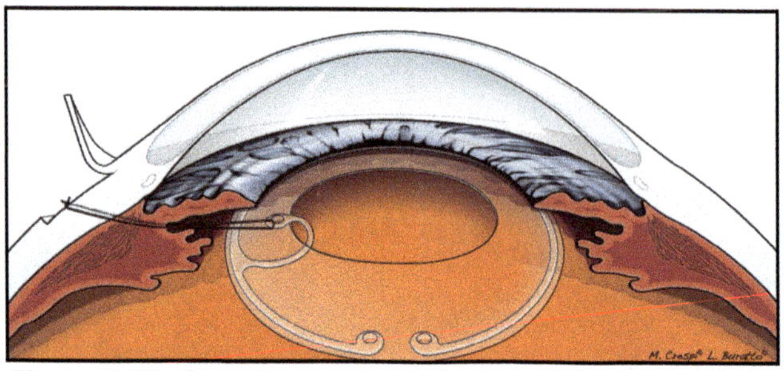

Figure 2-12. Centration and stabilization of the bag with the MCTR.

a study by Praveen et al[8] showed that this prevented implantation of a CTR in 2 eyes.

Postoperatively, possible complications include posterior capsule opacification (PCO), which is most frequently observed; breakage of sutures with dislocation of the IOL with reduction in visual acuity; corneal edema; mild iritis; an increase in intraocular pressure; and retinal detachment.

Konradsen et al[24] reported positive long-term results in a series of 37 eyes in children with nontraumatic ectopia lentis; they were treated with MCTR (33 eyes) and conventional CTR (4 eyes), all with an IOL. Twenty-six of the eyes required secondary surgery because of opacification of the visual axis. Sutures had to be replaced in 2 of the eyes (5.4%) due to dislocation of the IOL.

Vasavada et al[25] published findings on intraoperative and postoperative performance of CTRs in pediatric eyes with spontaneous or post-traumatic subluxation of the lens, with a range of 180 to 250 degrees. In all cases, a CTR and a one-piece AcrySof IOL (Alcon Laboratories) were placed in the bag. Clinically significant PCO developed in 19 eyes (54.3%). Postoperative decentration of the IOL occurred in 3 eyes (8.5%).

With the Cionni ring in position, onset of PCO appears to be accelerated by the ring fitted with a hook allowing the proliferation of the epithelial cells.[26]

Reports have shown that a CTR does not reduce the rate of PCO in young patients implanted with a round-edged or a square-edged IOL, even though some feel a square-edged CTR may delay the onset of PCO by blocking migration of lenticular epithelial cells.

Recent studies suggest delayed dislocation of the IOL associated with rupture of the polypropylene suture that fixed the IOL to the sclera, particularly in younger patients.[27,28] Asadi and Kheirkhah recently reported a similar delayed onset of dislocation of the IOL with scleral fixation in children. In this group, late dislocation of the IOL, associated with rupture of the polypropylene suture, was seen 10 years after surgery in 6 of 25 eyes (24%).[29] Despite the theoretically long lifespan of these sutures, Cionni et al reported an incidence of rupture of the suture in approximately 10% of patients after an average of 18 months; he recommended the use of more resistant sutures than 10-0 Prolene,[26] such as 9-0 Prolene or 8-0 Gore-Tex (W. L. Gore & Associates Inc, Flagstaff, AZ).

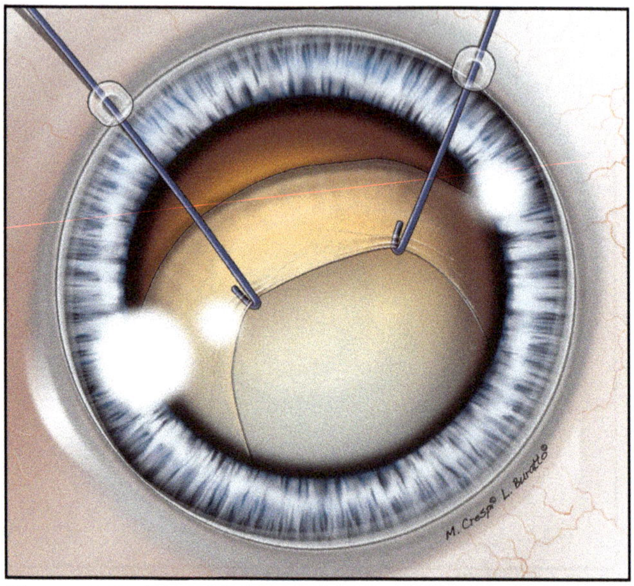

Figure 2-13. Use of 2 iris hooks to stabilize the subluxated capsular bag.

Thus, a situation that may develop over time is subluxation and consequent dislocation of the IOL-CTR-capsular bag complex. A vitrectomy may be necessary with complete removal of the complex and scleral fixation of a PC-IOL. It may sometimes be necessary to remove the CTR from the vitreous chamber, which may be difficult in the majority of cases and potentially be responsible for retinal damage.

Ma et al[30] described 2 techniques for removal of a CTR from the vitreous: the first involves removal of the CTR once it has been cut into 2 portions, while the second involves removing the CTR intact using an injector. Lang et al[31] suggest removing the CTR through a sclerotomy.

The surgical approach for the dislocated IOL-CTR-bag complex depends on the position of the CTR. If the complex has subluxated just behind the pupil, it can be sutured to the sclera using an anterior approach; however, if the complex is completely luxated in the vitreous, a pars plana vitrectomy is indicated with the CTR-IOL complex elevated using vitreous forceps.[32] In all of these cases, repositioning of the complex requires the CTR to be sutured to the sclera through the complex, or a CTS can be positioned in the bag and successively fixed to the sclera, or the IOL haptics can be sutured to the iris.

To provide support for the capsule during surgery with extreme laxity of the zonules, capsule retractors, such as iris hooks, are extremely helpful. These hook to the edge of the complete capsulorrhexis to stabilize the lens during phacoemulsification (Figure 2-13). These were introduced by John Merriam,[33] who showed efficacy of 3 or 4 of these flexible retractors through the paracentesis, positioning them to fix the capsulorrhexis. This system allows the surgeon to delay the insertion of the CTR until the cortex has been removed, as cortical removal with the CTR in place is difficult.

Once the nucleus has been removed, the insertion of the CTR is greatly simplified; leaving the capsule retractors in position, the risk of damaging the zonules during the CTR insertion is greatly reduced. The drawback is that the retractors do not expand the capsular equator, and consequently, the surgeon risks rupturing the capsule and causing iatrogenic zonular trauma during phacoemulsification and cortical removal. Most recommend 5 to 6 retractors for greater stabilization. The capsule retractors are removed once the CTR is in position.[33,34]

Richard Mackool designed titanium capsule retractors with hooks at the tips; they are long enough to support the peripheral capsular fornix and the capsulorrhexis.[35] In these cases, the retractors act as artificial zonules to stabilize the entire bag during phaco and cortical removal. As opposed to CTRs, the capsule retractors provide excellent support in the anterior-posterior direction without trapping cortex, each retractor creates just one pressure point on the capsular fornix without engaging the cortex. These hooks, called capsular support systems, are available as resterilizable instruments (Duckworth & Kent Ltd, Hertfordshire, England) and as disposables (Impex, Staten Island, NY). They can be inserted at any point of the surgery, even during capsulorrhexis. To stabilize the capsule against rotational forces, hydrodissection and rotation of the nucleus may also prove useful after capsulorrhexis. Some surgeons feel these are better than CTRs in preventing capsular rupture with generalized laxity; given that the CTR can only redistribute the capsular stress force to the remaining intact zonules, in the cases of large zonular defects, the CTR does not create bag stability.

It should be pointed out that these retractors may damage the margin of the capsulorrhexis during surgery. Moreover, as they are removed at the end of surgery, they do not resolve the problem of permanent capsular support for the IOL, a problem that can be managed with CTRs.

Ike Ahmed designed a CTS (Morcher GmbH) that combines the concept of the MCTR and a capsular retractor.[18] The Ahmed CTS is an incomplete, flexible 90-degree ring of PMMA; it has a radius of curvature of 5 mm, and similar to the Cionni MCTR, it has an eyelet for the iris hook (temporary, in that a single iris retractor can support the segment during surgery) or for scleral fixation (permanent). Different from the CTR, however, the surgeon can insert a CTS atraumatically in the bag in 1 or 2 areas of zonular weakness after having created the rhexis and prior to performing the phaco. Insertion is also easier than standard CTRs.

This provides intraoperative support of the bag, without making it difficult to remove the cortex. As these retractors are smooth, they should not induce any rupture of the capsulorrhexis. In cases of severe luxation, 2 or 3 CTSs may be required. At the end of surgery, they can either be removed or they can be sutured to the sclera to provide permanent support.

Like the Cionni MCTR, these are indicated with extensive zonular dialysis. They can also be used in the event of anterior or posterior capsular rupture.

An innovative alternative surgical device for subluxated lenses was used experimentally[36] and successively in humans.[37] This flat, intraocular PMMA implant (Capsular Anchor) is fixed to the anterior capsule to increase resistance. It consists of a central rod positioned in front of the anterior capsule and 2 side arms positioned behind the anterior capsule. The Anchor is sutured to the sclera with a single suture of 9-0 or 10-0 polypropylene. It can also be associated with implantation of a CTR. This new device appear to be effective in cases of significant zonular dehiscence.

With a subluxated lens, there are several alternatives to the insertion of the CTR or MCTR when the surgeon has been unable to perform a correct continuous curvilinear capsulorrhexis or if CTRs are not available. Instead of enlarging a small-diameter capsulorrhexis, the surgeon can create small relaxing incisions along the edge of the capsulorrhexis once the nucleus and the cortex have been removed and the IOL has been inserted into the bag. With a temporal main corneal incision, the haptics of the IOL are positioned along the horizontal axis (3 and 9 o'clock positions) and 2 opposite cuts are made in the edge of the capsulorrhexis at the vertical axis (6 and 12 o'clock positions). The cuts should not extend too far peripherally, as they serve simply to prevent contraction of the capsulorrhexis. The anterior capsular flap is flipped over to cover a zonular defect and is sutured to the scleral portion or a PC-IOL is implanted in the ciliary sulcus. In any case, it requires fixation in the sulcus in young patients with already compromised zonules, which may jeopardize the long-term stability of the IOL. With this technique, 10% of patients required a second surgery because of IOL decentration.

Some surgeons use the YAG laser after surgery to create relaxing incisions at the margin of the capsulorrhexis or straightforward implantation of the IOL in the sulcus, even though we feel that these options are not ideal.

Conclusion

Treatment of the congenital subluxated lens is probably the most difficult situation faced by an anterior segment surgeon. However, recently developed techniques and innovative surgical devices, particularly CTRs, give surgeons the chance to maintain the capsular bag, recentering the bag itself, and correctly position a PC-IOL inside the bag. This difficult surgery can be performed through a microincision (just 2 to 2.2 mm), allowing rapid visual recovery, particularly important in very young children because prolonged visual deprivation may result in serious amblyopia.

Two major problems remain with these patients, even after successful phacoemulsification and implantation of a CTR and an IOL: secondary capsular opacification and possible long-term dislocation of the IOL-CTR-capsular bag complex.

References

1. Jensen AD, Cross HE. Surgical treatment of dislocated lenses in Marfan's syndrome and homocystinuria. *Trans Am Acad Ophthalmol Otolaryngol.* 1972;76(6):1491-1499.
2. Varga B. The results of my operations improving visual acuity of ectopia lentis. *Ophthalmologica.* 1971;162(2):98-110.
3. Maumenee IH. The eye in the Marfan syndrome. *Birth Defects Orig Artic Ser.* 1982;18(6):515-524.
4. Straatsma BR, Allen RA, Pettit TH, Hall MO. Subluxation of the lens treated with iris photocoagulation. *Am J Ophthalmol.* 1966;61(5, pt 2):1312-1324.
5. Zetterström C, Lundvall A, Weeber H Jr, Jeeves M. Sulcus fixation without capsular support in children. *J Cataract Refract Surg.* 1999;25(6):776-781.
6. Cionni RJ, Osher RH. Endocapsular ring approach to the subluxed cataractous lens. *J Cataract Refract Surg.* 1995;21(3):245-249.
7. Jacob S, Agarwal A, Agarwal A, Agarwal S, Patel N, Lal V. Efficacy of capsular tension ring for phacoemulsification in eyes with zonular dialysis. J *Cataract Refract Surg.* 2003;29:315-321.
8. Praveen MR, Vasavada AR, Singh R. Phacoemulsification in subluxated cataract. *Indian J Ophthalmol.* 2003;51:147-154.
9. Maloney WF. Supracapsular phaco: achieving greater efficacy with phaco outside of the capsular bag—a 3 years experience. Presented at: the American Society of Cataract and Refractive Surgery; April 1999; Seattle, WA.
10. Osher RH. Slow motion phacoemulsification approach. *J Cataract Refract Surg.* 1993;19(5):667.
11. Gimbel HV. Divide and conquer nucleofractis phacoemulsification: development and variations. *J Cataract Refract Surg.* 1991;17(3):281-291.
12. Nagahara K. Video presentation. Presented at: American Society of Cataract and Refractive Surgery Film Festival; 1993; Seattle, WA.
13. Ursell PG, Spalton DJ, Pande MV, et al. Relationship between intraocular lens biomaterials and posterior capsule opacification. J *Cataract Refract Surg.* 1998;24(3):352-360.
14. Hollick EJ, Spalton DJ, Ursell PG, et al. The effect of polymethylmethacrylate, silicone, and polyacrylic intraocular lenses on posterior capsular opacification 3 years after cataract surgery. *Ophthalmology.* 1999;106(1):49-54; discussion 54-55.
15. Gimbel HV, Sun R, Heston JP. Management of zonular dialysis in phacoemulsification and IOL implantation using the capsular tension ring. *Ophthalmic Surg Lasers.* 1997;28(4):273-281.
16. Legler U, Wischel B. The capsular tension ring, a new device for complicated cataract surgery. Presented at the American Society of Cataract and Refractive Surgery;May 1993; Seattle, WA.
17. Nagamoto T, Bissen-Miyajima H. A ring to support the capsular bag after continuous curvilinear capsulorhexis. *J Cataract Refract Surg.* 1994;20(4):417-420.
18. Ahmed IK, Cionni RJ, Kranemann C, Crandall AS. Optimal timing of capsular tension ring implantation: Miyaki-Apple video analysis. *J Cataract Refract Surg.* 2005;31:1809-1813.
19. Osher RH. Synthetic zonules. *Video J Cataract Refract Surg.* 1997; 8(1).
20. Pfeifer V, Morela K. Ectopic lens extraction in children. *Coll Antropol.* 2001;25(suppl):37-41.
21. Cionni RJ, Osher RH. Management of profound zonular dialysis or weakness with a new endocapsular ring designed for scleral fixation. *J Cataract Refract Surg.* 1998;24(10):1299-1306.
22. Davison JA. Capsule contraction syndrome. *J Cataract Refract Surgery.* 1993;19(5):582-589.
23. Konradsen T, Kugelberg M, Zetterstrom C. Visual outcomes and complications in surgery for ectopia lentis in children. *J Cataract Refract Surg.* 2007;33:819-824.
24. Vasavada V, Vasavada VA, Hoffman RO, Spencer TS, Kumar RV, Crandall AS. Intraoperative performance and postoperative outcomes of endocapsular ring implantation in paediatric eyes. *J Cataract Refract Surg.* 2008;34:1499-1508.
25. Cionni RJ, Osher RH, Marques DM, et al. Modified capsular tension ring for patient with congenital loss of zonular support. *J Cataract Refract Surg.* 2003;29:1668-1673.
26. Vote BJ, Tranos P, Bunce C, Charteris DG, Da Cruz L. Long term outcome of combined pars plana vitrectomy and scleral fixated sutured posterior chamber intraocular lens implantation. *Am J Ophthalmol.* 2006;41:308-312.
27. Assia EI, Nemet A, Sachs D. Bilateral spontaneous subluxation of scleral fixated intraocular lenses. *J Cataract Refract Surg.* 2002;28:2214-2216.
28. Asadi R, Kheirkhah A. Long term results of scleral fixation of posterior chamber intraocular lenses in children. *Ophthalmology.* 2008;115:67-72.
29. Ma PE, Kaur H, Petrovic V, Hay D. Technique for removal of capsular tension ring from vitreous. *Ophthalmology.* 2003;110:1142-1144.
30. Lang Y, Fineberg E, Garzozi HJ. Vitrectomy to remove posteriorly dislocated endocapsular tension ring. *J Cataract Refract Surg.* 2001;27:474-476.
31. Ahmed IK, Chen SH, Kranemann C, Wong DT. Surgical repositioning of dislocated capsular tension rings. *Ophthalmology.* 2005;112:1725-1733.
32. Merriam JC, Zheng L. Iris hooks for phacoemulsification of the subluxated lens. *J Cataract Refract Surg.* 1997;23(9):1295-1297.
33. Lee V, Bloom P. Microhook capsule stabilization for phacoemulsification in eyes with pseudoexfoliation-syndrome-induced lens instability. *J Cataract Refract Surg.* 1999;25(12):1567-1570.
34. Mackool RJ. Capsule stabilization for phacoemulsification (letter). *J Cataract Refract Surg.* 2000; 26:629.
35. Ahmed II, Crandall AS. Ab externo scleral fixation of the Cionni modified capsular tension ring. *J Cataract Refract Surg.* 2001;27(7):977-981.
36. Ton Y, Michaeli A, Assia EI. Repositioning and scleral fixation of the subluxated lens capsule using an intraocular anchoring device in experimental models. *J Cataract Refract Surg.* 2007;33(4):692-696.
37. Assia EI, Ton Y, Michaeli A. Capsule anchor to manage subluxated lenses: initial clinical experience. *J Cataract Refract Surg.* 2009;35(8):1372-1379.

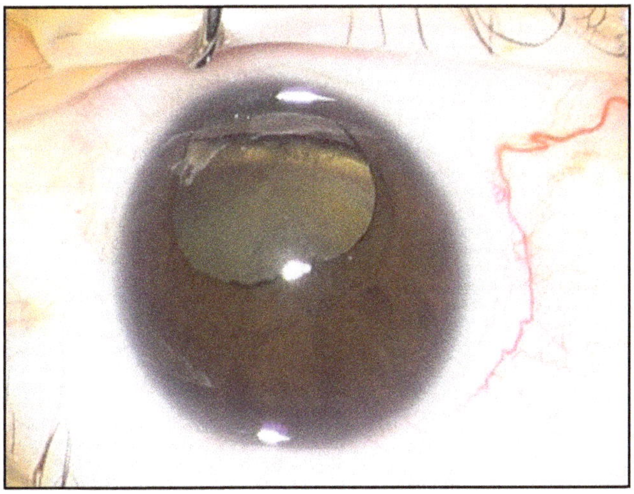

A-1. Brunescent cataract in microphthalmus with iris coloboma.

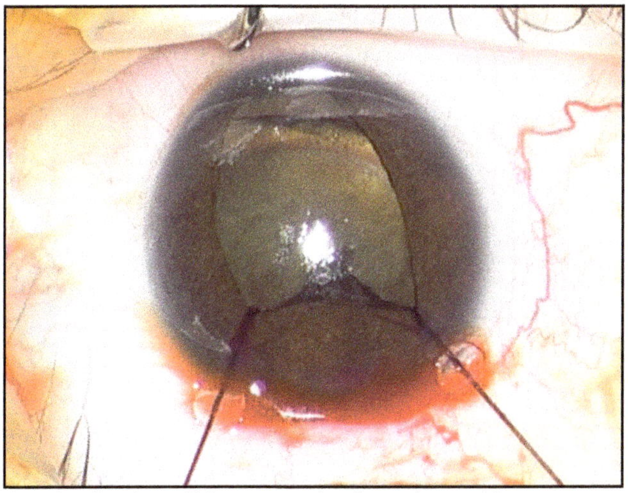

A-2. Application of iris retractor hooks and synechiotomy.

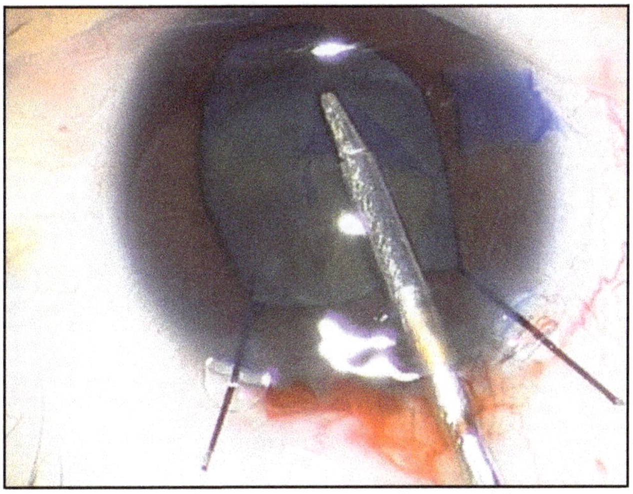

A-3. Capsulotomy following staining with trypan blue.

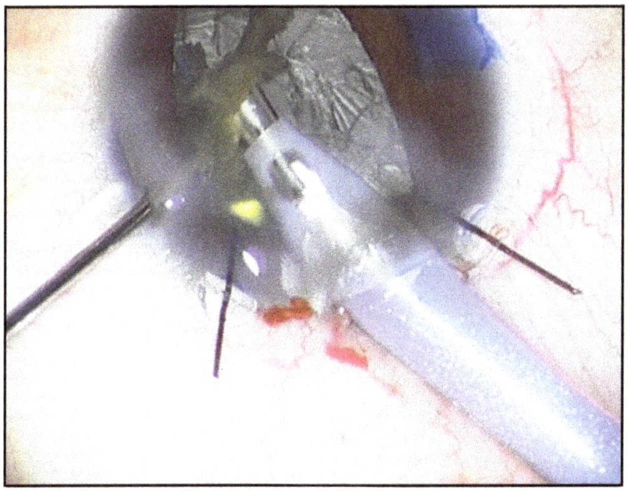

A-4. Phacoemulsification.

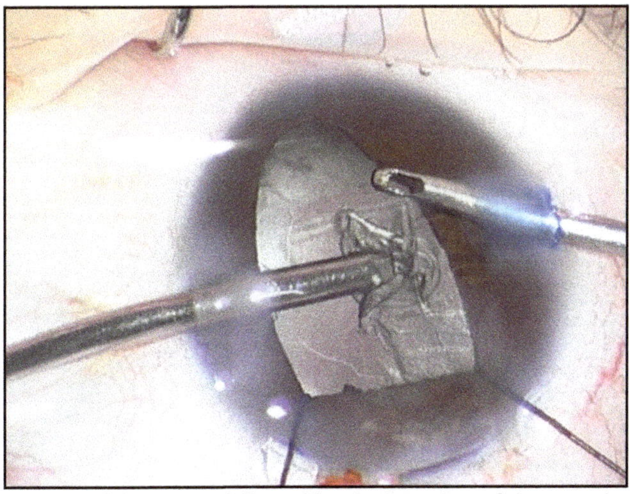

A-5. I/A of the cortex followed by the insertion of the capsular ring and the implantation of an IOL in the bag.

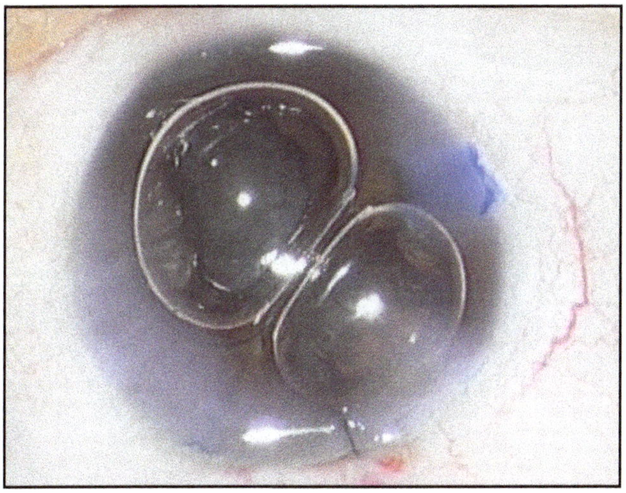

A-6. Some air is injected into the anterior chamber for a better closure of the all incisions.

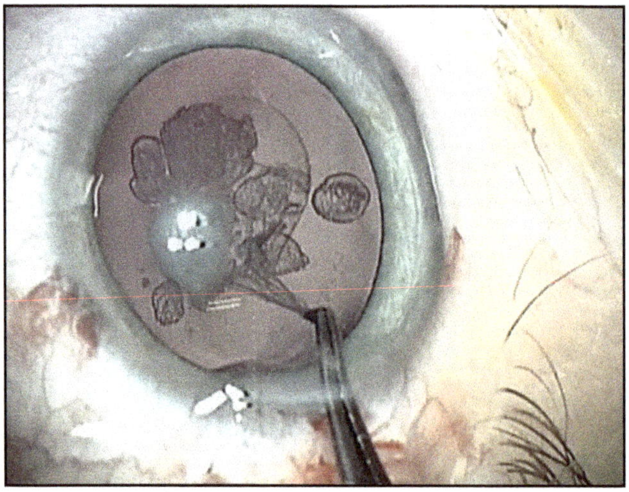

B-1. Congenital cataract: the capsulorrhexis is performed. Traditionally, this will tend to extend. (Reprinted with permission of Nikica Gabric.)

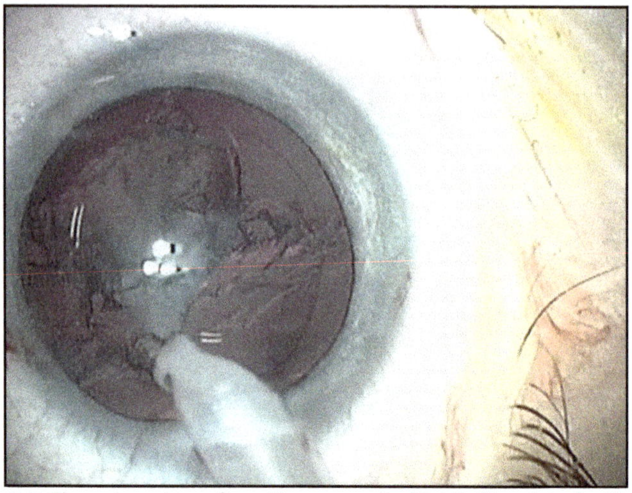

B-2. The cataract is soft and is removed with I/A. (Reprinted with permission of Nikica Gabric.)

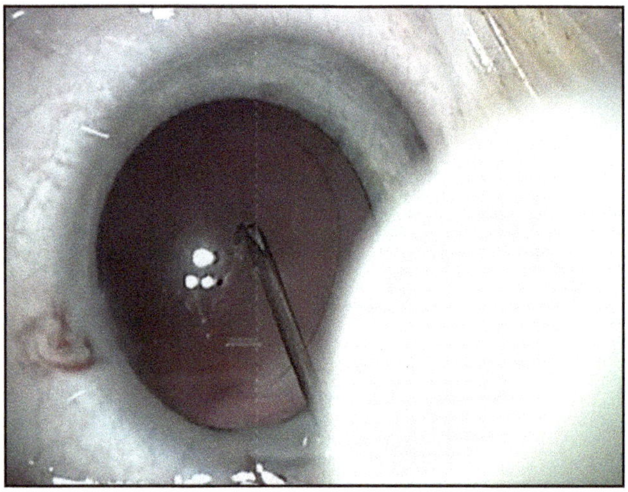

B-3. Posterior capsulorrhexis follows. (Reprinted with permission of Nikica Gabric.)

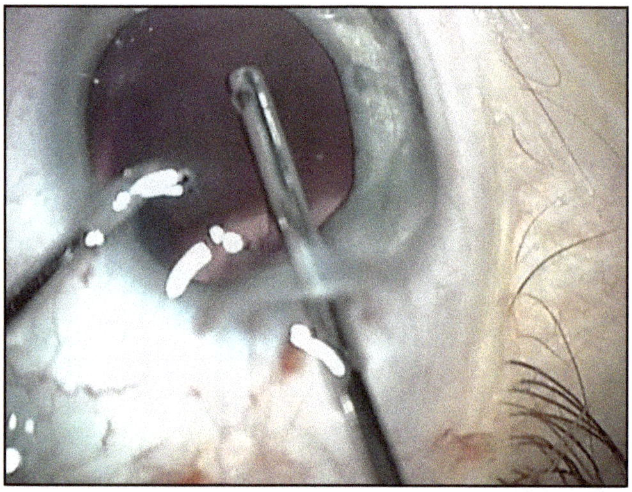

B-4. Then vitrectomy inside the rhexis. (Reprinted with permission of Nikica Gabric.)

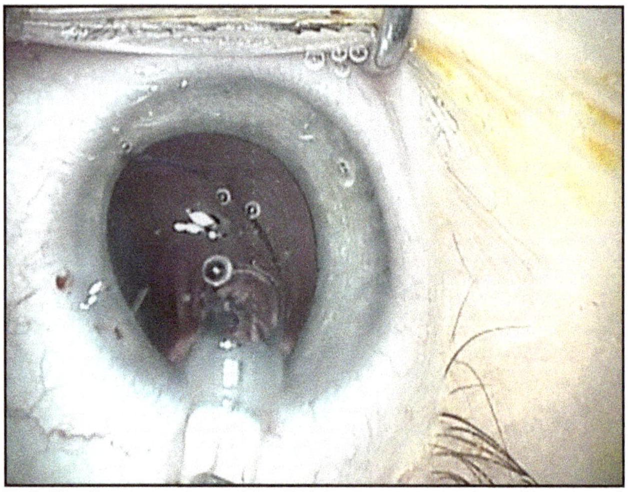

B-5. The implantation of the IOL in the capsular bag. (Reprinted with permission of Nikica Gabric.)

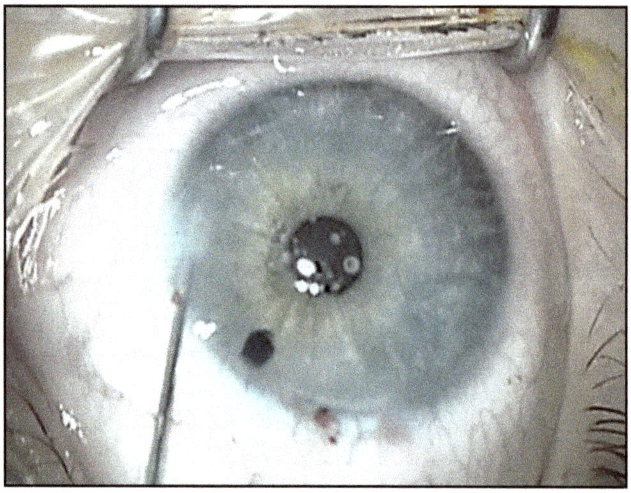

B-6. Iridectomy has been performed and pupil is constricted. (Reprinted with permission of Nikica Gabric.)

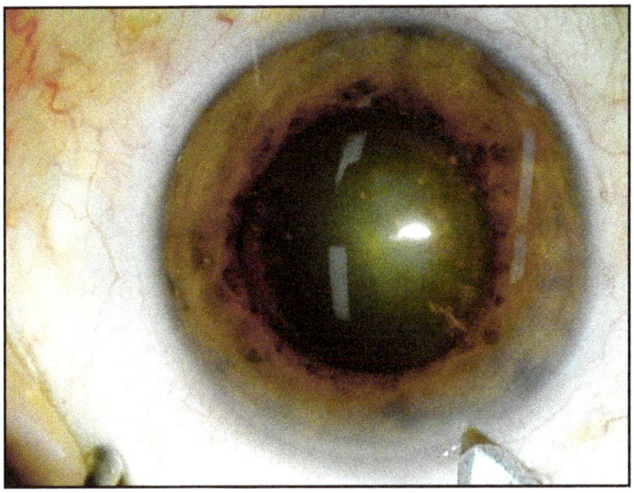

C-1. Luxated cataract. (Reprinted with permission of Josè Guell.)

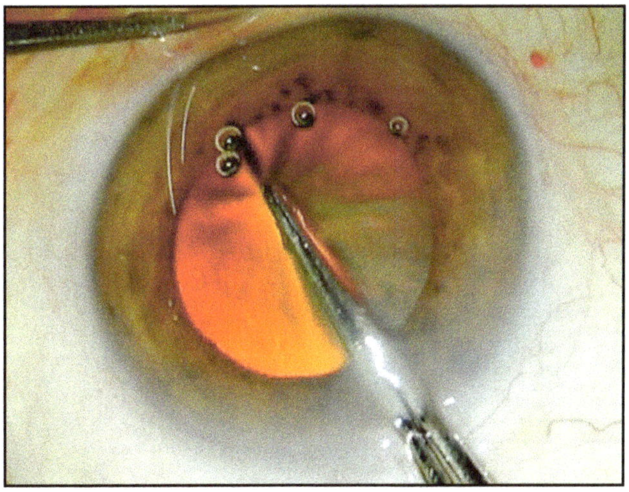

C-2. Attempt of incision of the anterior capsule. (Reprinted with permission of Josè Guell.)

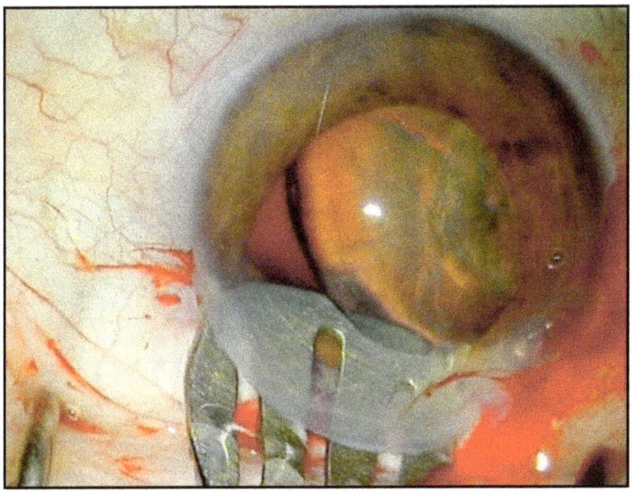

C-3. The surgeon decides to extract the cataract intact with a loop and extends the incision. (Reprinted with permission of Josè Guell.)

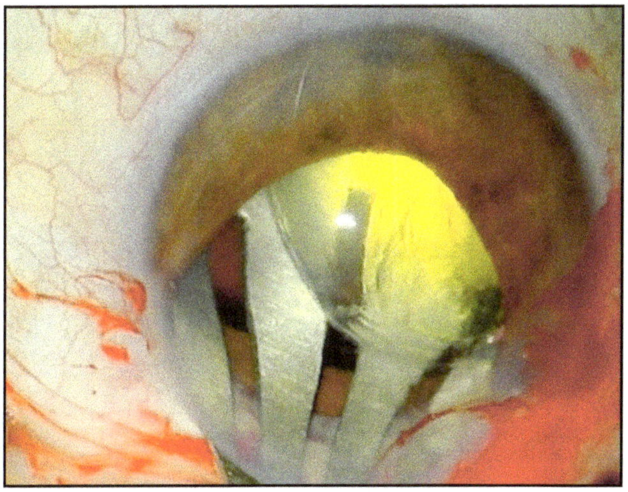

C-4. The loop penetrates the vitreous underneath the cataract. (Reprinted with permission of Josè Guell.)

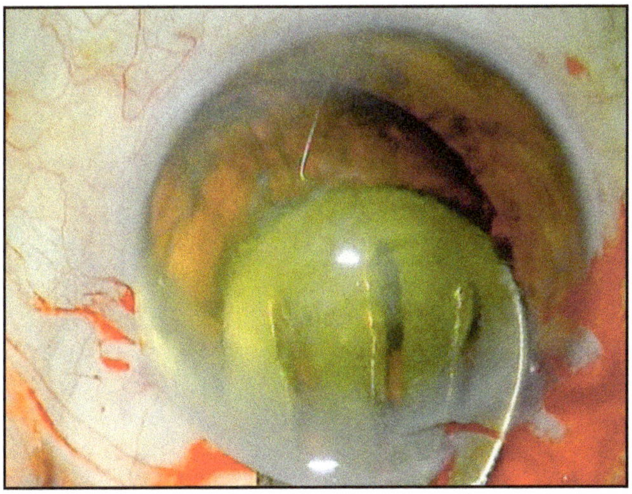

C-5. The cataract is removed intact with considerable displacement on the vitreous. (Reprinted with permission of Josè Guell.)

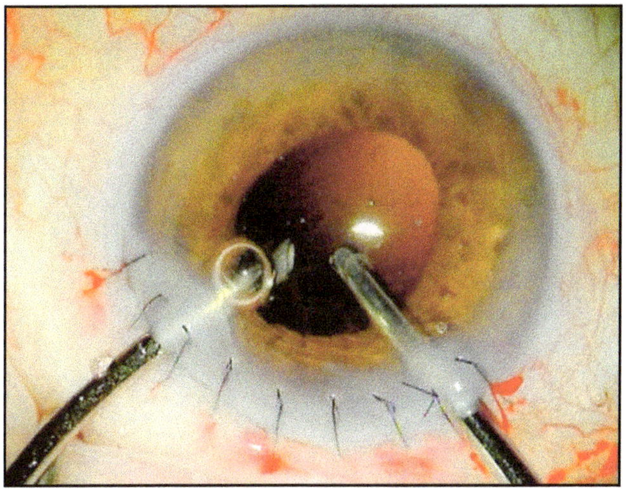

C-6. The anterior vitrectomy is performed followed by the secondary implant. (Reprinted with permission of Josè Guell.)

3

Cataract and Glaucoma

The incidence of cataracts with concomitant glaucoma is increasing. This increase is possibly due to better pressure control with currently available drugs and glaucoma treatments until the typical age of cataract development. Possible lens damage from laser treatments may also occur.[1,2] Moreover, the association of cataracts following filtration procedures is well known. Thus we recommend cataract surgery simultaneously with glaucoma surgery, even with only a slight opacity and particularly in patients aged 70 years and older.[3-5] An increasing number of surgeons are treating glaucoma associated with ectopic lentis and most forms of angle-closure glaucoma with lens removal.[6-9]

Phacoemulsification has encouraged increased use of combined cataract and glaucoma surgery[10]; all perforating and nonperforating glaucoma procedures can be combined with phacoemulsification. Extracapsular cataract extraction (ECCE) is not recommended because of increased incidence of intraoperative complications[11] resulting in poor vision and pressure control.[12-14]Better understanding of the various types of glaucoma has led to safer and more sophisticated surgery.

Cataracts and Glaucoma: Determining the Choice of Surgery

Determining indications and timing for glaucoma procedures is extremely complex. Generally speaking, glaucoma surgery is indicated for poor pressure control using topical medications and/or laser treatment, or with poor patient compliance. In making the best decision, the surgeon should consider the following[15-21]:

- Type of glaucoma
- Visual field changes
- Target intraocular pressure (IOP)
- Type of patient (age, complications, and risk factors for glaucoma)
- Degree of lens opacity
- Degree of safety and efficacy of the planned surgery

It is difficult to have general guidelines to follow, thus surgery should be made on a case-by-case basis.[13,14] The choice of surgery is based on visual acuity, field loss, and target IOP.

Cataract surgery alone is effective in all angle-closure glaucomas (treatable with pilocarpine alone). When the angle is free of synechiae, severe postoperative inflammation is not anticipated and there is minimal damage to the angle anatomy (Figure 3-1).

The importance of lens removal in angle-closure glaucoma was questioned by Friedman et al[16] in 2006 who could find no published evidence to support lens removal in primary chronic angle-closure glaucoma. However, efficacy was demonstrated in the results of 2 recently published studies[17,18] with a controlled randomized trial (Effectiveness in Angle-Closure Glaucoma of Lens Extraction [EAGLE] Study Group).[19]

With open-angle glaucoma, cataract removal alone can lower IOP 2 to 3 mm Hg (range 1.3 to 4.7 mm Hg) for several years.[20] This is unlikely to be enough with advanced glaucoma that is not controlled with maximal

Buratto L, Brint SF, Caretti L.
Cataract Surgery in Complicated Cases (pp 27-58).

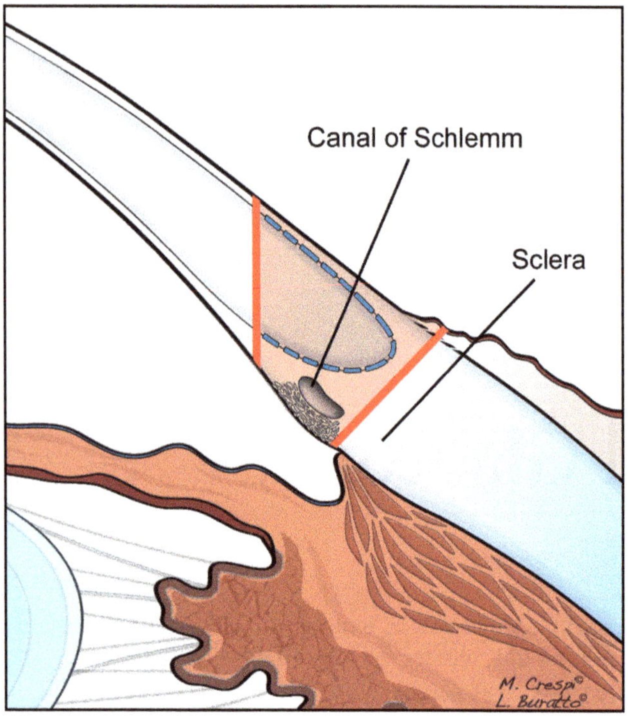

Figure 3-1. Anatomy: the red lines indicate the tissue block defined limbus; the broken line indicates the blue transition zone between the cornea and sclera. It is possible to observe a more regular arrangement of corneal collagen fibers.

therapy, though it may be adequate for mild glaucoma with well controlled pressures using a single agent.

The safety of phacoemulsification is excellent as it does not require conjunctival manipulation. With nonperforating glaucoma surgery, safety is good, though much less safe for perforating procedures.

It is possible for surgeons to combine phacoemulsification with glaucoma procedures whether perforating or nonperforating (combined surgery). Of the combined procedures, phacotrabeculotomy using mitomycin C (MMC) produces the greatest pressure reduction; however, it may also be associated with serious complications.

Surgical Options

Because surgical options for glaucoma and cataract differ in efficacy and complication rates, it is difficult to develop a strict treatment protocol. We will describe surgical options in which "compensated glaucoma" is defined as an IOP ≤20 mm Hg for at least 3 of 4 measurements during circadian tonometry.

For phacoemulsification only, the following apply:

- Angle-closure glaucoma controlled only with miotics
- Issue of acute glaucoma
- Phacolytic or phacomorphic glaucoma
- Open-angle glaucoma, if the following are present:
    - The IOP is <20 mm Hg using only a single drug
    - The visual field is normal or only minimally affected

For phacoemulsification with nonperforating surgery, the following apply:

- Angle-closure glaucoma controlled with a miotic or another drug
- Open-angle glaucoma controlled with 2 drugs (with a target pressure not extremely low)
- Glaucoma in which there is a risk of hypotony after filtration

For phacoemulsification combined with trabeculectomy, the following apply:

- Angle-closure or open-angle glaucoma controlled with more than 2 drugs (requiring a very low target pressure)
- Uncontrolled angle-closure or open-angle glaucoma

For phacoemulsification with trabeculectomy and antimetabolites, the following apply:

- Uncontrolled glaucoma in young patients (aged younger than 40 years)
- Post-traumatic glaucoma
- Glaucoma with prior unsuccessful surgery

Glaucoma drainage devices (GDDs) or shunts are available and are traditionally used in refractory glaucoma in which filtering procedures have a high risk of failure or have already been unsuccessful. Given the predictability of GDDs, their use in primary glaucoma has increased significantly. New surgical procedures have been developed that—while very promising and having a high safety profile—still have not been validated with controlled randomized studies.[20-23] These would be useful with high target pressure levels and using phacoemulsification.

Phacoemulsification in Glaucomatous Eyes

Phacoemulsification changes the anatomy of the eye with a potential effect on ocular hydrodynamics by removing the lens that has a central thickness of approximately 4 mm and inserting an intraocular lens (IOL) slightly thicker than 1 mm. Moreover, abundant irrigation of the anterior chamber (AC) and the angle may be a factor facilitating filtration. The following are reasons proposed for postsurgical reduction in IOP[24-29]:

- Increased outflow through the trabecular meshwork, increased AC depth, and increased depth of the angle
- Increased outflow due to trabecular stretching
- Reduced aqueous production having a direct and indirect effect on the ciliary body

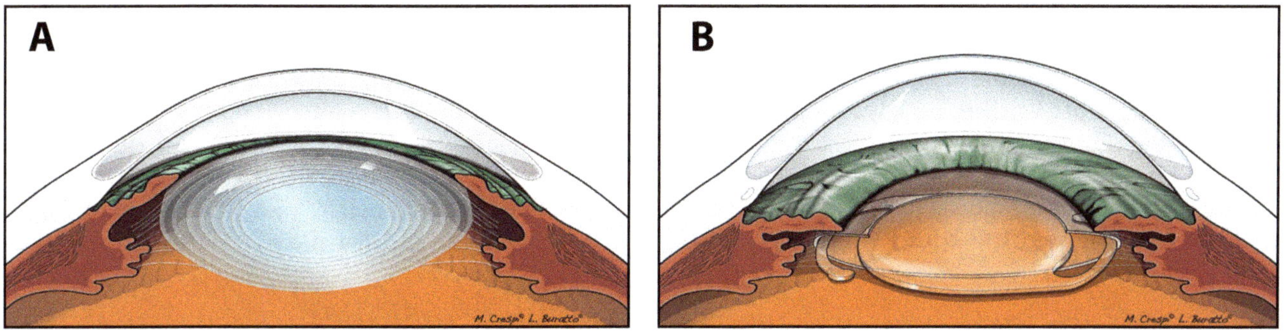

Figure 3-2. Angle-closure glaucoma and cataract removal. (A) The anterior chamber is shallow, especially in the periphery. (B) The anterior chamber is deepened significantly after surgery.

- Traction and opening of Schlemm's canal by the ciliary body, transmitting zonular traction
- Alteration of the blood aqueous barrier

It is reasonable to expect IOP reduction in eyes undergoing phacoemulsification. In normal eyes, 2 to 3 mm Hg is an expected pressure reduction initially after phacoemulsification, as has been reported[26,30-35]; this is a significant value, typically equal to that achieved with topical glaucoma therapy.

Cataract removal with phacoemulsification is sufficient to treat the mechanism of primary angle-closure glaucoma, regardless of starting IOP. Lens removal has been successful in glaucoma from ectopia lentis with angle-closure and in acute angle-closure glaucoma (Figure 3-2).[6-8] The surgical results are not impressive in terms of IOP, but allow abandonment of topical therapy, affecting 70% of patients.[6,36]

With open-angle glaucoma, cataract removal can result in a small improvement in pressure, between 1.3 and 4.7 mm Hg 6 months after surgery (though study results vary[6,12,37-39]). Pressure reduction does not differ greatly from eyes with normal IOP. It is important for incisions not to traumatize the conjunctiva for potential future glaucoma surgery; therefore, it is better to perform clear corneal phacoemulsification.[10]

Phacoemulsification alone is a good alternative to combined procedures for glaucoma with a small increase in IOP and minimal visual field changes. This is essentially true but may be misleading and it is dangerous not to consider the patient's specific type of glaucoma. It is also true that phacoemulsification alone, without trabeculectomy, increases the risk of increased IOP immediately after surgery (particularly with those who already have glaucoma), while phacotrabeculectomy reduces this risk.[35,40] As the relationship between pressure spikes and worsening of the visual field must still be carefully studied, combined procedures may be preferable, particularly in patients with significant visual field damage.

It is not clear whether the incision site (temporal or superior) influences IOP. Nevertheless, it is important to emphasize that in eyes with a superiorly located trabeculectomy, clear-corneal temporal phaco does not alter long-term IOP[41-50] and has advantages over ECCE, which can increase IOP in eyes with filtering blebs.[43]

Surgical Difficulties With Phacoemulsification in Glaucomatous Eyes

Although cataract surgery in eyes with glaucoma is frequently no different than standard cataract surgery, sometimes the lenses of glaucomatous eyes have characteristics that can complicate phacoemulsification. Loose zonules, shallow AC, and miotic pupils that are difficult to dilate are just some of the situations increasing the degree of difficulty of the operation (including low endothelial cell counts and vitreous pressure).

Surgery is more demanding if the eye has been through a procedure previously (trabeculectomy or deep sclerectomy) and if preserving the bleb is necessary (unsuccessful in 5.3% of eyes with phacoemulsification and 13.7% of eyes with ECCE).[44] In these eyes, bleb failure is caused by the normal scarring processes of the conjunctiva, Tenon's capsule, and episclera.

In this chapter we will examine individual steps of phacoemulsification, potential difficulties, and helpful tips.

Preoperative Intraocular Pressure Reduction

Opening the AC is an extremely dangerous moment in eyes with high IOP because of rapid pressure drop. The sudden drop in pressure (sometimes dropping to zero) occurs more frequently in ECCE, and always provokes dilatation of the choroidal vascular bed, often resulting in rupture of a choroidal vessel with choroidal hemorrhage and expulsive hemorrhage. The risk is greatly reduced with phacoemulsification performed with a basically closed system.

In combined surgery deep sclerectomy, viscocanalostomy, and canaloplasty contribute to a reduction of expulsive hemorrhage, at least in part. A sudden drop in pressure can still occur in a small number of eyes; therefore, it is advisable to attempt to reduce the IOP preoperatively, particularly when it is > 30 mm Hg. For this reason, when topical glaucoma drops and carbonic anhydrase inhibitors are insufficient, the surgeon should administer IV 20% mannitol (10 cc/kg) 1 hour prior to surgery.

Incision

With phacoemulsification, a properly created incision ensures greater safety during the procedure. The ideal incision allows better intra- and postoperative closure. Other factors important in the glaucomatous eye include minimized scarring of the conjunctiva, Tenon's, and episclera.

Paracentesis

The paracentesis is usually the first surgical step. To avoid aqueous escape and allow instrument maneuverability, the surgeon should create a paracentesis incision approximately 1 mm wide. Preservative-free 1% lidocaine for intracameral anesthesia and viscoelastic can be injected through the paracentesis. Deepening the AC with a viscoelastic substance (VES) is essential in glaucomatous eyes; in these eyes, a narrow angle and shallow AC occur frequently and may complicate subsequent maneuvers.

VES is injected using a cannula opposite the main incision. The injection begins opposite the paracentesis, gradually withdrawing the cannula, allowing the aqueous to escape from the paracentesis without creating localized pools that could cause unexpected collapse of the chamber if suddenly emptied. Therefore, VES is injected coaxially, maintaining the orientation of the cannula parallel to the longitudinal axis of the paracentesis, to allow escape of aqueous through the space between the cannula and the paracentesis tunnel. Viscoelastic should not be injected beneath the iris and should not increase IOP as this induces iris prolapse when the AC is later opened.

Position of the Incision

With combined cataract glaucoma surgery, the surgeon may use a single incision, creating a tunnel below the scleral opening, in association with trabeculectomy and nonpenetrating techniques. If phacoemulsification is performed in combination with a glaucoma procedure, the surgeon should use a lateral approach, the temporal approach being most popular,[47-49] avoiding unnecessary manipulation of the conjunctiva and bleb.

The incision may be clear corneal[46,47] or immediately in front of the vascular arcade (near clear).[48-52] In both cases, the advantage is decreased inflammatory stimulation from the incision. The increase in AC pressure during phacoemulsification almost never produces an increase in the size of an existing bleb, which confirms that a certain degree of fibrosis is always present in the conjunctiva of the bleb after filtering operations.

Even though Shea et al[53] reported increased IOP after phacoemulsification, others[41,42,54-56] demonstrated that phacoemulsification through a near clear temporal incision in eyes with a bleb does not affect pressure.

Incision Architecture

The use of micro-phaco tips with the latest ultrasonic (U/S) handpieces allows emulsification of the lens using 2.0- and 2.2-mm incisions. Small incisions have known advantages. Moreover, in a patient who has already had a filtering procedure or may in the future, small incisions lead to a reduction in inflammatory response.

Obviously, the size of the incision depends on the phaco tip/sleeve chosen; the length is also important in prevention of complications. A corneal tunnel length of 1.75 to 2 mm is a good compromise. In glaucomatous eyes, a more corneal incision and a tunnel that is slightly shorter than standard is created due to a shallow AC (which may be less than 2 mm), particularly with angle-closure glaucoma. The objective is to avoid damage to the iris, while allowing maneuvers in a restricted space.

Entrance to the Anterior Chamber

Penetration of the AC is a delicate moment, particularly in eyes with shallow chambers where the keratome can easily damage the iris or anterior capsule. This complication can be avoided if tunnel construction is preceded by VES injection through the paracentesis, to deepen the chamber.

If a bleb is present, the surgeon should avoid scleral fixation rings to avoid damaging the bleb and compromising its function. These instruments may lead to dangerous shallowing of the AC with excessive external pressure.

If the incision involving the iris is incorrect, it is useless to attempt repositing the iris as it results in iris damage with release of inflammatory mediators, possible bleeding, and pupillary defects. If the surgeon realizes that poor incision architecture allows iris prolapse, the incision should be sutured and a new tunnel made in a different location.

Small Pupils

Frequently, the pupil of a glaucomatous eye will often be difficult to dilate. Atrophy and/or sclerosis of the iris stroma, secondary to pseudoexfoliation, previous acute glaucoma attacks, or simply aging, create a situation in which mydriatics will not induce good dilation. The presence of irido lenticular synechiae from previous surgical procedures and/or from prolonged use of miotics create a fixed pupil and mydriatics are unable to induce even minimal mydriasis (see Chapter 5).

Preoperatively, the surgeon should not use sympathomimetic mydriatics, as they may cause damage leading to increased arterial blood pressure, dilating the choroidal bed, and increasing vitreous pressure.

Modern phacoemulsification techniques require the pupil to have a diameter of 4 to 5 mm to allow the procedure to be performed safely. This diameter allows the surgeon to create an adequate capsulorrhexis and to perform phacoemulsification without excessive risks. By using the chop technique or any of its variants such as quick chop, it is possible to bring the individual "chopped" fragments to the center of the pupil for emulsification, reducing the possibility of damaging the peripheral portion of the capsule.

The methods used to dilate the pupil differ depending on the reason for the miosis. However, the rules are always the same: rapid execution, maximum safety, and minimal invasiveness.

It is useful to remember that in previously filtered eyes, iris manipulation is associated with a loss of IOP control,[44] probably caused by rupture of the blood aqueous barrier.

The Under-Reactive Pupil

With under-reactive pupils, the surgeon can attempt to achieve mydriasis with good pharmacological preparation. The intraoperative addition of intracardiac epinephrine (1:1000, 0.1 to 0.5 mL in 500 cc) to the infusion bottle is useful.

After the primary incision, the surgeon may attempt to enlarge the pupil by injecting a high viscosity and high molecular weight VES such as Healon GV (Abbott Laboratories, Abbott Park, IL) or more recently, Healon 5 (Abbott Laboratories). Usually, this creates the 4 to 5 mm of dilation that is sufficient for the operation.

Fixed Pupil

A fixed pupil with a diameter of 1 or 2 mm is generally secondary to posterior synechiae.

The first step is lysis of the synechiae with a blunt spatula. The surgeon may then proceed with mechanical dilatation of the pupil with pupil stretching (mono- or bimanual), iris retractors, dilating rings, sphincterectomy, and sector iridectomy. Pupil stretching has proven to be effective even when the pupil is extremely small (1 to 2 mm) and can be done with a mono- or bimanual technique (see Chapter 5).

Capsulorrhexis

Capsulorrhexis may be more difficult in the glaucoma patient. With small pupils, the surgeon should attempt to create a rhexis that is as large as possible; forceps are used to follow the pupillary margin and eventually extend the edge of the rhexis slightly underneath the iris.

A capsulorrhexis of at least 5 mm will greatly facilitate all of the subsequent steps, from hydrodissection to removal of cataract and IOL. Capsulorrhexis is usually not difficult with miosis as rhexis escape is rare as the miotic pupil seems to confine it.

Greater attention is required with pseudoexfoliation syndrome (PEX) due to weak zonules. The diameter of the rhexis should be at least 5 mm to reduce later traction on the zonules; a larger diameter, moreover, helps to prevent contraction of the capsule, more frequently seen in PEX. The chamber depth, may be less than 2 mm, but can be deepened using high viscosity VES, such as Healon GV or Healon 5.

Implantation of a Capsular Tension Ring

A capsular tension ring (CTR) is a horseshoe-shaped polymethylmethacrylate (PMMA) device used in cases of zonular weakness, PEX, subluxed cataract (Marfan's syndrome, ectopia lentis, and Weill-Marchesani syndrome), elderly patients, traumatic cataracts, and intumescent cataract (see Chapter 2).

For glaucoma, implantation of a CTR should be considered with PEX glaucoma as the implantation of a CTR—an easy procedure if you have good visibility—may be impossible with miosis (see Chapter 4). The association of miosis and loose zonules is an extremely dangerous scenario affecting surgical outcomes that demands maximum caution even once the pupil has been dilated mechanically. The CTR places the capsular bag under tension and the ring counteracts the centripetal forces affecting the zonules. There are fewer complications related to loose zonules, despite cases of IOL decentration and postoperative fibrosis of the anterior capsule reported with CTRs.

Hydrodissection

In all eyes, not only those with glaucoma, the injection of balanced salt solution (BSS) during hydrodissection should not lead to increased IOP. This may induce 2 important complications: iris prolapse and pressure on the posterior capsule that could rupture.

When the cannula is inserted into the AC, the surgeon applies mild posterior pressure on the tunnel to allow some of the VES to escape, particularly if a dispersive VES has been used. This maneuver generally leads to expulsion of the central portion of the anterior capsule removed during capsulorrhexis, if the capsule has not been previously removed.

In glaucomatous eyes there are 3 other potential factors requiring caution during hydrodissection: loose zonules (particularly with pseudoexfoliation), overly small rhexis (due to poor dilation), and a large diameter nucleus. This combination makes the zonular capsular apparatus particularly sensitive to increases in pressure inside the capsular bag and can lead to capsular rupture. It is advisable to perform hydrodissection slowly with numerous small injections.

Phacoemulsification

Phacoemulsification in a glaucomatous eye may be complicated by a number of factors, including loose zonules, shallow chambers, pupils that are difficult to dilate, low endothelial cell count, and vitreous pressure. Speed, accuracy, and minimal invasiveness are essential for safety; surgeon experience with a specific procedure is also important. Regardless of technique, the following principles are standard:

- If dilation is not excellent, surgical maneuvers performed blindly behind the iris must be cautiously performed.
- Low ultrasound energy provides greater protection for the corneal endothelium. It should be remembered that the endothelial cell count may be very low in glaucomatous eyes, particularly with the angle-closure form often associated with a reduced AC depth. Cataract surgery must therefore be very delicate and the surgeon should use dispersive or viscoadaptive VES injected repeatedly into the AC during surgery.
- Particularly with shallow chambers, slower vacuum rise times (achieved by lowering aspiration flow rate) reduce the risk of engaging the iris or capsule with the tip.
- Bottle height should be low as the higher the bottle, the greater the infusion pressure into the AC. If IOP is greater than the vacuum in the aspiration line, passive vacuum will be generated (not created by the pump) engaging the iris or other structures.

Overall, phaco chop satisfies these needs, allowing rapid, safe completion of the surgery.

Irrigation/Aspiration

Cortical removal requires careful attention, particularly with loose zonules, where the surgeon may opt to implant a CTR. In eyes with a previous trabeculectomy, it is necessary to ensure that no nuclear or cortical material obstructs the trabeculectomy at the completion of irrigation/aspiration (I/A). In glaucomatous eyes, frequently I/A and lens implantation steps may be affected by vitreous pressure, particularly in angle-closure glaucoma. This creates shallowing of the chamber, increases surgical difficulty, and probability of capsular rupture. Eyes with shallow ACs, such as those with previous angle-closure glaucoma, are particularly prone to this complication.

That cataract surgery can be interrupted at any time is a big advantage of phacoemulsification. Prevention of posterior vitreous pressure means avoiding anything that causes it to develop (see Chapter 9).

Intraocular Lens Implantation

The use of a foldable lens is mandatory. Regardless of the material (ie, silicone or acrylic), the characteristics in terms of visual quality and incidence of posterior capsule opacification (PCO) do not vary significantly in the glaucomatous eye from normal eyes, even after filtering surgery.

The choice of implant must take special conditions into consideration. Pseudoexfoliation with its risk of phimosis of the anterior capsule, suggests implantation of lenses with PMMA haptics, providing greater resistance to capsular contraction. Silicone IOLs should be avoided as they create greater stimulation of capsular contraction (see Chapter 4).

In short eyes with IOLs of high dioptric power, a double or piggyback lens may be required so that the sum of the 2 powers is equivalent to the total power needed (see Chapter 9).

Final Steps of the Procedure

When the VES has been removed, injection of BSS into the AC can be used to test the survival of the bleb as it may have been damaged by direct trauma or by an intraoperative drop in IOP. If the bleb does not diffuse after BSS injection, the surgeon can attempt to reactivate it by introducing a cyclodialysis spatula through the opening of the sub-Tenon's space.[56] This maneuver, only possible in eyes after a trabeculectomy (not a deep sclerectomy), can be performed in eyes with a poorly filtering bleb prior to phacoemulsification.

Generally, coaxial microincision cataract surgery (C-MICS) incisions, if performed correctly, do not require sutures. It is advisable to place a single nylon 10-0 suture in the following situations:

- When there is intraoperative tendency for iris prolapse
- When there is capsular rupture with vitreous loss (even with a good anterior vitrectomy)
- Where there is a need for postoperative massage of the bleb

Postoperative Therapy

An antibiotic steroid combination is used 4 times per day for 15 days and then 2 times per day for an additional 15 days. The addition of nonsteroidal anti-inflammatory drug (NSAID) eyedrops may prove useful to reduce the onset of cystoid macular edema (CME). There is a tendency of glaucomatous eyes to develop increased IOP following cataract removal, requiring careful monitoring and administration of pressure-lowering drugs, if necessary.

Complications

Complications that may appear during surgery or postoperatively with phacoemulsification in cataract/glaucomatous eyes are usually the same as with standard cataract surgery, although more frequent. There are also complications in eyes with glaucoma such as malignant glaucoma, ciliary block glaucoma, and transitory postoperative pressure spikes. High

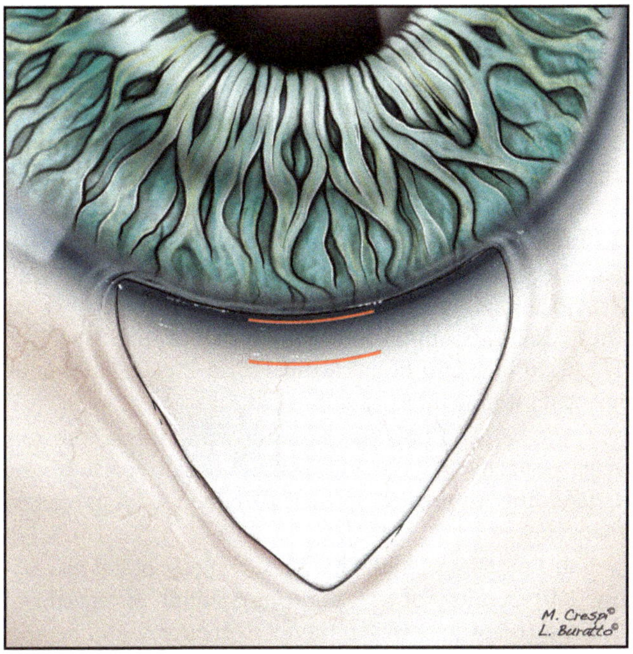

Figure 3-3. The surgical limbus is the area of blue-gray between the sclera and clear cornea and can be identified after removal of the conjunctiva and Tenon's capsule. Its posterior limit normally overlaps the front part of the trabecular meshwork.

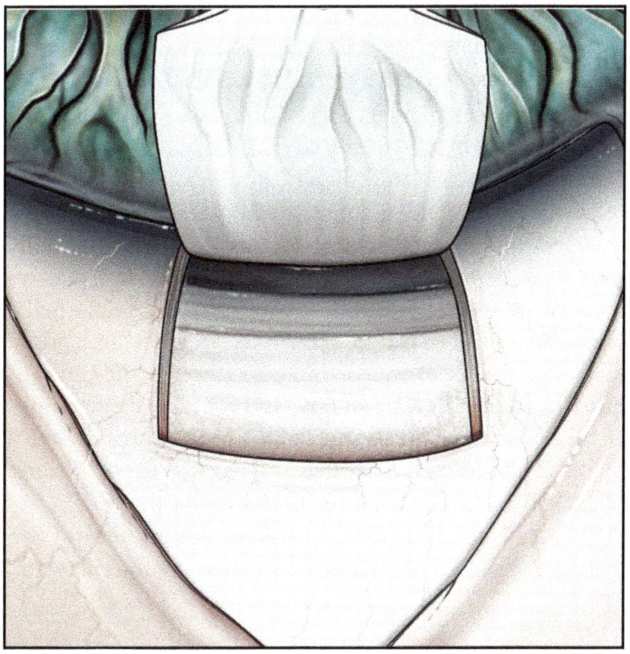

Figure 3-4. Display of the main landmarks in the dissection of a scleral flap at a depth of two-thirds the scleral thickness.

IOP deserves special mention as eyes with failed filters are particularly at risk of postoperative pressure spikes following phacoemulsification without combined glaucoma surgery. The increased IOP is almost always due to VES remaining in the eye after surgery. Although it has been shown that transitory high IOP does not cause further visual field damage,[57] elevated IOP should be addressed with AC decompression maneuvers using the side port incision depressed with a 30-gauge needle and repeating as necessary.

Combined Cataract and Glaucoma Surgery

The Limbus: Anatomical Description

The term *limbus* indicates the transition zone between the cornea and the sclera. Externally, it is characterized by the continuation of the conjunctival and corneal epithelial layers. Tenon's capsule is inserted on the episcleral surface about 1 to 2 mm posterior to the junction between the conjunctiva and cornea.

In anatomical terms, the limbus includes the block of tissue defined anteriorly by a line passing between Descemet's and Bowman's membranes and posteriorly, by a line starting from the scleral spur perpendicular to the external surface of the eye. Histologically, it is a continuation of scleral and corneal connective tissue; differentiation is possible by the varying thickness of the collagen fibers (600 Å for the cornea and 700 to 1000 Å for the sclera), by a more uniform arrangement, and less eosinophilia of the corneal fibers (Figure 3-3).

The surgical limbus is the blue-gray zone visible between the cornea and the sclera once the conjunctiva and Tenon's capsule have been removed (see Figure 3-3); the width is approximately 1.2 mm, and slightly larger in the vertical quadrants. The most important point that needs to be identified is the posterior limit, which normally corresponds to Schwalbe's line.

The creation of a groove extending approximately one-third of the scleral thickness, as in viscocanalostomy, deep sclerectomy, and canaloplasty, defines the posterior limit of the surgical limbus corresponding to the scleral spur (Figure 3-4). In front of the spur, the limbus is an opaque-gray color corresponding to the trabecular meshwork and transparent in front of Schwalbe's line where it continues into the cornea. The limbus contains the primary outflow of aqueous: the trabecular meshwork, Schlemm's canal, and the collecting canals.

The trabecular meshwork extends from the edge of the cornea to the scleral spur and has 3 main components: uveal, corneoscleral, and juxtacanalicular.

The uveal trabeculum is the innermost layer, and consists of strands of uveal tissue that extend from the scleral spur to the peripheral iris; generally, this does not resist aqueous outflow to any great degree.

The corneoscleral component, between the other 2 layers, forms the body of the trabeculum; it is a network of collagen fibers stretched between the scleral spur and the ciliary muscle on one side and Schwalbe's line on the other. The fibers are covered by a single layer of endothelial cells that produce the extracellular matrix and have a phagocytic activity.

The juxtacanalicular trabeculum (also called cribriform) consists of loose connective tissue lying immediately behind the interior wall of Schlemm's canal and appears to be largely responsible for resistance to aqueous outflow.

Schlemm's canal is a circular structure coated internally by a layer of endothellial cells. The internal wall has an irregular shape because of the partial overlap of endothelial cells and the presence of numerous vacuoles and pores, allowing passage of aqueous filtered through the trabeculum; the external wall is smooth and contains the openings of the collector channels. The lumen of Schlemm's canal is crossed by numerous partitions and has a reduced diameter in eyes with primary glaucoma.

The collector channels form an intrascleral plexus from which the aqueous flows into the episcleral venous network.

Phacoemulsification and Trabeculectomy

It is well known that trabeculectomy reduces IOP by allowing aqueous to flow into the subconjunctival space, or more precisely below Tenon's capsule. This filtration occurs through a continuous opening in the scleral wall at the trabeculum and is inevitably influenced by scarring that may involve conjunctiva and Tenon's capsule postoperatively.

Traditionally, a patient with cataracts and glaucoma was treated with a sequential approach: a trabeculectomy, followed by cataract surgery once the bleb had formed and the IOP had stabilized. Two separate procedures were performed because of poor results with combined ECCE/trabeculectomy.[11-13,54]

Sequential surgery, as it was performed until recently, had a number of drawbacks—mainly that 2 separate surgical procedures were required, which were inconvenient, increased costs, and delayed visual rehabilitation.

Phacoemulsification changed the mindset of the majority of surgeons and increased the use of combined surgery with pressure control similar to trabeculectomy alone.[55,56] The advantages of phaco as compared to ECCE are as follows:

- Less manipulation of the conjuntiva and corneoscleral tissue reducing scarring and fibrosis of the bleb
- The development of capsulorrhexis has led to greater stability of the capsular bag, leading to a decreased chance of vitreous plugging the opening
- Minimal invasiveness of phaco, particularly when a microincisional technique is used, creating less inflammation reducing synechia formation and release of pigments (with possible obstruction of the trabecular meshwork)
- Faster visual rehabilitation

Anesthesia

The choice of anesthesia depends largely on the surgeon. For trabeculectomy (either alone or in combination with phacoemulsification), general or local/regional anesthesia can be used (retrobulbar, peribulbar, or sub-Tenon's) and occasionally, the surgeon may choose topical anesthesia.

A retrobulbar block is the choice for the majority of surgeons as good akinesia and analgesia can be achieved with a small amount of anesthetic; when compared to peribulbar anesthesia, this option reduces the risk of increased IOP. The technique can be performed with 2 cc of anesthetic injected into the internal canthus.[61]

If the surgeon opts for peribulbar anesthesia, the surgeon performs 4 periconical injections in each of the 4 quadrants to ensure optimal distribution of the anesthetic.

Sub-Tenon's anesthesia has the advantage of not increasing IOP because of the reduced amount of anesthesic injected (1.5 mL); however, there is a greater risk of hemorrhage.[62] The agent should preferably be injected into the superior rectus muscle because it is not feasible to create more than one conjunctival opening and also because it is possible to pass the traction suture below the superior rectus muscle.

With all anesthetic injections, the block can be performed with 2% carbocaine (or 2% lidocaine) usually combined with 0.50% marcaine (in a 1:1 ratio) if the surgery is expected to take longer than normal (approximately 2 hours).

Compressing the eye allows better diffusion of the anesthetic solution and reduces IOP; this step is essential in the preparation of the patient, even though many surgeons do not use it because they believe that it increases IOP, a danger in patients with glaucoma. External pressure should be maintained for approximately 20 minutes between 30 and 40 mm Hg. If the surgeon wishes to achieve total akinesia of the eyelids, a facial nerve block should be used (Van Lint technique).

Some surgeons use topical anesthesia (4% xylocaine and 0.5% tetracaine hydrochloride); in addition to topical anesthesia, the surgeon should always do an intracameral injection of preservative-free 1% xylocaine. In the quadrant in which the scleral opening will be prepared, instillation of eyedrops may be combined with a sponge soaked in 4% xylocaine and applied to the conjunctiva for 30 seconds; alternatively, an injection of subconjunctival anesthetic may be used.[62,63] Good exposure of the surgical field can be obtained by asking the patient to look down.

Usually, a form of akinetic anesthesia is preferred, as the surgical dissection of the flap is a delicate procedure.

These techniques can be applied to the other surgeries described in this chapter.

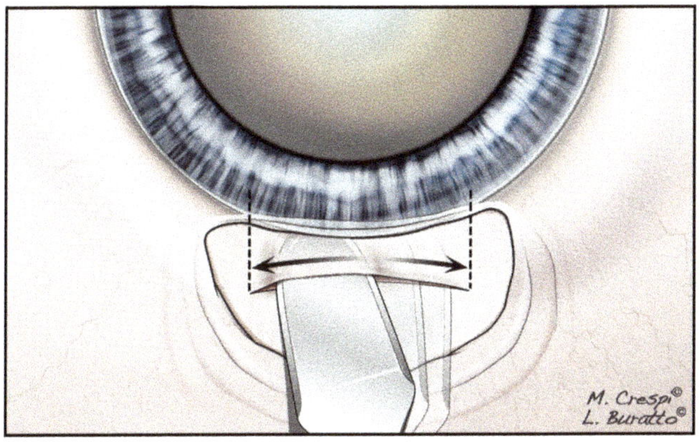

Figure 3-5. Phacotrabeculectomy in single incision; the scleral tunnel is extended to about 1 mm in clear cornea.

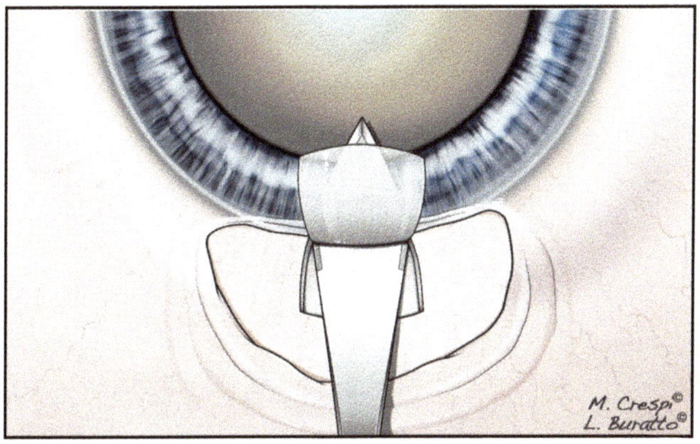

Figure 3-6. Phacotrabeculectomy in single incision: the AC will open with a knife calibrated to 2 to 2.2 mm.

Surgical Technique

There are numerous alternatives for phacotrabeculectomy. The first decision the surgeon must make is to choose the position for phaco; traditionally, this is performed superiorly, as part of the scleral incision used for trabeculectomy. Alternately, the 2 procedures can be performed through 2 separate incisions: a standard trabeculectomy is performed superiorly once the phaco procedure has been completed temporally. The technique can be modified based on the type of conjunctival flap, the use of antimetabolites, the method used to remove the corneoscleral block, and the type of lens implanted.

Phacotrabeculectomy With a Single Incision Superiorly

Preparation of the Scleral Bed

Once the eyelashes have been isolated from the operating field using an adhesive drape and after insertion of the lid speculum, if the surgeon is using local/regional anesthesia, it is necessary to place a traction suture under the superior rectus muscle, usually 4-0 silk; this will be taut for all of the surgical steps in the sclera and released during steps on the cornea or AC. Delicate forceps (Graefe [Arcrivet, Hennigsdorf, Germany] or Verzella [Janach, Como, Italy]) are generally used to grasp the muscle.

The next step is the preparation of the conjunctival flap at the 12 o'clock position, with a limbal or fornix base; the width of the incision should be 6 to 7 mm; if the conjuntival flap is limbal based, the incision is created 8 to 10 mm away from the limbus. The position of the hinge (at the limbus or at the fornix) depends largely on surgeon preference and requirements of the individual surgical case. There are no comparative studies that clearly demonstrate the superiority of one method over another.

Diathermy is used to stop any bleeding from the scleral surface; this must be relatively conservative to avoid damaging the sclera.

Scleral Tunnel

The creation of the scleral tunnel used to create the flap ensures that the AC is well sealed while phaco is being performed. A groove of 2 to 3 mm is created approximately 2 mm behind the limbus, at a depth approximately one-third scleral thickness; the sclera is dissected using a bevel-up knife, approximately 1 mm into clear cornea (Figure 3-5).

At this point, the surgeon creates a 1-mm side port incision, approximately at the 2 o'clock position from the tunnel and injects VES into the AC. Finally, the scleral tunnel is completed with a keratome, the width depending on the type of phacoemulsification tip being used (normally 2 to 2.2 mm; Figure 3-6).

Phacoemulsification and Implantation of the Intraocular Lens

The phacoemulsification technique is the same as previously described (see the Phacoemulsification in Glaucomatous Eyes section in this chapter) involving dilation of a small pupil, followed by a standard capsulorrhexis, hydrodissection, emulsification of the lens with a chop technique, and IOL implantation.

Protection of the delicate structures of the limbus suggests the implantation of foldable lenses with choice of material depending on surgeon preference. Acrylic lenses have numerous advantages in cataract surgery and these advantages also apply in combined surgery. If the tunnel is long enough (approximately 2 mm), the reduced size of the incision necessary for foldable IOLs ensures good closure of the tunnel with no need for sutures. If the surgeon elects to implant a rigid lens, it is possible to enlarge the tunnel to the desired dimensions and place 10-0 nylon sutures as needed at each end of the tunnel created for the phaco.

Following IOL implantation, residual VES is aspirated from the AC using a mono- or bimanual I/A system; the bimanual technique requires the creation of a second incision at the 10 o'clock position. It is essential to completely

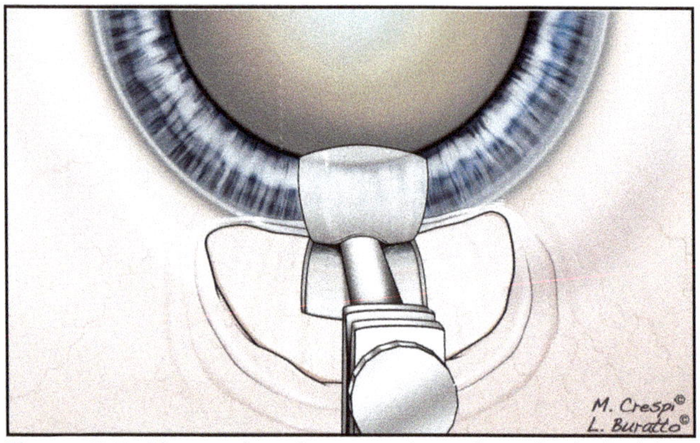

Figure 3-7. Phacotrabeculectomy through a single incision: maintaining the AC filled with viscoelastic pressure is applied to the punch for the removal of the scleral portion.

remove all VES (including behind the IOL) to reduce the risk of a pressure spike in the first hours after surgery.

The injection of acetylecholine into the AC at the end of phacoemulsification following aspiration of VES from the AC reduces the risk of involving the iris in successive steps of surgery.

Trabeculectomy

When phacoemulsification is complete, a small amount of cohesive VES is injected in a single spot onto the superior area of the iris in the position chosen for the trabeculectomy. Many surgeons believe that the VES should be left in the AC until the end of surgery to avoid sudden collapse of the AC following the trabeculectomy. At this point, the tunnel can be transformed into an L-shaped scleral flap using a radial incision (approximately 1.5 mm long) starting from one of the 2 posterior corners of the tunnel. Thus the points for the trabeculectomy are delineated.

In both combined procedures and in simple trabeculectomies, the section of trabeculum can be removed using several different methods, including blades, scissors, drills, or scleral punches (Figures 3-7 and 3-8).

According to Cairn's original technique, the surgeon creates an opening parallel to the limbus in clear cornea, below the scleral flap, and penetrates the AC. Starting from the ends of this incision, 2 further cuts are made in a radial direction to reach the posterior edge of the surgical limbus (corresponding to the scleral spur), outlining 3 sides of the tissue to be removed. This can be flipped over to visualize the structures present on the internal face and ultimately incised with Vannas scissors.[65] Clinical experience over the last 50 years has shown that trabeculectomy owes its success to aqueous filtration below Tenon's capsule through the fistula created. It is therefore essential that the portion of tissue excised is the correct size, allows a sufficient of filtration (to avoid risks of pressure drop), and does not create insufficient tissue ablation (to avoid residual high IOP).

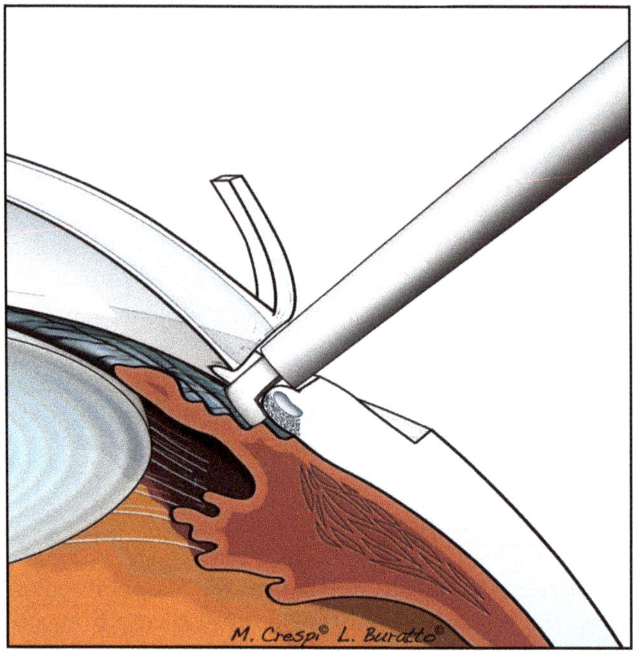

Figure 3-8. Phacotrabeculectomy in single incision: due to the depth of the inner edge of the tunnel meshwork, more than a bite of punch is needed to get a good result.

Over the years, the main variation observed in technique is the shape of the scleral flap (rectangular, square, triangular, or round) as in simple trabeculectomy. There have been a number of alternatives proposed for trabeculectomy including the use of different instruments for removal of the tissue such as the Elliot drill (with a diameter of 2 mm), Waalser emport-piece, and the Kelly Descemet's punch. Though instrument choice is surgeon preference, we recommend a scleral punch as it is more likely to produce the smoothest edges.

Other surgeons have gone even further and modified the technique for how the opening is created (ie, a technique invented by Phillips, Langerman's "reverse hinge" trabeculectomy, the inverted L-flap, and sutureless phacotrabeculectomy).[66-69]

Peripheral Iridectomy and Final Steps of Surgery

When the trabeculectomy has been completed, the surgeon performs a peripheral iridectomy; this must be large enough to prevent the iris occluding the opening. To ensure that the iridectomy is the correct size, it is recommended that the root of the iris be visible; for this reason, if the acetylcholine has not produced adequate miosis, the iris itself can be delicately manipulated away from the angle using a spatula. The iris is grasped with iris forceps through the scleral opening and brought slightly externally, to be cut peripherally with Vannas scissors. It is recommended to cut the basal iris by grasping it firmly with forceps held in the nondominant hand while simultaneously making a correct cut in the iris with scissors in the dominant hand (Figure 3-9). Residual VES can be then be aspirated.

A variation of this technique was proposed recently that suggested not performing an iridectomy as it is considered to be unnecessary as soon as the iris diaphragm has been pulled away from the cornea and from the area around the sclerectomy with removal of the lens. Although the iris and the internal scleral opening are displaced during phacotrabeculectomy, this variation is not very popular.

Sutures

Following VES aspiration, 1 or 2 10-0 nylon sutures are then placed in the flap, taking care to bury the knots. Alternately, surgeons may use absorbable sutures (10-0 Vicryl) to gradually increase filtration (10-0 polyglactin will reabsorb in 1 week)[70]; the conjunctiva and Tenon's are then sutured. Some surgeons prefer to place 5 sutures in the flap. Nylon lends itself to being cut using the laser when there is postoperative high pressures.

Some surgeons have suggested 2 adjustable sutures in the scleral flap to allow better postoperative IOP management and to minimize complications associated with excessive filtration.

An AC maintainer has recently been used to regulate the tension of the sutures; when the infusion bottle is positioned at a height of 30 cm, a one-drop flow rate should correlate to a postoperative IOP of 10 to 15 mm Hg.

With a fornix-based flap, 2 purse-string sutures (10-0 nylon or 8-0 silk) at the 11 and 1 o'clock positions will cover the entire scleral flap and allow good closure.

The creation of a limbal-based flap requires one separate suture for Tenon's capsule (preferably 8-0 Vicryl) and one for the conjunctiva (10-0 nylon).

The procedure concludes with injection of an antibiotic into the AC and with hydration of the paracenteses. The surgeon can then test the performance of the bleb, injecting a small amount of BSS into the AC through the paracentesis. The speculum should be removed very carefully to avoid creating undesired pressure on the globe, causing a flat chamber.

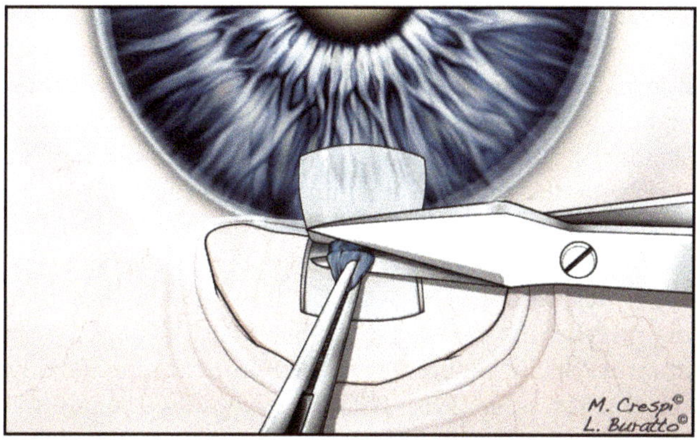

Figure 3-9. Phacotrabeculectomy in single incision: iridectomy-performance baseline.

Phacotrabeculectomy Using Separate Incisions

The use of a separate incision for temporal cataract surgery[69] has become very popular over the last 15 years because a 2-incision combined procedure is considered better than a single incision procedure. This approach does not differ greatly from the sequential technique. Prior to making the conjunctival and scleral flaps at the 12 o'clock position and before entering the AC, the surgeon moves temporally for phacoemulsification and IOL implantation, then returns to the 12 o'clock position to perform the trabeculectomy, peripheral iridectomy, flap, and conjunctival sutures. The rationale is performing the corneoscleral incisions with a closed globe having good pressure. The 2-incision technique is currently the most popular. The advantages of this technique include the following:

- Reduced manipulation of conjunctiva and sclera involving the bleb
- Nylon sutures closing the scleral flap can be cut with a laser postoperatively, scarring is not affected (important, particularly when antimetabilites are used)
- AC access is facilitated by greater visibility
- No need for compromising the 2 incisions

The advantages are countered slightly by loss of time necessary for surgical repositioning and the risk of tunnel leakage with serious postoperative hypotony. This risk is increased with phaco burns, an extremely rare occurrence with new instrumentation. Some surgeons recommend suturing the corneal incision just to be sure. Suturing the corneal tunnel is considered useful by many surgeons even with foldable MICS-IOL implantation because the surgeon may accidentally open the tunnel during successive surgical steps. A suture is mandatory in all cases in which antimetabolites are used.

Antimetabolites

Use of antimetabolites in phacotrabeculectomy has become popular over the last decade, to such an extent that most surgeons consider it essential. These agents reduce cell proliferation and subconjunctival scarring postoperatively. The best results have been achieved with intraoperative MMC[71-73]; the administration of 5-fluorouracil (5-FU; subconjunctival injection postoperatively) did not improve long-term success of filtration[74-76] and has been abandoned.

MMC is usually diluted to a concentration of 0.02 mg/mL. MMC is normally applied with a specific sponge (K Sponge [Katena Products Inc, Denville, NJ]), or a nonspecific sponge shaped and positioned between

Tenon's capsule and the superficial flap (and possibly below it, in a sandwich technique); the application usually lasts for 2 minutes. The sponge tip is cut creating a quadrangular or half-moon shaped fragment; once soaked, the sponge should be approximately 3×3 mm. Prior to placing the sponge on the episclera, it is necessary to check that there is no contact with the free-edge of the conjunctiva and Tenon's capsule. Once the sponge is positioned below Tenon's capsule, the risk of contact is reduced further when the surgeon lifts the edge of the flap with 2 forceps for the duration of the application of the antimetabolite. Finally, the area is irrigated with BSS; the forceps used to position the antimetabolite-soaked sponge fragment are also rinsed carefully.[71-73,77-83]

In combined surgery, MMC is applied once phacoemulsification is completed. We feel that MMC should be applied to the scleral bed prior to the trabeculectomy, allowing diffusion without seepage of the drug into the AC, as this can have a toxic effect on the endothelium. Conjunctival sutures must be placed carefully with needle passes that are close together. With a fornix-based flap, most surgeons use a continuous suture to securely fix the conjunctiva to the peripheral cornea.

Alternately, 5-FU can be administered postoperatively, particularly with a series of 5-mg subconjunctival injections; intraoperative use has also been suggested. The subconjunctival injections are repeated with 2 injections each week for 2 weeks. The injections can be used longer with greater intervals between them[74-76] however, this has not had encouraging results with phacotrabeculectomy.

Recently, some surgeons have advocated the use of antivascular endothelial growth factor (VEGF) drugs to control scarring of the bleb after trabeculectomy. Some studies[84] have used subconjunctival injections of bevacizumab (Avastin) with the trabeculectomy; however, the results are not as promising as with MMC.

Antibiotic Prophylaxis

There are many ways to administer intraoperative antibiotic prophylaxis. Gram-positive bacteria are responsible for the majority of endophthalmitis; these are from normal bacterial flora present on the eyelids and conjunctiva.[84,85] The risk of contamination by saprophytic bacterial flora can be reduced significantly by instilling a few drops of 5% povidone iodine a few minutes prior to surgery[85-88] and using an adhesive drape, excluding the eyelids and lashes from the operating field. Intraoperative antibiotics can be administered in the following 2 ways:

1. In the infusion bottle
2. Direct injection into the AC (through the paracentesis).

In any case, one should use prophylaxis covering Gram-positive and Gram-negative bacteria. The most popular combination is vancomycin and gentamycin.

Direct injection into the AC or better still, between the capsular bag and the IOL, offers—at least in theory—2 of the following advantages over infusion administration:

1. A precise amount of drug is injected into the eye (if antibiotics are in the bottle, it is impossible to know exactly how much has entered into the AC)
2. If the antibiotic is injected at the end of surgery, it persists longer and the concentration is greater

A number of antibiotics can be injected directly into the AC without damaging the endothelium

In 2007, ESCRS published the findings of an important multicenter study[89] that determined when cephuroxime (a second-generation cephalosporin) was administered at the end of cataract surgery, it reduced the risk of postoperative endophthalmitis. The dosage used was 1 mg in 0.1 mL of saline.

An alternative is intercameral injection of vancomycin (1 mg), combined with gentomycin in the irrigating solution (8 mg/L)[90]; otherwise the same dose of vancomycin can be injected with an aminoglycoside such as amikacin (0.4 mg).[91] Given the possible toxic effects of aminoglycosides, some surgeons have replaced amikacin with cephtazidime (a third-generation cephalosporin), which has a wide spectrum.

The protocols described above, developed for cataract surgery, can be used with phacoemulsification combined with glaucoma operations (ie, phacotrabeculectomy, phacoviscocanalostomy, deep phacosclerectomy, and phacocanaloplasty).

Postoperative Course

Fluctuations in the clinical picture in the first few days after phacotrabeculectomy demand careful follow-up by the surgeon. At each visit, the surgeon should check for perfect closure of incisions and exclude complications facilitating filtration, when necessary, with delicate bleb massage.

Pharmacological agents are very important in both trabeculectomy and phacotrabeculectomy. Normally, steroids are used for several weeks (4 times per day or more), tapering over the first month. Antibiotics are used at least during the first 10 to 15 days and in all cases when there is aqueous leak from the bleb. NSAID eyedrops can be used to reduce the risk of CME if trabeculectomy is combined with phacoemulsification (4 times per day for 2 weeks).

Indications

More than 50 years after the introduction of trabeculectomy, phacotrabeculectomy (particularly with antimetabolites) is still the gold standard in combined cataract and glaucoma procedures. Despite not being complication free, it produces excellent results in a large percentage of patients and in all types of glaucoma that respond to trabeculectomy.

On the other hand, the lower incidence of postoperative complications from deep sclerectomy, with viscocanalostomy and canaloplasty, appears to be enticing an increasing number of surgeons to abandon phacotrabeculectomy in favor of nonperforating techniques, particularly with open-angle glaucoma.

However, with narrow angle or angle-closure, phacotrabeculectomy is still the procedure of choice as the risk of Descemet's opening being occluded by the iris is high.

Results

Phacotraeculectomy allows excellent IOP control and good visual results in the majority of cases.

Effect of Phacotrabeculectomy on Intraocular Pressure

The combination of trabeculectomy and phacoemulsification in single surgeries is inviting. The results of phacotrabeculectomy with or without intraoperative MMC as reported in recent literature,[12,38,59,60,71-83,92-98] are good. Numerous controlled, randomized, prospective studies have demonstrated that MMC produces a decrease in pressure that is greater and longer lasting than in control eyes (without MMC), with good pressure control in approximately 90% of eyes.

The main problem is increased complications.[42,71-73,79,80] In a 2005 retrospective study, Wilkins et al[80] examined the results of 11 clinical trials having a total of 698 patients, with intraoperative use of MMC reducing the risk of surgical failure in eyes both without previous surgery and those with a high risk of failure. Compared with the placebo, the use of MMC reduces mean IOP after 12 months in all groups reviewed. Apart from increased risk of cataracts, the use of MMC did not increase postoperative complications.

Shin et al[92] identified factors jeopardizing filtration that include the following:

- Age < 40 years (more tissue reaction)
- Failure of previous filtering surgery
- Black patients
- Preoperative IOP greater than 20 mm Hg
- Preoperative use of at least 2 glaucoma eyedrops
- Persistent chronic uveitis
- Chronic conjunctival inflammation
- Pseudophakia

It was recently found that phacoemulsification with IOL implantation is a risk factor for trabeculectomy failure, with MMC in open-angle glaucoma.[81]

The debate on antimetabolites continues,[72,80,93-98] particularly regarding whether to use MMC in all eyes or just high risk eyes, as preferred by many surgeons. Many surgeons believe that there is a complex interaction of variables that when combined with the individual patient affects results; some surgeons believe there is no good scientific evidence supporting superiority of any MMC protocol, explaining its decreased use over the last 2 years.

There is no consensus on the results of combined versus sequential surgery, though as previously stated, pseudophakia is a risk factor that can lead to failure of the subsequent trabeculectomy. Considering that the surgeon desires a water-tight closure of the phaco incision with filtration through the trabeculectomy, if significant filtration is desired, the procedure should be performed through 2 separate incisions. Published results[99-102] indicate that filtration is better when there are separate incisions.

The position of the phaco incision (superior or temporal) does not seem to affect the pressure or visual results[103]; some surgeons report that the single-incision technique requires greater use of pressure-lowering drops postoperatively.[101]

The creation of a limbal-based flap leads to more complications during phacoemulsification, though with equal pressure results and formation of more cystic blebs as opposed to a fornix-based flap. Leakage from the bleb occurs more frequently in fornix-based flaps.[87,77,78,104-106]

The choice of foldable lenses does not appear to have any significant effect on the results of phacotrabeculectomy.[107,108]

Complications

Complications of phacotrabeculectomy can be divided into intraoperative, early postoperative, and late postoperative.

Intraoperative

Intraoperative complications can be attributed to the phaco and the trabeculectomy, with the most significant summarized in Table 3-1.

Early Postoperative

The majority of early postoperative complications of phacotrabeculectomy are similar to those of trabeculectomy alone and are related to hypotony, in that they create it (aqueous leak from the bleb and excess filtration) or depend on it (shallow/collapse AC and choroidal detachment). Antimetabolites have exacerbated this problem, particularly bleb leakage with an incidence of up to 40%.[109] Others report lower numbers, between 1% and 30%, and not all studies[57,71-73] have demonstrated increased leakage with MMC; its use requires extra caution when suturing the conjunctiva, Tenon's, and the scleral flap.

Primarily, treatment of leakage uses an application of large diameter soft contact lenses (or pressure patching using rolled-gauze compressing the upper eyelid and consequently the bleb) with instillation of antibiotic eyedrops; if the leakage has not resolved after a few days, surgical revision may be necessary using additional flap sutures.

Regardless of the cause, hypotony can lead to a shallow or collapsed AC, as seen in 1% to 5% of cases. Hypotony is

TABLE 3-1.

PRINCIPAL INTRAOPERATIVE COMPLICATIONS OF PHACOTRABECULECTOMY

COMPLICATION	CONSEQUENCE	TREATMENT
Phacoemulsification		
Wound burn	Poor wound closure (postoperative hyptony)	Change incision sites
PC rupture	Vitreous loss with possible vitreous incarceration in the opening	Good vitrectomy
Zonular dialysis	Vitreous presentation with possible occlusion in the opening	Good vitrectomy, tension ring
Trabeculectomy		
Conjunctival tear	Postoperative hypotony endophthalmitis	Suture or conjunctival surgery
Scleral flap tear	Postoperative hypotony	Suture
Hemorrhage	Hyphema-postoperative hypotony	Irrigation, cautery TPA

often associated with choroidal detachment with a variable incidence in phacotrabeculectomy of 0% to 26% without MMC and 2.4% to 21% with MMC.[71,72,104,106,109-112] It is the most serious complication in glaucoma surgery.

The transition from ECCE to phaco has reduced the frequency of complications, especially choroidal detachment.[100,112] For the same reason, hyphema is reduced as compared to ECCE-trabeculectomy, from about 30% to between 3% and 26%.[42,104,106,110,111] Hyphema is one of the most frequent complications of phacotrabeculectomy and usually resolves within 1 to 3 weeks.

Compared to ECCE, phaco in combined surgery also has fewer pressure spikes,[112-114] which could cause visual field loss in eyes with advanced glaucoma. Other possible early postoperative complications include a fibrinoid reaction in the AC (that is transitory and often related to iris manipulation), iris incarceration in the opening, choroidal hemorrhage, and corneal decompensation. A rare occurrence is endophthalmitis in the first 6 weeks postsurgery (approximately 1 case per 1000).[115]

Frequently, there is increased IOP immediately postoperative, due to lack of filtration; therefore, the surgeon must monitor the patient closely. If high pressure occurs in the first few days postoperatively (starting on day 1), treatment should include delicate massage of the bleb using 2 fingers; the lower portion of the globe is massaged with the patient looking upwards. Massage encourages filtration with swelling of the bleb (if the upper globe where the bleb is located is massaged, filtration is not encouraged).

The treatment of increased pressure a few days post-surgery consists of suture lysis (using an argon laser) or suture removal from the flap, creating immediate bleb enlargement. Even though there are no precise rules, suture lysis/removal is usually successful between 10 to 20 days postoperatively. It should not be performed earlier as this could lead to serious hypotony. Conversely, suture removal is generally useless after 20 days because scarring is more or less complete. Removal/lysis should be considered up to 20 days after the surgery if the bleb was present until a few days earlier.

Phacoemulsification has been significant in reduction of early postoperative complications in combined surgery as opposed to ECCE. These advantages are increased when phaco is combined with a nonpenetrating procedure such as deep sclerectomy, viscocanalostomy, or canaloplasty, allowing further reduction in complications traditionally associated with trabeculectomy.

Late Onset Complications

The most serious complication of filtering procedures is endophthalmitis.[116,117] MMC (and 5-FU) encourage development of a thin-walled bleb increasing the possibility of intraocular infection even several months after surgery[71,72,110,116]; streptococcus is most frequent. Fortunately, late-onset endophthalmitis is still very rare.

It is important to remember that a bleb is a permanent risk factor for infection. MMC has been associated with increased chronic hypotony, with possible maculopathy (incidence between 2% and 5%)[71,72,104,110]; fortunately, this is rare.

With scarring, the surgeon should use massaging or "needling" of the bleb; in untreatable cases, further surgery with MMC is inevitable.

Typically, PCO following combined procedures is the most common complication, having an incidence of between 7% and 25%,[57,104,106,110] though less frequent with acrylic lenses.[108] It has been shown that the need for yttrium-aluminum-garnet (YAG) capsulotomy is reduced with intraoperative MMC (0.5 mg/mL for 3 minutes), at least with PMMA lenses.[118]

Phacoemulsification and Trabeculotomy

Trabeculotomy was the first of the nonpenetrating antiglaucoma surgical techniques dating back to the 1960s.[119-124] The technique creates direct communication between the AC and Schlemm's canal, bypassing the main barrier to filtration, the trabecular meshwork. The procedure is similar to goniotomy, the difference being access to Schlemm's canal is ab externo as opposed to through the AC.

With combined surgery, phacotrabeculotomy has demonstrated reduction in IOP and is excellent for mild glaucoma. The technique is currently not very popular, except in congenital glaucoma.[39]

Technique

Anesthesia

Anesthesia is the same as with trabeculectomy.

Trabeculotomy

Preparation of the Scleral Bed

The conjunctiva and Tenon's capsule can be opened using either a fornix- or limbal-based flap, depending on surgeon preference. The surgeon creates a scleral flap approximately 4×4 mm, two-thirds scleral depth; dissection is extended forward to include the blue-gray area of the surgical limbus, with Schlemm's canal at the posterior edge.

Identification of Schlemm's Canal and Trabeculotomy

Once the side port is created, a radial incision is created in the scleral bed; this incision measures approximately 1 mm and is close to the surgical limbus. The incision is extended downward to allow identification of Schlemm's canal and when it is opened, a drop of aqueous will normally escape.

The objective is to open the external wall of the canal without perforating the internal wall, avoiding penetration into the AC. The surgeon can indirectly confirm the correct position of the canal by inserting a stiff, elastic 5-0 nylon suture; if this rebounds when grasped by the free end and then released suddenly, the elasticity of the suture ensures that it aligns with the canal if the other end remains inside the canal. Alternatively, the surgeon can create a deep scleral flap instead of a radial incision and identify Schlemm's canal using the same procedure used for viscocanalostomy, deep sclerectomy, and canaloplasty (each of these is detailed in relevant sections in this chapter).

Once the canal is identified, to facilitate successive introduction of the special canalicular probe, some surgeons recommend the creation of an incision parallel to the limbus by introducing the inferior edge of the Vannas scissors inside the canal.[125] Then a special probe (Harm's probe [Asico, Westmont, IL] or McPherson probe [Janach]) is inserted into the end of Schlemm's canal. These consist of a handpiece with 2 curved parallel arms. The inferior arm is inserted into the canal and the upper arm acts as a guide to permit indirect visualization of the position of the arm introduced into the canal; part of the trabeculum is incised (Figures 3-10 and 3-11). Leaving the distal end of the canalicular probe toward the center of the AC, the instrument is withdrawn from Schlemm's canal, opening the trabeculum as far as the insertion.

The trabeculotomy must extend to the left and right for a total length of approximately 120 degrees; however, it should not include the point where the scleral floor was cut. The internal wall of Schlemm's canal must be preserved, otherwise the procedure will perforate and require a peripheral iridectomy.

Suture of the Flap and Conjunctiva

The trabeculotomy does not involve filtration of aqueous into sub-Tenon's space and therefore a suture is needed to close the scleral flap. Normally 5 to 6 10-0-nylon sutures are sufficient. The conjunctiva and Tenon's are closed using the same technique used in viscocanalostomy (as discussed in the Phacoemulsification and Viscocanalostomy section).

Phacoemulsification

Trabeculotomy is ideal for a combined procedure with phacoemulsification. There are a number of options for creation of an access tunnel for the AC[126,127] using 1 or 2 scleral flaps.

There are no significant differences from viscocanalostomy, deep sclerectomy, and canaloplasty with regard to the steps of phacoemulsification.

Results

By reducing resistance to aqueous outflow, trabeculectomy leads to a drop in IOP with good results in primary open-angle, angle-closure, and even more so, in pseudoexfoliation glaucoma.[126,128-132] The hypotonic effect is also enhanced when combining phacoemulsification with trabeculotomy.[39] The advantage of this procedure is that it does not require formation of a filtering bleb and consequently is not associated with its long-term risks.

It is generally accepted that the IOP reduction with trabeculotomy is less likely than IOP reduction achievable with trabeculectomy. Consequently, even in combined surgical techniques, trabeculotomy should be reserved for eyes with mild glaucoma or high IOP, without visual field changes; here, phacotrabeculectomy is recommended.[126,127,133,134]

Complications

Complications are divided into 2 groups: intraoperative and postoperative.

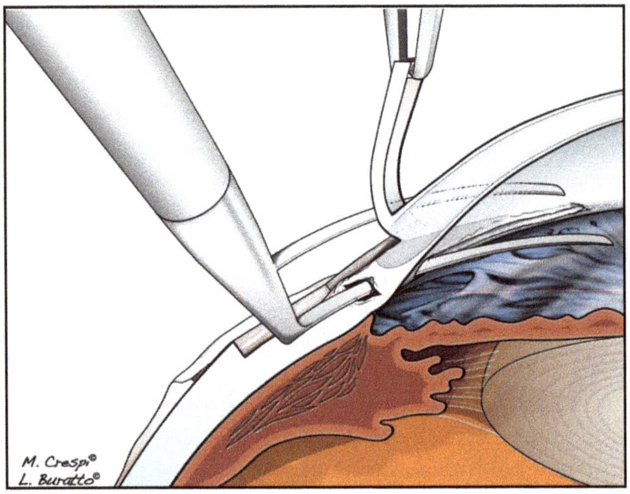

Figure 3-10. Trabeculotomy: the trabeculotome is rotated (gonioscopic view).

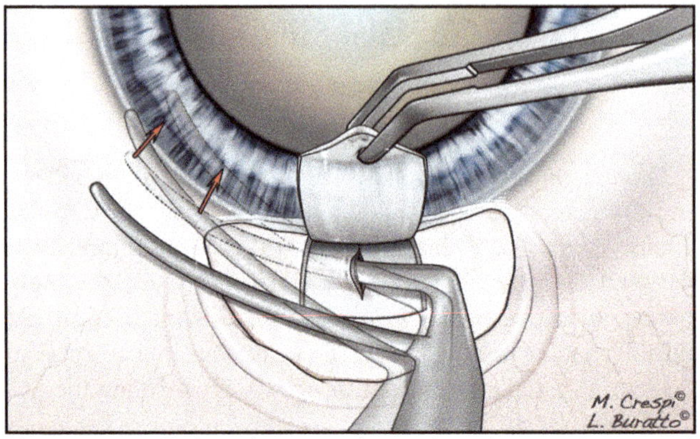

Figure 3-11. Trabeculotomy: the trabeculotome is rotated (external view).

Intraoperative

Mistakes may occur during preparation of the conjunctival and scleral flaps, including laceration of the conjunctiva, excessively superficial (or deep) flap creation, and these are the same as other antiglaucoma techniques. When these errors occur, the surgeon must suture the incisions and create another incision in a different location. Note that damage to the lens or iris is possible but rare.

Some complications are typical of trabeculotomy such as Descemet's detachment, caused when the instrument is rotated toward the AC with the tip facing the corneal endothelium. Another possible error resulting from the use of this instrument is the creation of a cyclodialysis that may occur due to lack of intubation of Schlemm's canal or a more posterior position of the canalicular probe. The resulting hypotony may require further surgery.

According to Tanihara et al,[133] in up to 84% of cases laceration of the trabeculum is accompanied by a mild hyphema (blood reflux from episcleral veins during the procedure when the IOP drops below the episcleral venous pressure). The clot normally re-absorbs in a matter of days.

Postoperative

The most frequent postoperative complications are the following:

- Residual increased IOP: If the IOP does not drop as desired, the surgeon must prescribe appropriate medical therapy or perform a second surgical procedure; sometimes, the option is enhancement of the trabeculotomy with a YAG laser.
- Formation of a conjunctival bleb: This requires suture placement to close a scleral flap with hypotony.

Overall, trabeculotomy is characterized by a lower incidence of postoperative complications (particularly those related to hypotony) as compared to trabeculectomy.[133]

Phacoemulsification and Viscocanalostomy

Viscocanalostomy is a nonperforating technique first described by Robert Stegmann[135] (Pretoria, South Africa) and was developed to avoid problems associated with scarring. Viscocanalostomy aims to restore the physiological conditions of aqueous outflow through Schlemm's canal and the venous collectors; filtration into sub-Tenon's space is absent.

An intrascleral space, called a "pool" or "lake," is created in which aqueous from the AC flows through a fine, specially prepared membrane: Descemet's window, consisting of anterior layers of the corneoscleral trabeculum and Descemet's. The aqueous is collected in the pool and then passes directly into the end of Schlemm's canal; the lumen has been cannulated and dilated with a VES injection. Aqueous flows from the canal into collector vessels and then into the episcleral venous network (Figure 3-12).

Aqueous from the pool spreading across the choroid is a situation that cannot be excluded, increasing the amount flowing along a uveoscleral pathway.[135] Viscocanalostomy has the following 2 advantages over trabeculectomy:

1. Elimination of the bleb will avoid all of its associated problems: failure from scarring of the conjunctiva, Tenon's, and sclera
2. The AC is not opened, and thus reduces the possibility of hypotony, phthisis, inflammation, and subsequent cataract formation

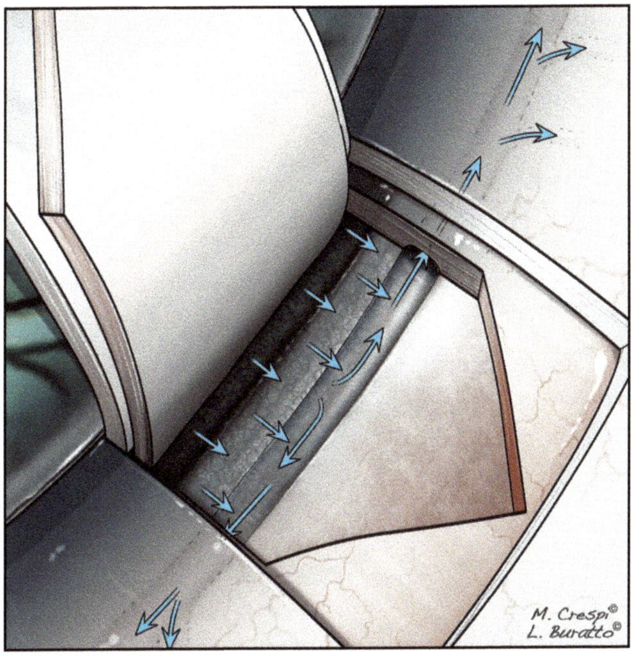

Figure 3-12. Presumed mechanism of action of viscocanalostomy. The aqueous humor filters through the trabecular meshwork and the Descemet's window and collects in the intrascleral lake. Then it flows into Schlemm's canal, whose lumen has been properly dilated with the viscoelastic. Finally the aqueous humor passes from Schlemm's canal into the collecting channels and episcleral veins.

The popularity of viscocanalostomy recently has convinced surgeons to try this technique even combined with phacoemulsification.

Technique

Anesthesia

Anesthesia is similar as described for trabeculectomy.

Viscocanalostomy

Preparation of Scleral Bed

A fornix-based conjunctival flap, 8 to 9 mm including Tenon's, is prepared at the 12 o'clock position. To keep the surgical field relatively free from blood, the surgeon may use an assistant or leave small segments of sponge on the sclera, replacing them continuously. The surgeon should try to minimize diathermy of scleral vessels, essential for outflow of aqueous. The main vessels should be identified and avoided, to prevent excessive bleeding. If diathermy cannot be avoided, the surgeon should use it minimally, coagulating the vessels one at a time.

Alternatively, good hemostasis can be achieved with topical ornipressin (L-ornitin 8-vasopressin, "POR 8 Ferring" [Sandoz, Switzerland]); a vasoconstrictor free from adrenergic action topically induces local ischemia for approximately 2 hours.

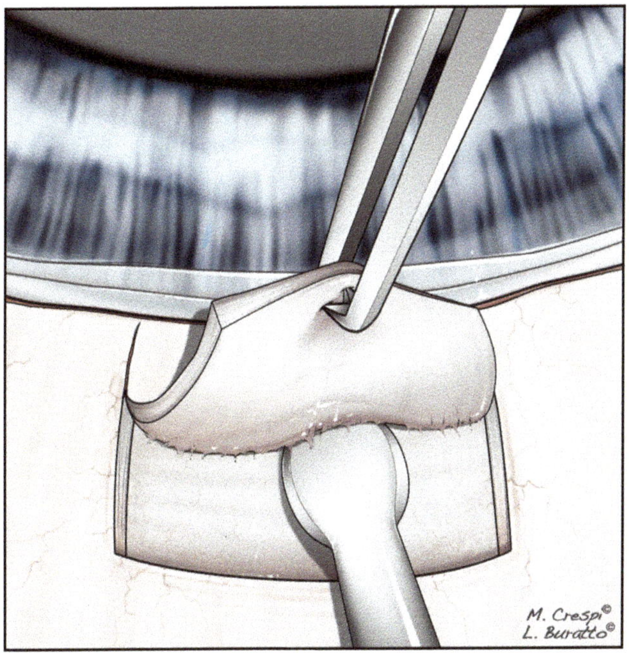

Figure 3-13. Viscocanalostomy: the flap is created using a crescent bevel-up or Grieshaber bevel-up blade.

Superficial Scleral Flap

Once the area between 2 venous collectors has been identified, a superficial scleral flap is created with a 1-mm incision into clear cornea. The flap may have various shapes and sizes though usually has a parabolic shape with dimensions between 5×5 mm and 4×3 mm, and a thickness of approximately 200 to 250 microns[135-141] (Figure 3-13).

Many instruments can be used to make the flap incisions such as a calibrated diamond blade or a 15- or 30-degree blade. A crescent bevel-up or Grieshaber bevel-up blade (Alcon Grieshaber, Schiffhausen, Switzerland) may be used for dissection as these blades have excellent dissecting ability.

Deep Scleral Flap

Preparation of a deep scleral flap is essential as Schlemm's canal can only be identified if the dissection plane is created at the correct depth. The edges of the deep flap are made approximately 0.5 mm inside the superficial flap to better seal when the superficial flap is sutured.

Considering variability in scleral thickness, it is difficult to determine appropriate depth. The use of a precalibrated blade is a relative contraindication. The correct approach requires that the blue-gray color be visible through the

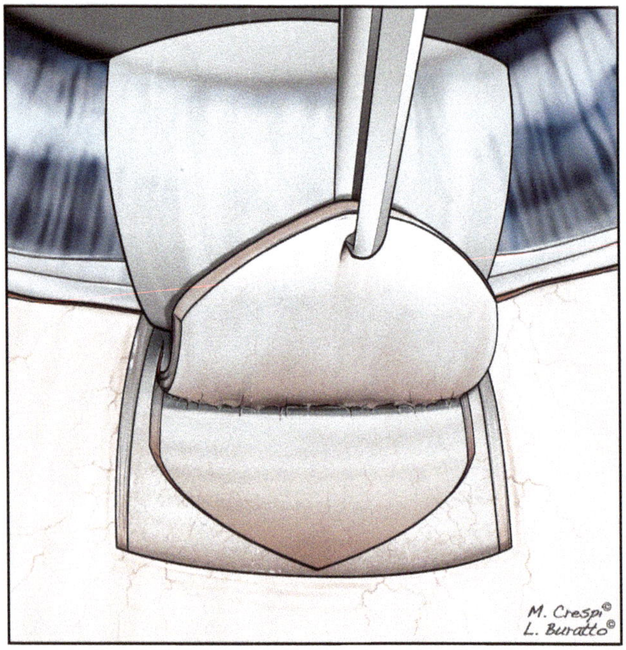

Figure 3-14. Viscocanalostomy: Schlemm's canal is identified and opened.

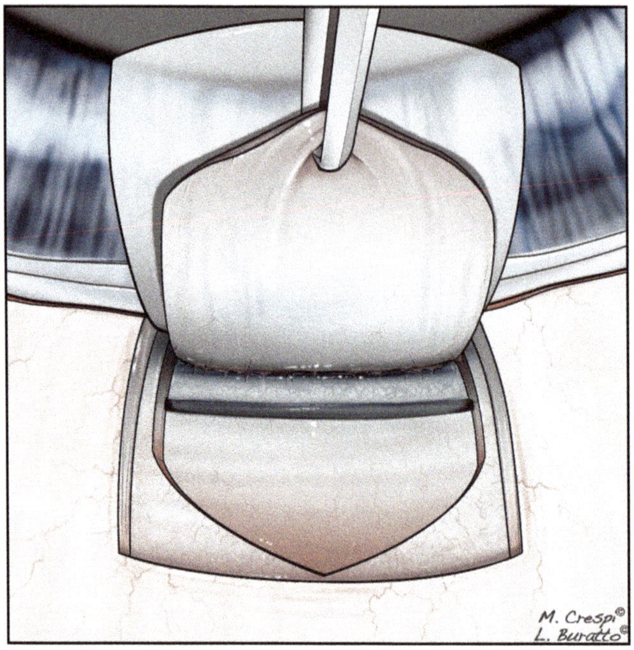

Figure 3-15. Viscocanalostomy: Schlemm's canal appears as a dark line, just anterior to the scleral spur.

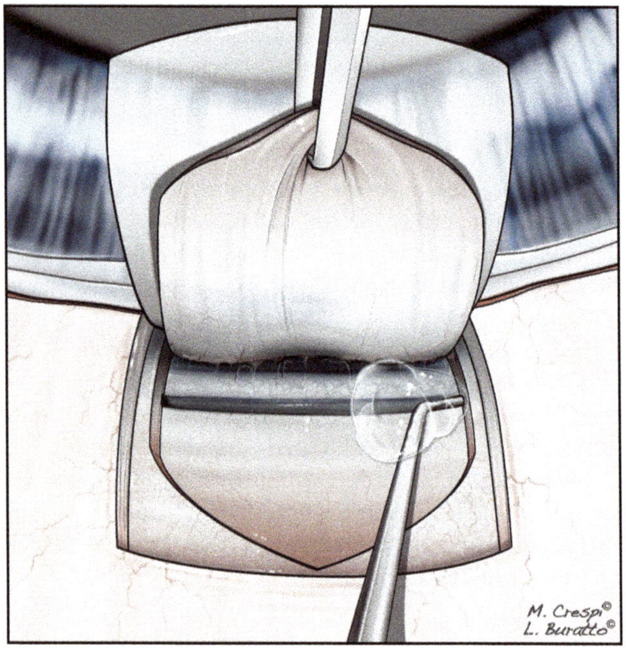

Figure 3-16. Viscocanalostomy: the viscoelastic is slowly injected into the opening cross-section of the Schlemm's canal. Simultaneously moderate traction is applied on the deep flap.

residual scleral lamellae.[135] The surgeon should use high magnification and instrumentation that will allow either a deeper or superficial dissection plane, depending on surgeon preference.

If the dissection is in the correct plane, Schlemm's canal will be unroofed as it is part of the deeper flap (Figure 3-14). Once open, Schlemm's canal appears as a dark line immediately in front of the scleral spur, defining the scleral bed anteriorly (Figure 3-15). Proceeding with centripetal dissection, the corneoscleral trabeculum is in front of Schlemm's canal with its typically granular appearance.

When viscocanalostomy is combined with phaco and the surgeon elects a single superior approach, the viscocanalostomy should be temporarily suspended. Once the deep flap has been formed, the surgeon creates the tunnel and proceeds with phacoemulsification. Viscocanalostomy or temporal phacoemulsification is then performed.

Dilation of Schlemm's Canal

Once Schlemm's canal is identified and opened, high viscosity sodium hyaluronic acid (Healon GV) is injected. A special Grieshaber cannula (Alcon Grieshaber) is used with an external diameter of 165 mm and an internal diameter of 90 microns (Figure 3-16).

The surgery should be atraumatic, inserting the cannula just 0.5 to 1 mm. Viscoelastic must be injected slowly, avoiding a sudden increase in pressure inside Schlemm's canal that could rupture the interior wall, creating an undesired trabeculectomy. VES mechanically dilates the lumen of the canal (pathologically reduced in primary open-angle glaucoma),[141] enlarging it from 25 to 30 microns to larger than 200 microns.[135] Immediately after injection, the episcleral collectors pale with the passage of VES through the canal. To achieve maximum dilation for the majority of Schlemm's, Stegmann recommended repeating the injection 2 or 3 times at both ends of Schlemm's.

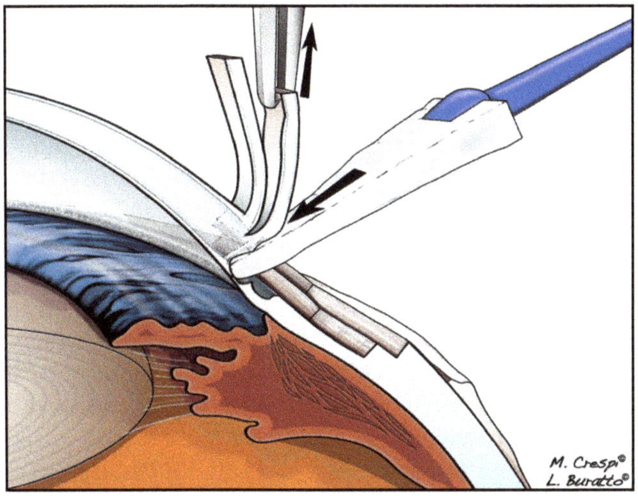

Figure 3-17. Viscocanalostomy: Descemet's window is created by applying gentle pressure on the Descemet's membrane with a sponge.

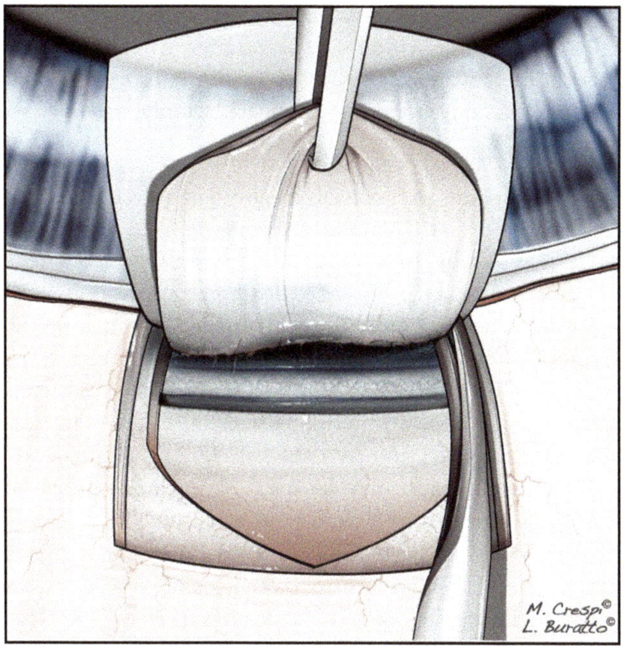

Figure 3-18. Viscocanalostomy: use of scissors to blunt the edges of the flap in order to extend deep.

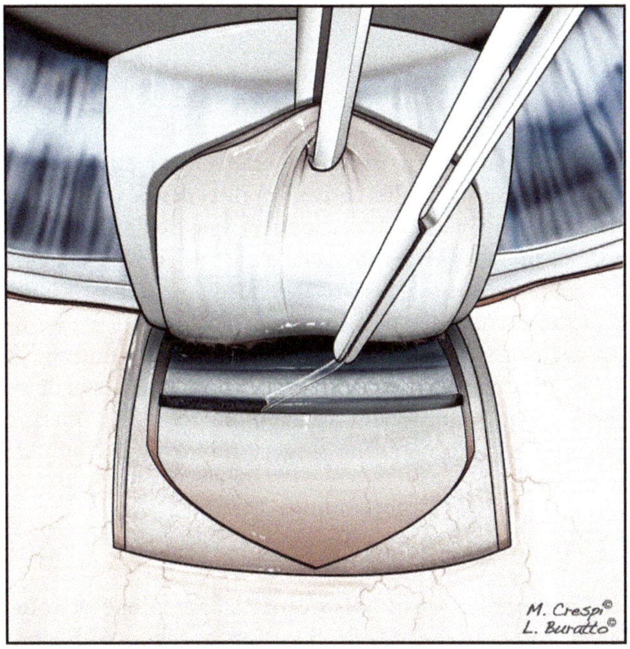

Figure 3-19. Viscocanalostomy: the stripping of the inner wall of Schlemm's canal increases the filtration through the Descemet's window.

Descemet's Window

The next step is creation of Descemet's window. Create a paracentesis at the 2 o'clock position; this reduces both the AC and posterior chamber (PC) pressure, reducing the risk of iris prolapse through the window. The drop in pressure frequently reduces the pressure gradient between the AC and venous collectors, creating an inversion of venous flow and blood reflux from Schlemm's canal, this slowly refluxes onto exposed trabecular meshwork. This indicates correct identification of the canal. With combined surgery, the paracentesis is used to introduce a second instrument.

Descemet's window is not created by dissection as moderately sharp instruments will increase the risk of AC penetration. The window should be created with blunt instruments, using a sponge to apply gentle pressure to the anterior limit of the trabeculum while simultaneously applying moderate, upward traction to the deep flap. Reduced IOP indicates success. This separates Descemet's membrane, still attached to the corneoscleral trabeculum, from the corneal stroma, continuing into the scleral tissue of the deep flap (Figure 3-17).

Descemet's of appropriate depth can be created when the sides of the deep flap are dissected approximately 1 mm into clear cornea, before exerting pressure on the trabecular meshwork with a sponge (Figure 3-18). Vannas scissors provide the best control during the cut as they have sharp tips and can perforate Descemet's membrane below. The use of scissors with long arms and blunt tips (Francesca scissors by Zanini [Janach]) reduce this risk.

Once Descemet's window is created, percolation of aqueous across Descemet's and the uncovered trabecular portion of the trabeculum typically occurs. When this percolation is insufficient or absent, the surgeon should remove any obstruction. The barrier is usually the juxtacanalicular trabeculum, the thin layer of connective tissue separating the endothelium of Schlemm's canal from the remaining trabecular layers. The juxtacanicular meshwork is removed along with the anterior wall of Schlemm's canal by "stripping" (Figure 3-19); Descemet's window will have been created in front of Descemet's membrane and behind the internal trabecular layers. The stripping can be repeated until good percolation is achieved.

These steps require great attention as there is a high risk of perforating the window. A perforation would eliminate most of the advantages associated with the procedure, and may require conversion into a trabeculectomy.

Excision of the Deep Flap and Sutures

Once aqueous percolation has been achieved, the deep flap can be excised. Vannas scissors are used once again as it is possible to accidentally perforate Descemet's window with sharp tips. Blunt-tipped surgical instruments available include the Pezzola scleral punch or the Francesca scissors by Zanini.

The superficial flap is sutured with 5 11-0 polyester sutures (Mersilene [Ethichon, Cornelia, GA])[135] to prevent aqueous filtration into the sub-Tenon's plane; alternatively, 10-0 nylon may be used.[136,137] It is important that the sutures induce closure to avoid bleb formation.

High-viscosity hyaluronic acid can then be injected into the intrascleral space to prevent collapse and reduce scarring during the early postoperative period. Mersilene or nylon sutures are also used to close the conjunctiva; 2 purse-string sutures are used on both sides of the conjunctival capsular flap. A subjconjunctival injection of a steroid antibiotic combination into the inferior fornix is made.

Phacoemulsification

Phacoemulsification can be performed using the viscocanalostomy access or a separate incision.

In the first case, the viscocanalostomy is commenced (and Schlemm's canal is identified), phaco is performed (through a tunnel below the superficial flap), and finally, the surgeon creates the Descemet's window and the viscocanalostomy is concluded.

In the second case, it is advisable to begin with phaco, complete the procedure, and then proceed with viscocanalostomy.

Incision

With a single approach (at the 12 o'clock position), the surgeon should create a tunnel that simultaneously satisfies the demands of phaco (intraoperative maintenance of chamber depth and incision closure at the end of the procedure) and of viscocanalostomy (demanding absolute integrity of the scleral flaps and Descemet's window). The tunnel for phacoemulsification is made after having identified Schlemm's canal but prior to creation of Descemet's window. The best position is the space between the superficial and deep flaps. As dissection of the deep flap is brought forward 1 mm into clear cornea, the tunnel is automatically created in clear cornea. It is approximately 2-mm long with the width depending on the tip selected.

There are advantages to a single approach as the surgeon does not have to change position. The risk of phacoemulsification close to the percolation site causing damage is reduced because the latest generation of phaco tips rarely cause wound burn; the small size of the tunnel and minimal trauma during IOL implantation are also important.

The phacoemulsification technique is as previously described: it may include dilatation of a small pupil, followed by standard capsulorrhexis, hydrodissection, phaco chop, and IOL implantation. It is important to avoid high IOP during phacoemulsification to avoid rupture of the filtering structures close to the sclerectomy.

Once the cataract is removed, the AC is filled with VES and the glaucoma procedure can resume with exposure and opening of Schlemm's canal. The surgeon will then notice aqueous percolation in phakic eyes, with minimal transudate in aphakic eyes.

At the end of phaco, once residual VES is aspirated, the eye should be left soft to reduce iris compressing Descemet's window. The injection of a miotic will reduce the risk of iris prolapse if there is perforation of Descemet's membrane (which would warrant conversion to a trabeculotomy). Finally, the surgeon hydrates the tunnel and paracentesis.

Indications

Viscocanalostomy, like deep sclerectomy and canaloplasty, is a surgical alternative for all types of open-angle glaucoma (primary or secondary), particularly with a normal pressure target (ie, glaucoma treated with a single drug). These techniques are indicated in cases of uveitic glaucoma (associated with low-grade postoperative inflammation) with high myopia and Sturge-Weber syndrome as these situations have a high risk of choroidal hemorrhage and subsequent postoperative hypotony following filtering surgery.[135] Nonpenetrating surgery improves the surgical safety profile.

Contraindications

Contraindications to viscocanalostomy (alone or combined with phacoemulsification) are absolute with neovascular glaucoma and iridocorneal sendothelial (ICE) syndrome; the contraindications are relative in chronic angle-closure or in eyes with extensive damage to the trabecular meshwork (such as post-traumatic angle recession, or previous laser trabeculoplasty).[138]

In neovascular glaucoma, the extensive fibrovascular phenomena blocking aqueous filtration cannot be corrected by dilation of Schlemm's canal.

In chronic narrow angle glaucoma, the advantages of viscocanalostomy are eliminated by the iris being close to the internal surface of the Descemet's window, leading to a postoperative filtration reduction. With narrow angle glaucoma, if the surgeon elects viscocanalostomy, a peripheral iridectomy or laser iridotomy is required.[139] Miotic eyedrops for the first 3 to 4 weeks postoperatively are required.

Results

Reports on viscocanalostomy and deep sclerectomy have recently increased. In viscocanalostomy (not combined with phaco), Stegmann et al[135] reported a success rate of 82.7% after 3 years. This refers to a relatively young, Black patient population (on average aged 54 years) with a high preoperative IOP (47 mm Hg), with results that are exceptional. Encouraging findings were also reported in Europe and America with success rates lower than trabeculotomy in the majority of cases.

When comparing trabeculectomy with nonpenetrating glaucoma surgery (deep sclerectomy, viscocanalostomy, and canaloplasty), the literature has conflicting results. While some have recently reported that these nonpenetrating techniques (with or without phacoemulsification) have produced comparable results in terms of IOP reduction, others have shown better results with trabeculectomy with or without MMC as compared to nonpenetrating techniques.[143-150]

Complications

Intraoperative

Procedures such as deep sclerectomy and canaloplasty thin the sclera without opening the AC and avoid rapid reduction of pressure seen with classic filtering surgeries. Thus complications associated with a drop in pressure are less frequent, such as intraoperative hemorrhage and postoperative choroidal detachment.

Perforation of Descemet's window is the most common intraoperative complication, particularly during the learning curve.[136] If microperforations can be ignored or even deliberately created to increase percolation, important continuity of the window will require conversion to trabeculectomy (or phacotrabeculectomy).

Perforation of the scleral bed from an excessively deep dissection, although rare, can have serious consequences, particularly if there is bleeding from the ciliary body. It is more likely to cause microperforations of the scleral bed, without uveal injury. When this occurs, the surgeon can complete the surgery and resume the dissection just in front of the microperforations more superficially.

Postoperative

Literature and surgeons have reported a very low incidence of complications early postoperatively after viscocanalostomy. Hyphema has been reported[135,136,143-146] though usually small (less than 4 mm) and even when severe, reabsorbs within 3 days. Sudden rises in pressure immediately after surgery are probably related to residual Healon GV in Schlemm's canal.

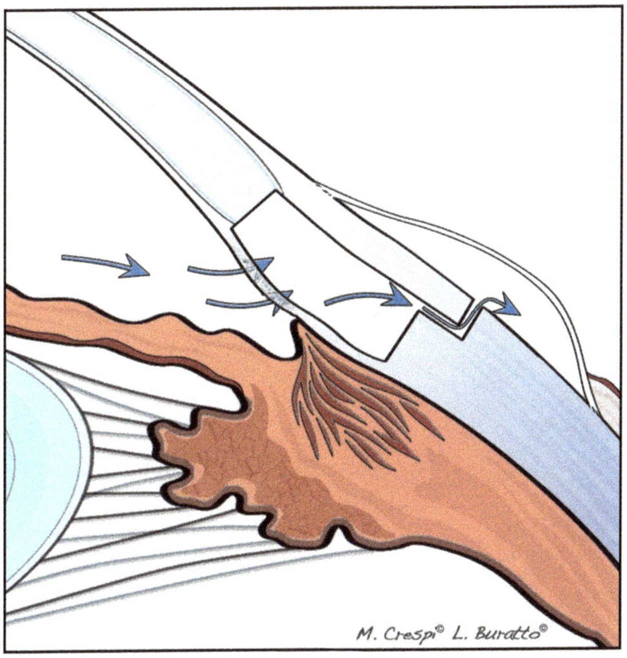

Figure 3-20. Deep sclerectomy: possible via filtration of aqueous humor in the intrascleral lake and here in the subconjunctival space.

Hypotony and all of its associated problems are rare, even considering that use of antimetabolites is not indicated with this surgery. Failure of viscocanalostomy and absence of IOP reduction may be caused by the following:

- Scarring leading to fibroblast proliferation on Descemet's window, obstructing filtration
- Failure of Schlemm's canal previously dilated
- Occlusion of the peripheral iris to the internal face of the window, seen more frequently in eyes with narrow angles[135]

Even the formation of a filtering bleb (5% of cases according to Stegmann[135]) can be considered to be a failure even though this is normally associated with excellent pressure control.

Phacoemulsification and Deep Sclerectomy

Deep sclerectomy is a nonpenetrating antiglaucoma procedure (such as viscocanalostomy and canaloplasty). It differs from viscocanalostomy as the objective is to filter aqueous in the sub-Tenon's space (not encouraging outflow by dilating Schlemm's canal with VES, as with viscocanalostomy) (Figure 3-20). The technique involves the removal of a portion of sclera that includes the part covering Schlemm's canal that is then opened, and a more anterior portion immediately above Descemet's membrane

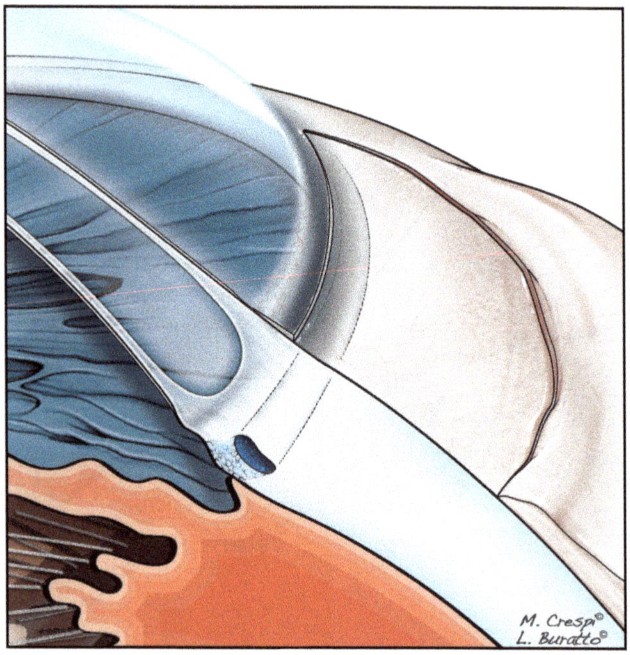

Figure 3-21. Deep sclerectomy: the waiting position of Schlemm's canal is scleral compared to the surgical limbus.

(Figure 3-21). The endothelial wall of the canal is also removed over the corneoscleral trabeculum. Consequently, an opening is not created between the AC and the subconjunctival space.

As with viscocanalostomy, drainage is encouraged by achieving outflow of aqueous humor through the thin ocular wall next to the corneo-scleral trabeculum. The aqueous is collected in an intrascleral outflow chamber and from there exits from the uveo-scleral outflow.

A bleb is an additional and unintentional way to reduce IOP, almost transforming the procedure into a classical bleb.[151-156] Like other glaucoma operations, deep sclerotomy can be combined with phacoemulsification.

Technique

Anesthesia

There are no major differences as compared to trabeculectomy.

Deep Sclerectomy

Preparation of the Scleral Bed

The conjunctiva and Tenon's capsule are generally incised at the limbus with the resulting flap being approximately 8 mm. Hemostasis of the episcleral vessels is achieved using bipolar cautery. It is important not to be too aggressive, to avoid inducing excessive scar reaction, with possible scleral retraction; however, it is not necessary to preserve the venous collectors as is the case in viscocanalostomy, as they do not play an essential role in the mechanism of deep sclerectomy.

Superficial Scleral Flap

The preparation of the superficial flap is essentially the same as described for viscocanalostomy.

The flap is normally square, approximately 4 × 4 mm; however, the surgeon may create a flap slightly larger or slightly smaller.[157]

When combined with phacoemulsification, the flap can be made superiorly, although some surgeons prefer a temporal incision; the deep sclerectomy is then created at the 12 o'clock position.[158]

Antimetabolites

With deep sclerectomy, as opposed to viscocanalostomy, intraoperative use of antimetabolites has a rationale in that the objective is filtration of aqueous into the sub-Tenon's space. Intraoperative use of antimetabolites is justified by the presence of one or more risk factors for bleb failure. With only deep sclerectomy, either 5-FU or MMC can be used. There are no studies that describe precise indications, dosages, or results with MMC or 5-FU with deep sclerectomy. The choice of antimetabolite, concentration, and application time depend on the associated risk factors.

In deep sclerectomy combined with phacoemulsification, MMC is preferred (0.03 mg/mL, 3-minute exposure time); its effect allows better long-term control of filtration.[71-73] Its application is similar to that described for phacotrabeculectomy.

Alternatively, 5-FU can be administered as a series of 5-mg subconjunctival injections, usually performed 180 degrees away from the sclerectomy[157]; however, in phacotrabeculectomy this has not been particularly successful and it is only used in selected deep sclerotomy cases and not combined with phacoemulsification.

Deep Scleral Flap

The deep flap is created using the same technique as in viscocanalostomy. For an easier grasp of the sclera, it is advisable that the deep flap be pentagonal pointing backwards (Figure 3-22).

If better control of filtration is needed, the deep flap can be made exactly the same way as with viscocanalostomy, with the edges approximately 0.5 mm inside the superficial flap to allow good closure once the sutures are complete. If the objective is greater filtration, it is possible to create a deep flap with the edges the same as those of the superficial flap.

Descemet's Window

After having identified Schlemm's canal and removing the posterior wall still adhered to the deep flap, Descemet's window can be created in deep sclerectomy.[159]

As this step has a high risk of accidental AC perforation, the surgeon should reduce AC pressure with a paracentesis, normally at the 2 o'clock position; with combined surgery, the paracentesis can be used for the second instrument.

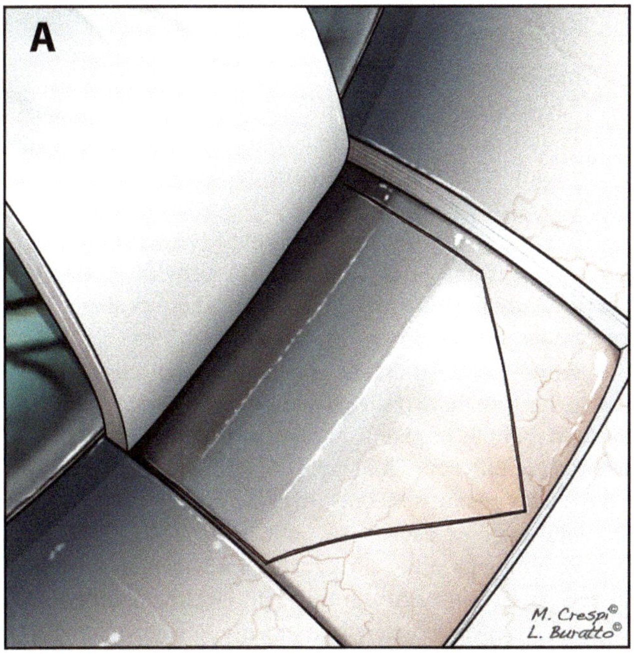

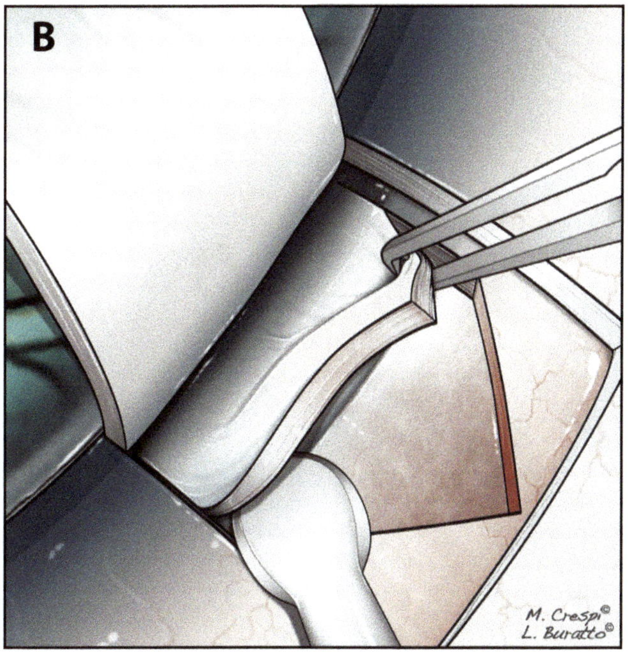

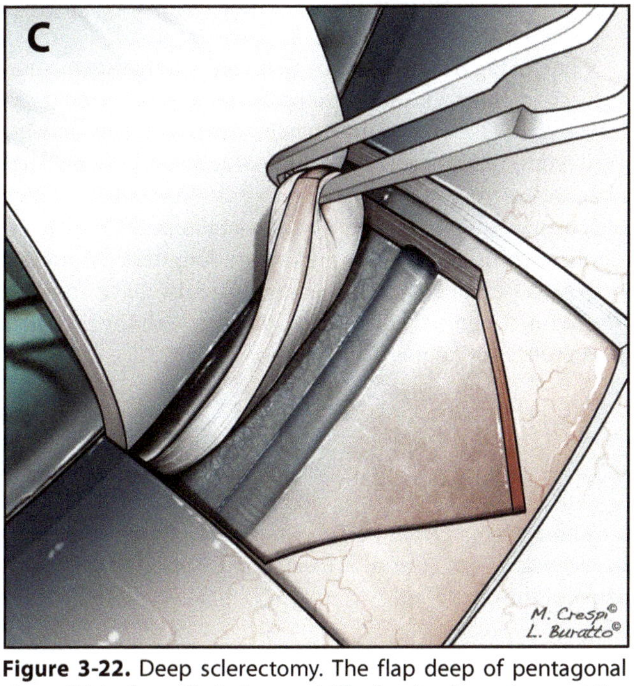

Figure 3-22. Deep sclerectomy. The flap deep of pentagonal shape (A) before, (B) during, and (C) after its dissection and the opening of Schlemm's canal.

Creation of Descemet's window is the same as described for viscocanalostomy.

Collagen and Hyaluronic Acid Inserts

To facilitate better medium- and long-term filtration, 2 inserts have been proposed, placed in the scleral space once the deep flap has been excised and contribute to maintaining intrascleral space, preventing occlusion from scarring. A collagen insert (Aqua-Flow [STAAR Surgical AG, CH-2560 Nidau, Switzerland]) is a cylinder of lyophylized pig collagen. This has great hydration and excellent biocompatibility.[156] The cylinder is positioned radially in the bottom of the scleral place, where it is sutured with 10-0 nylon (Figure 3-23); the anterior tip of the insert must be above Desecemet's window. The insert is slowly resorbed and persists for approximately 6 months. Despite not knowing the exact mechanism of action, its effect is probably maintenance of the intrascleral space and aqueous attraction by swelling; this increases its dimensions 2- or 3-fold.

The insert of reticulate hyaluronic acid (SK-Gel, Corneal, Paris, France) is a solid gel. Its mechanism of action is maintenance of the intrascleral space; the insert is placed at the bottom of this space before suturing the superficial flap. According to manufacturer's instructions, the insert stays in position for 2 to 3 months; degradation is slowed by the reticulant agent. In our experience, however, we have seen eyes in which the insert was still visible more than 2 years after surgery. There are 2 shapes of SK-Gel available: a trapezoid and an equilateral triangle. The reticulate hyaluronic acid insert is not particularly popular.

Excision of the Deep Flap and Suturing

The deep flap is removed using the same technique as described for viscocanalostomy. However, the suture of the superficial flap is different. It does not require good closure but must allow filtration in the sub-Tenon's space. Two or 3 10-0 nylon sutures are usually sufficient.

The conjunctiva and Tenon's capsule are closed with 2 10-0 nylon purse-string sutures, at the 2 ends of the

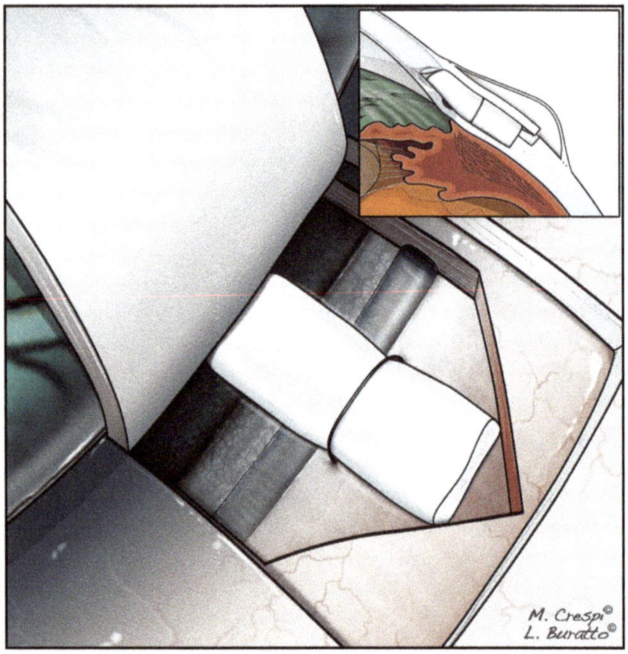

Figure 3-23. Deep sclerectomy: collagen device.

conjunctival flap. To allow good closure, when antimetabolites are used, it may be beneficial to add a running suture along the entire conjunctival flap.

Phacoemulsification

The phacoemulsification technique with deep sclerectomy is the same as previously described.

As with viscocanalostomy, it can be performed superiorly with the sclerectomy, or temporally; there are no significant differences in the pressure resulting from either superior or temporal incisions.[158]

Postoperative

As with viscocanalostomy, the postoperative course of deep sclerotomy is usually surprise-free in almost all patients. Good AC depth is maintained, inflammation is minimal, and visual aberrations are insignificant. If intraoperative percolation is sufficient, the bleb is flat. A standard steroid antibiotic combination is used for the first 3 to 4 weeks postoperatively (with or without phacoemulsification).

Indications

Deep sclerectomy is an alternative for all types of open-angle glaucoma.

Contraindications

These are the same as viscocanalostomy.

Results

Numerous studies have shown that deep sclerectomy, with or without phacoemulsification, can produce a satisfactory IOP with fewer complications, as opposed to trabeculectomy[143-150,159-176] (the same applies to viscocanalostomy and canaloplasty).

Nonpenetrating surgical techniques (viscocanalostomy, deep sclerectomy, and canaloplasty) provide good IOP control early postoperatively; however, there is also a high percentage of late failure.

Despite the fact that the efficacy of deep sclerotomy is felt to be less than trabeculectomy, intraoperative use of antimetabolites, implants, and laser goniopuncture appear to increase efficacy. The result of adding collagen to deep sclerectomy remains inconclusive.[147,157,161,164-166,174]

Meta-analyses have been published[147,173] on the efficacy of nonpenetrating surgery (deep sclerectomy, collagen inserts, insertion of hyaluronic acid, antimetabolites, and isolated viscocanalostomy) in open-angle glaucoma. All were felt to be successful when only moderate pressure reduction was desired.

Comparing trabeculectomy to nonpenetrating glaucoma surgery (with or without phacoemulsification), recent studies[145-148,158,166,173] continue to show contradictory results. With combined surgery, pressure reduction following deep phacosclerectomy appears to be slightly worse than that of phacotrabeculectomy without antimetabolites. There is no significant difference in visual acuity long-term; however, patients after phacotrabeculectomy usually have reduced visual function.[105] This is not surprising, with the minimal invasiveness of nonpenetrating surgery.

Complications

Intraoperative

The intraoperative complications are similar to those of viscocanalostomy and are primarily related to poor creation of the deep flap.

Postoperative

The incidence of early postoperative complications following deep sclerectomy is minimal when compared to perforating glaucoma surgery. A study[165] performed by laser flare meters show that during the first postoperative month deep sclerectomy causes less inflammation than trabeculectomy; the absence of a peripheral iridectomy and the nonpenetration are the primary factors.

On day 1, the condition of the eye is generally good, and hypotony and/or shallowing of the AC are extremely rare. Thus visual rehabilitation is rapid. The most frequent postoperative complication is hyphema, which usually resolves within a few days. In rare cases, deep sclerectomy may be complicated by malignant glaucoma caused by ciliary block.[171]

Even with combined surgery, there are few early postoperative complications, usually hyphema or an inflammatory reaction.[145-148,157,158,166,173] The major postoperative complication failure of the procedure is increased intraocular pressure. The barrier to filtration can be internal or external.

Yttrium-Aluminum-Garnet Laser Gonio-Puncture

Increased IOP may occur at any time after deep sclerectomy. Among possible causes is a barrier to outflow of aqueous through Descemet's window, related to intraoperative error (superficial dissection with poor percolation) or fibrosis of the window itself. In these cases, filtration can be increased by perforating Descemet's window internally with the YAG laser. YAG laser gonio-puncture may be necessary 40% to 50% of the time.[150,159,161,162,177]

IOP control following gonio-puncture is greater than 80% with the only complication being choroidal detachment (incidence rate of 4.8%) correlated to a sudden decrease in IOP following laser treatment. For this reason, the surgeon should reduce the pressure medically.[159] This can be performed early on postoperatively or 1 or 2 years later. As there is no clear indication of efficacy, surgeons are advised to wait 1 or 2 weeks following surgery to reduce the risk of hypotony.

Phacoemulsification and Canaloplasty

Canaloplasty was developed to improve aqueous outflow; it involves inserting a single or double Prolene suture into Schlemm's canal, dilated with a microcatheter. The suture attempts to stretch the juxtacanicular meshwork, improving circumferential outflow (Figure 3-24). This is a variation of viscocanalostomy with the addition of the following:

- Dilation of the canal using a catheter
- A permanent suture in the distended Schlemm's canal

The mechanism of action is therefore different from penetrating surgery. Rather than through the creation of an alternative pathway for aqueous escape, canaloplasty improves the efficiency of the natural pathway (trabecular meshwork) without interference with the subconjunctival space not normally used for this purpose. This is currently the favorite among the nonpenetrating procedures.

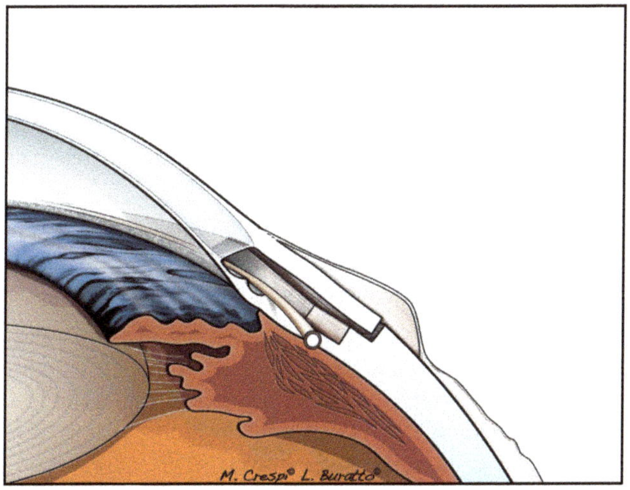

Figure 3-24. Canaloplasty: Schlemm's canal is cannulated with an optical fiber and a Prolene suture tensions the trabecular meshwork.

Surgical Technique

The surgical technique can be summarized in the following steps:

1. The first steps are the same as for the viscocanalostomy procedure: dissection of the conjunctiva with a fornix base, creation of a superficial flap with a parabolic shape, and a deep flap, paracentesis, excision of the deep flap to create the scleral space.
2. Enlargement of the canal using VES (Healon GV) with the objective of facilitating entrance of the microcatheter.
3. Insertion of a flexible microcatheter into Schlemm's canal. The catheter has a 250-micron tip with an internal lumen of 200 microns through which VES can be injected as needed. This device has an illuminated tip that assists correct insertion of the microcatheter as it is impossible to have direct vision. The illumination at the tip with reduction of the light of the microscope allows 360-degree control inside Schlemm's canal. This avoids moving in the wrong direction (ie, entering the AC on one hand or the suprachoroidal space on the other).
4. Once the microcatheter has reached the other hole of the canal, the end becomes the anchor for the 10-0 Prolene suture tied around it. When reversing direction, the surgeon should pay maximum attention to avoid damaging Schlemm's canal with the knot; a small amount of VES can be injected with a microcannula for the opposite pathway (every 2 hours for 360 degrees of Schlemm's canal). As the VES dilates the canal, it reduces the risk of damage. Once the microcatheter has been removed, the 10-0 Prolene suture is released (preferably single sutures, but double

sutures are acceptable) and the surgeon separates the 2 ends and completes the suture. The amount of suture tension is proportional to the stretching of Schlemm's canal and consequently the trabecular meshwork.

5. As this is an eye with extremely low IOP, it is easy to overdo the tension in the suture.
6. Once the Prolene suture has been tightened, the superficial flap is sutured and the surgeon confirms no filtration. Then the conjunctiva is sutured.

Canaloplasty can be used in open-angle glaucoma, pseudoexfoliative glaucoma, pigmentary glaucoma, and types of glaucoma in which the angle is greater than 25 degrees (when the angle is less, phacoemulsification must precede canaloplasty to open the angle); the target pressure is moderate to high.

Contraindications exist for certain types of glaucoma such as neovascular, narrow angle glaucoma, traumatic glaucoma with angle recession, and eyes having previous argon laser trabeculoplasty or trabeculectomy. The major advantage of canaloplasty is the circumferential treatment of Schlemm's canal with the possibility of intraoperative conversion to trabeculectomy. Possible disadvantages are difficulty with the external dissection (more difficult and longer than other angle surgeries) and conjunctival scarring increasing the risk of an unsuccessful trabeculectomy. Other potential risks are related to use of antimitotic agents and occasional bleb formation.

This procedure does not create direct access to the collector channels and IOP reduction is limited by resistance of Schlemm's and the pressure of the episcleral veins. Moreover, there are no reports of long-term effects caused by a foreign body (Prolene suture) in Schlemm's canal. As with other nonpenetrating glaucoma procedures, combined procedures with phacoemulsification are an option.

Results

The literature regarding canaloplasty does not provide much information. In 2008 Shingleton et al[22] analyzed 54 eyes with 1-year follow-up in a prospective, multicenter study. Recent long-term results from 2 different trials of open-angle glaucoma demonstrated that canaloplasty alone is able to provide IOP reduction for at least 3 years,[178,179] with few significant postoperative complications both short- and long-term. However, these studies also show that this procedure only provides modest IOP reduction, thus may be indicated only for patients with mild visual field changes and higher target pressures. Good results of combined results of combined canaloplasty and phacoemulsification were reported by Lewis.[179] These findings were not confirmed by Ayala et al[180] in which canaloplasty and trabeculectomy demonstrated significant IOP reduction that was only slightly greater for trabeculectomy, but not statistically significant.

Recently Koerber[181] presented a study in which he compared results of canaloplasty in one eye and viscocanalostomy in the other eye in patients with bilateral open-angle glaucoma. Koerber reported that both procedures have excellent safety profiles and that canaloplasty is superior to viscocanalostomy in terms of IOP reduction 18 months postoperatively. The use of MMC with canaloplasty is also safe and effective.[182] In a study by Grieshaber,[183] the use of 10-0 Prolene sutures has been shown to be slightly more effective in reducing IOP as opposed to 6-0 Prolene.

Complications

The surgery requires a certain degree of dexterity and may have both intra- and postoperative complications.

Intraoperative complications include the following:

- Lack of exposure of the canal
- During creation of Descemet's window:
  - Microperforation
  - Macroperforation without iris prolapse
- During catheterization and dilation of the canal:
  - Detachment of Descemet's membrane
  - Suprachoroidal pass

Postoperative complications include the following:

- The following are early onset (1 to 10 days postoperatively) complications:
  - Increased IOP (the following must be excluded: iris incarceration, angle-closure, peripheral iris synechiae, retained VES with combined procedures, and hyphema, steroid responders)
  - Visual acuity loss (more than 12% of patients initially lose 2 or more Snellen lines); this may be suture-induced astigmatism, which resolves within 6 to 10 weeks.
  - Hyphema: extremely frequent and may be considered to be physiological because of the retrograde reflux from Schlemm's canal (more frequently seen post laser procedures such as ALT or SLT)
  - Descemet's detachment: this may occur when Healon GV is injected.
  - Hypotony: a problem that usually quickly resolves.
- Late onset (2 to 5 weeks postoperative) complications include the following:
  - Increased IOP due to insufficient filtration due to micro- or macroperforations causing iris prolapse.

In conclusion, canaloplasty is a nonpenetrating glaucoma surgery that has the objective of restoring natural aqueous outflow without bleb formation. With canaloplasty, it is possible to significantly reduce IOP long-term with a moderate to high target pressure and a low complication rate.

Implants

Even though implants are not routine in combined procedures with phacoemulsification, recent findings deserve mention. Traditionally, GDDs are indicated in cases of uncontrolled glaucoma. These cases are at a high risk of failure following filtering surgery or when surgery has already failed. There are a number of different GDDs available; the most common are Molteno (Molteno Ophthalmic Ltd, Dunedin, New Zealand), Baerveldt (Abbott Laboratories), Krupin (Benson Hood Laboratories, Inc, Pembroke, MA), and Ahmed (New Medical Inc, Rancho Cucamonga, CA). Molteno and Baerveldt have no valves, while Krupin and Ahmed have valves.

The success rate for these 4 implants is approximately 70%, with a mean postoperative reduction in IOP of at least 50% from preoperative values.[182,183] Unfortunately, the failure rate is approximately 10% per year, with only 50% of the drainage devices functioning after 5 years. In a comparative trial of the Ahmed and Baerveldt devices, no clear superiority was seen at 1 year[184]; mean IOP is slightly greater with the Ahmed valve, but it has a lower incidence of early complications, which are less serious than those of the Baerveldt implants.

Recently, an update with 5-year follow-up was published in the Treatment Outcomes in Tube Versus Trabeculectomy Study (TVT)[188] showing that 5 years after the shunt procedure, IOP was slightly reduced (but not significantly) when compared to trabeculectomy. Postoperatively, both procedures have similar IOP reduction and use of topical glaucoma drops. GDDs have greater success when compared to trabeculectomy with MMC as the probability of failure over 5 years was 29.8% for GDDs and 46.9% with trabeculectomy; the incidence of repeat surgery was higher with trabeculectomy. Other trials have been reported with similar results.[185,186]

In regard to GGD complications, the results of another recent study with 5-year follow-up[187] stated that even with numerous complications, in the majority of cases they were temporary and resolved spontaneously. Moreover, as compared to trabeculectomy with MMC, there were fewer early onset complications. Both procedures had a similar incidence of late onset complications and repeat surgery secondary to complications and cataract surgery.

In 2008, a meta-analysis of shunts[187] demonstrated that long-term, the most serious complication involved corneal endothelium; the most frequent complication was conjunctival erosion over the GDD. The failure incidence in this study was approximately 10% per year, similar to that of trabeculectomy.

In conclusion, GDDs have good efficacy comparable, if not superior, to trabeculectomy in the management of complicated glaucoma. Traditionally, these devices are recommended in refractory cases, although they have always provided satisfactory results. They should probably be reconsidered in primary glaucoma management due to better predictability compared to trabeculectomy with MMC and fewer complications.

New Surgical Techniques for the Treatment of Glaucoma

Recently, new techniques have been advanced that are less invasive than trabeculectomy; they do not depend on bleb formation or the use of antifibrotic agents.[188]

The introduction and diffusion of these techniques have introduced a new era in glaucoma surgery. These new techniques have demonstrated excellent efficacy and a promising safety profile. Nevertheless, in order to demonstrate efficacy, randomized studies are needed with long-term follow up or a comparative trial with trabeculectomy.

The results of a recent trial by the American Academy of Ophthalmology (AAO)[188] showed that glaucoma procedures can be divided into the following 2 categories[188-195]:

1. Outflow surgeries developed to increase aqueous outflow from the eye
2. Inflow surgeries designed to reduce aqueous production

Outflow surgeries include trabeculectomy, shunts for aqueous, and their variants. This category can be subdivided into procedures that increase the following:

- Outflow by creating a new outflow channel
    - ExPRESS glaucoma shunt
    - Fugo knife transciliary filtration
- Outflow through the traditional (trabecular) pathway
    - Fugo knife goniotomy
    - Canaloplasty
    - Trabeculectomy
    - Excimer laser trabeculectomy (ELT)
    - Trabecular micro bypass stent
- Uveo-scleral outflow
    - SOLX Gold shunt

However, the results of the AAO study[188] did not demonstrate if these new procedures were superior, equal, or inferior to other surgical procedures such as trabeculectomy. All of these procedures can be combined with phacoemulsification.

In conclusion, both trabeculectomy and to a lesser extent, drainage devices are the gold standard of incisional glaucoma procedures. New surgical procedures that can effectively and safely reduce IOP are evolving.

Conclusion

An increasing number of surgeons treat glaucoma and cataracts with combined surgery, particularly to avoid the trauma resulting from 2 separate surgeries. This is made easier with constant improvements to surgical techniques. The surgeon must evaluate each case individually, considering a number of factors, including the risk/reward ratio. The surgeon's final choice of combined procedures must consider phacotrabeculectomy or phacoemulsification combined with nonpenetrating surgery. Phacotrabeculectomy is still the preferred procedure even though it has more frequent complications.

References

1. Greve EL, Wagemans MJU. Extracapsular cataract extraction in primary open-angle glaucoma. In: Greve EL, ed. *Surgical Managment of Coexisting Glaucoma and Cataract*. Amsterdam: Kugler Publisher;1987:51-57.
2. Raitta C, Tarkkanen A. Combined procedure for the management of glaucoma and cataract. *Acta Ophthalmol.* 1988;66:667-670.
3. Bonomi L, Marchini G, de Franco I, Perfetti S. Prospective study of lens changes after trabeculectomy. *Dev Ophthalmol.* 1989;17:97-100.
4. Bonomi L, Perfetti S, Bellocci R, De Franco I, Castellarin A. Il grado di opacità del cristallino come guida al tipo di intervento filtrante. *Boll Ocul.* 1993;72 (suppl 4):299-304.
5. Vesti E. Development of cataract after trabeculectomy. *Acta Ophthalmol (Copenh).* 1993;71(6):777-781.
6. Acton J, Salmon JF, Scholtz R. Extracapsular cataract extraction with posterior chamber lens implantation in primary angle-closure glaucoma. *J Cataract Refract Surg.* 1997;23:930-934.
7. Greve EL. Primary angle-closure glaucoma: extracapsular cataract extraction or filtering procedure? *Int Ophthalmol.* 1988;12:157-162.
8. Gunning FP, Greve EL. Uncontrolled primary angle-closure glaucoma: results of early intercapsular cataract extraction and posterior chamber lens implantation. *Int Ophthalmol.* 1991;15:237-247.
9. Wishart PK, Atkinson PL. Extracapsular cataract extraction and posterior chamber lens implantation in patients with primary chronic angle-closure glaucoma: effect on intraocular pressure control. *Eye (Lond).* 1989;3:706-712.
10. Samuelson T. Management of coincident cataract and glaucoma. *Curr Opin Ophthalmol.* 1998;9(1):33-38.
11. Kosmin AS, Wishart PK, Ridges PJ. Long-term intraocular pressure control after cataract extraction with trabeculectomy: phacoemulsification versus extracapsular technique. *J Cataract Refract Surg.* 1998;24(2):249-255.
12. Anand N, Menage MJ, Bailey C. Phacoemulsification trabeculectomy compared to other methods of combined cataract and glaucoma surgery. *Acta Ophthalmol Scand.* 1997;75(6):705-710.
13. Tezel G, Kolker AE, Kass MA, Wax MB. Comparative results of combined procedures for glaucoma and cataract: I. Extracapsular cataract extraction versus phacoemulsification and foldable versus rigid intraocular lenses. *Ophthalmic Surg Lasers.* 1997;28(7):539-550.
14. Bellucci R. Cataract e glaucoma. In: *Cataract, Relazione SOI.* Canelli, AT, Italy: Fabiano editore. 1999;447-473.
15. Crichton A. Management of coexisting cataract and glaucoma. *Curr Opin Ophthalmol.* 2010;21(2):129-134.
16. Friedman DS, Vedula SS. Lens extraction for chronic angle-closure glaucoma. *Cochrane Database Syst Rev.* 2006;19(3):CD005555.
17. Thomas R, Walland MJ, Parikh RS. Clear lens extraction in angle-closure glaucoma. *Curr Opin Ophthalmol.* 2011;22(2):110-114.
18. Thomas R, Walland MJ. Primary angle-closure glaucoma is a multifactorial disease. *Clin Experiment Ophthalmol.* 2011;39(7):593-594.
19. Azuara-Blanco A, Burr JM, Cochran C, et al; Effectiveness in Angle-Closure Glaucoma of Lens Extraction (EAGLE) Study Group. The effectiveness of early lens extraction with intraocular lens implantation for the treatment of primary angle-closure glaucoma (EAGLE): study protocol for a randomized controlled trial. *Trials.* 2011;12:133.
20. Vizzeri G, Weinreb RN. Cataract surgery and glaucoma. *Curr Opin Ophthalmol.* 2010;21(1):20-24.
21. Vass C, Menapace R. Surgical strategies in patients with combined cataract and glaucoma. *Curr Opin Ophthalmol.* 2004;15(1):61-66.
22. Shingleton B, Tezt M, Korber N. Circumferential viscodilation and tensioning of Schlemm's canal (canaloplasty) with temporal clear corneal phacoemulsification cataract surgery for open-angle glaucoma and visually significant cataract; one year results. *J Cataract Refract Surg.* 2008;34(3):433-440.
23. Francis BA, Minckler DS, Dustin L, et al; the Trabeculotomy Study Group. Combined cataract extraction and trabeculotomy by internal approach for coexisting cataract and open-angle glaucoma. *J Cataract Refract Surg.* 2008;34(7):1096-1103.
24. Dickens MA, Cashwell LF. Long-term effect of cataract extraction on the function of an established filtering bleb. *Ophthalmic Surg Lasers.* 1996;27:9-14.
25. Kooner KS, Dulaney DD, Zimmerman TJ. Intraocular pressure following extracapsular cataract extraction and posterior chamber intraocular lens implantation. *Ophthalmic Surg.* 1988;19:417-474.
26. Kooner KS, Cooksey JC, Perry P, Zimmerman TJ. Intraocular pressure following ECCE, phacoemulsification, and PC-IOL implantation. *Ophthalmic Surg.* 1988;19:643-646.
27. Miyake K, Asakura M, Kobayashi H. Effect of intraocular lens fixation on the blood-acqueous barrier. *Am J Ophthalmol.* 1984;98(4):451-455.
28. Stehul KP, Marahrens P, Frohn C, Frohn A. Intraocular pressure and anterior chamber depth before and after extracapsular cataract extraction with posterior chamber lens implantation. *Ophthalmic Surg.* 1992;23(4):233-237
29. Suzuki R, Tanaka K, Sagara T, Fujiwara N. Reduction of intraocular pressure after phacoemulsification and aspiration with intraocular lens implantation. *Ophthalmologica.* 1994;208(5):254-258.
30. Hansen TE, Naeser K, Rask KL. A prospective study of intraocular pressure four months after extracapsular cataract extraction with implantation of posterior chamber lenses. *J Cataract Refract Surg.* 1987;13(1):35-38.
31. Radius RL, Schultz K, Sobocinski K, Schultz RO, Easom H. Pseudophakia and intraocular pressure. *Am J Ophthalmol.* 1984;97:738-742.
32. Jahn CE. Reduced intraocular pressure after phacoemulsification and posterior chamber intraocular lens implantation. *J Cataract Refract Surg.* 1997;23:1260-1264.
33. Tennen DG, Masket S. Short- and long-term effect of clear corneal incisions on intraocular pressure. *J Cataract Refract Surg.* 1996;22:568-570.
34. Tezel JT, Miller KM. Intraocular pressure change after sutureless phacoemulsification and foldable posterior chamber lens implantation. *J Cataract Refract Surg.* 1998;24:256-262.
35. Peponis VG, Chalkiadakis SE, Katzakis MC, Parikakis EA. The effect of phacoemulsification on late bleb failure or intraocular pressure in patients with glaucoma: a systematic review. *Clin Ophthalmol.* 2012;6:1045-1049.
36. Bonomi L, Bellucci R, Pucci V, Morselli S, Morbio R. Risultati della surgery della cataratta in occhi affetti da glaucoma ad angolo stretto. *Boll Ocul.* 1995;74:51-57.

37. Peräsalo R. Phacoemulsification of cataract in eyes with glaucoma. *Acta Ophthalmo Scand.* 1997;75(3):299-300.
38. Yalvac I, Airaksinen PJ, Tuulonen A. Phacoemulsification with and without trabeculectomy in patients with glaucoma. *Ophthalmic Surg Lasers.* 1997;28(6):469-475.
39. Gimbel H, Meyer D, DeBroff B, Roux C, Ferensowicz M. Intraocular pressure response to combined phacoemulsification and trabeculotomy ab externo versus phacoemulsification alone in primary open-angle glaucoma. *J Cataract Refract Surg.* 1995;21(6):653-660.
40. Hopkins JJ, Apel A, Trope GE, Rootman DS. Early intraocular pressure after phacoemulsification combined with trabeculectomy. *Ophthalmic Surg Lasers.* 1998;29:273-279.
41. Park HJ, Kwann YH, Weitzman M, Caprioli J. Temporal corneal phacoemulsification in patients with filtered glaucoma. *Arch Ophthalmol.* 1997;115:1375-1380.
42. El-Sayyad FF, Helal MH, Khalil MM, El-Maghraby MA. Phacotrabeculectomy versus two-stage operation: a matched study. *Ophthalmic Surg Lasers.* 1999;30(4):260-265.
43. Wygnancsky-Jaffe T, Barak A, Melamed S, Glovinsky Y. Intraocular pressure increments after cataract extraction in glaucomatous eyes with functioning filtering blebs. *Ophthalmic Surg Lasers.* 1997;28(8):657-661.
44. Chun PP, Weaver YK, Budenz DL, Feuer WJ, Parrish RK 2nd. Trabeculectomy function after cataract extraction. *Ophthalmology.* 1998;105(10):1928-1935.
45. Cravy TV. Routine use of the lateral approach to cataract extraction to achieve rapid and sustained stabilization of postoperative astigmatism. *J Cataract Refract Surg.* 1991;17(4):415-423.
46. Fine IH. Corneal tunnel incision with a temporal approach. In: Fine IH, Fichman RA, Grabow HR, eds. *Clear Corneal Cataract Surgery and Topical Anesthesia.* Thorofare, NJ: SLACK Incorporated; 1993:xx-xx.
47. Grabow HB. The clear corneal incision. In: Fine IH, Fichman RA, Grabow HR, eds. *Clear Corneal Cataract Surgery and Topical Anesthesia.* Thorofare, NJ: SLACK Incorporated; 1993.
48. Zanini M, Tassinari G, Barboni P, Mularoni A, Della Pasqua V, Bellusci C. Induced astigmatism after near clear hinge incision. *J Cataract Refract Surg.* 1997;23(8):1190-1195.
49. Ernest PH, Neuhann T. Posterior limbal incision. *J Cataract Refract Surg.* 1996;22(1):78-84.
50. Langerman DW. Architectural design of a self-sealing corneal tunnel, single hinge incision. *J Cataract Refract Surg.* 1994;20(1):84-88.
51. Bonomi L, Bellucci R. Esperienze sull'procedure di cataract con impianto di lente intraoculare in occhi già operati per glaucoma. *Boll Ocul.* 1990;69(suppl 2):81-91.
52. Buratto L, Ferrari M. Extracapsular cataract surgery and intraocular lens implantation in glaucomatous eyes that had a filtering bleb operation. *J Cataract Refract Surg.* 1990;16(3):315-319.
53. Shea SLK, Jap A, Prata JA, et al. Cataract Surgery after trabeculectomy. *Ophthalmic Surg Lasers.* 1996;27(7):587-594.
54. Park HJ, Kwon YH, Weitzman M, Caprioli J. Temporal corneal phacoemulsification in patients with filtered glaucoma. *Arch Ophthalmol.* 1997;115(11):1375-1380.
55. Caprioli J, Park HJ, Kwon YH, Weitzman M. Temporal corneal phacoemulsification in filtered glaucoma patients. *Trans Am Ophthalmol Soc.* 1997;95:153-167.
56. Lu LW. Phacoemulsification in a previous functioning glaucoma surgery. In: Lu LW, Fine IH, eds. *Phacoemulsification in Difficult and Challenging Cases.* NY: Thieme;1999.
57. Lemon LC, Shin DH, Kim C, Bendel RE, Hughes BA, Juzych MS: Limbus based vs fornix based conjunctival flap in combined glaucoma and cataract surgery with adjunctive mitomycin C. *Am J Ophthalmol.* 1998;125(3):340-345.
58. Menezo JL, Maldonado MJ, Munoz G, Cisneros AL. Combined procedure for glaucoma and cataract: a retrospective study. *J Cataract Refract Surg.* 1994;20:489-503.
59. Stewart W, Crinkley C, Carlson A. Results of combined phacoemulsification and trabeculectomy in patients with elevated preoperative intraocular pressures. *J Glaucoma.* 1995;4(3):164-169.
60. Derick RJ, Evans J, Baker ND. Combined phacoemulsification and trabeculectomy versus trabeculectomy alone: a comparison study using mitomycin-C. *Ophthalmic Surg Lasers.* 1998;29:707-713.
61. Hustead RH, Hamilton RC, Loken RG. Periocular local anesthesia: medial orbital an alternative to superior nasal injection. *J Cataract Refract Surg.* 1994;20:197-201.
62. Greenbaum S. *Ocular Anesthesia.* Philadelphia, PA:WB Saunders;1997.
63. Vicari D, McLennan S, Sun XY. Topical plus subconjunctival anesthesia for phacotrabeculectomy: one year follow-up. *J Cataract Refract Surg.* 1998;24:1247-1251.
64. Cairns JE. Trabeculectomy. Preliminary report of a new method. *Am J Ophthalmol.* 1968;66(44):673-679.
65. Elder MJ, Molteno AC. Five year followup of clear cornea trabeculectomy. *Aust N Z J Ophthalmol.* 1992; 20(1):19-22.
66. Fahmy IA, Ali MA, Spaeth GL. Long term follow up of clear cornea trabeculectomy. *Ophthalmic Surg.* 1990;21:294-295.
67. Cairns JE. Clear-cornea trabeculectomy. *Trans Ophthalmol Soc U K.* 1985;104 (Pt 2):142-145
68. Keillor RB, Moleno AC. Twenty-two cases of clear cornea trabeculectomy. *Aust N Z J Ophthalmol.* 1986;14:339-342.
69. Vyas AV, Bacon PJ, Percival SB. Phacotrabeculectomy: comparison of results from 3.5- and 5.2-mm incisions. *Ophthalmic Surg Lasers.* 1998;29:227-233.
70. Weitzman, Caprioli J. Temporal corneal phacoemulsification combined with separate incision superior trabeculectomy. *Ophthalmic Surg Lasers.* 1995;26(3):271-273.
71. Shin DH, Kim YY, Sheth N, et al. The role of adjunctive mitomycin C in secondary glaucoma triple procedure as compared to primary glaucoma triple procedure. *Ophthalmology.* 1998;105:740-745.
72. Carlson DW, Alward WL, Barad JP, Zimmerman MB, Carney BL. A randomized study of mitomycin augmentation in combined phacoemulsification and trabeculectomy. *Ophthalmology.* 1997;104:719-724.
73. Cohen JS, Greff LJ, Novack GD, Wind BE. A placebo-controlled, double-masked evaluation of mitomycin C in combined glaucoma and cataract procedures. *Ophthalmology.* 1996;103(11):1934-1942.
74. Gandolfi SA, Vecchi M. 5-fluorouracil in combined trabeculectomy and clear-cornea phacoemulsification with posterior chamber intraocular lens implantation. A one-year randomized, controlled clinical trial. *Ophthalmology.* 1997;104:181-186.
75. Hurvitz LM, 5-FU-supplemented phacoemulsification, posterior chamber intraocular lens implantation, and trabeculectomy. *Ophthalamic Surg.* 1993;24;674-680.
76. O'Grady JM, Juzych MS, Shin DH,et al: Trabeculectomy, phacoemulsification, and posterior chamber lens implantation with and without 5-fluorouracil. *Am J Ophthalmol.* 1993;116(5):594-599.
77. Berestka JS, Brown SV. Limbus- versus fornix-based conjunctival flaps in combined phacoemulsification and mitomycin C trabeculectomy surgery. *Ophthalmology.* 1997;104(2):187-196.
78. Belya DA, Dan JA, Lieberman MF, Stamper RL: Midterm follow-up results of combined phacoemulsification, lens implantation, and mitomycin-C trabeculectomy procedure. *J Glaucoma.* 1997;6(2):90-98.
79. Cohen JS, Greff LJ, Novack GD, Wind BE: A placebo-controlled, double-masked evaluation of mitomycin C in combined glaucoma and cataract procedures. *Ophthalmology.* 1996;103(11):1934-1942.
80. Wilkins M, Indar A, Wormald R. Intraoperative mitomycin C for glaucoma surgery. *Cochrane Database Syst Rev.* 2005;(4):CD002897.
81. Stead RE, King AJ. Outcome of trabeculectomy with mitomycin C in patients with advanced glaucoma. *Br J Ophthalmol.* 2011;95(7):960-965

82. Cheng JW, Cai JP, Li Y, Wei RL. Intraoperative mitomycin C for nonpenetrating glaucoma surgery: a systematic review and meta-analysis. J Glaucoma. 2011;20(5):322-326.
83. Nilforushan N, Yadgari M, Kish SK, Nassiri N. Subconjunctival bevacizumab versus mitomycin C adjunctive to trabeculectomy. *Am J Ophthalmol.* 2012;153(2):352-357.
84. Results of the Endophthalmitis Vitrectomy Study. A randomized trial of immediate vitrectomy and of intravenous antibiotics for the treatment of postoperative bacterial endophthalmitis. Endophthalmitis Vitrectomy Study Group. Arch Ophthalmol. 1995;113:1479-1489.
85. Ariyasu RG, Nakamura T, Trousdale MD, Smith RE. Intraoperative bacterial contamination of the aqueous humor. *Ophthalmic Surg.* 1993;24(6):373-374.
86. Klie F, Boge-Rasmussen I, Jensen OL. The effect of polyvinylpyrrolidone-iodine as a disinfectant in eye surgery. *Acta Ophthalmol (Copenh).* 1986;64:67-71.
87. Boes DA, Lindquist TD, Fritsche TR, Kalina RE. Effects of povidone-iodine chemical preparation and saline irrigation on the perilimbal flora. *Ophthalmology.* 1992; 99(10):1569-1574.
88. Dereklis DL, Bufidis TA, Tsiakiri EP, Palassopoulos SI. Preoperative ocular disinfection by the use of povidone-iodine 5%. *Acta Ophthalmol (Copenh).* 1994;72(5):627-630.
89. Endophthalmitis Study Group, European Society of Cataract & Refractive Surgeons. Prophylaxis of postoperative endophthalmitis following cataract surgery: results of the ESCRS multicenter study and identification of risk factors. *J Cataract Refract Surg.* 2007;33(6):978-988.
90. Gimbel HV, Sun R, De Brof BM. Prophylactic intracameral antibiotics during cataract surgery: the incidence of endophthalmitis and corneal endothelial cell loss. *Eur J Implant Ref Surg.* 1994;6:280-285.
91. Teichmann KD. Antibiotic supplementation of intraocular irrigation solutions. *Ophthalmology.* 1997;104:900-901.
92. Shin DH, Huges BA, Song MS, et al. Primary glaucoma triple procedure with or without adjunctive mitomycin. Prognostic factors for filtration failure. *Ophthalmology.* 1996;103:1925-1933.
93. Takihara Y, Inatani M, Seto T, et al.Trabeculectomy with mitomycin for open-angle glaucoma in phakic vs pseudophakic eyes after phacoemulsification. *Arch Ophthalmol.* 2011;129(2):152-7.
94. Shin DH, Ren J, Juzich MS, et al. Primary glaucoma triple procedure in patients with primary open-angle glaucoma: the effect of mitomycin C in patients with and without prognostic factors for filtration failure. *Am J Ophthalmol.* 1998;125:346-352.
95. Bellucci R, Perfetti S, Babighian S, Morselli S, Bonomi L. Filtration and complication after trabeculectomy and after phacotrabeculectomy. *Acta Ophthalmol Scand Suppl.* 1997;(224):44-45.
96. Mamalis N, Lohner S, Rand AN, Crandall AS. Combined phacoemulsification, intraocular lens implantation, and trabeculectomy. *J Cataract Refract Surg.* 1996;22(4):467-473.
97. Perasolo R, Flink T, Lehtosalo J, Ralli R, Sulonen J. Surgical outcome of phaco-emulsification combined with trabeculectomy in 243 eyes. *Acta Ophthalmol Scand.* 1997;75(5):581-583.
98. Park HJ, Weitzman M, Caprioli J. Temporal corneal phacoemulsification combined with superior trabeculectomy. A retrospective case-control study. *Arch Ophthalmol.* 1997;115:318-323
99. Bellucci R, Luraschi M. Trabeculectomy and phacoemulsification: one way and two way approach compared after one year. *Acta Ophthalmol Scand Suppl.* 1998;(227):50-51.
100. Rossetti L, Bellucci R, Miglior S, Orzalesi N. Temporal corneal phacoemulsification combined with separate incision superior trabeculectomy vs standard phacotrabeculectomy. A comparative study. *Acta Ophthalmol Scand Suppl.* 1997;(224):39.
101. Wyse T, Meyer M, Ruderman JM, et al. Combined trabeculectomy and phacoemulsification a one site versus a two site approach. *Am J Ophthalmol.* 1998;125(3):334-339.
102. Cotran PR, Roh S, McGwin G. Randomized comparison of 1-Site and 2-Site phacotrabeculectomy with 3-year follow-up. Ophthalmology. 2008;115(3):447-454.
103. el Sayyad F, el-Maghraby A. The contribution of phacoemulsification to combined cataract and glaucoma surgery. *Curr Opin Ophthalmol.* 1998;92): 95-100.
104. Tezel G, Kolker AE, Kass MA, Wax MB. Comparative results of combined procedures for glaucoma and cataract: II. Limbus based versus fornix based conjunctival flaps. *Ophthalmic Surg Lasers.* 1997;28(7):551-557.
105. Lederer CM Jr. Combined cataract extraction with intraocular lens implant and mitomycin-augmented trabeculectomy. *Ophthalmology.* 1996;103(7):1025-1034.
106. Shingleton BJ, Chaudhry IM, O'Donoghue MW, Baylus SL, King RJ, Chaudhry MB. Phacotrabeculectomy: limbus-based versus fornix-based conjunctival flaps in fellow eyes. *Ophthalmology.* 1999;106(6):1152-1155.
107. Sanchez E, Schnyder CC, Mermoud A. Résultats comparatifs de la sclérectomie profonde transformée en trabéculectomie et de la trabéculectomie classique. *Klin Monatsbl Augenheilkd.* 1997;210:261-264.
108. Lemon LC, Shin DH, Song MS, et al. Comparative study of silicone versus acrylic foldable lens implantation in primary glaucoma triple procedure. *Ophthalmology.* 1997;104(10):1708-1713.
109. Zacharia PT, Shuman JS. Combined phacoemulsification and trabeculectomy with mitomycin C. *Ophthalmic Surg lasers.* 1997;28:739-744.
110. Yang KL, Moster MR, Azura-Blanco AA, Wilson RP, Araujo SV, Schmidt CM. Mitomycin-C supplemented trabeculectomy, phacoemulsification, and foldable lens implantation. *J Cataract Refract Surg.* 1997;23:565-569.
111. Wishart PK, Austin MA. Combined cataract extraction and trabeculectomy: Phacoemulsification compared with extracapsular technique. *Ophthalmic Surg.* 1993;24:814-821.
112. Stewart W, Crinkley C, Carsol A. Results of trabeculectomy combined with phacoemulsification versus trabeculectomy combined with extracapsular cataract extraction in patients with advanced glaucoma. *Ophthalmic Surg.* 1994;25:621-627.
113. Wedrich A, Menapace R, Radax U, Papapanos P. Long-term results of combined trabeculectomy and small incision cataract surgery. *J Cataract Refract Surg.* 1995;21(1):49-54.
114. Goug PNJ, Roux P. Preliminary report of sutureless phacotrabeculectomy through a modified self sealing scleral tunnel incision. *J Cataract Refract Surg* 1995;21(2):160-169.
115. Aaberg TM Jr, Flynn HW Jr, Schiffman J, Newton J. Nosocomial acute-onset postoperative endophthalmitis survey. A 10-year review of incidence and outcomes. *Ophthalmology.* 1998;105:1004-1010.
116. Kangas TA, Greenfield DS, Flynn HW Jr, Parrish RK 2nd, Palmberg P. Delayed-onset endophthalmitis associated with conjunctival filtering blebs. *Ophthalmology.* 1997;104:746-752.
117. Greenfield DS, Suner IJ, Miller MP, Kangas TA, Palmberg PF, Flynn HW Jr. Endophthalmitis after filtering surgery with mitomycin. *Arch Ophthalmol.* 1996;114(8):943-949.
118. Shin DH, Kim YY, Ren J, et al. Decrease of capsular opacification with adjunctive mitomycin C in combined glaucoma and cataract surgery. *Ophthalmology.* 1998;105(7):1222-1226.
119. Smith R. A new technique for opening the canal of Schlemm. Preliminary report. Br J Ophthalmol. 1960;44:370-373.
120. Allen L, Burian HM. Trabeculotomy ab externo. A new glaucoma operation: technique and results of experimental surgery. *Am J Ophthalmol.* 1962;53:19-26.
121. Burian HM. A case of Marfan's syndrome with bilateral glaucoma. With description of a new type of operation for developmental glaucoma (trabeculotomy ab externo). *Am J Ophthalmol.* 1960;50:1187-1192.

122. Harms H. Glaukomoperationen am Schlemm'schen Kanal. *Ber Vers Ver Rhein-Westf Augenarzte.* 1966;994:93-100.
123. Harms H, Dannheim R. Epicritical consideration of 300 cases of trabeculotomy "ab externo." *Trans Ophthalmol Soc U K* 1969;89:491-499.
124. McPherson SD Jr. Results of external trabeculotomy. *Am J Ophthalmol.* 1973;76:918-920.
125. Dannheim R. Symposium: microsurgery of the outflow channels. Trabeculotomy. *Trans Am Acad Ophthalmol Otolaryngol.* 1972;76:375-383.
126. Honjio M, Tanihara H, Negi A, et al. Trabeculotomy ab externo, cataract extraction and intraocular lens implantation: preliminary report. *J Cataract Refract Surg.* 1996;22:601-606.
127. Honjio M, Tanihara H, Inatani M, et al. Phacoemulsification, intraocular lens implantation, and trabeculectomy to treat pseudoexfoliation syndrome. *J Cataract Refract Surg.* 1998; 24;781-786.
128. Chiara E, Nishida A, Kodo M, et al. Trabeculotomy ab externo: an alternative treatment in adult patients with primary open-angle glaucoma. *Ophthalmic Surg.* 1993;24:735-739.
129. Wada Y, Nakatsu A, Kondo T: Long-term results of trabeculotomy ab externo. *Ophthalmic Surg* 1994;25:317-320.
130. Tanihara H, Negi A, Akimoto M, et al. Surgical effects of trabeculotomy ab externo in adult eyes with primary open-angle glaucoma and pseudoexfoliation with primary open-angle glaucoma and pseudoexfoliation syndrome. *Arch Ophthalmol.* 1993;111:1653-1661.
131. Akimoto M, Tanihara H, Negi A, Nagata M. Surgical results of trabeculotomy ab externo for developmental glaucoma. *Arch Ophthalmol.* 1994;112:1540-1544.
132. Tanihara H, Negi A, Akimoto M, Nagata M. Long term results of non filtering surgery for the treatment of primary angle-closure glaucoma. *Graefes Arch Clin Exp Ophthalmol.* 1995;233:563-567.
133. Tanihara H, Negi A, Akimoto M, Nagata M. Long-term surgical results of combined trabeculotomy ab externo and cataract extraction. *Ophthalmic Surg.* 1995;26:316-324.
134. Tanihara H, Honjo M, Inatani M, et al. Trabeculotomy combined with phacoemulsification and implantation of an intraocular lens for the treatment of primary open-angle glaucoma and coexisting cataract. *Ophthalmic Surg Lasers.* 1997;28:810-817.
135. Stegmann R, Pienaar A, Miller D. Viscocanalostomy for open-angle glaucoma in black African patients. *J Cataract Refract Surg.* 1999;25:316-322.
136. Carassa RG, Bettin P, Fiori M, Brancato R. Viscocanalostomy: a pilot study. *Eur J Ophthalmol.* 1998;8:57-61.
137. Stegmann R. Visco-canalostomia. *Highlights of Ophthalmology.* 1996;10(4):67-70.
138. Sharaawy T, Bhartiya S. Surgical management of glaucoma: evolving paradigms. Indian J Ophthalmol. 2011;59(suppl):S123-130.
139. Sarodia U, Shaarawy T, Barton K. Nonpenetrating glaucoma surgery: a critical evaluation. Curr Opin Ophthalmol. 2007;18(2):152-158.
140. Kratz RP. Viscocanalostomy shows high success in difficult cases. *Eye World.* 1997;2(7):32-33.
141. Singer HW. Viscocanalostomy: effective glaucoma technique without troublesome blebs. *Ocular Surgery News (Int. Ed.)* 1998;9(3):18.
142. Wishart MS, Dagres E. Seven-year follow-up of combined cataract extraction and viscocanalostomy. *J Cataract Refract Surg.* 2006;32(12):2043-2049.
143. Drolsum L. Longterm follow-up after deep sclerectomy in patients with pseudoexfoliative glaucoma. *Acta Ophthalmol Scand.* 2006; 84(4):502-506.
144. Reekonen P, Kannisto T, Puustjarvi T, Terasvirta M, Uusitalo M. Deep sclerectomy for the treatment of exfoliation and primary open-angle glaucoma. *Acta Ophthalmol Scand.* 2006;84(4):507-511.
145. Cillino S, Pace FD, Casaccio A, Calvaruso L, et al. Deep sclerectomy versus punch trabeculectomy with or without phacoemulsification: a randomized clinical trial. *J Glaucoma.* 2004;13(6):500-506.
146. Wishart MS, Shergill T, Porooshani H. Viscocanalostomy and phacoviscocanalostomy: long-term results. *J Cataract Refract Surg.* 2002;28(5):745-751.
147. Hondur A, Onol M, Hasanreisoglu B. Nonpenetrating glaucoma surgery: meta-analysis of recent results. *J Glaucoma.* 2008;17(2):139-46.
148. Chai C, Loon SC. Meta-analysis of viscocanalostomy versus trabeculectomy in uncontrolled glaucoma. *J Glaucoma.* 2010;19(8):519-527.
149. Gilmour DF, Manners TD, Devonport H, Varga Z, Solebo AL, Miles J. Viscocanalostomy versus trabeculectomy for primary open-angle glaucoma: 4-year prospective randomized clinical trial. *Eye (Lond).* 2009;23(9):1802-1807.
150. Anand N, Pilling R. Nd:YAG laser goniopuncture after deep sclerectomy: outcomes. *Acta Ophthalmol.* 2010;88(1):110-115.
151. Zimmerman TJ, Kooner KS, Ford VJ, et al: Effectiveness of nonpenetrating trabeculectomy in aphakic patients with glaucoma. *Ophthalmic Surg.* 1984;15(1):44-50.
152. Zimmerman TJ, Kooner KS, Ford VJ, et al: Trabeculectomy vs. nonpenetrating trabeculectomy: a retrospective study of two procedures in phakic patients with glaucoma. *Opthalmic Surg.* 1984;15(9):734-740.
153. Arenas E. Trabeculectomy ab externo. *Highlights of Ophthalmology.* 1991;19:60-65.
154. Tavano G, Chabin T, Barrut JM. Hemitrabeculectomie ab externo non invasive. *Bull Soc Ophthalmol Fr.* 1993;93:749-750.
155. Fyodorov SN, Kozlov VI, Timosckina NT, et al. Nonpenetrating deep sclerectomy in open-angle glaucoma. *Ophthalmosurgery.* 1990;3:52-55.
156. Kozlov VI, Bagarov SN, Anisimova SY, et al. Nonpenetrating deep sclerectomy with collagen. *Ophthalmosurgery.* 1990;3:44-46.
157. Mermoud A, Schnyder CC, Sickenburg M, Chiou AG, Hediguer SEA, Faggioni R. Comparison of deep sclerectomy with collagen implant and trabeculectomy in open-angle glaucoma. *J Cataract Refract Surg.* 1999;25(3):323-331.
158. Gianoli F, Schnyder CC, Bovey E, Mermoud A. Combined surgery for cataract and glaucoma: phacoemulsification and deep sclerectomy campared with phacoemulsification and trabeculectomy. *J Cataract Refract Surg.* 1999;25(3):340-346.
159. Mermoud A, Karlen ME, Schnyder C, et al. Nd:YAG goniopuncutre after deep sclerectomy with collagen implant. *Ophthalmic Surg Lasers.* 1999;30:120-125.
160. Chiou AGY, Mermoud A, Hediguer SEA, Sachnyder CC, Faggioni R. Ultrasound biomicroscopy of eyes undergoing deep sclerectomy with collagen implant. *Br J Ophthalmol.* 1996;80:541-544.
161. Karlen ME, Sanchez E, Schnyder CC, Sickenberg M, Mermoud A. Deep sclerectomy with collagen implant: medium term result. *Br J Ophthalmol.* 1999;83:6-11.
162. Demailly PH, Jeantur-Lunel MN, Berkani M, et al. La sclérectomie profonde non perforante associée à la pose d'un implant de collagène dans le glaucome primitif à angle ouvert. Résultats rétrospectifs à moyen terme. *J Fr Ophthalmol.* 1996;19(11):659-666.
163. Massi J, Gruber D, Muraine M, Brasseur G. Non-penetrating deep sclerectomy in the surgical treatment of chronic open-angle glaucoma. Mid-term result [in French]. *J Fr Ophthalmol.* 1999;22(3):292-298.
164. Demailly P, Lavat P, Kretz G, Jeanteur-Lunel MN. Non-penetrating deep sclerectomy (NPDS) with or without collagen device (CD) in primary open-angle glaucoma: middle-term retrospective study. *Int Ophthalmol.* 1996-1997;20(1-3):131-140.
165. Sanchez E, Schnyder CC, Sickenberg M, Chiou AG, Hediguer SE, Mermoud A. Deep sclerectomy: results with and without collagen implant. *Int Ophthalmol.* 1996-1997;20(1-3:157-162.

166. Cillino S, Di Pace F, Casuccio A, et al. Deep sclerectomy versus punch trabeculectomy with or without phacoemulsification: a randomized clinical trial. *J Glaucoma.* 2004;13(6):500-506.
167. Shaarawy T, Mermoud A. Deep sclerectomy in one eye vs deep sclerectomy with collagen implant in the contralateral eye of the same patient: long-term follow-up. *Eye (Lond).* 2005;19(3):298-302.
168. Sourdille P, Santiago PY, Villani F, et al. Reticulated hyaluronic acid implant in nonperforating trabecular surgery. *J Cataract Refract Surg.* 1999;25:332-339.
169. Sanchez E, Schnyder CC, Mermoud A. Resultas comparatifs de la sclerectomie profonde transformèe en trabèculectomie et de la trabèculectomie classique. *Klin Monatsbl Augenheilkd.* 1997;210(5):261-264.
170. Chiou AG, Mermound A, Jewelewicz DA. Post-operative inflammation following deep sclerectomy with collagen implant versus standard trabeculectomy. *Graefes Arch Clin Exp Ophthalmol.* 1998;236(8):593-596.
171. Chiou AG, Mermoud A, Hediguer SE. Glaucome malin par blocage ciliare après sclèrectomie profonde. Imagerie par biomicroscope à ultrasons. *Klin Monatsbk Augenheilkd.* 1996;208(5):279-281.
172. Khairy HA, Green FD, Nassar MK, Azuara-Blanco A. Control of intraocular pressure after deep sclerectomy. *Eye (Lond).* 2006;20(3):336-340.
173. Cheng JW, Ma XY, Wei RL. Efficacy of non-penetrating trabecular surgery for open-angle glaucoma: a meta-analysis. *Chin Med J (Engl).* 2004;117(7):1006-1010.
174. Ollikainen ML, Puustjärvi TJ, Rekonen PK, Uusitalo HM, Teräsvirta ME. Mitomycin C-augmented deep sclerectomy in primary open-angle glaucoma and exfoliation glaucoma: a three-year prospective study. Acta Ophthalmol. 2011;89(6):548-555.
175. Mielke C, Dawda VK, Anand N. Deep sclerectomy and low dose mitomycin C: a randomised prospective trial in west Africa. *Br J Ophthalmol.* 2006;90(3):310-313.
176. Choudhary A, Wishart PK. Nonpenetrating glaucoma surgery augmented with mitomycin C or 5-fluorouracil in eyes at high risk of failure of filtration surgery: long-term results. *Clin Experiment Ophthalmol.* 2007;35(4):340-347.
177. Mansouri K, Mendrinos E, Shaarawy T, Dosso AA. Visualization of the trabeculo Descemet's membrane in deep sclerectomy after Nd:YAG goniopuncture: an in vivo confocal microscopy study. *Arch Ophthalmol.* 2011;129(10):1305-1310.
178. Bull H, von Wolff K, Körber N, Tetz M. Three year canaloplasty outcomes for the treatment of open-angle glaucoma: European study results. *Graefes Arch Clin Exp Ophthalmol.* 2011;249(10):1537-1545.
179. Lewis RA, von Wolff K, Tetz M, et al. Canaloplasty: Three year results of circumferential viscodilation and tensioning of Schlemm's canal using a microcatheter to treat open-angle glaucoma. *J Cataract Refract Surg.* 2011;37(4):682-690.
180. Ayyala RS, Chaudhry AL, Okogbaa CB, Zurakowski D. Comparison of surgical outcomes between canaloplasty and trabeculectomy at 12 months' follow-up. *Ophthalmology.* 2011;118(12):2427-2433.
181. Koerber NJ. Canaloplasty in one eye compared with viscocanalostomy in the contralateral eye in patients with bilateral open-angle glaucoma. *J Glaucoma.* 2012;21(2):129-134.
182. Barnebey HS. Canaloplasty with intraoperative low dosage mitomycin C: a retrospective case series. *J Glaucoma.* In press.
183. Grieshaber MC, Pienaar A, Olivier J, Stegmann R. Comparing two tensioning suture sizes for 360 degrees viscocanalostomy (canaloplasty): a randomised controlled trial. *Eye (Lond).* 2010;24(7):1220-1226.
184. Patel S, Pasquale LR. Glaucoma drainage devices: a review of the past, present, and future. *Semin Ophthalmol.* 2010;25(5-6):265-270.
185. Budenz DL, Barton K, Feuer WJ, et al; Ahmed Baerveldt Comparison Study Group. Treatment outcomes in the Ahmed Baerveldt Comparison Study after 1 year of follow-up. *Ophthalmology.* 2011;118(3):443-52.
186. Gedde SJ, Schiffman JC, Feuer WJ, Herndon LW, Brandt JD, Budenz DL; Tube versus Trabeculectomy Study Group. Treatment outcomes in the Tube Versus Trabeculectomy (TVT) Study after five years of follow-up. *Am J Ophthalmol.* 2012;153(5):789-803.
187. Gedde SJ, Herndon LW, Brandt JD, Budenz DL, Feuer WJ, Schiffman JC; Tube Versus Trabeculectomy Study Group. Postoperative complications in the Tube Versus Trabeculectomy (TVT) Study during five years of follow-up. *Am J Ophthalmol.* 2012;153(5):804-814
188. Minckler DS, Francis BA, Hodapp EA, et al. Aqueous shunts in glaucoma: a report by the American Academy of Ophthalmology. *Ophthalmology.* 2008;115(6):1089-1098.
189. Barton K, Heuer DK. Modern aqueous shunt implantation: future challenges. *Prog Brain Res.* 2008;173:263-276.
190. Francis BA, Singh K, Lin SC, et al. Novel glaucoma procedures: a report by the American Academy of Ophthalmology. *Ophthalmology.* 2011;118(7):1466-1480.
191. Minckler DS, Baerveldt G, Alfaro MR, Francis BA. Clinical results with the Trabectome for treatment of open-angle glaucoma. *Ophthalmology.* 2005;112(6):962-967.
192. Liu J, Jung J, Francis BA. Ab interno trabeculotomy: Trabectome surgical treatment for open-angle glaucoma. *Expert Rev Ophthalmol.* 2009;4(2):119-128.
193. Minckler D, Mosaed S, Dustin L, Ms BF; Trabectome Study Group. Trabectome (trabeculectomy internal approach): additional experience and extended follow-up. *Trans Am Ophthalmol Soc.* 2008;106:149-59; discussion 159-60.
194. Jea SY, Francis BA, Vakili G, Filippopoulos T, Rhee DJ. Ab interno trabeculectomy versus trabeculectomy for open-angle glaucoma. *Ophthalmology.* 2012;119(1):36-42.
195. Ting JL, Damji KF, Stiles MC. Trabectome Study Group. Ab interno trabeculectomy: outcomes in exfoliation versus primary open-angle glaucoma. *J Cataract Refract Surg.* 2012;38(2):315-323.

4

Pseudoexfoliation Syndrome

Pseudoexfoliation syndrome (PEX) is an age-related systemic pathology. It is caused by the production and accumulation of abnormal extracellular fibril material in the tissues.

In the eye, it affects the entire anterior segment, including conjunctiva and periorbital tissues. PEX is characterized by deposits of amyloid pseudoexfoliative material on the anterior capsule of the lens, ciliary body, zonules, margins of the iris, corneal endothelium, anterior vitreous, and the trabecular meshwork. PEX is associated with glaucoma and cataract, which are more common in these patients.

Presently, this syndrome is still not completely defined and a range of clinical scenarios occur. Fibril material similar to that seen in the eye also occurs in the skin and in the connective tissue of internal organs (heart, lungs, liver, kidney, meninges).[1] Along with others, Dvorak-Theobald suggested that the multiple locations of this material indicate multiple production sights. The term *pseudoexfoliation* was proposed to distinguish PEX from the pathology of exfoliation of the lens occurring in eyes undergoing prolonged exposure to high temperatures (eg, molten glass blowers or boiler specialists).[2]

Epidemiology

Frequency Observed in the General Population

PEX has been seen in all populations and races; however, the incidence varies widely and may differ 10-fold. In the Inuit Eskimo population,[3] the incidence is close to zero; for the Navajo Indians, the incidence is 38%.[4] The incidence in a specific population or country may vary up to 3-fold.

This variability occurs because of a number of issues: age, sex, hereditary factors, environmental factors, clinical criteria used for the diagnosis, and ability of the observer to diagnose cases early on. The incidence of PEX increases in patients over 50 years of age; with high intraocular pressure (IOP); and having had glaucoma surgery or absolute glaucoma.

In Italy, the incidence varies between 0.8% (80 cases for every 10,000 people)[5] and 2.5% (180 cases for every 7000 people).[6] Thus, PEX is relatively frequent.

Factors Frequently Associated With Pseudoexfoliation Syndrome

Age

All articles report age-related increase in cases of PEX. The increase is so proportional to age that Forsius et al[3] estimated that the incidence in patients over 50 years of age doubled with every decade. An increase in the incidence of PEX in patients over 50 years of age was confirmed by a recent Japanese study.[7]

Sex

There was no clear dominance of male or females with PEX; however, because females tend to live longer, there is an increased incidence in females.

Hereditary Factors

This aspect of PEX has been precisely defined due to genetic studies; however, a clear hereditary pattern has not been defined, even though autosomal dominance with incomplete penetrance is suspected.[8,9] Aasved reported an incidence of 9.4% in 25 families having PEX, compared to 1% of the controls.[8] In a subset of the Finnish population,

Buratto L, Brint SF, Caretti L.
Cataract Surgery in Complicated Cases (pp 59-75).

Forsman et al estimated that the percentage with PEX was 16% if one parent had it and 18% if both parents did.[10]

Recently, 2 studies[9,11] of molecular genetics focused attention on hereditary aspects of this pathology. Even though the results were not conclusive, these 2 studies created a beginning for understanding the molecular genetics of PEX, an important step in the understanding of treatment for the syndrome with gene therapy. In one of these studies, it was demonstrated that PEX is correlated with polymorphism of a single nucleotide in the 15q24.1 region, more precisely with 2 nonsynonomous polymorphisms in the axon 1 of the gene LOXL1.[11] Twenty-five percent of the general population is homozygous for high-risk aplotype, with the probability of developing PEX 100 times more than patients with low-risk aplotype. It should be pointed out that the gene LOXL1 produces a protein that catalyzes formation of elastin fibers, identified as one of the major components in PEX. Another study, restricted to a specific group (islanders from the Finnish archepelagos, probably with a higher percentage of blood relatives than the general public), illustrated a higher probability of linkage of PEX with the locus 18q12.1-21.33 and a lower yet statistically significant probability of linkage with the chromosomes 2q, 17p, and 19q.[9]

Uni- or Bilateral Ocular Involvement

According to Ritch and Schlotzer-Shrehardt, the term *unilateral PEX* is incorrect. This is because in almost all biopsied cases, PEX changes were seen in otherwise healthy eyes.[1] It is therefore more appropriate to speak of asymmetry. The frequency of bilateral PEX is greater in Europe compared to elsewhere, with a bilateral frequency of 75%[12-15]; in the United States and Japan, the frequency is just the opposite (75% monocular).[16-18] Patients with monocular pathology tend to be slightly younger than patients with bilateral involvement.[19]

Association of Cataract and Pseudoexfoliation Syndrome

Anterior segment surgeons are familiar with the association between PEX and cataracts because of the difficulties and complications that may occur during surgery. It has been reported as between 23% and 61% (depending on patient groups).[1] Unilateral cataracts are often associated with unilateral PEX.[1]

Association of Glaucoma and Pseudoexfoliation Syndrome

Twenty percent to 25% of patients with PEX also have glaucoma (usually open-angle). Moreover, patients with PEX but no glaucoma when diagnosed have a 40% risk of developing glaucoma within 10 years, because the trabecular meshwork is blocked by pseudoexfoliative material and melanin.

The frequency of PEX in patients with glaucoma is significantly higher than similar patients without glaucoma; it is greater in Scandinavian countries and populations of Celtic descent, and lower in the United States.[16,19,20]

There is a specific problem associated with the frequency of PEX in patients with closed-angle glaucoma. Some feel this does not differ greatly from the frequency in the general population; however, others report a much higher frequency ranging from a minimum of 10% to a maximum of 32%. An Italian study reported a frequency of 21% of closed angles in 233 pseudoexfoliation glaucoma patients.[21]

Pathogenesis

A number of theories regarding the origin of the PEX material and its pathogenesis exist. These include the following[1,2,22-24]:

- Secondary deposits from aqueous components
- Deposits from pigmented iris epithelium
- Production by lens epithelial cells (LECs)
- Localized degeneration of lens capsule or zonule lamellae

More recently, deposits of clinically visible material have been identified as a passive process that originates in the aqueous and on the iris, while material visible microscopically on the pre-equatorial zonules appears to be produced by LECs.[1,25] Subsequent macroscopic deposits (central or paracentral) are caused by pupil movement.

Moreover, pseudoexfoliation phenomena may coexist with true exfoliation phenomena as surface layers of the capsule may be ruptured with secondary loss of capsular material.[1,26]

Regarding the pathogenesis, the origins of PEX still have not been identified; however, the presence of pseudoexfoliative material in an organ other than the eye suggest that this pathology is systemic.

Histopathology and ultrastructural analysis of the chemical composition of the material in PEX (observing reaction to specific different dyes) have given rise to 3 main theories of pathogenisis. A fourth has recently been added, based on epidemiological and clinical considerations; nevertheless the exact nature of psuedoexfoliation material is still unclear.

Theory of Amyloid Substance

This is probably the oldest of the theories and is based on marking of the exfoliative substance with anti-amyloid serum. Few surgeons support this theory as more sophisticated tests (using monoclonal antibodies against beta amyloid, light chain immunoglobulin, etc) do not confirm it.[27]

Theory of the Basal Membrane

Dvorak-Theobald identified a positive reaction of PEX material with periodic acid Schiff (PAS) stains, suggesting the presence of glycoprotein, typical components of the basal membranes.[2] Frequent association of PEX with altered basal membranes in various cell types and the immunohistochemical detection of epitomes of the basal membrane (laminin, nidogen, and heparan sulfate proteoglycans) support the idea that the pseudoexfoliative deposits are produced by a modified basal membrane.[28]

Elastic Microfibrils Theory

The strongest theory is that there is abnormal production of elastic material (elastosis) with subsequent abnormal aggregation. Microscopically, Garner and Alexander determined that the substance produced in PEX consisted of microfibrils similar to those found in elastic fibers.[29] Since this is also found in zonules (the main component of these fibers is oxytalan), researchers have examined the possibility that this substance is a major component of the microfibrils.[30] Consequently, close association between the pseudoexfoliative material and the main components of the elastic system (zonules, elastic fibers, elastic microfibrils [oxytalan], and other elastic material) suggested that PEX is a form of elastosis that selectively affects elastic microfibrils. As the exact nature of pseudoexfoliative material is still unknown, immunohistochemical and electron microscopic evidence suggests the presence of elastic epitomes (elastin, vitronectin, amyloid P, and fibrillin). In particular, the electronic immunomicroscopic detection of fibrillin-1 and protein binding type-1 latent transforming growth factor (LTBP-1) in microfibril subunits of intra- and extraocular exfoliative material suggests that PEX is caused by excessive production and abnormal aggregation of elastic microfibrils. (LTBP-1 is a marker for diagnosis of PEX even in extraocular tissues).[1,31,32] This finding agrees with the polymorphism of the LOXL1 gene that regulates the formation of elastin fibers. Zenkel et al studied genes expressed differently in anterior segment tissues and concluded that PEX is a stress-induced elastic microfibrillopathy.[33]

Infective Theory

A greater incidence of PEX in couples as compared to control groups and a large number of cases in younger patients with PEX following intraocular surgery suggests that this pathology could have infectious origins.[34-36] This is reinforced by great structural similarity between fibrillary material that deposits during episodes of "scrapie" (sheep spongiform encephalopathy) and the PEX fibrils.[37]

Others detected increased levels of malondialdehyde and glutathione in the LECs of PEX eyes, indicating an important oxidative response suggesting that oxidative stress plays a role in the pathogenesis and progression of PEX.[38]

In conclusion, most studies report that PEX material comes from disorders in synthesis of the extracellular matrix, since it consists of glycoprotein and glycosaminoglycan molecules with structural components belonging to both basal membranes and elastic tissues.[14,29-31]

According to Ritch and Schlotzer-Shrehardt, the fact that a unilateral cataract is frequently associated with clinically unilateral PEX suggests there is a common pathogenetic origin, chronic ocular ischemic syndrome.[1]

Histopathological and Ultrastructural

Currently, from the analysis of different histopathological and ultrastructural studies, it is clear that PEX is a systemic pathology characterized by the production of fibrillary material of unknown origin, deposited in the extracellular matrix of various tissues and organs.

The eye is unquestionably the elective site for PEX and the organ that has the greatest damage; the iris and the pre-equatorial epithelium of the lens are the main production sites for the fibrillary material. This syndrome is characterized by pseudoexfoliative material depositing on the anterior capsule of the lens, the ciliary body, the zonules, the pupillary edge of the iris, the corneal endothelium, the anterior vitreous, and on the trabecular meshwork.

Aside from the iris and pre-equatorial epithelium of the lens and possibly the angle, all other sites with PEX examined under the slit lamp are secondary deposits that develop following dispersion of primary deposits in the aqueous humor.

Lens

Under the microscope, the anterior surface of a normal lens has a stratified appearance with a thin external layer, the precapsular layer, another layer, the pericapsular membrane, and the zonular lamellae, becoming strongly colored following various staining techniques (hematoxylin/eosin, Masson's trichrome stain, Mallory's connective tissue stain, Van Gieson's stain). There is an internal layer that absorbs less color; this is called the fibrillary layer, with a variable thickness. It forms the true anterior capsule of the lens.

In a PEX lens, an additional layer has been seen between the previous two. It is an amorphous layer[24] defined by Bertelsen et al. Using Masson's trichrome stain, there is a clear distinction between the amorphous layer, which is an intense blue color, and the fibrillary layer, which is orange. The amorphous layer under low magnification electron microscopy appears to be a highly electrodense fibrogranular stripe, more abundant in the pre-equatorial region, giving the anterior capsule a disorganized and sponge-like appearance.[39]

Given that this material, consisting of PEX fibrils, is more abundant below the pre-equatorial capsule, in relationship with the germination zone of the lens, the pathogenetic theory is plausible; according to this theory the PEX material is produced by the pre-equatorial epithelium of the lens.[2,14,16,24,30]

Using ultrasound biomicroscopy (UBM), it has been demonstrated that the anterior capsule in PEX eyes is thicker than in normal eyes.[40]

Under the slit lamp, the material of the central disk has a scaly appearance; however, under the optical microscope, it appears to consist of branched filaments that extend over the anterior capsule of the lens, posterior surface of the iris, zonules, and the ciliary body.

Ciliary Body and Zonules

Observation of ciliary bodies in PEX eyes reveals a material with identical histological affinities as other sites, deposited in small clusters on the basal membrane of the nonpigmented epithelial cells. Under high magnification, the PEX material appears to be stratified on the epithelial cell surfaces and on the zonules, appearing as filaments arranged perpendicular to the surface.[2,36] The PEX material stratifies on the basal membrane of the epithelium, emerging on the surface through tiny intraepithelial spaces.

There are deposits of fibrillary material on the zonules, and under UBM, these have a nodular appearance.[40] A number of studies[17,18,41] detected deposits of this material in 3 different locations:

1. Origin of the zonules on the ciliary body, where the fibers appear to be separated from the basal membrane of the nonpigmented epithelium
2. Pars plicata, where the material covers the surface without affecting its ultrastructure
3. Anchor site of the zonules on the anterior capsule of the lens

These findings are of considerable clinical importance and may explain the high incidence of zonular instability of the lens and the complications that may develop in individuals with PEX.

Using UBM, some authors[42] demonstrated bilateral involvement of the zonules in patients with unilateral PEX: the zonule changes of the contralateral eye can be extensive even when there is no clinically evident PEX material. Consequently, the authors suggested possible clinical relevance of an UBM examination of the zonules as part of the preoperative workup of a patient with PEX scheduled for cataract surgery.

Iris

Regarding the iris, PEX is characterized by scale-like deposits on the pupillary margin and a fibrotic, rarefied appearance of the pupil. Physiological rubbing of the iris against the anterior surface of the lens will "scrape" PEX material from the anterior capsule of the lens and deposit scale-like material on the pupillary margin of the iris. There is also secondary pigment dispersion with loss of melanin from the pigmented epithelium from the margin of the pupil and the accumulation of melanin granules in the trabecular meshwork and on the corneal endothelium.

Examination of the iris under the optical microscope again revealed PEX material on both the posterior surface as clusters and on the anterior surface, deposited in the grooves, the crypts, and on the pupil sphincter. The proximity of the iris to the anterior surface of the lens suggests that it deposits the material on the surface; then when the capsule is rubbed, the deposits are transported toward the pupil and accumulate to form the central disk that is seen at the slit lamp.

Ultrastructural studies have confirmed that the posterior surface of the iris appears to be covered with disorganized fibrillary material that deposits between the pigmented cells and extends as far as the basal membrane where it then stratifies.[43] This material does not appear to affect the cell ultrastructure even though some have seen ruptured pigmented cells containing fibrils similar to those present in PEX material.[26]

Fibrillary material has also been seen in the iris stroma; in this case, it is mixed with collagen fibers particularly around the adventitia or external wall of the blood vessels.[37,43] The capillaries appear to be contracted and sometimes obliterated (iris vasculopathy). The iris of a patient with PEX is therefore poorly nourished; this combined with the degenerative process described above for the pigmented epithelium may explain the dispersion of the pigment in the aqueous and its deposit on the corneal endothelium and in the intratrabecular spaces.

The Angle

As mentioned before, it is not clear whether the angle is another production site; nevertheless, progressive involvement of this structure frequently leads to development of secondary open-angle glaucoma.

Ultrastructural studies on the trabecular meshwork[31,37] are interesting. Most of the PEX material was detected in the subendothelial space of Schlemm's canal and in the juxtacanalicular tissue.

PEX material is always extracellular; it also appears to have a fibrillary appearance and tends to organize into thin highly electrodense fibers. Accumulation of PEX material has also been found in the uveal portion of the trabecular

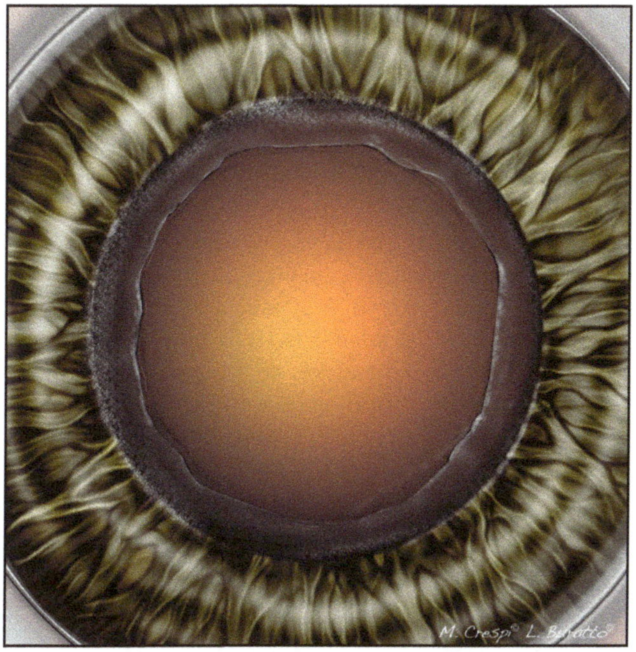

Figure 4-1. Deposits of pseudoexfoliative material on the anterior capsule of the crystalline of an eye affected by PEX on the periphery of the anterior capsule.

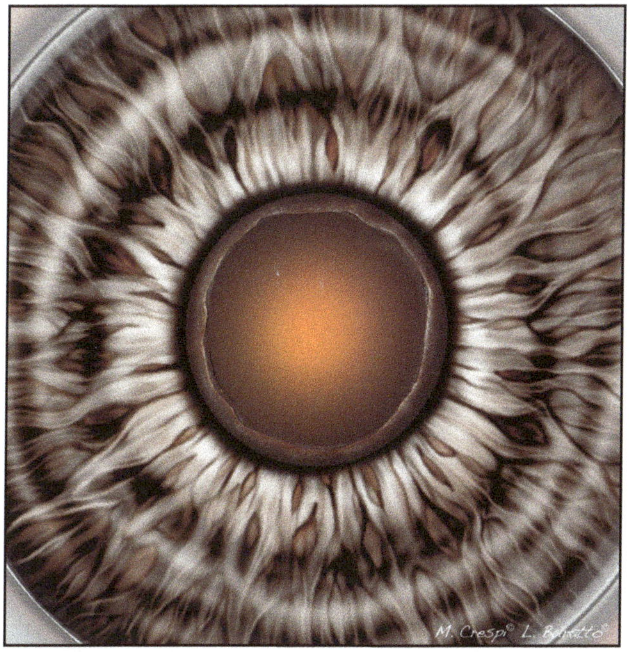

Figure 4-2. Reduced dilation of the pupil and deposits on the anterior surface of the iris in an eye affected by PEX.

meshwork and inside the trabecular endothelial cells that appear to be "dusted" with this material. Ultrastructural examination of eyes with glaucoma detects this material inside Schlemm's canal and in the openings in its walls. These elements explain the association between PEX and chronic glaucoma; this illustrates the frequently seen trabecular block to aqueous outflow. Finally, deposits of PEX material have also been seen around the collection ducts of Schlemm's canal and the aqueous veins.

Clinical Aspects

PEX is often found on a routine exam with a lack of symptoms. Thus, the diagnosis is based on recognition of specific signs that are detected during a routine examination.

By examining the anterior capsule of the lens, when dilated, 3 areas may be identified (Figure 4-1):

1. A central homogeneous disk around the circular zone of whitish gray PEX material
2. An intermediate wrinkled area, occasionally with radial striations, resulting from mechanical friction between the pupil margin and anterior capsule
3. A peripheral granular area that is white at the center, another deposit site for this material

The most characteristic aspect can be seen on the anterior edge of the more peripheral area; it appears to be uneven and wrinkled, as though the capsule is peeling back in this area.

The PEX material can also be found at the edge of the pupil (where it has a scale-like appearance) as well as on the anterior surface of the iris (Figure 4-2). The anterior surface of the iris must be transilluminated to allow detection of signs of atrophy that are expressed as radial intrastromal defects at the sphincter portion. It is well known that the iris of individuals with this syndrome have poor mydriasis, even after the instillation of mydriatic eyedrops (see later in this chapter).

Examination of the anterior chamber (AC) sometimes reveals moderate cellularity, the origin of which can be linked to a break in the uveal blood-aqueous barrier rather than an inflammatory reaction. If there are iridocapsular synechiae (another occasional finding of this pathology), it explains why some define this as a pseudo-uveitis.

Dispersion of pigment is another situation that is also seen in PEX eyes. The origin of this dispersion is also controversial.

Under gonioscopy, small bluish gray clusters can be observed in the trabecular meshwork; these are deposits of the PEX material (Figure 4-3). Actually, the angle appears to be hyperpigmented because of deposits on the meshwork and on the anterior edge of Schwalbe's line, forming the so-called Sampaolesi line, commonly seen in these eyes.

Pigment deposits can also be found on the corneal endothelium and rarely will form a Krukenberg spindle. The endothelium often has a dotted appearance created by fine, nonpigmented deposits that are the in situ formations of PEX material. Acquired endothelial dysfunction has been suggested in PEX patients, given that over time some of these patients develop keratopathy caused by endothelial failure with pleomorphism and polymegathism,

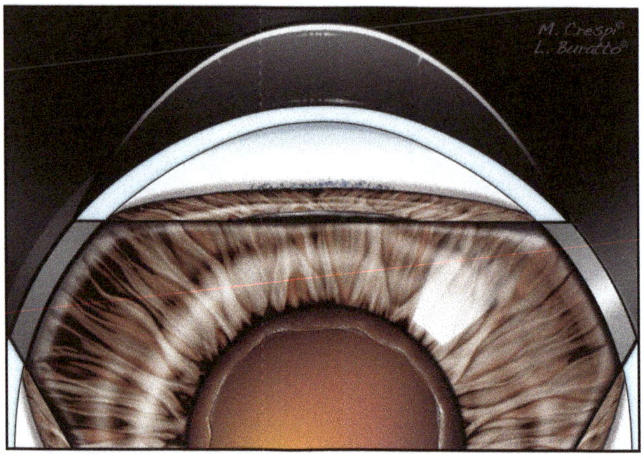

Figure 4-3. Gonioscopic examination of an eye affected by PEX. Note the small deposits of gray-blue material on the trabecular meshwork.

clearly distinguished from Fuchs or bullous keratopathy in pseudophakic patients,[1,44] even though some studies do not confirm this, demonstrating that PEX does not increase endothelial cell loss.[45,46]

Less common sites for deposits of PEX material are the ciliary body, the zonules, and the anterior hyaloid face (more evident in pseudophakic eyes).

Another aspect of this syndrome is the presence of zonular instability that explains the tendency toward partial or total luxation of the lens that frequently occurs spontaneously; there is also a greater risk of complications during cataract surgery.

Recently, electron microscopy and immunohistochemical examinations allow the analysis of other tissues in PEX patients: the orbit and eyelid skin, the liver, the meninges, skin, kidneys, bladder, lungs, and the myocardium. Tissue structurally identical to PEX was seen in these locations.[32,46-51] Moreover, there is increasing interest in the correlation between PEX and pathologies affecting these organs. Some publications document association of PEX with ischemic cardiopathy, transitory ischemic attacks, Alzheimer's disease, and alterations of blood values (eg, the metabolic disorder hyperhomocysteinemia). This explains why PEX is considered to be a systemic disease with the eye being the predominant site.

Risk Factors in Cataract Surgery

As mentioned, there may be changes of the AC, considered to be risk factors for complications during and after cataract surgery.

In the past, with extracapsular cataract extraction (ECCE), many studies reported increased phacodonesis and zonular dialysis, increase in the hardness of the nucleus, poor mydriasis, posterior capsule ruptures, vitreous loss, and postoperative inflammation.[52-62] In particular, in patients having ECCE, the percentage of anterior capsulorrhexis escape was 27%, posterior capsule rupture or zonular dialysis between 13% and 28%, and a vitreous loss rate of between 5% and 12%. These studies showed zonular dialysis 10 times higher and vitreous loss 5 times greater than normal.[62-68]

With the use of phacoemulsification, the frequency of serious intraoperative complications was lower in all patients and particularly in PEX patients.[54,69-72] In patients having phacoemulsification, there is a frequency of vitreous loss of between 0% and 5%. In the newest studies,[73-76] results of phacoemulsification in eyes with PEX are almost identical to those of normal eyes when preoperative preparation and necessary precautions were taken.

Moreover, in some recent studies, there was no statistical difference in the complication rate in PEX patients as compared to normals.[77-80]

A reduction in complications has been seen because phacoemulsification reduced the surgical risks associated with PEX; however, it has also reduced because of better pre- and intraoperative understanding of potential problems by the surgeon. New technology (phacoemulsifiers, instruments, and viscoelastic substance [VES]) have made important contributions allowing the surgeon to prevent many of the problems.

Preoperative Diagnosis

The pathogenesis of the PEX cataract explains the decisions required when dealing with this type of cataract both pre- and intraoperatively, facilitating some of the intra- and postoperative decisions required for good outcomes.

With these patients, problems may occur at any time during surgery. By systematizing the more important complications, the PEX cataract can be divided into the following 2 groups:

1. Iris-related problems
2. Problems associated with the anterior capsule, the capsular bag, and the zonules[81,80]

For each of these situations, surgeons should evaluate the degree of intra- and postoperative risk to allow less experienced colleagues to understand and reduce the potentially negative aspects of PEX on good surgery. Iris involvement and the capsule-zonules in PEX can have different degrees of expression that can influence the surgery. The syndrome can manifest itself in many ways, with a clinical picture ranging from similar to a normal cataract to extremely difficult.

Iris Problems

The examination of the iris should be done prior to dilation, when it is possible to evaluate the stability of the iris (iridodonesis), changes in the pupil margin, ranging from straightforward deposits of PEX material (scale-like deposits on the sphincter) to partial or total atrophy of the pupillary margin with atrophic membranes on the iris margin. This range of conditions is the first evaluation of pseudoexfoliative expression, and dynamic pupillography provides information on pupil mobility determining possible multifocal intraocular lens (IOL) implantation (a highly controversial subject). Iridodonesis should be evoked by asking the patient to perform rapid repeated eye movements.

The objective of the second part of the preoperative evaluation of the iris is to measure its mydriatic response to drugs to determine if surgery can be safely performed. The more time or drugs needed to achieve "good" mydriasis, the greater the risk of PEX damage affecting the iris and entire lens-zonular apparatus.

Regarding movement and pupil size, it should be stressed that preoperative evaluation of the eye's response to mydriatics is one of the most important parts of the preoperative examination for every cataract operation. However, with PEX cataracts, this evaluation is much more important and provides useful information for surgery as regards the pre- and intraoperative drug administration.

Patients with PEX usually have partial iris atrophy, characterized by defects of the iris collar highlighted with transillumination; this is sometimes associated with posterior synechiae. Prior to surgery, it may prove difficult to induce sufficient mydriasis. Poor mydriasis may be linked to alteration of the microfibril structures and deposits of PEX material. Deposits of PEX material will also be responsible for the reduced consistency and decreased tone of the iris due to loss of pigment from the pigmented pupillary epithelium.

In most cases of PEX, the pupil will have less response to mydriatics as compared to normal; however, surgery can usually be performed with no significant problems. Sometimes the mydriasis is poor, and surgical manipulation will be required for surgery. Lack of mydriasis can be managed in a number of ways, allowing surgery to be continued with security. When synechiae, membranes, or sector atrophy occurs and prevents dilation, techniques including viscodilation, synechotomy, iris hooks or expansion rings, sphincterotomies, or stretching may be considered.[83,84] (These are described in detail in Chapters 2 and 5.)

Problems Associated With the Anterior Capsule, the Bag, and the Zonules

One should evaluate the structure of the anterior capsule (elasticity and thickness) and resistance of the capsule-zonules. It is well known that in the normal eye, the zonules are a system of very fine fibrils stretching between the lens and the ciliary body, radiating from the lens equator, separated from the hyaloid face by a virtual canal (Hannover's canal). The zonules are unquestionably thicker and more elastic in children, thinner and more fragile in the elderly.

With PEX deposits between the anterior capsule and pars plicata of the ciliary body, degeneration of the zonules with their consequent ciliary disinsertion is associated with the risk of subluxation of the lens. In PEX, lysosomial proteinase destroys the normal structure of the basal membrane of the nonpigmented epithelium of the ciliary body and the anterior capsule. The rupture of the basal membrane alters the zonular-capsule complex and creates adhesions between the zonules and the nonpigmented epithelium. As a result, the forces of rotation and anterior posterior movements that are generated during the surgery can rupture the zonules with vitreous loss.

Zonular dialysis is the most significant complication; the surgeon must use all the maneuvers for the so-called immobile cataract surgery (this will be discussed later in more detail).

The degree of lens mobility (varying considerably from case to case), as seen preoperatively, determines the choice of surgery: intracapsular cataract extraction or phacoemulsification.

Surgical Technique

When the surgeon elects phacoemulsification, he or she first performs a clear corneal incision, as opposed to a scleral incision, to avoid eliminating a future trabeculectomy if required because of the high incidence of PEX glaucoma. The corneal incisions should be slightly longer to reduce the risk of iris prolapse.

Regardless of the surgical technique, the introduction of capsulorrhexis was an important step for these patients as zonular stress is limited.

In general, the capsulorrhexis should be 5 to 5.5 mm, just slightly smaller than the diameter of the optic to avoid damaging the zonules that extend on to the anterior capsule for approximately 2 mm. The surgeon should create a uniform rhexis that is well centered, circular with smooth edges. This is even more important with PEX as the capsulorrhexis should not pass through the areas containing PEX deposits. The iris will scrape PEX material on the central part of the anterior lens. PEX material then deposits on the central and peripheral portions, leaving the intermediate part free from deposits. The peripheral band, observed only after mydriasis, is identifiable by irregular radial striations and granular deposits that may allow the rhexis to escape. The surgeon may decide to make the capsulorrhexis smaller, as this reduces the risk. This maneuver, however, should be avoided to prevent capsular phimosis, leading to zonular dialysis with a possibility of late-onset luxation of the bag. The surgeon must ensure that the rhexis is large enough because the centripetal force created with contraction of the bag may play an important role in late-onset damage to the zonules (this will be addressed further in the following sections).

Problems during the capsulorrhexis include the following:

- Formation of small folds
- Dropped lens
- Dislocated lens
- Folds around the rhexis
- Escape of the rhexis

It is advisable to use special rhexis forceps in these patients to ensure good control. A high-viscosity viscoelastic substance (VES; eg, Healon GV [Abbott Laboratories, Abbott Park, IL]) should be used, allowing transparency and pseudoplasticity.

For PEX patients, a reduction in AC depth will allow relaxation of the zonules, encouraging forward movement of the lens. This is an additional risk factor for rhexis escape.

When the surgeon performs the rhexis, the direction is influenced by 2 forces: the first is centrifugal, transmitted to the edge of the rhexis by the tension of the zonules; the second is centripetal, transmitted by the surgeon to the flap. The combination of these 2 forces determines the direction of the capsulorrhexis. In patients with forward displacement of the lens as in PEX, the zonules are stretched, allowing a greater possibility of escape. This is why a high molecular weight VES should be used; as it increases AC depth, it will relax the zonules.

The capsulorrhexis may not be straightforward in these patients due to pupillary miosis.

If the capsulorrhexis is impossible because of excessive mobility of the lens (lateral and anterior-posterior movements), the surgeon should proceed with an intracapsular approach (ie, intracapsular cataract extraction) preoperatively; this should be anticipated if phacodenesis is seen at the slit lamp. If the capsulorrhexis can be completed, with the lens moving laterally, the surgeon can cautiously proceed. A large rhexis should be created to allow hydroluxation into the AC, with phacoemulsification at the iris plane (supracapsular phacoemulsification). If the zonular stability is good and no movements of the lens are detected during capsulorrhexis, the surgeon can proceed with traditional in-the-bag phacoemulsification, with good hydrodissection. The degree of lens mobility determines the location for emulsification, taking into account preoperative phacodonesis and intraoperative zonular stability allowing formation of folds from a lack of zonular tension during the rhexis. The folds, lens density, and condition of the endothelium determine the option of performing supracapsular phacoemulsification with zonules that are severely compromised.

Hydrodissection must always be performed accurately, delicately, and completely with the surgeon paying special attention to breakage of the capsular-cortical adhesions with minimal rotation of the nucleus. He or she should push down on the peripheral areas allowing balanced salt solution (BSS) to escape. Rotation of the nucleus should be minimal, and in high-risk cases, the nucleus should not be rotated at all.

Hydrodelineation should always be performed. In some cases, the surgeon may find it useful to perform viscodelineation with a low molecular weight VES.

Particularly during phacoemulsification, forces of rotation and anterior-posterior movement can create stress on the zonules. The surgeon should be extremely delicate; he or she can convert to a quick chop technique (centrally) aspirating the cortex in a tangential direction rather than perpendicular to reduce trauma to the zonules.

During phacoemulsification, it is essential to use a flow rate that will avoid fluctuations of the AC with trampolining of the iridolenticular diaphragm. The surgeon must avoid high settings and continuous irrigation with bottles that are too high. The flow rate should be low to avoid pressure surges or excess pressure in the AC, reducing zonular stress further. The flow rate should be set to avoid sudden occlusion that could bring the nucleus toward the incision.

Modern machines with sophisticated software create stability of the AC, allowing us to work under safe conditions, using a slightly higher flow rate.

The fact that PEX also leads to reduced iris tone and greater sensitivity to flow in the AC during surgery is another good reason for setting the phaco parameters, reducing iris movements (low bottle height and lower values of flow rate and vacuum). This reduces the risk of aspirating the iris with the phaco, a complication that can have serious consequences. If there is limited dialysis as opposed to zonular relaxation, some have suggested bimanual cataract extraction—having the irrigation probe separate from the aspiration probe, allowing the surgeon to use the irrigation probe as a surgical instrument.

The infusion can be directed inside the bag at the dialysis point to stabilize the bag, allowing easier lens removal.

After IOL implantation, aspiration of residual cortex that could not be aspirated previously can be done.

Other Problems

At the completion of surgery, it is essential to accurately remove the VES to avoid or at least reduce postoperative pressure spikes. At the corneal level, the white-gray extracellular material typical of PEX may deposit on the endothelium along with pigment. This may lead to endothelial cell loss with pleomorphism and polymegatism.

Following cataract surgery, there is an increased risk of corneal decompensation, from the intraocular maneuvers, energy levels, and possible postoperative IOP increase. This has not been confirmed by the findings of a recent study[86] that reported no statistically significant differences in terms of endothelial cell density, pleomorphism, polymegatism, and increased corneal thickness in eyes with or without PEX.

Another important factor is greater postoperative inflammation and a greater risk of intra- and postoperative hemorrhage.

Electron microscopy and immunohistochemical examinations have shown that immediately following the operation, there may be increased Tyndall scattering, fibrin in the AC, and formation of posterior synecchiae.[54,86-89] These are caused by surgical trauma of pathological iris vessels (characterized by accumulation of PEX material in the subendothelial area) causing rupture of the blood-aqueous barrier and miosis, requiring mechanical dilation.

The greater inflammatory reaction may be responsible for an increased incidence of posterior capsule opacity and contraction of the anterior capsule.

Intraocular Lens Choice

With PEX cataracts, the IOL selection is determined by 2 peculiar conditions of this syndrome:

- Uveal and capsular tissue reactivity
- Vulnerability of the capsular bag and its suspension apparatus

These have an extremely important role in some of the early- or late-onset complications, and the choice of a suitable IOL is a major factor in reducing later complications.

In PEX eyes, deposits of fibrillary material on the walls of the vessels of the iridociliary microcirculation creates increased permeability of the blood-aqueous barrier with increased postoperative inflammation.[22,26] Many studies have demonstrated that these eyes are unusually susceptible to surgical trauma, with increased cellular and fibrin reaction in the AC and greater incidence of posterior synechiae.[54,86-89]

More recently, studies of biocompatibility of IOLs have demonstrated their relation to postoperative inflammation,[90-93] in particular, the chemical-physical characteristics of the surface and the reactivity of the inflammatory cells on the IOL surface.[94,95] First, small inflammatory cells in the aqueous deposit on the surface of the IOL. These macrophages will remove residual postsurgical debris, cells, and pigment. The cells can change and increase in size, giving rise to gigantic epithelioid cells that are the expression of foreign body reaction against the IOL. The attempt to "digest" the foreign body is accompanied by release of inflammatory mediators.[96] The presence of inflammatory cells on the IOL surface creates a secondary inflammatory reaction. There are 2 main factors that determine the permanence of these cells on the surface of the IOL: first, the severity of the postoperative inflammation, and second, the biocompatibility of the IOL.[97,98]

Just a few hours after lens implantation, a protein film covers the surface of the IOL. The protein layer consists of albumin, immunoglobulin, complement fractions, fibrin, type IV collagen, fibronectin, laminin, and vitronectin that bind to the lens surface to varying degrees.[99-102] The composition of the protein film depends on the chemical-physical characteristics of the IOL material showing variable affinity for different proteins.

This layer becomes the mediator of the interaction between the IOL surface and the inflammatory cells, therefore increasing or limiting the permanence of the cellular deposits on the IOL. The greater biocompatibility of a specific material depends on its ability to bind proteins inhibiting cell adhesion. Numerous studies have demonstrated greater inflammatory response with hydrophobic lenses as opposed to hydrophilic lenses.[90,91,103,104] Biocompatibility of hydrophilic acrylic lenses is greater than silicone lenses or hydrophobic acrylic lenses.[105] This has been shown in normal eyes and eyes with a high risk of postoperative inflammation and confirmed in eyes with PEX.[90,91,106] Hydrophilic acrylic lenses are indicated in cases with a tendency to postoperative inflammation, as is the case with PEX.

The implantation of an IOL induces a reactive response of the LECs, persisting until after the surgery. The early response derives from the lens cells that persist under the part of the anterior capsule that remains following capsulorrhexis. It appears as an opacification of the anterior capsule and the growth of cell membranes that start from the edge of the rhexis and extend above the optic plate of the IOL. Histopathological studies demonstrated that the opacification of the anterior chamber is due to fibrous metaplasia of the LECs.[107] The membrane growth at the edge of the rhexis is linked to phenomena of cell proliferation and migration that give rise to a layer of cells and an extracellular matrix.[108,109]

The late response is associated with equatorial cell activity giving rise to posterior capsule opacification with the same mechanism of proliferation and migration and, to a lesser degree, fibrous metaplasia.

While posterior capsule opacification has multifactorial origins, including systemic and ocular factors, and depending on the IOL itself, the early response of the lens depends largely on the cellular response to the material (or capsular biocompatibility) and to a lesser degree on other factors such as the diameter of the rhexis, the degree of postoperative inflammation, and associated conditions such as PEX.[110,111]

Both lens reactions (early and late) play an important role in dislocation of the IOL and the capsular bag, exacerbating the loose zonules, characteristic of PEX.

With time, progressive loss of zonular support in PEX may lead to total dislocation of the bag, the so-called *in-the-bag dislocation*. This is closely related to the development of the capsular contraction syndrome. This condition was first described by Davison in 1993 and was defined as progressive and excessive decrease in the capsulorrhexis size[80] phimosis of the rhexis coming from fibrotic anterior capsule contraction.

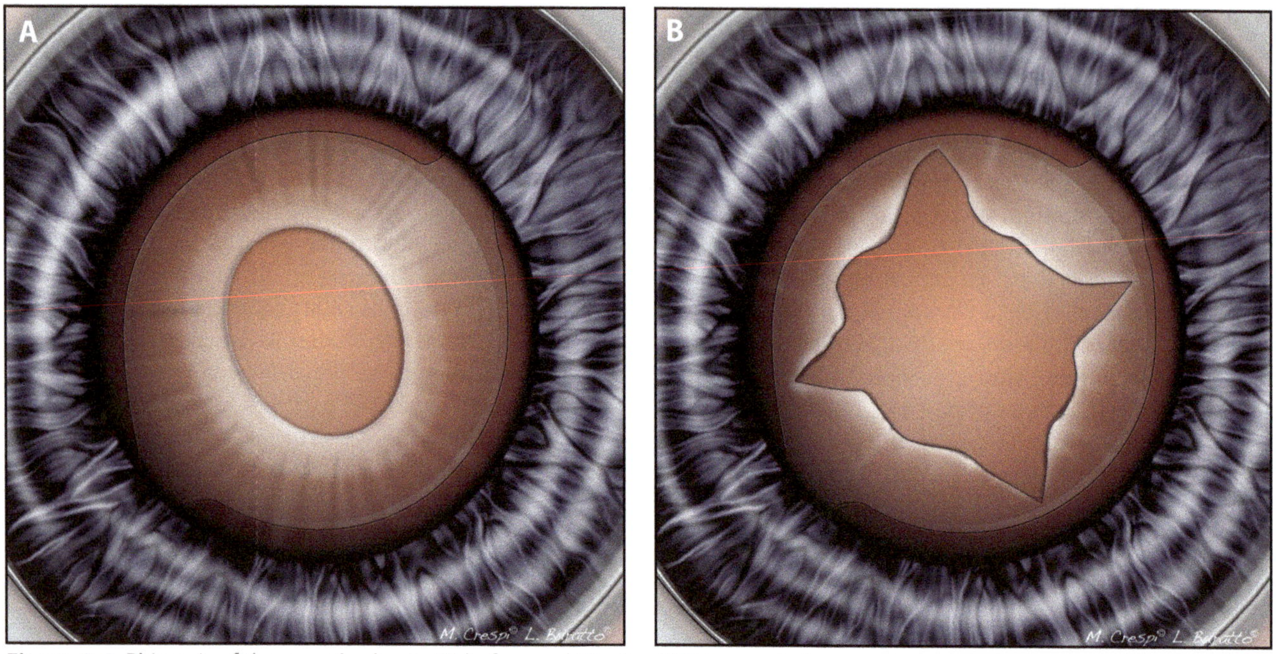

Figure 4-4. Phimosis of the capsulorrhexis: (A) before and (B) after YAG laser anterior capsulotomy.

This problem is associated with several factors, the most important of which is capsular biocompatibility. The behavior of the LECs, like the inflammatory response, depends on their interaction with the protein film covering the biomaterial and the degree of activation.[102,112]

A number of clinical studies demonstrate that some biomaterials stimulate cell proliferation and fibrous metaplasia to a greater degree than others and therefore will lead to opacification of the anterior capsule.[106,113-115] In normal patients, it was reported that silicone and hydrophilic acrylic lenses more frequently produce opacification of the anterior capsule as compared to hydrophobic acrylic lenses. Hydrophilic acrylic lenses also induce cell membrane growth on the IOL surface more frequently than lenses of other materials.[85,86,106,115,116] The contraction of the anterior capsule generates traction on the equator of the capsular bag and therefore on the zonules. The traction is proportional to the extent of the fibrosis. In addition to the biomaterial, the latter is assisted by contact between the anterior capsule and the surface of the IOL. It has been shown that silicone plate haptic lenses are associated with frequent and severe opacification of the anterior capsule.[116]

To reduce contact between the anterior capsule and the IOL, and to prevent fibrosis, the surgeon should perform a capsulorrhexis just smaller than the optic of the IOL; he or she should avoid an excessively small rhexis. Nevertheless, this may not be easy in patients with PEX due to a small pupil diameter. This may also interfere with complete cortex and LEC removal, facilitating the formation of a Soemmering's ring.

The increased weight of the IOL capsular bag complex may be an additional factor contributing to further weakening of the already weakened zonules.

The traction on the capsular bag created by contraction of the rhexis is countered to a certain degree by the tension of the lens haptics or from the presence of a capsular tension ring (CTR) that distributes centripetal forces over the circumference of the bag. Polymethylmethacrylate (PMMA) haptics are more rigid and provide greater resistance as compared to the haptics of acrylic or silicone lenses.[117-119]

With capsular phimosis, the surgeon may find it useful to perform a posterior capsulotomy and also relaxing incisions on the margin of the rhexis with either surgery or the yttrium-aluminum-garnet (YAG) laser (Figure 4-4).[79-86]

Loose zonules are the primary factor determining choice of IOL in the PEX patient with 2 additional conditions determining the IOL to be implanted:

1. Increased risk of capsule rupture
2. Increased risk of dislocation of the entire IOL capsular bag complex, a phenomenon described as in-the-bag dislocation[119]

Increased Risk of Capsule Rupture

The risk of capsule rupture associated with PEX does not come from thinning of the posterior capsule; on the contrary, it appears to be thicker though this is due to excessive intraoperative fluctuation because of lack of zonular tension.[26]

Capsule rupture resulting in insufficient capsular support creates the choice between an IOL with scleral fixation or an angle, or iris supported AC-IOL. A recent review of this subject shows no evidence to support the superiority of one option over the other.[120] The incidence of glaucoma, endothelial decompensation, and cystoid macular edema is similar following implantation of an IOL in the AC or with scleral fixation. Nevertheless, this technique is associated with possible additional complications such as suture exposure, increased risk of endophthalmitis, intraocular hemorrhage, tilt, and dislocation of the IOL.[120]

If the capsule support is sufficient for implantation of an IOL in the posterior chamber, the surgeon must decide on implanting an IOL in the capsular bag or in the ciliary sulcus. Bag implantation is preferable if the capsule rupture is small and allows secure implantation in the bag without risk of dislocation. If there is capsule rupture and the remnants allow implantation in the sulcus, following vitrectomy, the choice is an IOL of 13 mm overall length, with a 6-mm optic plate of 6 mm, preferably with rigid haptics (PMMA).

Some surgeons prefer one-piece PMMA IOLs because of the greater compression force from the haptics to the sulcus. However, new IOL designs with more biocompatible materials appear to have comparable results.

In-the-Bag Dislocation

One consequence of IOL implantation in the bag with bag dehiscence will be development of capsular folds encouraging migration of LECs and increase in fibrous and myofibrous pseudometaplasia causing capsular phimosis, with the subsequent possibility of IOL decentration (the elastic action of the IOL haptic will be insufficient).

The decentration of the IOL depends on the overall length of the lens and the material of the loops. A more rigid material such as PMMA, despite being more reactive than other materials, will withstand a greater force than softer materials.

With partial or total dehiscence less than 90 degrees, the force from the IOL haptics may be sufficient to distend the capsular bag. Implantation of an IOL in the bag should parallel the subluxed region; the surgeon should avoid rotating the lens as this will create trauma to the zonules adjacent to the dialysis.

With zonular dehiscence between 90 and 120 degrees, the IOL alone cannot stabilize the bag as the haptic action is sectorial. Here, the surgeon should implant a CTR, which will have a 360-degree action and will better counter the centripetal forces from the bag. In patients with loose zonules, CTRs prevent IOL decentration by distending and reducing opacification of the capsular bag. However, CTRs do not ensure stability of the IOL/bag complex over the years. A number of cases of late luxation of the bag-IOL-CTR complex have been described. Modified CTRs that can be sutured to the sclera will reduce phacodonesis and decentration in PEX patients (refer to Chapters 2 and 20).

With significant capsular dehiscence, a CTR is valuable in preventing IOL decentration. These include the following:

- Expansion and stabilization of the bag
- Reduction in posterior capsule opacity due to prevention of capsular folds and creation of a barrier effect opposing the migration of the LECs
- Containment of the vitreous following contraction of the bag itself

The limitations include the following:

- Difficulty with the implant
- Risk of increasing the dehiscence
- The need for an expert surgeon

In-the-bag dislocation is a late onset complication; risk factors are PEX,[121-125] advanced age, severe myopia, previous posterior vitrectomy, previous trauma, uveitis, and some forms of collagenopathies (Ehlers-Danlos syndrome, Marfan's syndrome, Weill-Marchesani syndrome, homocystinuria, and hyperlysinemia).[126] Apart from the presence of PEX, the common element in all of these conditions in zonular weakness.

The IOL-capsular bag complex can partially dislocate (Figure 4-5) or totally with complete luxation in the vitreous chamber (Figure 4-6). The exact incidence of this type of dislocation is not known; there is no doubt that it is a late-onset complication that has been more frequently reported in recent years. The increase is related to the use of capsulorrhexis and the ability to complete the surgery even with marked phacodonesis.[122] Stabilizing the capsular bag with a CTR and iris retractor hooks used on the margin of the rhexis have made it possible to implant an IOL in the bag even with marked phacodonesis. Improvements in operative techniques have shifted the onset of this complication from during surgery to the postoperative period.

The fact that the dislocation may occur even many years after surgery suggests that weakening of the zonules is a process that continues for a long time after capsular contraction has occurred.

In conclusion, the preferred implant for a PEX patient should be hydrophobic acrylic because of its capsular biocompatibility and the possibility of preventing complications arising from the contraction of the capsular bag.

An IOL with PMMA haptics with an overall length of 13 mm is preferable to allow distension of the capsular bag and to facilitate the repositioning process of the lens in the event of dislocation. The resistance to compression is greater with a one-piece PMMA lenses as compared to (in descending order) a 3-piece PMMA lens, a foldable 3-piece lens, and finally a foldable one-piece lens. Yet despite all of this, at the end of surgery, the surgeon may still have an oval rhexis or folds in the posterior capsule. A larger optic (6 to 6.5 mm) will prevent edge diffraction if there is decentration.

It is essential that the choice of the IOL is accompanied by precise surgery combining the management of the pupil and rhexis with the complete removal of lens material and an accurate evaluation of capsular stability.

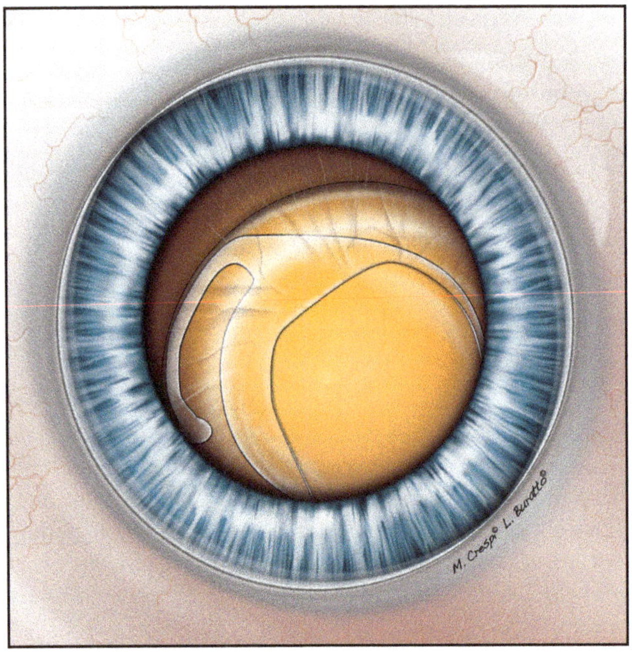

Figure 4-5. Partial dislocation of the IOL-capsular bag complex.

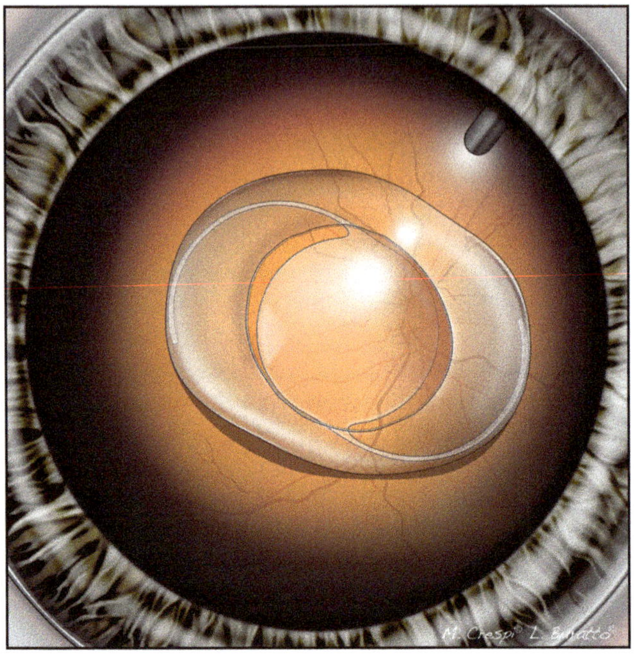

Figure 4-6. Total dislocation of the IOL-capsular bag complex.

Finally, with PEX, different authors recommend avoiding the use of multifocal IOLs (because of altered pupil kinetics and instability of the zonules) and accommodative lenses because of the rigidity of the haptics.

Surgical Management of the Dislocated Lens

Dislocation of the lens is not uncommon. The surgeon can use a surgical solution, even with PEX, that varies with each case in terms of lens removal and the primary or secondary implantation of the IOL.

Surgical Technique

Techniques that can be used to treat luxation of the lens vary depending on the surgeon's experience and on the characteristics of the lens itself.[127-133]

Surgery to remove the dislocated lens is not urgent, and it may be useful to delay surgery by a few days or weeks to allow the degree of inflammation of the eye to decrease or allow better visibility of the posterior segment. The onset of increased IOP or phacolytic uveitis will determine the need for a timeless surgery.

For surgery, posterior vitectomy should be available, preferably with an endophaco tip, and appropriate ability to examine the retina, particularly with panoramic-type lenses (Figure 4-7). Perfluorocarbonate liquid (PFCL) is essential; VES is also useful. Cryo and lasers are essential when there may be retinal damage.

Pars plana vitrectomy is a fundamental technique in this pathology; it depends on the lens density.

Once 3 sclerotomies have been prepared and the infusion tip has been placed, the surgeon proceeds with accurate removal of the posterior vitreous and the vitrectomy around the luxated nucleus. The vitrectomy must extend to the vitreous base to avoid successive contraction of the peripheral vitreous with the formation of retinal tears.

Once the primary vitrectomy has been performed, the nucleus can be approached using 3 different techniques, determined by the density of the nucleus.

1. If the nucleus is very soft, as with young patients and spontaneous luxation caused by the absence of or loose zonules, the nucleus can be removed using the vitectomy with a low cut rate. This should never be performed close to the posterior pole until PFCL or VES has been injected (Figure 4-8) to protect the macula. Recently, with soft nuclei, some surgeons have opted for mini-invasive surgery via pars plana—23 or 25 gauge—however, with this approach, the endophacoemulsification tip cannot be used.
2. When the lens is harder, due to the patient's age or the presence of a cataract, the nucleus should be approached using the endophacoemulsification tip, using vitrectomy to remove small residual fragments. Again in this case, the procedure must follow an injection of PFCL, pushing the nucleus up into the anterior part of the vitreous chamber in a safer position away from the retina.
3. If the lens is mature and denser, the surgical strategy must be different. The surgeon must remove the lens

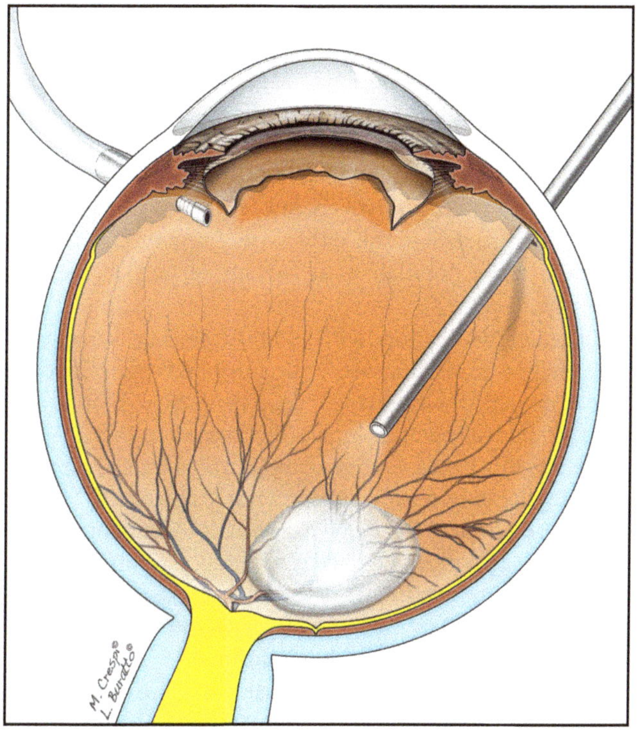

Figure 4-7. Nucleus is visible in the vitreous chamber.

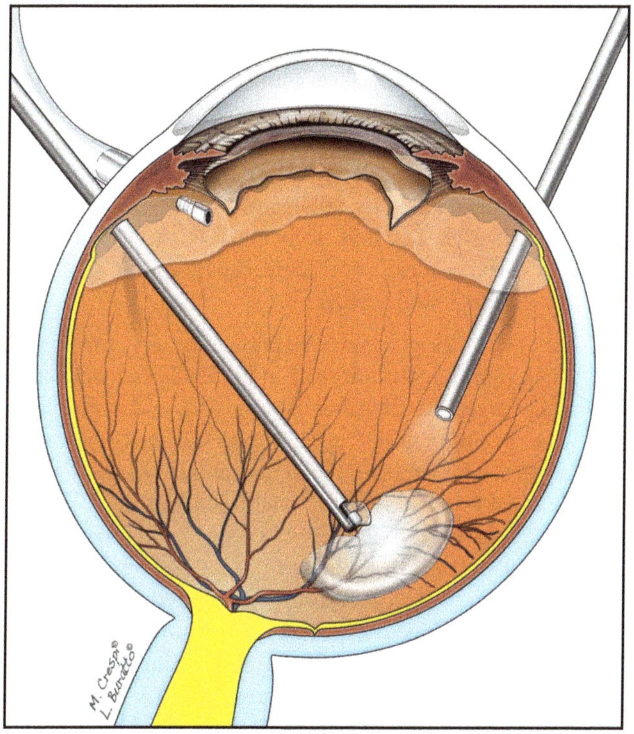

Figure 4-8. Removal of the nucleus using the vitrectomy device.

as a whole via the limbus (ie, anterior). Once the vitreous has been removed as far as the base, the posterior chamber is filled with PFCL as far as the iris to elevate the entire lens for removal through the limbus with a loop or cryoprobe used for cataracts.

In any case, once the luxated lens has been removed, the PFCL is removed and the peripheral retina is managed. With rhegmatogenous lesions, the surgeon can use cryo spots or, better still, the endolaser.

At the conclusion of the pars plana vitrectomy, the surgeon can decide to fill the vitreous cavity with air, gas, or polydimethylsiloxane (PDMS), then the IOL is implanted.

Management of Glaucoma Associated With Cataract

In patients with PEX, glaucoma is often associated with the cataract. In order to treat the glaucoma, the surgeon must always consider the characteristics of the 2 pathologies: the risk profiles and priorities (reduction in IOP versus visual rehabilitation).

The 2 clinical conditions (glaucoma and cataract) mutually interact. The cataract (and surgical/interventions) can cause or aggravate glaucoma; vice versa, worsening glaucoma and/or therapy (prolonged use of IOP-reducing drops, parasurgical surgical treatments) can induce cataract formation.

Pathogenesis of Glaucoma and Therapeutic Approach

In patients with PEX, glaucoma can be caused by 3 different mechanisms:

1. The most frequent PEX glaucoma is trabecular block, due to presence of PEX material in the AC, depositing in the trabecular meshwork.
2. Cases of pupillary block have also been described, caused by posterior synechiae, forward displacement of the lens due to zonular weakness, and increased rigidity of the iris with a tendency for miosis. These may lead to an acute glaucoma attack; synechiae in the angle may lead to narrow- or closed-angle glaucoma.
3. There have also been reports of pupillary block induced by contraction of the ciliary muscle due to loose zonules allowing forward lens movement.

Progression and prognosis of PEX glaucoma is worse than straightforward chronic open-angle glaucoma. In PEX patients, early surgical treatment is the norm, as pretreatment IOP will be higher and medical treatment will be less successful.

In these patients, medical treatment is typically poor, laser trabeculoplasty has a temporary effect, and surgical complications are greater and more frequent.

There are 3 conditions that should be managed differently:

1. Patients with good IOP and insignificant cataract. In these cases, the management is on a case-by-case

basis with medical treatment and laser treatment for glaucoma. There are several drugs available, each having a different action. The surgeon should opt for drugs that will increase the trabecular flow. Medical treatment can be combined with argon laser trabeculoplasty (ALT) or selective laser trabeculoplasty (SLT) treatments producing satisfactory results immediately postoperative; however, they are less successful long-term. Fifty percent of the time, the treatment will have lost its effect after 5 years.

2. Patients with glaucoma needing surgery for visual rehabilitation. With narrow-angle PEX glaucoma, cataract surgery may correct the pupillary and angle block with reduction in IOP up to 7 mm Hg even 2 years after surgery. Thus, in these patients cataract surgery alone should be performed as it will produce long-lasting reduction of the IOP. In patients with open-angle PEX glaucoma, an IOP less than 20 mm Hg and good tolerance to topical therapy, combined surgery will not be necessary. Phacoemulsification allows visual rehabilitation with moderate IOP reduction 15% to 20% of the time. Findings reported years ago[134] confirmed by more recent clinical studies[47,63,74,135,136] demonstrated significant long-term IOP reduction (after 6, 12, and 24 months) in PEX patients after cataract surgery. The mean reduction is significantly greater in PEX eyes compared to chronic open-angle glaucoma; phacoemulsification with bag IOL implantation can be considered a form of IOP treatment in PEX patients. Moreover, postoperative reduction of IOP is proportional to the preoperative value: the greater the preoperative IOP, the greater the reduction in IOP.
3. Patients with cataract and uncontrolled glaucoma, with visual field loss. In these cases, the priority is to reduce the IOP.
   - Any glaucoma treatment will accelerate cataract formation; the patient will probably require cataract surgery; in turn, this may compromise the survival of the bleb and IOP control.
   - It is unlikely that the cataract surgery alone will resolve the problem of high IOP.

Thus, the surgeon should avoid the risks associated with sequential surgery and use a combined approach. However, this also has potential complications, as combined surgery may not be as effective as trabeculectomy alone (refer to Chapter 3). Combined surgery reduces the trauma from 2 sequential surgeries; however, one should consider patient characteristics (age, compliance, personal requirements, risk factors for glaucoma), amount of glaucoma-related damage, the target IOP (estimated case by case), degree of lens opacification, and the degree of safety and efficacy of the surgery.

Given the multiple factors whether combined surgery is indicated and the surgery used, it is difficult to provide general guidelines. The surgeon must make the choice on an individual basis.

The best surgical option is the standard phacotrabeculectomy; it is the most popular of the combined glaucoma and cataract procedures. The reason for its popularity is its excellent functional results, in terms of IOP reduction, visual recovery, and relatively low incidence of complications. The procedure can either use 2 separate incisions, which is more popular, or it can be performed using a single incision.

Phacoemulsification with nonpenetrating surgery is indicated in cases that are well controlled (eg, glaucoma that is managed with a single drug or in cases that have a low risk of postoperative high IOP). Even though this technique has less postoperative complications than the previous one, the long-term results are less satisfactory.[137,138] If the surgeon desires a very low target IOP (in patients with a cataract and poorly controlled glaucoma), phacotrabeculectomy with mitomycin C[139] or a trabeculectomy with mitomycin C followed by cataract surgery if necessary, waiting at least 6 to 12 months, can be performed.

Recently, more surgeons are opting for a combined technique avoiding the trauma resulting from 2 separate surgeries. This decision is encouraged by ongoing improvements in surgical techniques for glaucoma and cataracts. The success of combined surgery has been confirmed in numerous studies reporting safety and efficacy, particularly in terms of postoperative complications.

References

1. Ritch R, Schlotzer-Schrehardt U. Exfoliation syndrome. *Surv Opthtalmol.* 2001;45(4):265-315.
2. Dvorak-Theobald G. Pseudoexfoliation of the lens capsule: relation to true exfoliation of lens capsule as reported in the literature and role in the production of glaucoma capsulocuticulare. *Am J Ophthalmol.* 1954;37:1-12.
3. Forsius H, Forsman E, Fellman J, et al. Exfoliation syndrome: frequency, gender distribution and association with clinically induced alterations of the cornea and conjunctiva. *Acta Ophthalmol Scand.* 2002;80(5):478-484.
4. Friederich R. Eye disease in the Navajo Indians. *Ann Ophthalmol.* 1982;14(1):38-40.
5. Gorgonie G, Spina F, Amantia L. La pseudoesfoliazione capsulare. Rassegna bibliografica con contributo personale alla conoscenza della sua associazione con il glaucoma. VI Conv. S.O.Si. 202-81 Cl Oc 1, 75, 1982.
6. Tripodi G, cit da Ponte F, Scullica L, Bisantis C. I glaucomi secondari. Pag. 172. Ed. S.O.I. Società Oftalmologia Italiana-Editrice Plurigrafica Sicula, Massina, 1983.
7. Miyazaki M, Kubota T, Kubo M, et al. The prevalence of pseudoexfoliation syndrome in a Japanese population: the Hisayama study. *J Glaucoma.* 2005;14(6):482-484.
8. Aasved H. Study of relatives of person with fibrillopathia epitheliocapsularis (pseudoexfoliation of lens capsule). *Acta Ophthalmol (Copenh).* 1975;53(6):879-886.
9. Lemmela S, Forsman E, Sistonen P, et al. Genomewide scan of exfoliation syndrome. *Invest Ophthalmol Vis Sci.* 2007;48(9):4136-4142.

10. Forsman E, Cantor RM, Lu A, et al. Exfoliation syndrome: prevalence and inheritance in a subisolate of the Finish population. *Acta Ophthalmol Scand.* 2007;85(5):500-507.
11. Thorleifsson G, Magnusson KP, Sulem P, et al. Common sequence variants in the LOXL 1 gene confer susceptibility to exfoliation glaucoma. *Science.* 2007;317(5843):1397-1400.
12. Ruprecht KW, Hoh G, Guggenmoos-Holzamann T, et al. Pseudoexfoliation syndrome. Clinical and statistical studies. *Klin Monatsbl Augenheilkd.* 1985;187(1):9-13.
13. Moreno Montane EJ, Alcolea Paredes A, Campos Garcia S. Prevalence of pseudoexfoliation syndrome in the northwest of Spain. *Acta Ophthalmol (Copenh).* 1989;67(4):383-385.
14. Dirvela H, Luukinen H, Laatikainen L. Prevalence and risk factors of lens opacities in the elderly in Finland. A population-based study. *Ophthalmology.* 1995;102(1):108-117.
15. Kozobolis VP, Papatzanaki M, Vlachonikolis IG, et al. Epidemioligy of pseudoexfoliation in the island of Crete (Greece). *Acta Ophthalmol Scand.* 1997;(6):726-729.
16. Layden WE, Shaffer RN. Exfoliation syndrome. *Am J Ophthalmol.* 1974;78(5):835-841.
17. Henry JC, Krupin T, Schmitt M, et al. Long-term follow-up of pseudoexfoliation and the development of elevated intraocular pressure. *Ophthalmology.* 1987;94(5):545-552.
18. Shimizu K, Kimura Y, Aoki K. Prevalence of exfoliation syndrome in the Japanese. *Acta Ophthalmol.* 1988;184(suppl):112-115.
19. Roth M, Epstein DL. Exfoliation syndrome. *Am J Ophthalmol.* 1980;89(4):477-481.
20. Cashwell LF Jr, Shields MB. Exfoliation syndrome in the southeastern United States. I. Prevalence in open-angle glaucoma and non-glaucoma populations. *Acta Ophthalmol.* 1988;184(suppl):99-102.
21. Brusini P, Tosoni C, Miani P. Increased prevalence of occludable angles and angle-closure glaucoma in patients with pseudoexfoliation. *Am J Ophthalmol.* 1994;118(4):540.
22. Dickson DH, Ramsey MS. Symposium on pseudocapsular exfoliation and glaucoma. Fibrillopathia epitheliocapsularis: review of the nature and origin of pseudoexfoliative deposits. *Trans Ophthalmol Soc UK.* 1979;99:284-292.
23. Ashton N, Shakib M, Collier R. Electron microscopic study of pseudoexfoliation of the lens capsule. I. Lens capsule and zonular fibers. *Invest Ophthalmol Vis Sci.* 1965;4:141-153.
24. Bertelsen TI, Drablos PA, Flood PR. The so-called senile exfoliation (pseudoexfoliation) of the anterior lens capsule, a product of the lensepithelium. Fibrillopathia ephitheliocapsularis. *Acta Ophthalmol (Copenh).* 1964;42:1096-1113.
25. Schlotzer-Schrehardt U, Naumann GO. Ocular and systemic pseudoexfoliation syndrome. *Am J Ophthalmol.* 2000;141(5):921-937. Review.
26. Morrison JC, Green WR. Light microscopy of the exfoliation syndrome. *Acta Ophthalmol.* 1988;184(suppl):5-27. Review.
27. Meretoja J, Tarkkanen A. Occurrence of amyloid in eyes with pseudo-exfoliation. *Ophthalmic Res.* 1977;9:80-91.
28. Eagle RC Jr, Front RL, Fine BS. The basement membrane exfoliation syndrome. *Arch Ophthalmol.* 1979;97(3):510-515.
29. Garner A, Alexander RA. Pseudoexfoliative disease: histochemical evidence of an affinity with zonular fibres. *Br J Ophthalmol.* 1984;68(8):574-580.
30. Streeten BW, Dark AJ, Barnes CW. Pseudoexfoliative material and oxytalan fibers. *Exp Eye Res.* 1984;38(5):523-531.
31. Scholzer-Schrehardt U, Vin der Mark K, Sakai LY, et al. Increased extracellular deposition of fibrillin-containing fibrils in pseudoexfoliation syndrome. *Invest Ophthalmol Vis Sci.* 1997;38(5):970-984.
32. Schlotzer-Schrehardt U, Kuchle M, Hofmann-Rummelt C, et al. Latent TGF-beta 1 binding protein (LTBP-1): a new marker for intra- and extraocular PEX deposits. *Klin Monatsbl Augenheilkd.* 2000;216(6):412-419.
33. Zenkel M, Poschl E, Von Der Mark K. Differential gene expression in pseudoexfoliation syndrome. *Invest Ophthalmol Vis Sci.* 2005;46(10):3742-3752.
34. Horven I, Hutckinson BT. Exfoliation syndrome. Case report of 31 and 35 years old patients. *Acta Ophthalmol (Copenh).* 1967;45:294-298.
35. Kostas AG, Williamson TH. Co-existence of exfoliation syndrome, previous iris surgery, and heterochromia. *Acta Ophthalmol (Copenh).* 1993;71:850-852.
36. Sampaolesi R, Casiraghi JF, Geria R. The occurrence of exfoliation syndrome after penetratine keratoplasty: a report of three cases. *Klin Monatsbl Augenheilkd.* 1995;206(suppl 2):8-9. Abstract.
37. Ringvold A. Exfoliation syndrome immunological aspects. *Acta Ophthalmol.* 1988;184(suppl):35-43.
38. Gartaganis SP, Patsoukis NE, Nikolopoulos DK, Georgiou CD. Evidence for oxidative stress in lens epithelial cells in pseudoexfoliation syndrome. *Eye (Lond).* 2007;21(11):1406-1411.
39. Ashton N, Shakib M, Collyer R, Blach R. Electron microscopic study of pseudo-exfoliation of the lens capsule I. Lens capsule and zonular fibers. *Invest Ophthalmol Vis Sci.* 1965;4(2):141-153.
40. Guo S, Gewirtz M, Thaker R, Reed M. Characterizing pseudoexfoliation syndrome through the use of ultrasound biomicroscopy. *J Cataract Refract Surg.* 2006;32(4):614-617.
41. Conway RM, Schlötzer-Schrehardt U, Küchle M, Naumann GO. Pseudoexfoliation syndrome: pathological manifestations of relevance to intraocular surgery. *Clin Exp Ophthalmol.* 2004;32(2):199-210.
42. Sbeity Z, Dorairaj SK, Reddy S, Tello C, Liebmann JM, Ritch R. Ultrasound biomicroscopy of zonular anatomy in clinically unilateral exfoliation syndrome. *Acta Ophthalmol.* 2008;86(5):565-568.
43. Shakib M, Auhton N, Blach R. Electron microscopic study of pseudo-exfoliation of the lens capsule II. Iris and ciliary bodies. *Invest Ophthalmol Vis Sci.* 1965;4(2):154-161.
44. Wali UK, Bialasiewicz AA, Rizvi SG, Al-Belushi H. In vivo morphometry of corneal endothelial cells in pseudoexfoliation keratopathy with glaucoma and cataract. *Ophthalmic Res.* 2009;41(3):175-179.
45. Quiroga L, Lansingh VC, Samudio M, Peña FY, Carter MJ. Characteristics of the corneal endothelium and pseudoexfoliation syndrome in patients with senile cataract. *Clin Exp Ophthalmol.* 2010;38(5):449-455.
46. Kaljurand K, Teesalu P. Exfoliation syndrome as a risk factor for corneal endothelial cell loss in cataract surgery. *Ann Ophthalmol (Skokie).* 2007;39(4):327-333.
47. Amari F, Umihira J, Nohara M, et al. Electron microscopic immunohistochemistry of ocular and extraocular pseudoexfoliative material. *Exp Eye Res.* 1997;65(1):51-56.
48. Bojic L, Ermacora R, Polic S, et al. Pseudoexfoliation syndrome and asymptomatic myocardial dysfunction. *Graefes Arch Clin Exp Opthtalmol.* 2005;243(5):446-449.
49. Mitchell P, Wang JJ, Smith W. Association of pseudoexfoliation syndrome with increased vascular risk. *Am J Ophthalmol.* 1997;124(5):685-687.
50. Linner E, Popovic V, Gottfries CH, Jonsson M, Sjogren M, Wallin A. The exfoliation syndrome in cognitive impairment of cerebrovascular or Alzheimer's type. *Acta Ophthalmol Scand.* 2001;79(3):238-235.
51. Vessani RM, Ritch R, Liebmann JM, Jofe M. Plasma homocysteine is elevated in patients with exfoliation syndrome. *Am J Ophthalmol.* 2003;136(1):41-46.

52. Alfaiate M, Leite E, Mira J, Cunha-Vaz JG. Prevalence and surgical complications of pseudoexfoliation syndrome in Portuguese patients with senile cataract. *J Cataract Refract Surg.* 1996;22:972-976.
53. Guzek JP, Holm M, Cotter JB, et al. Risk factors for intraoperative complications in 100 extracapsular cataract cases. *Ophthalmology.* 1987;94:461-466.
54. Drolsum L, Haaskjold E, Davanger M. Pseudoexfoliation syndrome and extracapsular cataract extraction. *Acta Ophthalmol.* 1993;71:765-770.
55. Drolsum L, Haaskjold E, Sandvig K. Phacoemulsification in eyes with pseudoexfoliation. *J Cataract Refract Surg.* 1998;24:787-792.
56. Goder GJ. Our experiences in planned extracapsular cataract extraction in the exfoliation syndrome. *Acta Ophthalmol.* 1988;184(suppl):126-128.
57. Lumme P, Laatikainen L. Exfoliation syndrome and cataract extraction. *Am J Ophthalmol.* 1993;116:51-55.
58. Naumann GOH. Exfoliation syndrome as a risk factor vitreous loss in extracapsular cataract surgery (preliminary report): the "Erlanger augenblatter-Group." *Acta Ophthalmol.* 1988;184(suppl):129-131.
59. Moreno J, Duch S, Lajra J. Pseudoexfoliation syndrome (clinical factors related to capsular rapture in cataract surgery). *Acta Ophthalmol.* 1993;71:181-184.
60. Zetterstrom C, Olivestedt G, Lundvall A. Exfoliation syndrome and extracaspular cataract extraction with implantation of posterior chamber lens. *Acta Ophthalmol.* 1992;70:85-90.
61. Avramides S, Traiandis P, Sakkias G. Cataract surgery and lens implantation in eyes with exfoliation syndrome. *J Cataract Refract Surg.* 1997;23:583-587.
62. Hovding G. The association between fibrillopathy and posterior capsular/zonular breaks during extracapsular cataract extraction and posterior chamber IOL implantation. *Acta Ophthalmol.* 1988;66:662-666.
63. Chitkara DK, Smerdon DL. Risk factor, complication, and result in extracapsular cataract extraction. *J Cataract Refract Surg.* 1997;23:570-574.
64. Shingleton BJ, Heltzer J, O'Donoghue MW. Outcomes of phacoemulsification in patients with and without pseudoexfoliation syndrome. *J Cataract Refract Surg.* 2003;29:1080-1086.
65. Osher RH, Cionni RJ, Gimbel HV, Crandall AS. Cataract surgery in patients with pseudoexfoliation syndrome. *Eur J Implant Refract Surg.* 1993;5:46-50.
66. Shastri L, Vasavada A. Phacoemulsification in Indian eyes with pseudoexfoliation syndrome. *J Cataract Refract Surg.* 2001;27:1629-1637.
67. Jehan FS, Mamalis N, Crandall AS. Spontaneous late dislocation of intraocular lens within the capsular bag in pseudoexfoliation patients. *Ophthalmology.* 2001;108:1727-1731.
68. Nagashima RJ. Decreased incidence of capsule complications and vitreous loss during phacoemulsification in eyes with pseudoexfoliation syndrome. *J Cataract Refract Surg.* 2007;30:127-131.
69. Chang DF. Prevention of bag-fixated IOL dislocation in pseudoexfoliation. *Ophthalmology.* 2002;109:1951-1952. Letter.
70. Gross JG, Kokame GT, Weinberg DV. In-the-bag intraocular lens dislocation: the Dislocated In-the-Bag Intraocular Lens Study Group. *Am J Ophthalmol.* 2004;137:630-635.
71. Sherme M, Bertelmann E, Rieck P. Late spontaneous in-the-bag intraocular lens and capsular tension ring dislocation in pseudoexfoliation syndrome. *J Cataract Refract Surg.* 2006;32:672-675.
72. Cionni RJ, Osher RH. Management of profound zonular dialysis or weakness with a new endocapsular ring designed for scleral fixation. *J Cataract Refract Surg.* 1998;24:1299-1306.
73. Belovay GW, Varma DK, Ahmed II. Cataract surgery in pseudoexfoliation syndrome. *Curr Opin Ophthalmol.* 2010;21(1):25-34.
74. Shingleton BJ, Crandall AS, Ahmed II. Pseudoexfoliation and the cataract surgeon: preoperative, intraoperative, and postoperative issues related to IOP, cataract, and intraocular lenses. *J Cataract Refract Surg.* 2009;35(6):1101-1120.
75. Drolsum L, Ringvold A, Nicolaissen B. Cataract and glaucoma surgery in pseudoexfoliation syndrome: a review. *Acta Ophthalmol Scand.* 2007;85(8):810-821.
76. Akinci A, Batman C, Zilelioglu O. Phacoemulsification in pseudoexfoliation syndrome. *Ophthalmologica.* 2008;222(2):112-116.
77. Ahmed IIK, Crandall AS. Ab externo fixation of the Cionni modified capsular tension ring. *J Cataract Refract Surg.* 2001;27:977-981.
78. Spinelli D, De Felice GP, Vigasio F, Coggi G. The iris vessels in the exfoliation syndrome: ultrastructural changes. *Exp Eye Res.* 1985;41:449-455.
79. Kaiya T. Observation of blood-aqueous barrier function after posterior chamber intraocular lens implantation. *J Cataract Refract Surg.* 1990;16:320-324.
80. Davison JA. Capsule contraction syndrome. *J Cataract Refract Surg.* 1993;19:582-589.
81. Aldakaf A, Bakir H, Almogahed A, Carstocea B. Evaluation of different surgical techniques in the management of subluxated cataractous lens. *Oftalmologia.* 2007;51(1):80-94.
82. Menkhaus S, Motschmann M, Kuchenbecker J, Behrens-Baumann W. Pseudoexfoliation (PEX) syndrome and intraoperative complications in cataract surgery. *Klin Monbl Augenheilkd.* 2000;216(6):388-392.
83. Nichamin LD. Enlarging the pupil for cataract extraction using flexible nylon iris retractors. *J Cataract Refract Surg.* 1993;19:793-796.
84. Dupps WJ, Oetting TA. Diamond iris retractor configuration for small-pupil extracapsular or intracapsular cataract surgery. *J Cataract Refract Surg.* 2004;30:2473-2475.
85. Venkatesh R, Tan CS, Veena K, Ravindran RD. Severe anterior capsular phimosis following acrylic intraocular lens implantation in a patient with pseudoexfoliation. *Ophthalmic Surg Lasers Imaging.* 2008;39(3):228-229.
86. Ostern AE, Drolsum L. Corneal endothelial cells 6-7 years following cataract surgery in patients with pseudoexfoliation syndrome. *Acta Ophthalmol.* 2010;90(5):408-411
87. Dubois VD, Ainsworth G, Liu CS. Unilateral capsular phimosis with an acrylic IOL and two capsular tension rings in pseudoexfoliation. *Clin Exp Ophthalmol.* 2009;37(6):631-633.
88. Dosso AA, Bonvin ER, Leuenberger PM. Exfoliation syndrome and phacoemulsification. *J Cataract Refract Surg.* 1997;23:122-125.
89. Colin J. Exfoliative syndrome and phacoemulsification. *J Fr Ophthalmol.* 1994;17:465-469.
90. Richter-Mueksch S, Kahraman G, Amon M, Schild-Burggasser G, Schauersberger J, Abela Formanek C. Uveal and capsular biocompatibility after implantation of sharp-edged hydrophilic acrylic, hydrophobic acrylic, and silicone intraocular lenses in eyes with pseudoexfoliation syndrome. *J Cataract Refract Surg.* 2007;33(8):1414-1418.
91. Abela-Formanek C, Amon M, Schauersberger J, et al. Uveal and capsular biocompatibility of 2 foldable acrylic intraocular lenses in patients with uveitis or pseudoexfoliation syndrome: comparison to a control group. *J Cataract Refract Surg.* 2002;28(7):1160-1172.
92. Werner L. Biocompatibility of intraocular lens materials. *Curr Opin Ophthalmol.* 2008;19(1):41-49.
93. Saika S. Relationship between posterior capsule opacification and intraocular lens biocompatibility. *Prog Retin Eye Res.* 2004;23(3):283-305.
94. Yamanaka A, Kazusa R, Takayama S. Cells on the varius kinds of intraocular lens implants. *Eur J Implant Refract Surg.* 1989;1:15-17.
95. Amon M, Menapace R. In vivo documentation of cellular reactions on lens surfaces for assessing the biocompatibility of different intraocular implants. *Eye.* 1994;8:649-656.
96. Wenzel M, Reim M, Heinze M, Bocking A. Cellular invasion on the surface of intraocular lenses. In vivo cytological observation following lens implantation. *Grafes Arch Clin Exp Ophthalmol.* 1988;226:449-454.
97. Amon M, Menapace R. In vivo observation of surface precipitates of 200 consecutive hydrogel intraocular lenses. *Ophthalmologica.* 1992;204:13-18.

98. Ravalico G, Baccara F, Lovisato A, Tognetto D. Postoperative cellular reaction on various intraocular lens materials. *Ophthalmology.* 1997;104:1084-1091.
99. Cunanan M, Tarbaux NM, Knight PM. Surgace properties of intraocular lens material and their influence on in vitro cell adhesion. *J Cataract Refract Surg.* 1991;17:767-773.
100. Wolter JR. Lens implant cytology. *Ophthalmic Surg.* 1982;13:939-942.
101. Fabrizius-Homan DJ, Cooper SL. Competitive absorption of vitronectin with albumin, fibrinogen and fibrinectin on polymeric biomaterials. *J Biomed Mater Res.* 1991;25:953-971.
102. Versura P, Torreggiani A, Cellini M, Caramazza R. Adhesion mechanism of human lens epithelial cell on 4 intraocular lens materials. *J Cataract Refract Surg.* 1999;25:527-533.
103. Hollick EJ, Spalton DJ, Ursell PG, Pande MV. Biocompatibility of poly(methylmethacrylate), silicone and Acrysof intraocular lenses: randomized comparison of the cellular reaction on the anterior lens surface. *J Cataract Refract Surg.* 1998;24:361-366.
104. Hollick EJ, Spalton DJ, Ursell PG. Surface cytology features on intraocular lenses: can increased biocompatibility have disadvantages? *Arch Ophthalmol.* 1999;117:872-878.
105. Linnola RJ, Sund M, Ylonen R, Pihhlajaniemi T. Adhesion of soluble fibronectin, laminin and collagen type IV to intraocular lens materials. *J Cataract Refract Surg.* 1999;25:1486-1491.
106. Ravalico G, Tognetto D, Baccara F. Heparin-surface-modified intraocular lens implantation in eyes with pseudoexfoliation syndrome. *J Cataract Refract Surg.* 1994;20:543-549.
107. Caporossi A, Casperini F, Tosi GM, Balestrazzi A, Stampo M, Tom P. Histology of anterior capsule fibrosis following phacoemulsification. *J Cataract Refract Surg.* 1998;24:1343-1346.
108. Nagamoto T, Hara E. Postoperative membranous proliferation from the anterior capsulotomy margin onto the intraocular lens optic. *J Cataract Refract Surg.* 1995;21:208-211.
109. Wolter JR. Continuous sheet of lens epithelium on an intraocular lens: pathological confirmation of specular microscopy. *J Cataract Refract Surg.* 1993;19:789-792.
110. Gonvers M, Sickenberg M, Van Melle G. Change in capsulorexis size after implantation of three types of intraocular lenses. *J Cataract Refract Surg.* 1997;23:231-238.
111. Kato S, Suzuki T, Hayashi Y, et al. Risk factors for contraction of the anterior capsule opening after cataract surgery. *J Cataract Refract Surg.* 2002;28:109-112.
112. Olivero DK, Furcht LT. Type IV collagen, laminim, and fibronectin promote the adhesion and migration of rabbit lens epithelial cells in vitro. *Invest Ophthalmol Vis Sci.* 1993;34(10):2825-2834.
113. Mullner-Edienbock A, Amon M, Schauersberger J, et al. Cellular reaction on the anterior surface of types of intraocular lenses. *J Cataract Refract Surg.* 2001;27:734-740.
114. Tognetto D, Sanguinetti G, Ravalico G. Tissue reaction to hydrophilic intraocular lenses. *Export Rev Med Dev.* 2005;2:57-60.
115. Tognetto D, Toto L, Ballone E, Ravalico G. Biocompatibility of hydrophilic intraocular lenses. *J Cataract Refract Surg.* 2002;28:644-651.
116. Tognetto D, Toto L, Sanguinetti G, et al. Lens epithelial cell reaction after implantation of different intraocular lens material. Two-year results of a randomized prospective trial. *Ophthalmology.* 2003;110:1935-1941.
117. Werner L, Pandey SK, Escobar-Gomez M, Visessook N, Peng Q, Apple DJ. Anterior capsule opacification: a histopathological study comparing different IOL styles. *Ophthalmology.* 2000;107:463-471.
118. Gallagher SP, Pavilack MA. Risk factors for anterior capsule contraction syndrome with polypropylene or poly(methylmethacrylate) haptics. *J Cataract Refract Surg.* 1999;25:1356-1361.
119. Gross JG, Kokame GT, Weinberg DV. For the Dislocated In-the-Bag Intraocular Lens Study Group. In-the-bag intraocular lens dislocation. *Am J Ophthalmol.* 2004;137:630-635.
120. Wagoner MD, Cox TA, Ariyasu RG Jacobs DS, Karp CL; American Academy of Ophthalmology. Intraocular lens implantation in the absence of capsular support; a report by America Academy of Ophthalmology. *Ophthalmology.* 2003;110:840-853.
121. Basket S, Osher R. Late complications with intraocular lens dislocation after capsulorhexis in pseudoexfoliation syndrome. *J Cataract Refract Surg.* 2002;28:1481-1484.
122. Gimbel HV, Condon GP, Kohen T, Olson RJ, Halkiadakis I. Late in-the-bag intraocular lens dislocation: incidence, prevention and management. *J Cataract Refract Surg.* 2005;31:2193-2204.
123. Balestrazzi A, Tosi GM, Alegente M, et al. Spontaneous in-the-bag intraocular lens luxation into the vitreous cavity: last-stage complication of pseudoexfoliative syndrome after phacoemulsification. *Ophthalmologica.* 2009;223(5):339-342.
124. Davis D, Brubaker J, Espandar L, et al. Late in-the-bag spontaneous intraocular lens dislocation: evaluation of 86 consecutive cases. *Ophthalmology.* 2009;116(4):664-670.
125. Scherer M, Bertelmann E, Rieck P. Late spontaneous in-the-bag intraocular lens and capsular tension ring dislocation in pseudoexfoliation syndrome. *J Cataract Refract Surg.* 2006;32(4):672-675.
126. Hayashi K, Hirata A, Hayashi H. Possible predisposing factors for in-the-bag and out-the-bag intraocular lens dislocation and outcomes of intraocular lens exchange surgery. *Ophthalmolgy.* 2007;114:969-975.
127. Giuliari GP, Cortez MA, Ubiera J. Perfluorocarbon liquid left in vitreous cavità after recovery of dropped nuclei by anterior segment surgeons after cataract surgery. *Can J Ophthalmol.* 2007;42(4):617-619.
128. Arbisser LB, Charles S, Howcroft M, Werner L. Management of vitreous loss and dropped nucleus during cataract surgery. *Ophthalmol Clin North Am.* 2006;19(4):495-506. Review.
129. Kaynak S, Celik L, Kocak N, Oner FH, Kaynak T, Cingil G. Staining of vitreous with triamcinolone acetonide in retained lens surgery with phacofragmentation. *J Cataract Refract Surg.* 2006;32(1):56-59.
130. Misra A, Burton Rl. Incidence of intraoperative complications during phacoemulsication in vitrectomized and nonvitrectomized eyes: prospective study. *J Cataract Refract Surg.* 2005;31(5):1011-1014.
131. Lifshitz T, Levy J. Posterior assisted levitation: long-term follow-up data. *J Cataract Refract Surg.* 2005;31(3):499-502.
132. Lal H, Sethi A, Bageja S, Popli J. Chopstick technique for nucleus removal in an impending dropped nucleus. *J Cataract Refract Surg.* 2004;30(9):1835-1839.
133. Arbisser LB. Managing intraoperative complications in cataract surgery. *Curr Opin Ophthalmol.* 2004;15(1):33-39. Review.
134. Merkur A, Damji KF, Mintsioulis G, et al. Intraocular pressure decrease after phacoemulsification in patients with pseudoexfoliation syndrome. *J Cataract Refract Surg.* 2001;27:528-532.
135. Mamalis N. Exfoliation syndrome: effects of cataract surgery on glaucoma. *J Cataract Refract Surg.* 2008;34(11):1813-1814.
136. Damji KF, Konstas AG, Liebmann JM, et al. Intraocular pressure following phacoemulsification in patients with and without exfoliation syndrome: a 2 year prospective study. *Br J Ophthalmol.* 2006;90(8):1014-1018.
137. Drolsum L. Long-term follow-up after deep sclerectomy in patients with pseudoexfoliative glaucoma. *Acta Ophthalmol Scand.* 2006;84(4):502-506.
138. Reekonen P, Kannisto T, Puustjarvi T, Terasvirta M, Uusitalo M. Deep sclerectomy for the treatment of exfoliation and primary open-angle glaucoma. *Acta Ophthalmol Scand.* 2006;84(4):507-511.
139. Landa G, Pollack A, Rachmiel R, Bukelman A, Marcovich A, Zalish M. Result of combined phacoemulsification and trabeculectomy with mitomicyn-C in pseudoexfoliation versus non-pseudoexfoliation glaucoma. *Graefes Arch Clin Exp Ophthalmol.* 2005;243(12):1236-1240.

5

Phacoemulsification With a Small Pupil

In cataract surgery, good mydriasis is essential for safe surgery. Presently, cataract extraction can be completed with a small pupil, as long as the surgeon takes necessary surgical precautions and uses appropriate technology. Phacoemulsification with a small pupil is one of the most common moderately difficult procedures, with an incidence of approximately 1.5%.

A small pupil is an important risk factor in cataract surgery. Consequently, the surgeon should plan the operation very carefully, taking into consideration all possible situations he or she may encounter, to minimize complications, avoid iris deformation, and overcome obstructions created by the miotic pupil.

Methods used with this type of surgery must attempt good return of pupil function, not causing esthetically poor results or functional problems such as photophobia and diplopia. The postoperative esthetic results of this type of surgery are potentially disturbing for the patient; any surgical alteration of the pupil may have a significant effect on its function with side effects such as iatrogenic glare that can be debilitating.[1]

During the preoperative evaluation of patients with a miotic pupil, the surgeon must always consider potential intraoperative complications, the need to maintain the esthetic appearance of the iris, and that surgery must maintain pupil function.

A small pupil is defined as having a diameter equal to or less than 4 mm; in these cases, the surgeon must enlarge the pupil prior to beginning phacoemulsification.

Preoperative Evaluation

Presence of iridocorneal or iridolenticular synechiae, iris atrophy, fibrosis of the edge, and paralysis of the iris muscle most frequently prevent good mydriasis. Consequently, the eyes must be carefully examined at the slit lamp and any problems noted. The surgeon must ensure that sufficient mydriasis can be achieved following instillation of mydriatic drops (10% phenylephrine and 1% tropicamide, one drop instilled twice 30 minutes prior to observing the dilated eye). The degree of dilation can be classified as excellent, good, sufficient, or poor. Inflamed pupillary membranes, posterior synechiae, and pseudoexfoliation will be evident, and a surgical plan can be formulated. Occasionally, the surgeon may see nonspecific resistance to pupil dilation.

Basically, there are 2 types of small pupils: hyporeactive (functional) and fixed (anatomical).

The hyporeactive pupil is the condition under which the pupil dilates with mydriatics, but dilation is not satisfactory; this is seen in hyperopic patients and in patients treated with chronic antiglaucoma medication.

The fixed pupil (anatomical) is characterized by anatomical alterations of the iris, largely induced by posterior synechiae resulting from uveitis, trauma, neurological diseases, iatrogenic origins (the chronic use of parasympathetic-mimetics for glaucoma), in response to closed-angle glaucoma, anterior or posterior segment procedures, including retinal laser procedures or deterioration associated with old age (atrophy of the iris dilator muscle).

Poor mydriasis can also be seen with other conditions, such as Marfan's syndrome, pseudoexfoliation (atrophy and sclerosis of the iris stroma and the iris sphincter), diabetes, previous ocular surgery (eg, vitrectomy and trabeculectomy), intraoperative trauma, or it can be idiopathic.

The etiology of iris atrophy will determine the choice of pupil dilation technique and can affect the behavior of the iris tissue following expansion maneuvers; the surgical approach differs depending on the reason for the

Buratto L, Brint SF, Caretti L.
Cataract Surgery in Complicated Cases (pp 77-91).

presurgical miosis. Preoperatively, the surgeon decides from the following techniques, individually or combined:

- Pharmacological treatment
- Techniques for pupil expansion
- Iris surgery

Viscoelastic substance (VES) injection into the anterior chamber (AC) also allows the surgeon to achieve better pupillary dilation.

The choice of procedure is also influenced by the capsular extraction technique (extracapsular extraction or phacoemulsification). Phacoemulsification is now the preferred method with poor mydriasis.

Pharmacological Treatment

If the patient has had prolonged use of miotics for the treatment of glaucoma, the drugs should be discontinued for a washout period normally of 10 to 15 days. If necessary, the intraocular pressure can be treated with alternative drugs, as long as there are no contraindications.

Mydriatic drug treatment is essential in an atonic pupil (eg, small globes of hyperopic or extremely elderly patients). Poor mydriasis affects intraoperative management of the nucleus, with a greater incidence of capsular rupture; the capsulorrhexis will often be too small, implanting the intraocular lens (IOL) will be difficult, and phimosis is more frequent.

Optimal dilation of the pupil is achieved by using 3 topical agents: a cycloplegic, a mydriatic, and a nonsteroidal anti-inflammatory drug (NSAID). Mydriasis is commonly achieved using 3 different eye drops: 1% cyclopentolate, 10% phenylephrine, and 1% tropicamide (mydriatics) + 0.03% flurbiprofen (NSAID), all instilled 3 times during the hour immediately preceding surgery.

Presently, the following cycloplegic drugs are available:

- 1% cyclopentolate hydrochloride is the most commonly used cycloplegic. It provides good pupillary dilation in addition to cycloplegia. It is long acting, and the pupil may remain dilated for up to 36 hours after surgery.
- 1% tropicamide hydrochloride can also produce excellent mydriasis though its duration is shorter than cyclopentolate. It does not produce the same degree of cycloplegia.
- 1% atropine sulfate is extremely long acting, and the pupil may be dilated for up to 1 week after surgery. It is not used frequently and should be considered only for cases of chronic uveitis or when there is chronic alteration of the blood-eye barrier (previous surgery [eg, postvitrectomy or diabetes with iris rubeosis]).

The mydriatic drugs are the following:

- 2.5% phenylephrine hydrochloride is the most commonly used mydriatic agent, and when combined with a cycloplegic agent, it produces excellent pupil dilation for surgery.
- 10% phenylephrine hydrochloride is also used when the pupil is not well dilated. The risks may outweigh the benefits associated with the increased concentration, as 10% phenylephrine can induce a significant rise in blood pressure in some individuals and will commonly induce keratopathy, making the surgeon's operating view more difficult.
- Mydriasert[2] is a compact insoluble ophthalmic insert; it is sterile and biocompatible and is used to provide slow release of low doses of 2 mydriatic agents, namely phenylephrine hydrochloride (5.376 mg) and tropicamide (0.280 mg). The use of this insert produces maximum, long-lasting mydriasis in normal cataract cases. Moreover, the combination of the effect of the 2 active ingredients and their synergism allows a reduction in the amount of each agent used, with a lower probability of side effects (possible episodes of accumulation and inflow into the nasal-lacrimal canal associated with repeated instillations, systemic side effects, and individual sensitivity). It is quick and easy to use.[3-6] The main disadvantage is the cost of the product.

In a controlled, randomized, single-blind trial that examined traditional mydriasis (1% tropicamide, 2.5% phenylephrine, 0.1% sodium diclofenac) and mydriasis achieved with slow-release mydriatic drugs prior to cataract surgery, no significant difference in the pupil diameter was observed between the 2 groups.[7]

When NSAIDS are used preoperatively in addition to cycloplegics and mydriatics, they reduce the probability of pupil constricted during the operation. They may be even more useful in the event of prolonged surgery or in eyes with rupture of the blood-ocular barrier. The first NSAIDs approved by the US Food and Drug Administration (FDA) specifically as intraoperative antimiotics were 1% suprofene, 1% and particularly 0.03% sodium flurbiprofen; these inhibit synthesis of prostaglandins by blocking the cyclooxygenase pathway responsible for miosis. Subsequently, 0.4 to 0.5% ketorolac proved to be safe and efficacious in maintaining intraoperative mydriasis.[8-10] Other types of NSAIDs are useful—0.1% nepafenac has greater efficacy in rabbit eyes than flurbiprofen[11] and ketorolac[12] in reducing intraoperative miosis.

Another option is 0.5 mL of 1:1000 preservative-free adrenaline diluted in 10 mL of balanced salt solution (BSS); this is injected at the beginning of surgery, through the side-port incision or added to the infusion bottle (4 IU of 1:1000 adrenaline in 500 cc).[13,14]

Recently, a study[15] on pig eyes was published. The results showed that N-methyl-3,4-dihydroxyphenylalanine (epinephrine) injected into the AC is a more efficacious mydriatic than phenylephrine (at various concentrations) in addition to being safe for the corneal endothelium. Consequently, epinephrine can be used to achieve good mydriasis in ocular surgery.[15]

Surgical Methods to Expand the Pupil

Following presurgical pharmacological dilation, the pupil may still not be large enough to allow safe surgery. Even though there is no such thing as an absolutely safe pupil size, a number of factors affect the confidence of the surgeon: the surgeon's experience, the characteristics of the cataract (some cataracts require a larger pupil diameter than others), the general ocular anatomy, and the condition of the anterior segment. The surgeon would always like to use the simplest, quickest, least invasive, and most financially attractive method for expanding the pupil diameter, meeting the surgical objectives. Moreover, the method used should not affect the choice of anesthesia for that specific patient. In general, if the mydriasis allows creation of an adequate capsulorrhexis, it should be sufficient for the remaining steps of the surgical procedure.

The following methods are used to expand the pupil:

- Techniques that do not specifically alter the iris sphincter
- Techniques that alter the iris sphincter

The first group includes techniques such as viscomydriasis, synechiolysis, and pupil membrane stripping.

Alternatively, if the initial methods are inappropriate or inadequate, the pupil sphincter can be enlarged with a variety of techniques, such as pupil stretching, mini-sphincterotomies, and pupil-expanding devices. These techniques have the common objective of enlarging the pupil to allow surgery to be performed, with the pupil returning to its normal diameter, shape, and function following surgery, with the sphincter modified as little as possible.[16]

Viscomydriasis

For a number of years, injections of VES have been used to achieve intraoperative pupil dilation.[17,18] The product should have a high or a very high molecular weight, be transparent to allow optimal visibility, with no air bubbles and no cleavage lines created with the aqueous humor or the BSS. The VES must not interfere with the capsulorrhexis, hydrodissection, and phacoemulsification. We recommend high molecular weight cohesive products, such as Healon GV or Healon 5 (Abbott Laboratories, Abbott Park, IL). These compounds also have a "soft and permanent spatula" capacity that allows excellent control during capsulorrhexis. When the surgeon depresses the posterior lip of the surgical wound, a cohesive product may escape from the AC and may need to be replaced.

The VES must be injected into the AC in a specific direction because it has a purely mechanical action. The VES is injected toward the iris with the AC closed, causing a peripheral displacement of the central portion of the iris and a corresponding expansion of the pupil (viscomydriasis; Figure 5-1).

Moreover, the VES will maintain space during the capsulorrhexis, and it will counterbalance positive vitreous pressure, reducing the possibility of rhexis escape. It also allows

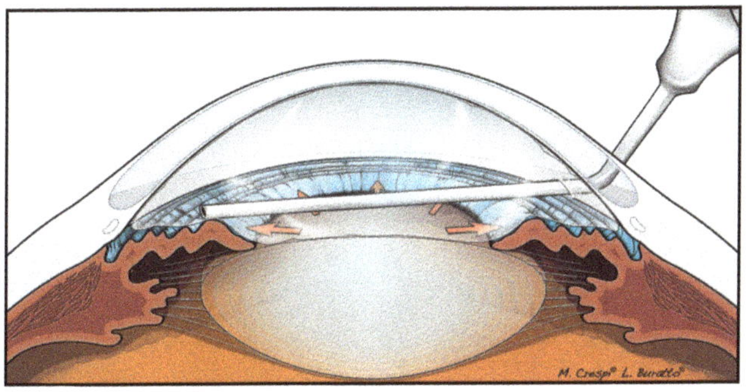

Figure 5-1. Viscomydriasis.

the surgeon to push against the iris tissue when this is lax or when it tends to prolapse in the surgical opening, arresting any bleeding that may originate from the iris vessels.

It should be remembered that the VES will enlarge the pupil only initially; the effect of VES is less in the successive steps of phacoemulsification.

Synechiolysis

Synechiolysis is indicated when a pupil is fixed or anchored by variable amounts of posterior synechiae (adhesions between the iris and the underlying lens capsule) and must always be performed to achieve greater or more uniform mydriasis.

The posterior synechiae are usually limited to the pupillary margin and normally do not extend to the root of the iris. Frequently, by resolving the problem of posterior synechiae, the pupil diameter will be adequate for cataract surgery. Synechiae must be evaluated carefully preoperatively (ie, depth, shape, and extension of the synechiae and duration).

Synechiae must be broken, with the AC filled with VES; a blunt spatula is used (eg, Buratto's button spatula to avoid damaging the anterior capsule; a fine 25-gauge cohesive VES cannula can also be used) inserted through a paracentesis. Excessive traction may cause bleeding (Figure 5-2A). In phacoemulsification, through the tunnel incision, the tip of the spatula should be passed underneath the iris with gentle, fan-shaped tangential movements to the left and to the right; this will detach the synechiae approximately 180 degrees. The residual posterior synechiae can be detached in a similar fashion through a corneal incision created on the opposite side.

The use of VES has made this much easier, as it allows detachment of the synechiae through the pressure created by the VES injected underneath the iris; the synechiae are gently detached and may be facilitated by mechanical action of the injection cannula. During this maneuver, the surgeon must continually inject VES to avoid damaging adjacent structures.

Frequently after synechiolysis, the addition of cohesive VES in the pupil will create a pupil diameter that will allow the surgery to continue.

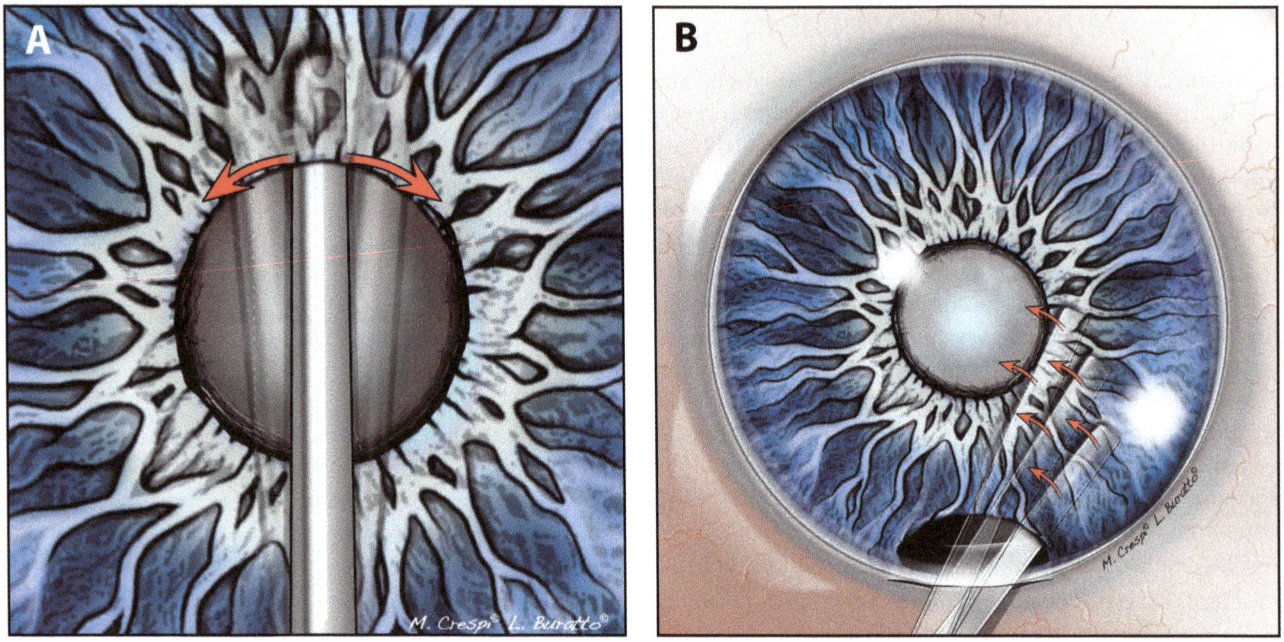

Figure 5-2. Posterior synechiolysis. (A) The problem of the synechiae is resolved with a spatula inserted below the iris and moved in a centripetal direction. (B) The problem of the synechiae is resolved with a spatula inserted below the iris through a peripheral iridectomy.

With a peripheral iridectomy from previous surgery, the surgeon may opt to insert the spatula here and slide it below the iris to detach the posterior synechiae (Figure 5-2B). In the event the adhesions extend toward the iris root, it is advisable to inject small quantities of VES underneath the iris, to enlarge the extension, stretch them, and block any bleeding.

Synechiolysis should not be performed when the capsular bag is partially disinserted or when there are areas of zonular weakness. The additional support, from the posterior synechiae, will provide greater stability to a poorly anchored capsular bag.

At the end of synechiolysis, if the VES has not produced adequate mydriasis, the surgeon will have to directly address the sphincter.

Removal of the Pupil Rim

Sufficient mydriasis can often be achieved simply by removing the fibrous pupillary band using the technique developed by Robert Osher.[19] This technique engages the pupillary fibrous band with forceps (for capsulorrhexis, vitreoretinal surgery, or angled iris forceps), tearing it gently around the circumference. The tearing maneuvers must be slow and delicate to avoid excessive damage of the iris or the more serious iridodialysis. This maneuver is facilitated by a partial sphincterotomy using microscissors initially and repeated if necessary at a different position, allowing a better grip by the forceps (Figure 5-3).

The frequent bleeding is well controlled by injection of a VES; the VES also facilitates good viscomydriasis. The surgeon must check that the result achieved by removing the pupillary fibrosis is sufficient for surgery.

This technique produces limited enlargement of the pupil; however, it can be combined with other dilatation maneuvers.

Pupil Stretching

Pupil stretching was introduced by Miller and Keener[20]; this maneuver is helpful with sclerosis of the pupillary rim. It induces numerous, very fine partial ruptures of the sphincter that induce mydriasis. On some rare occasions, this maneuver will create a deformed pupil postoperatively with consequent esthetic issues.

Many surgeons are often surprised to learn that pupil stretching can be performed under topical anesthesia with or without the addition of intracameral lidocaine[21]; this maneuver has little effect on the total surgical time and involves no additional cost.

This procedure can be performed with 1 of 2 systems: bimanual or monomanual. The most straightforward method is the 2-handed or bimanual pupil stretching. It can be performed with 2 separate push-pull instruments or with special instruments (hooks), designed specifically to stretch the pupil sphincter.[22-24]

A number of hooks are available (Osher iris retractors [Amann Ophthalmic Instruments, Liptingen, Germany] and Graether collar button [Amann Ophthalmic Instruments]). Their common surgical objective is to stretch the pupillary margin with the least possible trauma.

Pupil stretching must be performed under VES protection to maintain AC depth and protect the other structures in the anterior segment. The 2 hooks are introduced into the AC; the pupil is engaged at 2 opposite points; and the surgeon applies peripheral pressure, sufficient to ensure moderate and controlled relaxation of the pupil edge to increase mydriasis.

Repetitive gentle and progressive "push-pull" movements of the instruments are recommended to enlarge the pupillary opening (Figure 5-4). With this, rupture of the sphincter is minimized. Vice versa, rapid stretching with rapid movements may cause serious damage to the sphincter.

The hook should not be large, as it must be inserted through the side-port incision and through the main incision; it is used to stretch the pupil in several different and opposite directions (initially at the 12 and 6 o'clock positions and then at the 3 and 9 o'clock positions). This will result in less pushing toward the iris root, with less trauma and more uniform stretching of the iris in various directions. The Osher hook is commonly used in vertical stretching; this instrument pushes the pupil margin toward the iris root with pressure on the point that lies opposite the entrance incision. A blunt iris hook engages the pupil edge just in front of the incision itself. For the horizontal stretching, the surgeon uses 2 Osher hooks (Duckworth & Kent, Ltd, Baldock, England) positioned at the pupil margin, opposite the first stretching direction. The surgeon can then stretch obliquely and pull the iris in any direction.

The side port is slightly larger than standard to allow easy access and to facilitate the intraocular maneuvers of the instruments. During these maneuvers, a small amount of VES may escape from the AC. The surgeon should replace it immediately to ensure adequate space for the surgical maneuvers, maintain the AC, and protect the capsule from possible trauma.

Several one-handed dilators are available (Beehler [Rhein Medical Inc, St. Petersburg, FL], Keuch [Katena Products Inc, Denville, NJ], Zanini)[25]; inserted through the main incision, these stretch the pupil with a single maneuver (Figure 5-5). These instruments have been designed as a handpiece with a narrow cannula containing several hooks (between 2 and 4), with a fixed hook on its outside edge. The fixed hook engages the pupil edge at the main incision and pulls it toward the edge; light pressure applied to the plunger of the handpiece push the remaining hooks that engage the pupil edge in other positions and stretch it. So, similar to the bimanual dilators, the objective of this maneuver is to engage the edge of the pupil and push it peripherally.

There is greater VES loss with the monomanual dilators compared to bimanual; in our opinion, there are fewer possibilities for adjustment with this technique. When the dilator acts on a single meridian, its action will sometimes be excessively aggressive as it is not possible to distribute the push evenly in several directions.

Pupil stretching almost always achieves a satisfactory degree of mydriasis; there is little bleeding and the maneuvers are usually well controlled, allowing a return to good pupil function and appearance. Good stretching of one meridian with 1 or 2 instruments may be adequate, but it

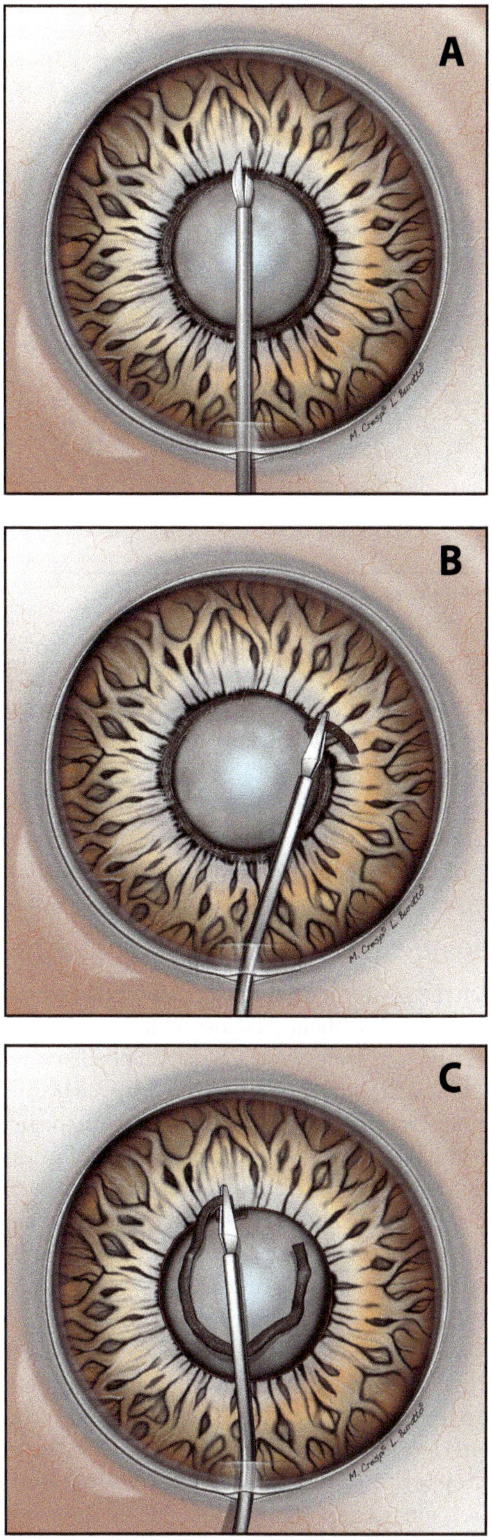

Figure 5-3. Removal of fibrotic pupillary membrane with microscissors and removal of the fibrotic pupil ring with forceps.

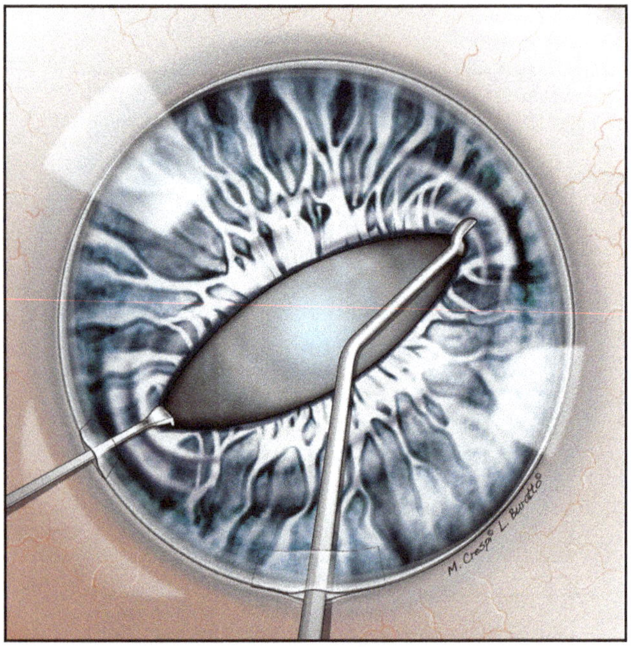

Figure 5-4. Bimanual pupillary stretching.

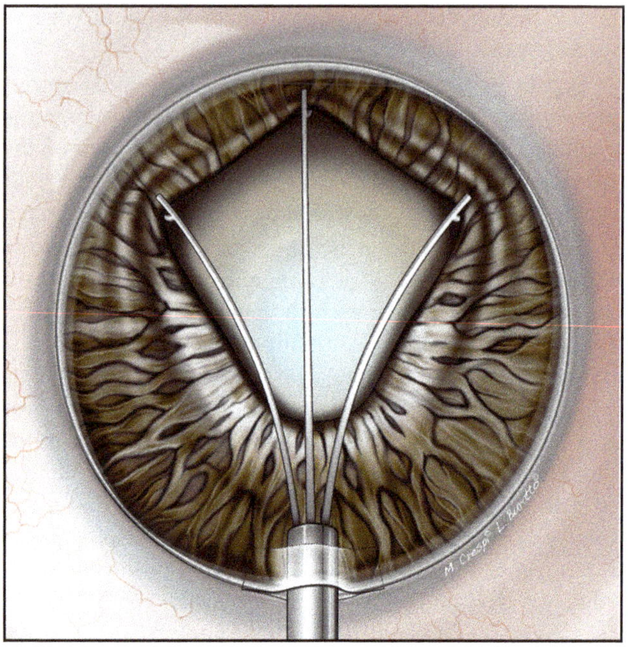

Figure 5-5. Beehler's one-handed pupil dilator.

may be necessary to stretch several meridians. It should be pointed out that contact with the anterior capsule, lesions to the pupil sphincter that are deeper than desired, and bleeding may result from the use of this technique.[26]

However, in the majority of cases, this method is usually safe and rapid. The surgeon must be careful in his or her selection of the appropriate mono- or bimanual surgical instruments.

Sphincterotomy and Sphinterectomy

Sphincterotomy (or partial radial iridotomy) can produce moderate mydriasis without total loss of the pupillary sphincter, preserving satisfactory postoperative pupillary motion and minimal inflammation. Mydriasis is achieved because the sphincter muscle fibers form tight adhesions with the fibers of the adjacent iris stroma. Sphincterotomy is useful in cases in which the sclerosis of the iris tissue is restricted to the central zone, typical of the senile pupil, capsular pseudoexfoliation, postinflammatory miosis, or iatrogenic inflammation resulting from the prolonged use of miotics.

The micro-incisions (mini-sphincterotomies), usually 6 to 8, are created using fine microscissors. Those for vitreoretinal surgery are ideal; the incisions continue radially for approximately two-thirds of the length of the iris sphincter (Figure 5-6). The surgeon starts with the easiest position, opposite the main surgical opening, and uses straight scissors to perform the cuts. He or she continues with the lateral incisions and completes the operation with the more difficult proximal incisions that require angled instruments.[27] The length of the corneal incision through which the scissors are inserted determine the degree of circumferential extension of the incisions. The sphincterotomies proximal to the main incision, particularly when this incision has a limited size, will require additional limbal paracentesis incisions, created with a self-sealing incision at the limbus.

Eight equidistant sphincterotomy cuts are considered ideal; however, it is possible to achieve good pupillary dilation with 6 or even 4 cuts. It should be pointed out that a reduction in the number of cuts should not be associated with an increase in the length of the cut, as this would compromise the sphincter's action.

Space maintenance is achieved with VES injected, repeatedly if necessary, to block any bleeding and to achieve viscomydriasis at the end of the sphincterotomy. Additional stretching maneuvers can also be performed.

If the surgeon creates a greater number of small incisions in the sphincter, the pupil will function normally and the esthetic appearance of the eye will not be compromised.

Partial sphincterotomies involve incomplete separation of the iris sphincter, after having engaged it with a hook and pulled it into a position for cutting with microscissors. In this case, the iris will have an oval shape, depending on the cut of the iris tissue.

Pupil Dilators (Mechanical Retractors or Expanders)

In some cases, even after pupil stretching, mydriasis may still not be sufficient. Iris laxity may risk repeated aspiration of the iris tissue itself by the phaco tip.

In these cases, mechanical hook retractors (dilator hooks) or iris rings may be used. Iris rings are only indicated when the iris tissue is sufficiently elastic to allow distention without causing lacerations (see Chapters 2, 12, and 15).

Surgeons will be most familiar with the De Juan (Alcon Grieshaber, Schffhausen, Switzerland) and the Mackool (Janach, Como, Italy) iris dilator hooks. The De Juan hooks were designed for complex surgery of the posterior segment; however, they can be used in cataract surgery.[28,29] These instruments consist of segments of single nylon or 5-0 Prolene hooks with a curved hook at one end. A small piece of silicone is transfixed in the segment, allowing it to be secured at the required length (Figure 5-7). The technique for positioning the De Juan hooks involves the creation of one or more limbal paracenteses for the insertion of the hooks (see the following sections), under protection of VES. The hooks engage the pupil margin and pull it in a centrifugal direction; the silicone fragment is engaged in the desired position at the limbus. Normally, 4 hooks are positioned, producing a square-shaped iris (Figure 5-8). The position of the limbal paracenteses, and consequently the hooks themselves, are important to ensure the successive surgical steps. These incisions are created at 4 equidistant points, allowing for the main and side incisions. With the square shape created, the iris below lies parallel to the main incision, with a reduced risk of accidentally engaging the iris. For correct pupil stretching, the hook should pull in a direction parallel to the iris plane, and the iris must not be elevated. This can be achieved by creating the incisions as close as possible to the limbus with an appropriate orientation. Once the hooks have been positioned, the surgeon cuts the excess to avoid displacement of the hooks in the event the patient moves his or her eye. The hooks are removed quite easily through the insertion incisions. Occasionally, one of the hooks is dislocated during the surgical maneuvers; however, this situation is easy to correct.

The hooks designed by Richard Mackool[30] are titanium and available in a sterilizable version (Duckworth & Kent Ltd, Hertfordshire, England) and as disposables (Impex, Staten Island, NY).

The technique with the Mackool hooks is similar to the previous one (De Juan); however, as the titanium hooks are supplied protruding a fixed distance, once they have been introduced through a limbal paracentesis, the surgeon must engage them at the pupil margin by pushing them through a counterpositioned opening using a second instrument (Figure 5-9).

Using either of these hooks will create ample adjustable mydriasis. Hooks should be used to create mydriasis that is adequate for the surgical maneuvers yet not excessively large to avoid the risk of a lax pupil postoperatively.

Positioning these hooks is sometimes not easy and may be time consuming. The hooks must be used with caution to prevent iris lacerations during phacoemulsification: they can displace the iris anteriorly, resulting in chafing and mechanical damage during emulsification.[31,32] Damage to the iris can be prevented if the hooks are positioned parallel to the iris plane through small, short peripheral paracenteses (at the limbus and not in clear cornea) or by

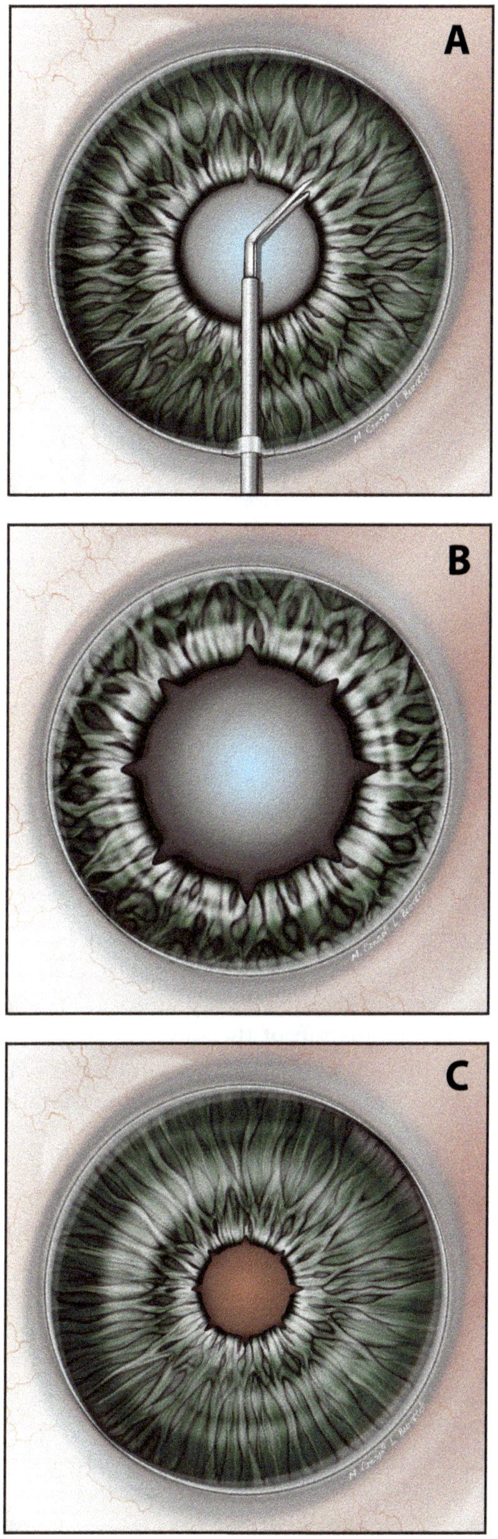

Figure 5-6. Multiple partial sphincterotomies. (A-C) Cuts in the sphincter that are equidistant from each other.

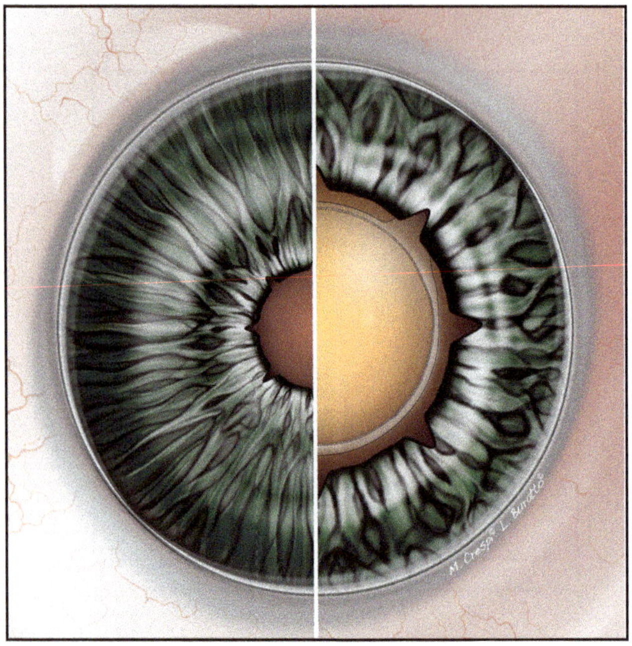

Figure 5-7. Postoperative miosis, secondary to the preservation of the sphincter's function.

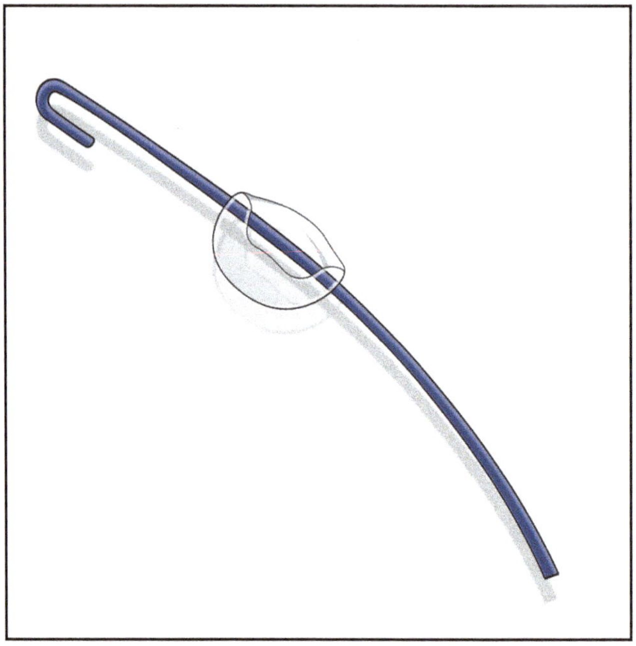

Figure 5-8. Disposable hook to enlarge the pupil.

releasing the hooks following capsulorrhexis and prior to phacoemulsification.[33,34]

As with pupil stretching, gradual enlargement of the pupil is preferred to a rapid and immediate tear. Even though the use of iris hooks can increase operating costs and surgical time, they are ideal for the surgeon who requires a relatively large pupil, and they can be used advantageously when a pupil becomes miotic during surgery.

An alternative use of the hooks is the stabilization of the capsular bag during surgery. The surgeon positions the hooks around the margin of the anterior capsulorrhexis, even though this procedure does not eliminate the problems associated with potential postoperative dislocation of the IOL-capsular bag complex (Figure 5-10).

Recently, Bohm described an irrigating iris retractor for cataract surgery in small pupils. The retractor, a modified irrigation handpiece, consists of 2 standard irrigation ports with a blunt button iris hook at the front. The hook is inserted at the edge of the pupil and pulls the pupil peripherally to allow visualization of residual cortex in the equatorial area of the capsule. The surgeon can then safely clean the capsule with the aspiration handpiece held in his or her other hand.[35]

Pupil expansion rings are another group of instruments designed to enlarge the miotic pupil without damaging the sphincter, creating mydriasis through iris retraction (Figure 5-11). These can be complete or incomplete rings; some are manufactured in polymethylmethacrylate (PMMA), others are silicone or expandable hydrogel (ie, Perfect Pupil, Morcher, Graether, and Siepser; details provided for each option in this section).[36] Surgeons are probably most familiar with the hydrogel ring by Siepser. When dehydrated, it has an irregular oval shape and is easily inserted through a 3-mm opening. Hydrated inside the AC, it expands to form a circle and positions on the pupil edge with the help of a positioning hook. Its feet engage the pupil and expand it. It can be removed through the same tunnel (Figure 5-12).

The Perfect Pupil (Milvella, Savage, MN) is a ring in polyurethane with a central groove and a diameter of 7 mm. The iris is engaged by small wings at the edges of the groove. At one end of this ring, there is an arm that is positioned outside the corneal incision and facilitates the removal. The ring is unfolded at 45 degrees to facilitate the straightforward introduction. An injector is not essential; however, there is one available (Geuder, Heidelberg, Germany).

The maximum pupil diameter obtained with Perfect Pupil was 7.8 mm; the mean pupil diameter following surgery was approximately 1 mm more than preoperatively. No cases of intraoperative iris rupture, bleeding, or capsular ruptures were reported.

The Morcher pupil dilator ring (diameter 7.5 mm; FCI Ophthalmics, Pembroke, MA) is manufactured in PMMA (Figure 5-13). An injector facilitates introduction of this ring. Due to its PMMA structure and its stiffness, many surgeons consider the Morcher to be more difficult to insert through a small incision, compared to the Perfect Pupil. This device has no arms, and this makes the introduction and removal less efficient. The maximum iris width obtained with this type of ring was an average of 5.9 to 6.0 mm. There was a 10% incidence of sphincter rupture.

The Arpa ring (internal diameter of approximately 7 mm; FCI Ophthalmics) is produced in silastic. The

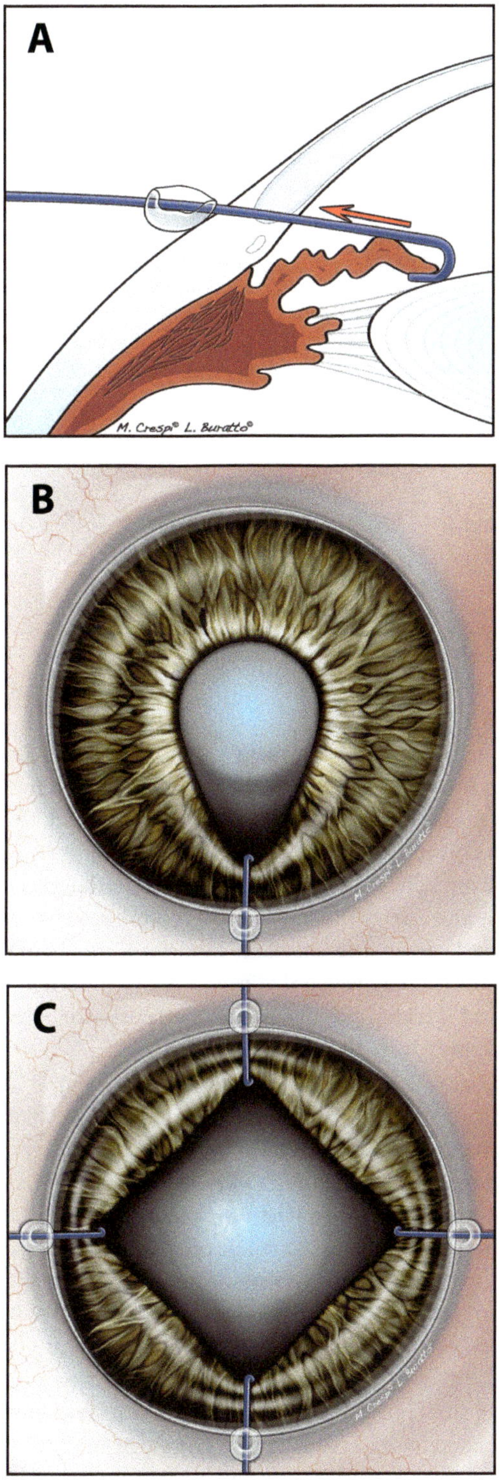

Figure 5-9. Positioning of De Juan iris retractors.

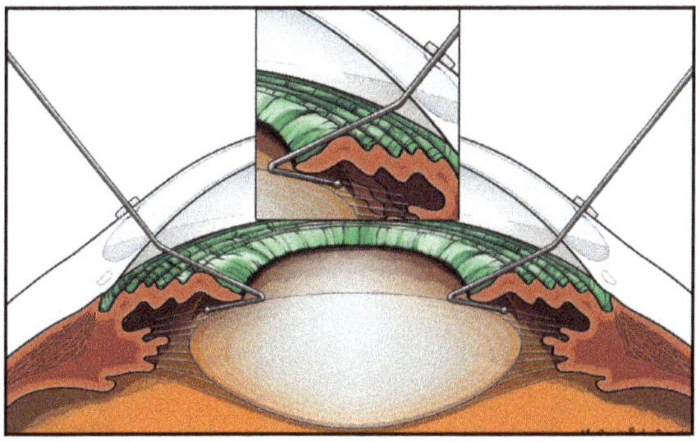

Figure 5-10. Positioning of Mackool iris hooks.

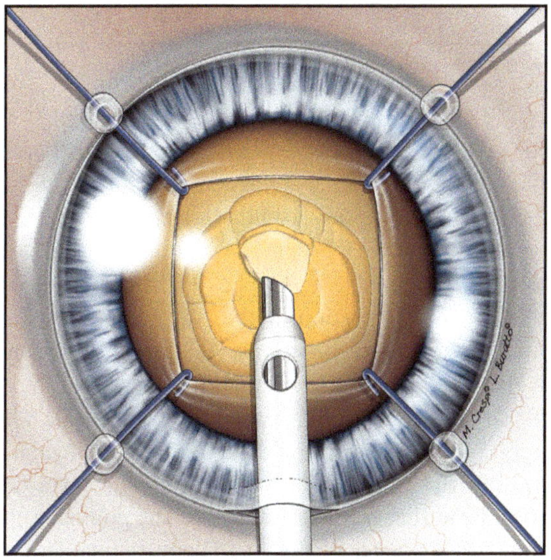

Figure 5-11. Stabilization of the capsulorrhexis with 4 iris hooks during phacoemulsification.

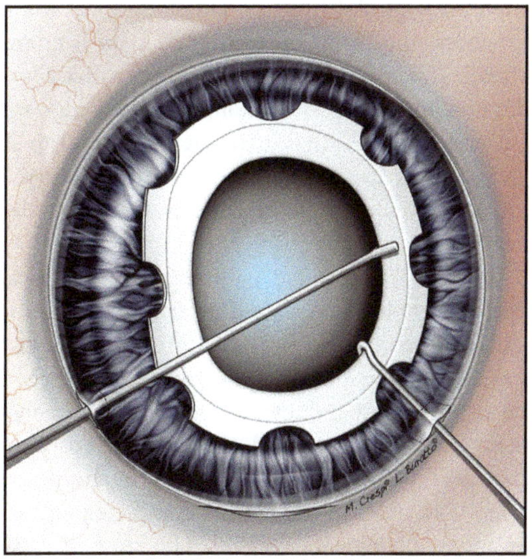

Figure 5-12. Positioning of the iris protection ring and its expansion to dilate the pupil.

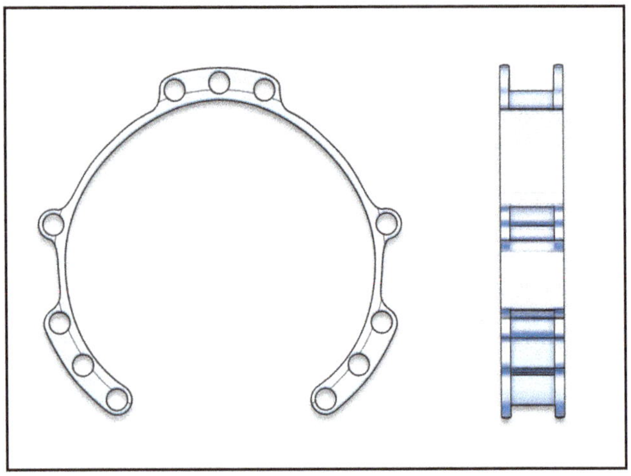

Figure 5-13. Morcher's PMMA pupil expansion ring.

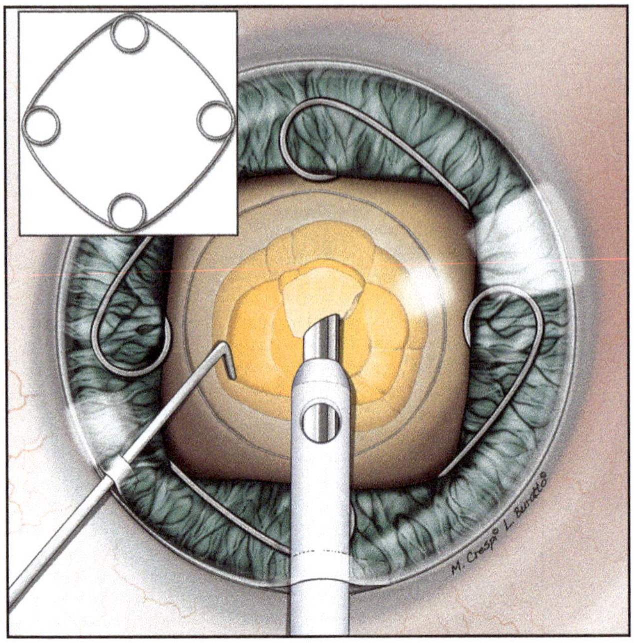

Figure 5-14. Malyugin's pupil expander.

outside edge has a concave shape to engage the pupillary edge of the iris. The ring is introduced into the AC with McPherson forceps (Storz Ophthalmics) through an incision of approximately 2 mm at the limbus.

Recently, incomplete C-shaped PMMA dilating rings were developed. A portion of the ring is not closed; this is where the phaco tip functions. As opposed to complete rings, the incomplete ring will not be engaged.

The Graether 2000 pupil expander system (Eagle Vision, Memphis, TN) is an incomplete ring in soft silicone. The aperture of the ring is 3.75 mm, and this is surmounted by a fine strap that facilitates access to the pupillary space. The internal diameter of the ring is approximately 7 mm, and the external circumference is grooved to engage the iris. This device is inserted with an iris retractor to hold the iris sphincter at the internal edge of the incision and is preloaded on a special inserter. Differing from the previous 2 devices, the insertion technique is of fundamental importance; this ring lacks any real rigidity that allows the introduction and progression along the pupil edge without the assistance of additional instruments. The strap should be removed prior to commencing the capsulotomy. Small tears in the sphincter have been observed when this ring has been used.

The advantage associated with expansion rings is that they produce stable and uniform mydriasis throughout the procedure. However, the introduction and removal processes are often long and difficult, particularly if the AC is shallow and the pupil diameter is less than 4 mm, there may be contact with the corneal endothelium or the capsule. The entire surgery will be slower and there is additional risk associated with a device remaining completely intraocular for the entire duration of surgery. The rings increase the cost of surgery; however, they produce a pupil of maximum dilatation with less tendency to sphincter rupture, given that the rings do not create pressure points on the pupillary margin. These rings will wrap around the sphincter for approximately 300 degrees. Moreover, the surgeon must pay maximum attention when the device is removed from the eye to avoid damaging the pupillary edge. These instruments can be cumbersome, time is required to position them correctly, and they can interfere with the phacoemulsification. These instruments have been improved over the years, and currently, they are used more frequently than in the past, given the excellent mydriasis they can produce. Previously there was only limited use of the rings, and they enjoyed greater popularity in the posterior segment for which they were designed.

Recently, Malyugin presented a new pupil expander (Microsurgical Technology, Redmond, WA)[37-39]; the use of this device also appears to be easier and faster compared to iris hooks and other pupil expansion rings. This development would appear to be an excellent and much safer strategy for dealing with a small pupil, particularly in eyes with intraoperative floppy iris syndrome. This device is roughly rectangular in shape; it is a one-piece device of 5-0 Prolene. There are 4 circular buttonholes positioned at equidistant points; these engage the pupil edge and expand the pupil to 6 mm (Figure 5-14). Its main advantage is low trauma associated with engaging the iris edge and the excellent control of the pupil stretching. It is manufactured in 2 sizes with 2 different internal diameters (6.2 or 7 mm). There is a greater tendency to use the smaller ring in surgery; the 6.2-mm ring is usually sufficient. Surgeons normally use the 7-mm ring only in special cases (eg, when he or she has to implant an unusually large IOL). The newest disposable ring is inserted and removed with an injector through a 2.2-mm corneal incision. This ring is associated with a number of advantages: it is easy to implant and induces very little trauma as the ring is free from sharp edges and the stretching pressure is evenly distributed over the pupil edge; the stretching is not excessive, something that occurs frequently when the iris hooks are positioned incorrectly.

This device exerts uniform generalized pressure on the iris sphincter, preventing structural damage, like the other rings described and completely opposite to iris hooks. This is particularly useful in patients in which cutting the iris tissue should be avoided (eg, iris rubeosis, chronic iritis, or systemic coagulopathies). Following surgery, the appearance of the majority of pupils is more or less the same as preoperatively, and functional activity is preserved. The iris rim is fixed securely by the loops of the ring, creating a large surgical working area. The risk of engaging the iris is greatly reduced. Compared to other devices, additional corneal incisions are not necessary. The device is inserted through the main incision using an injector; this reduces surgical trauma, the risk of contamination, and postoperative inflammation. The surgeon also avoids the risk of iris prolapse, a real possibility when traditional iris hooks are used to create a square-shaped pupil.

This is particularly true in the case of excessively large paracenteses and in the presence of atonic and atrophic irises (intraoperative floppy iris syndrome).

Regardless of the method used to expand the pupil, at the end of surgery the pupil must be constricted to avoid it being captured by part of the optic, adhering to the capsule, or other deformities.

Iris Surgery

Iris surgery provides other alternatives. In addition to sphincterotomy, sphincterectomy, and removal of the pupil rim, options available include iridectomy and the placement of iris sutures.

All of these methods have specific indications (eg, in iris atrophy); however, they are associated with the disadvantages of bleeding, postoperative inflammation, iris traction, and permanent iris sutures.

Iridectomy

An iridectomy can produce a pupil opening when the iris tissue is excessively atrophic and sclerotic and it is the only option for mydriasis. This situation may follow an acute attack of glaucoma or with chronic inflammation of the iris.

The iridectomy may be performed in a proximal or distal position. With the proximal position, the radial cut progresses as far as the pupil edge with microscissors, starting from the previously made peripheral iridectomy or from a new peripheral iridectomy (Figures 5-15A and 5-15B). Iridectomies are greatly facilitated by VES initially injected into the AC to create and maintain space and then to separate the cut sections of the iris.

The technique can be combined with others in an attempt to achieve better mydriasis. In addition to the iridectomy, the surgeon can create a series of partial sphincterotomies or extend the iris incision at the base.

If the iridectomy is created distally from the surgical access, it simply involves cutting the iris radially from the pupil opening and proceeding toward the iris base for a length needed to achieve the desired mydriasis.[40] This technique is indicated when the surgeon wishes to sculpt the nucleus; thus, he or she works in a position opposite the surgical access. This type of iridectomy is rarely used because of the difficulty of suturing. Whenever an iridectomy is required, the surgeon must pay maximum attention to avoid engaging the fragmented iris tissue in the phaco tip. Also, abundant VES is required to stop the bleeding when the iris tissue is cut.

At the end of surgery, iris plastic surgery techniques are used that involve the placing of one or two 10-0 Prolene sutures (Figure 5-15C).

Iris Sutures for Pupil Expansion

These sutures are rarely used to obtain mydriasis with a triangular, square, or hexagonal shape, depending on the number of sutures used. This procedure is part of vitreoretinal surgery but rarely used in phacoemulsification.[41]

The techniques have in common a suture passed from the anterior to the posterior chamber, transfixed through the pupil, and pulled radially toward the outside and tied.

The risk of damage to the anterior capsule is high during the suture pass; moreover, the suture can actually split the iris tissue (particularly if it is sclerotic), damaging it permanently with irregularity of shape and motion, requiring the surgeon to apply sutures. Bleeding may also occur from the ciliary body or loss of VES from overly large paracentesis sites

Steps of the Operation

Expansion of the pupil as described allows the surgeon to proceed with the surgery (extracapsular cataract extraction [ECCE] or phacoemulsification).

If an ECCE is required, it should be remembered that this is associated with significant risk with small pupils. It requires a large anterior capsulotomy, difficult with existing miosis. The pupil dilation techniques required will be more invasive as maximum pupillary dilation is essential to allow the nucleus to be expressed through the pupil. This is associated with risk of vitreous loss or a deep laceration of the sphincter; serious damage is induced to the iris, often requiring sutures.

Phacoemulsification is really preferred for this type of eye. However, it should be remembered that miosis may be present preoperatively and may also occur intraoperatively because the iris is being touched, because of repeated instability of the AC, or because of excessive duration of surgery. In any case, pure preservative-free adrenaline is recommended, used intracameral or diluted in the infusion liquid, as previously mentioned.

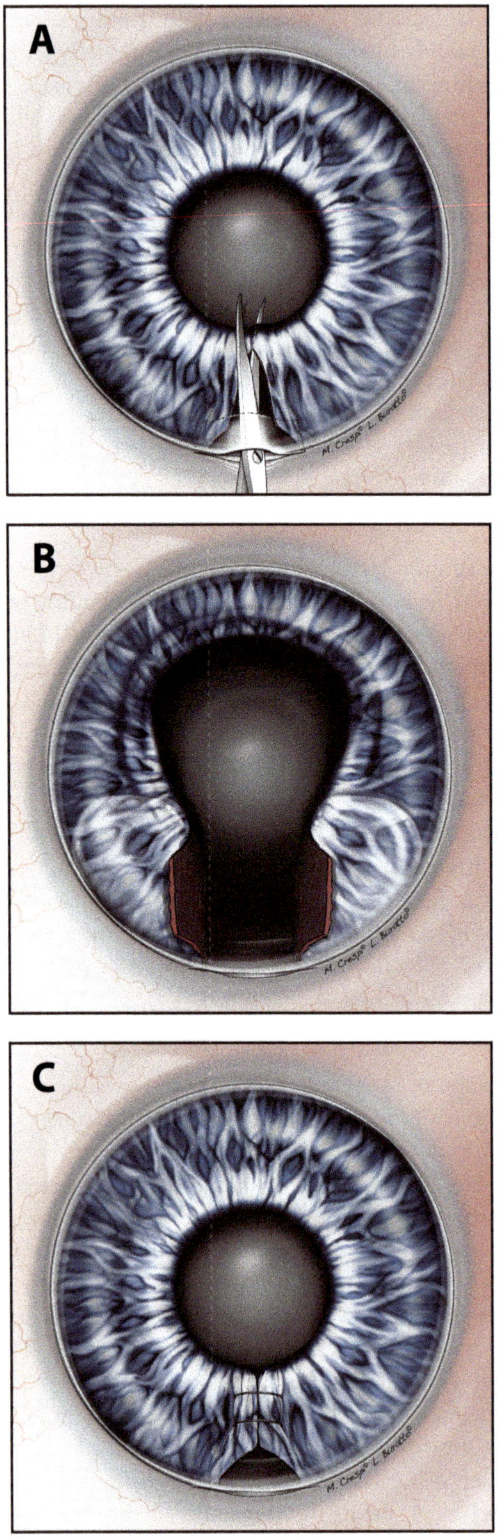

Figure 5-15. (A) Radial iris incision with scissors. (B) Exposure of the lens plane. (C) Iris suture.

Given that mydriasis obtained with the dilation techniques described will never reach maximum size, during surgery the surgeon must always prepare for a certain degree of pupil constriction with increased mobility of the iris diaphragm caused by the inevitable loss of tension and stability.

Corneal Incisions

The corneal tunnel created is slightly longer to reduce the risk of iris prolapse. The paracentesis incisions should likewise be small and carefully placed.

Anterior Capsulotomy

The continuous circular capsulotomy is a routine procedure if the pupil expansion allows a diameter of 5 mm. It can be extended beyond the pupil opening if the surgeon carefully tears the capsular flap that extends underneath the iris.

To improve visualization of the rhexis, the surgeon can retract the iris edge into the desired area with an iris hook ("push and pull," Osher hooks, etc) introduced through the sideport incision.

Hydrodissection

If the size of the pupil is sufficient for visualization of the edge of the capsulorrhexis, the maneuver should not pose a problem. If not, an irrigation cannula can be introduced blindly underneath the anterior capsule, based on the distance from the iris surface and from the anterior cortex. If the procedure is unsuccessful, it can be repeated in other areas until the fluid wave is seen. The injection of liquid is continued even after the wave has passed the microscope view, reduced by miosis, to allow complete cleavage of the cortex; the surgeon should decompress the bag to allow any excess liquid to escape and to increase the effect of the separation.

A combination of hydrodelineation and hydrodissection is very useful when a miotic pupil limits visibility; it will facilitate the successive maneuvers to remove the lens fragments (greater safety with an epinuclear bowl).

Phacoemulsification

For a number of years, phacoemulsification has been the preferred method with poor mydriasis. Technological progress and improvements in surgical technique have resulted in considerable benefits for surgeon and patient outcomes. Microcoaxial phacoemulsification considerably reduces the risk of intraoperative complications. The possibility of operating through incisions measuring just 2 to 2.2 mm with a 21-gauge phaco tip adds considerable precision (with greater movement of the small instruments) during all steps of the operation, with greater safety compared to the traditional coaxial system. Also, the stability of the AC is better, and the surgeon can achieve a reduction of intraocular flow (reducing the parameters of infusion and aspiration) and lower intraocular turbulence with less iris stimulation inducing miosis.

In our opinion, the techniques with minimal horizontal excursion (eg, "chop" or "quick chop") have undeniable advantages. The surgeon uses the instruments at the center of the pupil allowing constant visualization of the phaco tip and associated with few risks of engaging the structures of the anterior segment.

The phaco tip and the chopper are placed into the center of the nucleus, avoiding excessive movements underneath the rhexis, as has been described.

This technique is indicated for nuclei of moderate or high density. The nucleus is fragmented into small pieces that can be easily removed through a small pupil; very large, hard nuclei can therefore be extracted through a small capsulorrhexis.

When the pupil is very small and the surgeon opts for a grooving technique, difficulties may arise. This technique is indicated for nuclei of moderate or minimal density. A central groove is created, the length limited by the visualization. It should be as deep as possible to allow easy fracture of the nucleus into 2 halves. The groove should be created with the aspiration at zero and with a reduced flow rate to avoid engaging the iris; the surgeon can then create a deep groove with no risk of breaking the posterior chamber. Once the first fracture has been completed, the nucleus is rotated and split into 4 or 6 pieces depending on how dense it is. The nuclear fragments can be aspirated in the center of the pupil, inside the capsular bag in a position avoiding adjoining structures.

Irrigation/Aspiration

The greatest difficulty of this step is the poor visualization of the peripheral cortex. With coaxial irrigation/aspiration technique, the peripheral areas of the bag can be exposed with the use of a number of iris hooks attached to the pupil edge and pulling toward the base. The bimanual irrigation/aspiration technique may prove useful as it allows greater expansion of the bag and displacement of the pupil edge with the infusion cannula.

Insertion of the Intraocular Lens

Here, the greatest difficulties are poor visualization of the capsular edge, interfering with the safety of inserting a lens in the capsular bag. The success is facilitated by the exact inclination during the lens insertion, which must be downward until the optic enters the capsular opening. A tilting movement parallel to the iris plane facilitates the introduction.

If an IOL with 2 haptics is used, the second haptic is positioned in the bag by dialing with a Sinskey hook (Asico, Westmont, IL) on the surface of the optic. The certainty of position should be checked by retracting the iris with push-pull hooks to ensure the entire lens is in the bag

Conclusion

Cataract surgery with small pupils is one of the most difficult situations for the surgeon, requiring special attention, experience, and great skill to avoid serious complications. The combination of microcoaxial phacoemulsification, continuous circular capsulotomy, and techniques of nucleofracture will minimize complications and safeguard the shape and function of the pupil. This is made possible by the use of pupil expansion techniques that cause less damage to the integrity of the iris.

Preoperative presence of miosis is evaluated to determine its etiology, as the small pupil inhibits successive surgical maneuvers. Miosis caused by posterior synechiae or fibrosis of the pupil margin can be resolved by mechanical dilation early in the operation; miosis caused by structural deficiencies of the iris (atonic) that occasionally appear during surgery must be addressed with permanent systems for dilation (hooks and/or expansion rings).

It should be pointed out that only pupils with a diameter of less than 4 mm should require artificial expansion.

The techniques of pupil dilation have consequences, proportionate to the aggressiveness of the maneuvers. The surgeon must be familiar with these and be able to manage them: pupil deformation, loss of some or all of the sphincter function (particularly in cases that require iris sutures), bleeding, breaks in the blood-ocular barrier, inflammation possibly inducing cystoid macular edema, an increase in the frequency of posterior capsule opacity and postoperative infections, formation of posterior synechiae, fibrosis, and the retraction of the anterior capsule.

Thoughtful drug therapy is recommended, both preoperatively (suspension of miotic drugs 10 to 15 days prior to surgery, NSAID eyedrops and agents to stabilize the mydriasis), intraoperatively (adrenaline and antibiotics in the infusion), and finally, postoperatively (anti-inflammatory steroid and antibiotic eye drops for up to 3 weeks after surgery, possibly in combination with mydriatic, cycloplegic, and NSAID eyedrops for a long period following the suspension of steroids).

References

1. Masket S. Relationship between postoperative pupil size and disability glare. *J Cataract Refract Surg.* 1992;18(5):506-507.

2. Morgado G, Barros P, Martins J, Lima A, Martins N. Comparative study of mydriasis in cataract surgery: topical versus Mydriasert versus intracameral mydriasis in cataract surgery. *Eur J Ophthalmol.* 2010;20(6):989-993.
3. Korobelnik JF, Tavera C, Renaud-Rougier MB, El Meski S, Colin J. The Mydriasert insert: an alternative to eye drops for preangiographic mydriasis. *J Fr Ophthalmol.* 2004;27(8):897-902.
4. Levet L, Touzeau O, Scheer S, Borderie V, Laroche L. A study of pupil dilation using the Mydriasert ophthalmic insert. *J Fr Ophtalmol.* 2004;27(10):1099-1108.
5. Caruba T, Couffon-Partant C, Oliary J, Tadayoni R, Limelette N, Gaudric A. Efficacy and efficiency of preoperative mydriasis: drops versus ocular insert. *J Fr Ophtalmol.* 2006;29(7):789-795.
6. Mouly S, Mahé I, Haouchine B, et al. Pharmacodynamics of a new ophthalmic mydriatic insert in healthy volunteers: potential alternative as drug delivery system prior to cataract surgery. *Basic Clin Pharmacol Toxicol.* 2006;98(6):547-554.
7. Dubois V, Wittles N, Lamont M, Madge S, Luck J. Randomised controlled single-blind study of conventional versus depot mydriatic drug delivery prior to cataract surgery. *BMC Ophthalmol.* 2006;6:36.
8. Solomon KD, Turkalj JW, Whiteside SB, Stewart JA, Apple DJ. Topical 0.5% ketorolac vs 0.03% flurbiprofen for inhibition of miosis during cataract surgery. *Arch Ophthalmol.* 1997;115:1119-1122.
9. Stewart R, Grosserode R, Cheetham JK, Rosenthal A. Efficacy and safety profile of ketorolac 0.5% ophthalmic solution in the prevention of surgically induced miosis during cataract surgery. *Clin Ther.* 1999;21:72-732.
10. Donnenfeld ED, Perry HD, Wittpenn JR, Solomon R, Nattis A, Chou T. Preoperative ketorolac tromethamine 0.4% in phacoemulsification outcomes: pharmacokinetic-response curve. *J Cataract Refract Surg.* 2006;32(9):1474-1482.
11. Yoon MK, Naseri A, Porco T, McLeod SD. Nepafenac-assisted mydriasis in a rabbit model. *J Cataract Refract Surg.* 2010;36(10):1779-1782.
12. McCulley JP. Ketorolac versus nepafenac in cataract surgery. *J Cataract Refract Surg.* 2008;34(3):345-346; author reply, 346.
13. Liou SW, Chen CC. Maintenance of mydriasis with one bolus of epinephrine injection during phacoemulsification. *J Ocul Pharmacol Ther.* 2001;17(3):249-253.
14. Lundberg B, Behndig A. Intracameral mydriatics in phacoemulsification cataract surgery. *J Cataract Refract Surg.* 2003;29(12):2366-2371.
15. Lundberg B, Behndig A. The mydriatic effect of intracameral epinine hydrochloride. *Invest Ophthalmol Vis Sci.* 2009;50(11):5336-5338.
16. Akman A, Yilmaz G, Oto S, Akova YA. Comparison of various pupil dilatation methods for phacoemulsification in eyes with a small pupil secondary to pseudoexfoliation. *Ophthalmology.* 2004;111(9):1693-1698.
17. Tognetto D, Cecchini P, Ravalico G. Survey of ophthalmic viscosurgical devices. *Curr Opin Ophthalmol.* 2004;15(1):29-32.
18. Dick HB, Krummenauer F, Augustin AJ, Pakula T, Pfeiffer N. Healon 5 viscoadaptive formulation: comparison to Healon and Healon GV. *J Cataract Refract Surg.* 2001;27(2):320-326.
19. Osher RH. Pupillary membranectomy. *Video Journal of Cataract and Refractive Surgery.* 1991;7(7).
20. Miller KM, Keener GT Jr. Stretch pupilloplasty for small pupil phacoemulsification. Am J Ophthalmol. 1994;117:107-108. Letter.
21. O'Brien PD, Fitzpatrick P, Power W. Patient pain during stretching of small pupils in phacoemulsification performed using topical anesthesia. *J Cataract Refract Surg.* 2005;31(9):1760-1763.
22. Shepherd DM. The pupil stretch technique for miotic pupils in cataract surgery. *Ophthalmic Surg.* 1993;24(12):851-852.
23. Osher RH. Pupil stretch technique. *J Cataract Refract Surg.* 2007;33(3):362; author reply, 362.
24. Dinsmore SC. Modified stretch technique for small pupil phacoemulsification with topical anesthesia. *J Cataract Refract Surg.* 1996;22(1):27-30.
25. Barboni P, Zanini M, Rossi A, Savini G. Monomanual pupil stretcher. *Ophthalmic Surg Lasers.* 1998;29(9):772-773.
26. Fine IH. Pupilloplasty for small pupil phacoemulsification. *J Cataract Refract Surg.* 1994;20(2):192-196.
27. Shingleton BJ, Campbell CA, O'Donoghue MW. Effects of pupil stretch technique during phacoemulsification on postoperative vision, intraocular pressure, and inflammation. *J Cataract Refract Surg.* 2006;32(7):1142-1145.
28. de Juan E Jr, Hickingbotham D. Flexible iris retractor. *Am J Ophthalmol.* 1991;111(6):776-777.
29. Sethi HS, Sinha A, Pal N, Saxena R. Modified flexible iris retractor to retract superior iris and support inferior capsule in eyes with iris coloboma and inferior zonular deficiency. *J Cataract Refract Surg.* 2006;32(5):715-716.
30. Mackool RJ. Small pupil enlargement during cataract extraction. A new method. *J Cataract Refract Surg.* 1992;18(5):523-526.
31. Tognetto D, Agolini G, Grandi G, Ravalico G. Iris alteration using mechanical iris retractors. *J Cataract Refract Surg.* 2001;27(10):1703-1705.
32. Birchall W, Spencer AF. Misalignment of flexible iris hook retractors for small pupil cataract surgery: effects on pupil circumference. *J Cataract Refract Surg.* 2001;27(1):20-24.
33. Masket S. Avoiding complications associated with iris retractor use in small pupil cataract extraction. *J Cataract Refract Surg.* 1996;22(2):168-171.
34. Nichamin LD. Enlarging the pupil for cataract extraction using flexible nylon iris retractors. *J Cataract Refract Surg.* 1993;19(6):793-796.
35. Böhm P, Horvath J, Zahorcova M. Irrigating iris retractor for complicated cataract surgery. *J Cataract Refract Surg.* 2009;35(3):419-421.
36. Goldman JM, Karp CL. Adjunct devices for managing challenging cases in cataract surgery: capsular staining and ophthalmic viscosurgical devices. *Curr Opin Ophthalmol.* 2007;18(1):52-57.
37. Malyugin B. Small pupil phaco surgery: a new technique. *Ann Ophthalmol.* 2007;39(3):185-193.
38. Chang DF. Use of Malyugin pupil expansion device for intraoperative floppy-iris syndrome: results in 30 consecutive cases. J *Cataract Refract Surg.* 2008;34(5):835-841.
39. Agarwal A, Malyugin B, Kumar DA, Jacob S, Agarwal A, Laks L. Modified Malyugin ring iris expansion technique in small-pupil cataract surgery with posterior capsule defect. J *Cataract Refract Surg.* 2008;34(5):724-726.
40. Masket S. Preplaced inferior iris suture method for small pupil phacoemulsification. *J Cataract Refract Surg.* 1992;18(5):518-522.
41. Freitas LL, Casanova FH, Bonomo PP. Small pupil phacoemulsification using iris sutures: a new method? *Ophthalmic Surg Lasers Imaging.* 2004;35(5):434-437.

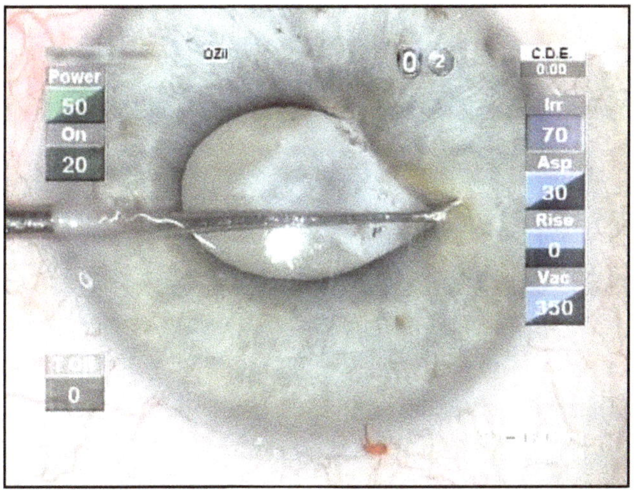

D-1. Hard/mature cataract and small pupil with posterior synechias and fibrotic capsule.

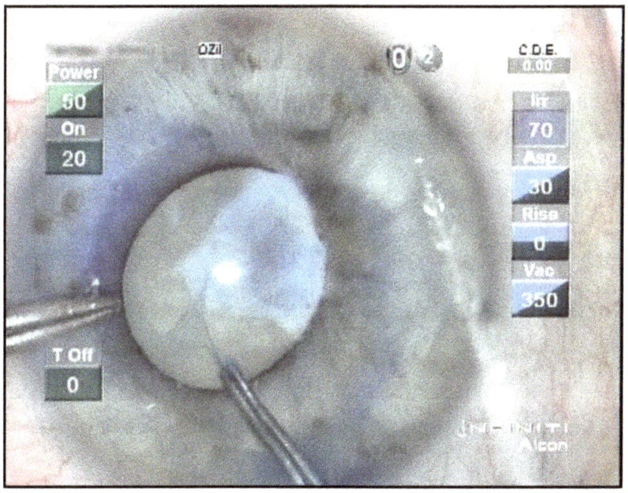

D-2. Staining with trypan blue and anterior capsulotomy.

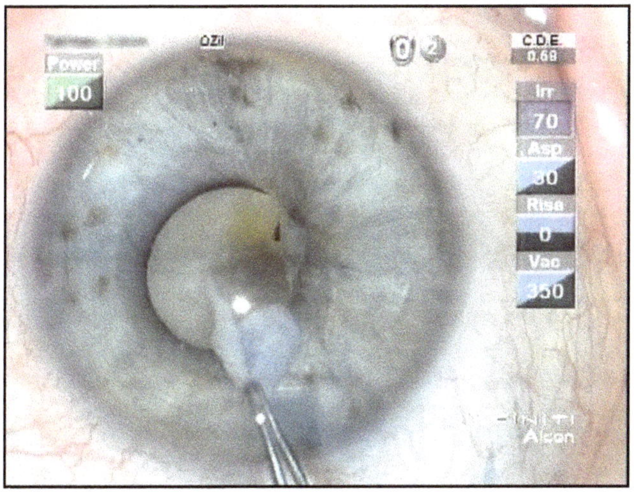

D-3. Removal of the fibrotic capsule.

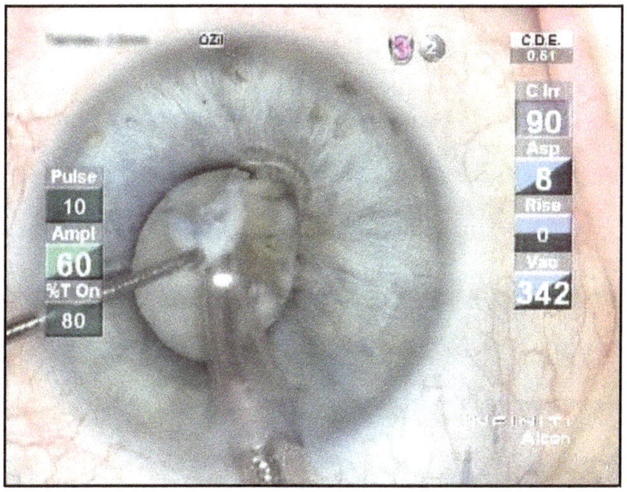

D-4. Phacoemulsification follows; the posterior capsule is opaque and disinserted.

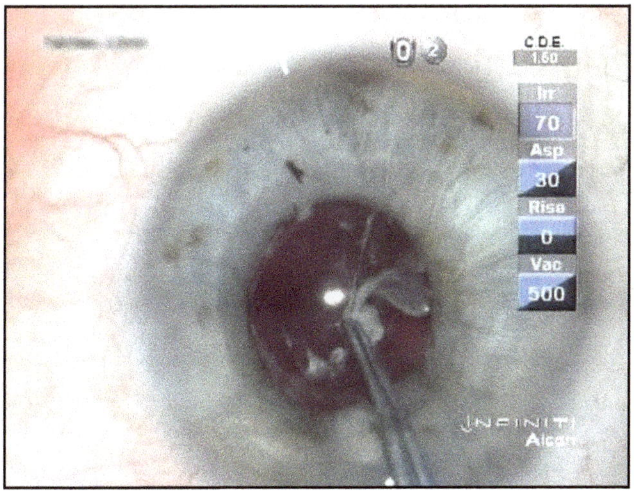

D-5. The entire capsule is then removed.

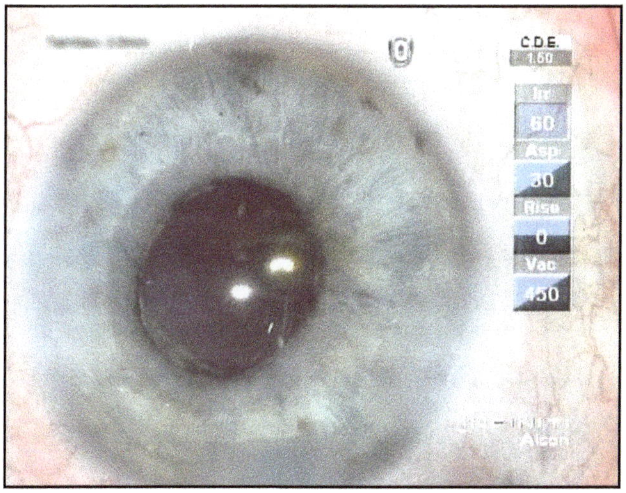

D-6. Once the intracapsular removal of the cataract has been performed through a 2.75-mm incision, the surgeon will perform a secondary implant.

6

Cataract Surgery in Age-Related Macular Degeneration

Cataract and age-related macular degeneration (AMD) are 2 very common causes of reduced visual acuity. Worldwide, cataract is the largest cause of blindness in the world, totaling 17.6 million cases (approximately 48%).[1] AMD is the most frequent cause of blindness in the over-65 adult population in Western countries (Table 6-1).[2,3] Given that both conditions are age related, many cataract patients also show signs of AMD. It is still not clear whether there is a direct connection between the 2 conditions.[4-7]

In view of the frequency of these 2 conditions, when performing cataract surgery in an elderly patient, the surgeon also has to consider AMD.

The literature evaluates whether cataract surgery (the most frequent surgery worldwide) may cause progression of non-neovascular AMD[8-12]; this topic is of great interest to ophthalmologists, leading to scientific studies (eg, case series, epidemiological studies, and autopsy studies).

Forms of Age-Related Macular Degeneration

There are 2 forms of AMD, as defined by the Beaver Dam Eye Study[13]—early and late.

Early AMD is defined as the presence of drusen, the degeneration of retinal pigment epithelium (RPE), or an increase in macular pigment. This form is associated with minimal reduction in visual acuity (Figure 6-1).

Late AMD is defined as the presence of geographical atrophy (dry or nonexudative form) and/or neovascularization (wet or exudative form) that may be choroidal (choroidal neovascularization [CNV]; Figure 6-2) or, less frequently, retinal (retinal angiomatous proliferation). The atrophic form is more frequent, with a prevalence that can reach 90%; the exudative form is more uncommon (10% to 15%) but more important in blindness associated with AMD.

All studies indicate that the prevalence and incidence of all forms of AMD increase with age.[13-24] In addition to the age factor and an important genetic component, there are a number of different risk factors associated with progression of the maculopathy[25-29]: lifestyle, demographic factors, and cardiovascular and ocular conditions. In relation to lifestyle, apart from smoking, there are suggestions that excessive exposure to sunlight (of short wavelength) can potentially damage the retina.[19] It has been suggested that when the natural crystalline lens is removed, a colored artificial lens should be implanted to recreate the eye's natural barrier to light rays.[30]

The Macular Photocoagulation Study group has identified risk factors associated with development of CNV in an eye, with existing CNV in the other eye.[31] These include the presence of 5 or more drusen, focal hyperpigmentation, one or more large drusen (> 63 microns), and systemic hypertension. With juxtafoveal CNV in one eye, there is an incidence of CNV in the other eye of 87% after 5 years if all 4 risk factors are present. Lanchoney et al reported that the risk of patients with soft bilateral drusen developing CNV after 10 years increases from 8.6% to 15.9%.[32] Hyperopia has a greater association with AMD, while a dark iris may be a form of protection against the development of AMD.[25,33]

Physiopathological Mechanisms

Retinal carotenoids, including the xantophyllic yellow pigments lutein and zeaxantine, protect the macula from dangerous blue light rays, because their absorption

Buratto L, Brint SF, Caretti L.
Cataract Surgery in Complicated Cases (pp 93-98).

Table 6-1.

Definition of Blindness According to Italian Law[a]

TOTAL BLINDNESS IS DEFINED AS THE FOLLOWING:
• A total lack of sight in both eyes
• The mere perception of light and darkness and hand movement in both eyes or in the better eye
• Residual peripheral binocular vision of less than 3%
PARTIAL BLINDNESS IS DEFINED AS THE FOLLOWING:
• Residual vision not exceeding 1/20 in both eyes or in the better eye, even with correction
• Residual peripheral binocular vision of less than 10% (ie, between 3% and 10%)
[a]Classification and quantification of visual impairment and rules on inspections eye, law 138, Official Gazette no. 93 of 04.21.2001 [in Italian].

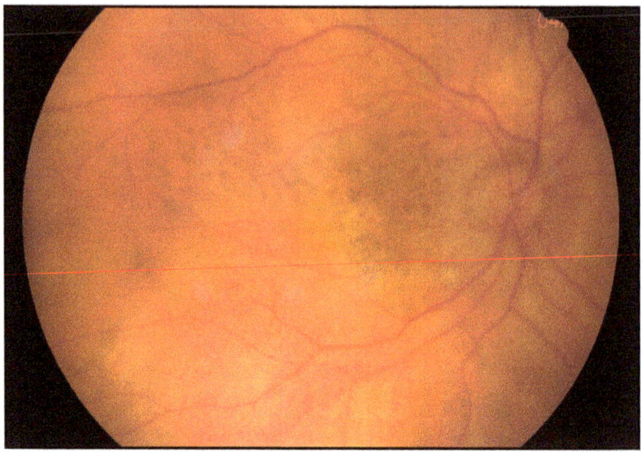

Figure 6-1. Early stages of AMD.

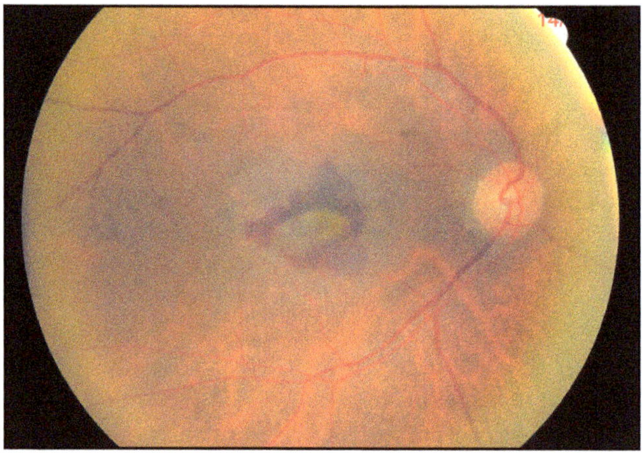

Figure 6-2. Active CNV in AMD.

spectrum is greatest for the shortest wavelengths. At the shortest absorption wavelengths, the xantophyllic pigments protect the photoreceptors from heat damage. When the molecules in the RPE absorb blue light, free radicals will form and these can damage the cell.[34]

The natural crystalline lens is the best protective barrier against light rays close to the ultraviolet (UV) spectrum (between 300 and 400 nm). Yellowing of the natural lens will lead to greater light absorption at the shorter wavelengths (eg, blue light).[35]

Findings from the Framingham Eye Study showed that patients with a nuclear cataract had a slightly lower incidence of macular changes (from mild to severe) as compared to patients with cortical cataracts.[36] The macular changes have been defined as mild if there are changes to the pigment or less than 10 small drusen. The changes have been defined as moderate to severe if more than 10 small drusen, large drusen, or hemorrhagic or exudative pathologies are present. Cortical cataracts are associated with a small increase in the risk of changes to the macula.[37]

Because of these observations and other scientific evidence illustrating that maculopathy deteriorates following cataract surgery (discussed in the following section), ophthalmology has shown greater interest in the use of intraocular lenses (IOLs) that can block the passage of harmful light rays into the eye.

In brunescent nuclear cataracts, insoluble proteins accumulate, possibly due to photo-oxidation by the UV rays. One suggestion is that their yellow filter protects the retina against damage from blue light in the visible spectrum. If this natural filter is replaced with an IOL, there may be subsequent damage to the retina caused by radiation close to the wavelengths of UV and blue light, depending on the transmission spectrum of the IOL.[38]

In recent years, a number of companies have developed IOLs that block UV and blue radiation.[39] Researchers have shown that yellow-filter IOLs reduce the damage to the RPE associated with lipofuscin fluorophore A2E.[40] Moreover, the incidence of CNV in patients with bilateral drusen and pigmentary changes was much higher in eyes implanted with nonfiltering IOLs compared to phakic eyes.[10] Nevertheless, the use of filtering IOLs is still a subject for debate. It has been suggested that these can decrease the patient's scotopic vision and color detection, particularly in more elderly patients.[41] However, at the time of writing, no study has been able to clearly document these phenomena. Age-related reduced visual capacity under scotopic conditions has been attributed by some researchers to an age-related reduction in the function of the retinal rods[42] and to a dysfunction of the central visual pathway.[43] Braunstein and Sparrow[44] therefore caution use of an IOL that blocks blue radiation, similar to a cataractous lens in adults.

In conclusion, removal of the natural lens unquestionably increases the exposure of the retina to light waves of short wavelengths and may increase the incidence of some macular changes, even if the relationship between cataract surgery and late AMD is still not clear.

Three mechanisms have been suggested for damage to the macula. The first is retinal toxicity; this may be caused by UV light and even light from the operating microscope used during the cataract operation. In addition to the problems caused by light rays, damage may also be caused by inflammation and retinochoroidal trauma.

Intraocular inflammation caused by surgery activates macrophages that increase the frequency of neovascularisation in subjects so inclined. The postoperative inflammatory reaction depends on the surgical technique. Inflammation is greater with extracapsular cataract extraction compared to phacoemulsification. It is well known that inflammation, even subclinical, is very frequent; in almost all eyes undergoing phacoemulsification (97%), angiography reveals ruptures in the blood-eye barrier.[45] Finally, retinochoroidal trauma may be associated with intraoperative intraocular pressure fluctuations. This can damage the fragile Bruch's membrane in patients with AMD.

Age-Related Macular Degeneration and Cataract Surgery

As mentioned previously, there is great debate on the role of cataract surgery in the progression of AMD. While some observed a higher incidence of late AMD cases in eyes undergoing cataract surgery,[46-49] others report a clear association with progression to forms of neovascular AMD, with a subsequent reduction in visual acuity after surgery.[4,8,10,13,50-53] Van der Schaft et al[46] observed more frequent formation of a disk-shaped scar secondary to AMD in pseudophakic eyes postmortem as compared to phakic eyes in patients of the same age. A population study[48] reported a higher incidence of late AMD (neovascular and geographic) in aphakic eyes. Freeman et al[48] believe that cataract surgery may be associated with an increased incidence of late AMD; we believe that severe cataracts were associated with a not statistically significant increase in the prevalence of late AMD. Recently, results from a study on 810 patients by Mönestam and Lundqvist[49] suggested that in the long-term (5 to 10 years), patients with AMD have poorer visual acuity than patients not affected by AMD. Pollack et al[10,54] followed 47 patients with symmetrical bilateral non-neovascular AMD undergoing extracapsular surgery in just one eye. The percentage of patients that progressed to neovascular AMD in the year following surgery was greater in eyes having surgery (19%) compared to the contralateral eye used as a control (4.3%). Nevertheless, the selection of the eye to be operated had not been randomized. The researchers who worked on the Beaver Dam Eye Study[4] and the Blue Mountain Eye Study[5] concluded cataract surgery increased 3- to 10-fold the risk of developing late AMD after 5 years.[50] The Blue Mountain Eye Study also reports a positive association between cataract surgery and the incidence of late neovascular AMD after 10 years,[52] but no increase in geographic atrophy. The authors believe that surgery carries risks for both the patient and concerns for the surgeon and consequently have identified restrictive indications for cataract surgery in patients with AMD.

All of these studies have led many eye surgeons to suspect a causal relationship between cataract surgery and the incidence of neovascular AMD. However, it should be remembered that observational studies have greater structural methodology limitations compared to prospective studies.

Vice versa, some studies do not support the hypothesis that cataract surgery negatively affects the condition of the macula.[37,55-57] Armbrecht et al[55] performed a retrospective study for 1 year on 2 groups of patients affected by AMD. The study group included 40 eyes that underwent surgery and a control group of 43 patients not having surgery. No progression to the neovascular form was observed in the study group, with 2 cases of progression observed in the control group. The Age-Related Eye Disease Study (AREDS) compared phakic eyes with non-neovascular lesions undergoing cataract surgery with a group not having surgery (a total of 342 subjects). Again in this study, no increase of the progression to the neovascular form of AMD was observed following surgery, compared to those that remained phakic; however, there was a risk of geographic atrophy.[38]

In a case control study on 499 patients with neovascular maculopathy associated with recent onset, Sutter et al did not observe any differences between the phakic eyes with neovascular AMD compared to the contralateral eye not having neovascular AMD.[56] Even in a recent retrospective case control study, no difference was detected between phakic and pseudophakic eyes with early AMD in the development of neovascular AMD in the year following cataract surgery.[57]

Even in a population study in Australia, the Visual Impairment Project, it was shown that cataract surgery is not associated with the progression of AMD.[58]

The only randomized clinical trial was performed by Hooper et al.[59] The trial included 56 eyes and suggested that there is no increased risk in the short-term (6 months) for progression of high-risk forms of AMD to the neovascular form following uncomplicated phacoemulsification surgery. Consequently, surgery is considered to be efficacious in these patients.

Moreover, a recent prospective study demonstrates a low percentage of progression of AMD in 108 subjects during the first postoperative year. During this period, only 3 of 65 eyes (4.6%), with no signs of neovascular AMD prior to or 1 week after surgery developed neovascularization.[60] These findings do not support the hypothesis that surgery increases the risk of progression of AMD. No case of geographic atrophy was observed again after 1 year in the 59 eyes in which atrophy was not detected prior and 1 week after surgery. The authors suggested that the previous studies showing an association or progression of the non-neovascular form to late AMD after surgery could be clouded by the absence of a detailed examination (optical coherence tomography or retinochoroidal angiography) of the neovascular or atrophic macular condition immediately pre- or postoperatively. It is possible that the macular changes existed prior to surgery and had not been adequately documented because of opacity of the media.

Additional data have been supplied in a recent report by the AREDS group (report no. 25).[61] In this prospective study, the group included 4577 patients (8050 eyes). The fundus was photographed every year and examined for the appearance of late AMD. This is one of the few prospective studies in which the severity of the AMD is documented before and after surgery in a large number of cases with a follow-up of years. According to the results of this study, there is inconclusive evidence to show that cataract surgery increases the risk of progression to late AMD.

A more recent report by the AREDS group (report no. 27)[62] describes the visual results for the largest group of patients recorded in the literature (4757 patients). The patients had AMD and underwent cataract surgery. The participants benefited from the cataract surgery with a statistically significant mean increase in visual acuity. This persisted for at least 8 months after surgery. The mean improvement in vision was seen in all the different degrees of severity of AMD including extremely advanced cases.

Moreover, Rosenfeld at al[63] demonstrated that cataract surgery is safe and useful in patients affected by AMD, including those affected by the neovascular form, treated with intravitreal injections of Lucentis (ranibizumab injection), with a mean increase in visual acuity of 2 Snellen lines.

Currently, it is not possible to state whether cataract surgery is useful or should be avoided in patients affected by AMD. This is supported by the recent study by Cochrane[64] in 2009, which reviewed a large number of articles relative to different research trials published between 1982 and 2004 including The Cochrane Central Register of Controller Trials, Medline, Embase, and Latin American and Caribbean Literature of Health Sciences. The trials were all nonrandomized, prospective, and case controlled. No randomized studies were included.

Concluding from careful analysis of recent literature, it is clear that cataract surgery in patients with AMD may be useful.

Surgery

From a strictly surgical point of view, the degree of difficulty of cataract surgery in patients with AMD is the same as that of a standard cataract operation. The only relative problem may be associated with poor visibility of the anterior capsule during the capsulorrhexis procedure, due to the reduced or absent red reflex in cases of late AMD.

The surgeon must always use modern techniques of phacoemulsification, using minimal quantities of ultrasound and without inducing complications. The surgical times must be short with less postoperative inflammation, and when possible, the surgeon must implant filtering IOLs. In theory, this type of lens will protect the macula from the retinotoxic effects of UV light, meaning sunlight or the light from the operating microscope. The surgeon must always use coaxial light, reduce the light intensity to a minimum, use obscuring spots following the implantation of the IOL, and ensure that the surgery is as short as possible.

The surgeon must also attempt to minimize intraoperative fluctuations of the intraocular pressure to reduce stress on the fragile Bruch's membrane. The progress on the first eye should be monitored before peforming surgery on the second eye.

Finally, it should be remembered that at the end of uncomplicated phacoemulsification surgery in patients with neovascular AMD, the surgeon may decide to perform an intravitreal injection of anti-angiogenic drugs for the treatment of the macular pathology. Reports in the literature would suggest that this treatment is beneficial for the patient.[65]

Conclusion

The scientific literature provides contradictory information on the relationship between cataract surgery and the progression to late AMD. Today, however, thanks to the most recent scientific literature, we can be more confident in performing cataract surgery on patients with AMD. The visual results should be extremely satisfactory.

References

1. World Health Organization. *Magnitude and Causes of Visual Impairment: Fact Sheet No. 282*. Geneva: WHO; 2004.
2. Bressler NM. Age-related macular degeneration is the leading cause of blindness. *JAMA*. 2004;291(15):1900-1901.
3. Friedman DS, O'Colmain BJ, Muñoz B; et al, Eye Diseases Prevalence Research Group. Prevalence of age-related macular degeneration in the United States. *Arch Ophthalmol*. 2004;122(4):564-572.
4. Klein R, Klein BE, Jensen SC, Cruickshanks KJ. The relationship of ocular factors to the incidence and progression of age-related maculopathy. *Arch Ophthalmol*. 1998;116:506-513.

5. Wang JJ, Mitchell PG, Cummings RG, Lim R. Cataract and age-related maculopathy: the Blue Mountains Eye Study. *Ophthalmic Epidemiol.* 1999;6:317-326.
6. Klein R, Klein BE, Wang Q, Moss SE. Is age-related maculopathy associated with cataracts? *Arch Ophthalmol.* 1994;112:191-196.
7. Liu IY, White L, LaCroix AZ. The association of age-related macular degeneration and lens opacities in the aged. *Am J Public Health.* 1989;79:765-769.
8. Blair CJ, Ferguson J Jr. Exacerbation of senile macular degeneration following cataract extraction. *Am J Ophthalmol.* 1979;87(1):77-83.
9. Shuttleworth GN, Luhishi EA, Harrad RA. Do patients with age related maculopathy and cataract benefit from cataract surgery? *Br J Ophthalmol.* 1998;82(6):611-616.
10. Pollack A, Marcovich A, Bukelman A, Oliver M. Age-related macular degeneration after extracapsular cataract extraction with intraocular lens implantation. *Ophthalmology.* 1996;103(10):1546-1554.
11. Armbrecht AM, Findlay C, Kaushal S, Aspinall P, Hill AR, Dhillon B. Is cataract surgery justified in patients with age-related macular degeneration? A visual function and quality of life assessment. *Br J Ophthalmol.* 2000;84(12):1343-1348.
12. Smith BT, Belani S, Ho AC. Light energy, cataract surgery, and progression of age-related macular degeneration. *Curr Opin Ophthalmol.* 2005;16(3):166-169.
13. Klein R, Klein BE, Linton KL. Prevalence of age-related maculopathy. The Beaver Dam Eye Study. *Ophthalmology.* 1992;99:933-943.
14. Leibowitz HM, Krueger DE, Maunder LR, et al. The Framingham Eye Study monograph: an ophthalmological and epidemiological study of cataract, glaucoma, diabetic retinopathy, macular degeneration, and visual acuity in a general population of 2631 adults, 1973-1975. *Surv Ophthalmol.* 1980;24(suppl):335-610.
15. The AREDS2 Research Group; Chew EY, Clemons T, et al. The Age-related Eye Disease Study 2 (AREDS2): study design and baseline characteristics (AREDS2 report number 1). *Ophthalmology.* 2012;119(11):2282-2289.
16. Klein R, Rowland ML, Harris MI. Racial/ethnic differences in age-related maculopathy. Third National Health and Nutrition Examination Survey. *Ophthalmology.* 1995;102:371-381.
17. Vingerling JR, Dielemans I, Hofman A, et al. The prevalence of age-related maculopathy in the Rotterdam Study. *Ophthalmology.* 1995;102:205-210.
18. Mitchell P, Smith W, Attebo K, Wang JJ. Prevalence of age-related maculopathy in Australia. The Blue Mountains Eye Study. *Ophthalmology.* 1995;102:1450-1460.
19. Klein R, Klein BE, Jensen SC, Meuer SM. The five-year incidence and progression of age-related maculopathy: the Beaver Dam Eye Study. *Ophthalmology.* 1997;104:7-21.
20. Piguet B, Wells JA, Palmvang IB, et al. Age-related Bruch's membrane change: a clinical study of the relative role of heredity and environment. *Br J Ophthalmol.* 1993;77:400-403.
21. Seddon JM, Ajani UA, Mitchell BD. Familial aggregation of age-related maculopathy. *Am J Ophthalmol.* 1997;123:199-206.
22. Hamdi HK, Kenney MC. Age-related macular degeneration: a new viewpoint. *Front Biosci.* 2003;8:305-314.
23. Zareparsi S, Reddick AC, Branham KE, et al. Association of apolipoprotein E alleles with susceptibility to age-related macular degeneration in a large cohort from a single center. *Invest Ophthalmol Vis Sci.* 2004;45:1306-1310.
24. Seddon JM, Cote J, Page WF, et al. The US Twin Study of Age-Related Macular Degeneration: relative roles of genetic and environmental influences. *Arch Ophthalmol.* 2005;123:321-327.
25. Age-Related Eye Disease Study Research Group. Risk factors associated with age-related macular degeneration. A case-control study in the age-related eye disease study: AREDS report number 3. *Ophthalmology.* 2000;107:2224-2232.
26. Tomany SC, Wang JJ, Van Leeuwen R, et al. Risk factors for incident age-related macular degeneration: pooled findings from 3 continents. *Ophthalmology.* 2004;111:1280-1287.
27. Klein R, Peto T, Bird A, Vannewkirk MR. The epidemiology of age-related macular degeneration. *Am J Ophthalmol.* 2004;137:486-495.
28. Age-Related Eye Disease Study Research Group. A randomized, placebo-controlled, clinical trial of high-dose supplementation with vitamins C and E, beta carotene, and zinc for age-related macular degeneration and vision loss: AREDS report number 8. *Arch Ophthalmol.* 2001;119:1417-1436.
29. Galan A, Ferlin A, Caretti L, Buson G, Sato G, Frigo AC, Foresta C. Association of age-related macular degeneration with polymorphisms in vascular endothelial growth factor and its receptor. *Ophthalmology.* 2010;117(9):1769-1774.
30. Okuno T, Saito H, Ojima J. Evaluation of blue-light hazards from various light sources. *Dev Ophthalmol.* 2002;35:104-112.
31. Macular Photocoagulation Study Group. Risk factors for choroidal neovascularization in the second eye of patients with juxtafoveal or subfoveal choroidal neovascularization secondary to age-related macular degeneration. *Arch Ophthalmol.* 1997;115:741-747.
32. Lanchoney DM, Maguire MG, Fine SL. A model of the incidence and consequences of choroidal neovascularization secondary to age-related macular degeneration. Comparative effects of current treatment and potential prophylaxis on visual outcomes in high-risk patients. *Arch Ophthalmol.* 1998;116:1045-1052.
33. Sandberg MA, Gaudio AR, Miller S, Weiner A. Iris pigmentation and extent of disease in patients with neovascular age-related macular degeneration. *Invest Ophthalmol Vis Sci.* 1994;35:2734-2740.
34. Sparrow JR, Zhou J, Ben Shabat S, et al. Involvement of oxidative mechanisms in blue-light-induced damage to A2E-laden RPE. *Invest Ophthalmol Vis Sci.* 2002;43:1222-1227.
35. Mellerio J. Yellowing of the human lens: nuclear and cortical contributions. *Vision Res.* 1987;27:1581-1587.
36. Sperduto RD, Hiller R, Seigel D. Lens opacities and senile maculopathy. *Arch Ophthalmol.* 1981;99:1004-1008.Guttman C, Ferris FL. No link between cataract surgery, AMD, study shows. *Ophthalmology Times.* 2003;28(5).
37. Guttman C, Ferris FL. No link between cataract surgery, AMD, study shows. *Ophthalmology Times.* 2003;28(5).
38. Mainster MA. Spectral transmittance of intraocular lenses and retinal damage from intense light sources. *Am J Ophthalmol.* 1978;85:167-170.
39. Niwa K, Yoshino Y, Okuyama F, et al. Effects of tinted intraocular lens on contrast sensitivity. *Ophthalmic Physiol Opt.* 1996;16:297-302.
40. Sparrow JR, Miller AS, Zhou J. Blue light-absorbing intraocular lens and retinal pigment epithelium protection in vitro. *J Cataract Refract Surg.* 2004;30:873-878.
41. Mainster MA. Intraocular lenses should block UV radiation and violet but not blue light. *Arch Ophthalmol.* 2005;123:550-555.
42. Curcio CA, Owsley C, Jackson GR. Spare the rods, save the cones in aging and age-related maculopathy. *Invest Ophthalmol Vis Sci.* 2000;41:2015-2018.
43. Schefrin BE, Tregear SJ, Harvey LO, Werner JS. Senescent changes in scotopic contrast sensitivity. *Vision Res.* 1999;39:3728-3736.
44. Braunstein RE, Sparrow JR. A blue-blocking intraocular lens should be used in cataract surgery. *Arch Ophthalmol.* 2005;123:547-549.
45. Lobo CL, Faria PM, Soares MA, Bernardes RC, Cunha-Vaz JG. Macular alterations after small-incision cataract surgery. *J Cataract Refract Surg.* 2004;30(4):752-760.
46. Van der Schaft TL, Mooy CM, de Bruijn WC, Mulder PG, Pameyer JH, de Jong PT. Increased prevalence of disciform macular degeneration after cataract extraction with implantation of an intraocular lens. *Br J Ophthalmol.* 1994;78(6):441-445.

47. Chaine G, Hullo A, Sahel J; et al, France-DMLA Study Group. Case-control study of the risk factors for age related macular degeneration. *Br J Ophthalmol.* 1998;82(9):996-1002.
48. Freeman EE, Munoz B, West SK, Tielsch JM, Schein OD. Is there an association between cataract surgery and age-related macular degeneration? Data from three population-based studies. *Am J Ophthalmol.* 2003;135(6):849-856.
49. Mönestam E, Lundqvist B. Long-term visual outcome after cataract surgery: comparison of healthy eyes and eyes with age-related macular degeneration. *J Cataract Refract Surg.* 2012;38(3):409-414.
50. Kaiserman I, Kaiserman N, Elhayany A, Vinker S. Cataract surgery is associated with a higher rate of photodynamic therapy for age-related macular degeneration. *Ophthalmology.* 2007;114(2):278-282.
51. Klein R, Klein BE, Wong TY, Tomany SC, Cruickshanks KJ. The association of cataract and cataract surgery with the long-term incidence of age-related maculopathy: the Beaver Dam Eye Study. *Arch Ophthalmol.* 2002;120(11):1551-1558.
52. Wang JJ, Klein R, Smith W, Klein BE, Tomany S, Mitchell P. Cataract surgery and the 5-year incidence of late-stage age-related maculopathy: pooled findings from the Beaver Dam and Blue Mountains Eye studies. *Ophthalmology.* 2003;110(10):1960-1967.
53. Cugati S, Mitchell P, Rochtchina E, Tan AG, Smith W, Wang JJ. Cataract surgery and the 10-year incidence of age-related maculopathy: the Blue Mountains Eye Study. *Ophthalmology.* 2006;113(11):2020-2025.
54. Pollack A, Bukelman A, Zalish M, Leiba H, Oliver M. The course of age-related macular degeneration following bilateral cataract surgery. *Ophthalmic Surg Lasers.* 1998;29(4):286-294.
55. Armbrecht AM, Findlay C, Aspinall PA, Hill AR, Dhillon B. Cataract surgery in patients with age-related macular degeneration: one-year outcomes. *J Cataract Refract Surg.* 2003;29(4):686-693.
56. Sutter FK, Menghini M, Barthelmes D, et al. Is pseudophakia a risk factor for neovascular age-related macular degeneration? *Invest Ophthalmol Vis Sci.* 2007;48(4):1472-1475.
57. Baatz H, Darawsha R, Ackermann H, et al. Phacoemulsification does not induce neovascular age-related macular degeneration. *Invest Ophthalmol Vis Sci.* 2008;49(3):1079-1083.
58. McCarty CA, Mukesh BN, Fu CL, et al. Risk factors for age-related maculopathy: the Visual Impairment Project. *Arch Ophthalmol.* 2001;119:1455-1462.
59. Hooper CY, Lamoureux EL, Lim L, et al. Cataract surgery in high-risk age-related macular degeneration: a randomized controlled trial. *Clin Experiment Ophthalmol.* 2009;37(6):570-576.
60. Dong LM, Stark WJ, Jefferys JL, et al. Progression of age-related macular degeneration after cataract surgery. *Arch Ophthalmol.* 2009;127(11):1412-1419.
61. Chew EY, Sperduto RD, Milton RC, et al. Risk of advanced age-related macular degeneration following cataract surgery in the Age-Related Eye Disease Study. AREDS report number 25. *Ophthalmology.* 2009;116(2):297-303.
62. Forooghian F, Agrón E, Clemons TE, Ferris FL 3rd, Chew EY for the AREDS Research Group. Visual acuity outcomes after cataract surgery in patients with age-related macular degeneration: Age-Related Eye Disease Study report number 27. *Ophthalmology.* 2009;116(11):2093-2100.
63. Rosenfeld PJ, Shapiro H, Ehrlich JS, Wong P; MARINA and ANCHOR Study Groups. Cataract surgery in ranibizumab-treated patients with neovascular age-related macular degeneration from the phase 3 ANCHOR and MARINA trials. *Am J Ophthalmol.* 2011;152(5):793-798.
64. Casparis H, Lindsley K, Bressler NB. Surgery for cataracts in people with age-related macular degeneration. *Cochrane Database Syst Rev.* 2009;21(1):CD006757.
65. Jonas JB, Spandau UH, Schlichtenbrede F, Libondi T, Vossmerbaeumer U, von Baltz S. Intravitreal bevacizumab combined with cataract surgery for treatment of exudative macular degeneration. *J Ocul Pharmacol Ther.* 2007;23(6):599-600.

7

Brunescent Cataract

Extremely dense cataracts have always been considered more challenging in phacoemulsification, not only because of their frequency, but also because of their real management difficulties.

In our opinion, it is essential to match the correct surgical technique (phacoemulsification, extra- and intracapsular cataract extraction) in relation to the patient's clinical history, the characteristics of the cataract, and the surgeon's experience. In order to plan the surgical approach correctly and to predict the emulsification of the nucleus in an acceptable period of time, it is essential to evaluate the type and the degree of hardness of the nucleus. The development of phacoemulsification devices and techniques that are increasingly more efficient has considerably reduced the difficulties and complications associated with this type of surgery, limiting it particularly to nuclei of truly leather-like hardness (called the *nigra cataract*) and in those cases when the hard nucleus is associated with other alterations of the anterior segment.

The problems encountered in this type of surgery are determined not just by the hardness and the dimensions of the nucleus, but also by the poor degree of hydration of the lens (the protein has been denatured), absence of the red reflex, a capsule that is thin and fragile, and weak or absent zonules. We, however, remain convinced that these surgeries should be performed under topical anaesthesia, using phacoemulsification equipment with a micro-incisional coaxial technique (an incision of 2.0 or 2.2 mm), enhancing these operations that are associated with a high degree of difficulty.

Difficulties and Solutions

Apart from the hardness of the nucleus, it is essential to take other aspects into consideration to ensure a good surgical outcome. We will analyze the individual difficulties that the surgeon may face and suggest the most appropriate solutions.[1]

Tunnel

The corneal tunnel created should be slightly shorter and larger; this will reduce the danger of wound burn, given that the quantity of ultrasound and energy used in the treatment is likely to be much greater than that of a standard cataract. It also allows greater freedom of movement of the tip that will probably have to work longer. An additional advantage of a shorter tunnel will be lower traction on the adjacent tissue.

Capsulorrhexis

Visibility is probably the most critical aspect. A reduced or absent red reflex associated with the density of this type of cataract greatly reduces the visualization of the anterior capsule. The capsulorrhexis should ideally be intact if the surgeon wishes to perform phacoemulsification with the implantation of an intraocular lens (IOL) in the capsular bag. A useful tip is to change the angle of the microscope's coaxial light beam to produce better visibility of the capsule itself. In the event the visibility remains insufficient, the use of vital dyes (such as trypan blue; refer to Chapters 1 and 15) may prove useful. In addition to improving visibility of the capsule during capsulorrhexis, it improves visibility during phacoemulsification, helping the surgeon avoid traumatizing the edge of the capsulorrhexis with the phaco tip or the chopper (Figure 7-1).

Regardless of whether the capsule is treated with dye or not, the next step is the injection of a high viscosity sodium hyaluronate (eg, Viscoat [Alcon Laboratories, Fort Worth, TX] and Healon 5 [Abbott Laboratories, Abbott Park, IL]) into the anterior chamber (AC); this has dispersive and

Buratto L, Brint SF, Caretti L.
Cataract Surgery in Complicated Cases (pp 99-104).

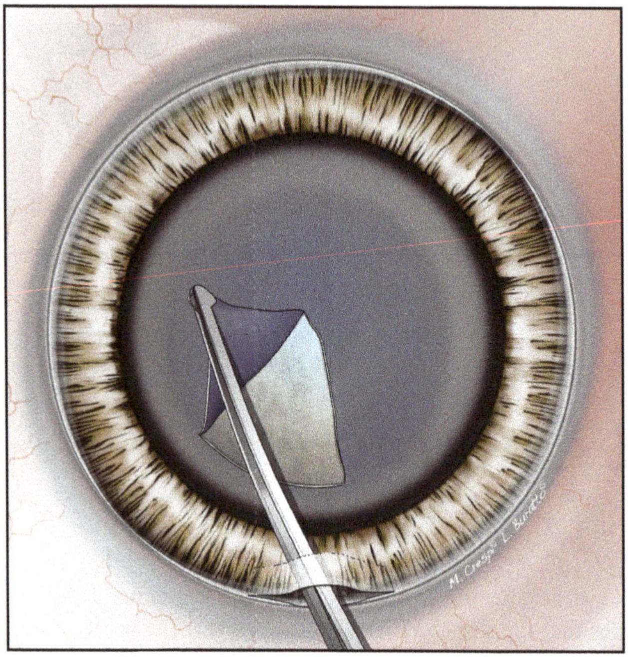

Figure 7-1. Capsulorrhexis of a brunescent cataract with the help of trypan blue.

cohesive properties and has the advantage of flattening the convex shape of the anterior lens surface, increasing AC depth (which has been reduced due to the large volume of the crystalline lens) to reduce zonular stretch and orient the rhexis in the desired direction.[2] When the contents of the lens are liquefied and an appropriate viscoelastic has not been injected, typically the nucleus may ooze in the AC as soon as the anterior capsule is perforated and the white cortex will obscure the surgeon's view. In this case, the surgeon should interrupt the capsulorrhexis procedure and, to improve visibility, add viscoelastic substance (VES) to the AC and remove the cloudy liquid by infusion/aspiration, taking care to avoid the capsule.

Capsulorrhexis is a difficult procedure not just because of poor visibility; normally, with a very hard, mature cataract the anterior capsule becomes extremely fragile and will tend to rupture in inappropriate areas. The addition of a pseudo-adaptive VES will lead to a reduction in the centrifugal forces of the open capsule, facilitating the completion and the positioning of the rhexis flap. A large rhexis (5.5 to 6.0 mm or larger) is advisable for a number of reasons. There is greater freedom of movement of the phaco tip with less risk of damaging components of the AC, important considering that manipulations inside the capsular bag will be prolonged and traumatic; this will also reduce capsular contraction syndrome. In the event of difficulties, a large rhexis can allow luxation of the nucleus in the AC and its subsequent removal with a hook once the corneal incision has been extended. In extremely mature cataracts, the anterior capsule may contain deposits of calcium or dense focal plaques that interfere with the normal rhexis procedure. The surgeon must therefore guide the cut around it, or if this is not possible, he or she should use Gills-Vannas scissors (Katena Eye Instruments, Denville, NJ) or curved vitreal scissors to cut through these dense areas.

Hydrodissection and Hydrodelineation

Before proceeding, it may prove useful to remove a small amount of VES from the AC by exerting moderate pressure on the tunnel with a hydrodissection cannula; this maneuver will prevent any excessive increase to the intraocular pressure during hydrodissection.

Hydrodissection separates the capsule from the external cortex of the hard nucleus and should be performed with maximum caution. A 26-gauge cannula is used to raise the anterior capsule; the surgeon carefully, delicately, and progressively injects balanced salt solution (BSS) below the capsule, close to the equator, to shift the large nucleus slightly forward; this shift must be stopped by the surgeon as soon as the nucleus moves toward the capsulorrhexis to avoid capsule-lenticular blockage.

Repeated and extremely delicate hydrodissection maneuvers are recommended. More specifically, half of the hydrodissection should be completed, then the center of the raised nucleus should be pushed with the cannula to depress the nucleus posteriorly; a further cautious hydrodissection is performed on the opposite side (if required, the surgeon can combine a limited viscodissection procedure to rotate the nucleus). This is important as the anterior shift of the large brunescent nucleus during hydrodissection may lead to a capsule-lenticular blockage. In this case, if the surgeon proceeds with further and aggressive injections of liquid below the nucleus, the posterior capsule may be distended and rupture. Another aspect that can increase the complexity of this operation is the presence of strong corticocapsular adhesions that interfere with rotation of the nucleus; this procedure must be performed delicately without excessive force being applied. Before the surgeon begins ultrasound, it is essential that the nucleus rotate freely inside the capsular bag.

In addition to the hardness of the nucleus and increase in volume of the lens with these very hard cataracts, the fibers of the lens are often modified. These will be very compact, cohesive, and tenacious, making hydrodelineation and the formation of an epinuclear shell almost impossible (a procedure that is not recommended). Moreover, they absorb the phaco energy and make division a more difficult procedure.

Zonular Fragility

It is important to remember that zonular weakness or the complete absence of some zonules is a major problem for the surgeon. This may be associated with the advanced age of these patients, with previous traumatic episodes that may have gone unnoticed, or with a chronic cumulative weakening of the zonules associated with microtrauma that the enormous mass of the cataractous nucleus induces by friction over time. Zonular fragility is particularly problematic in the absence of an epinucleus; the posterior capsule will have a greater tendency to shift toward the phaco tip even with a minimal degree of postocclusion surge.

Severe capsular laxity, induced by the zonular weakness, increases the risk of capsular rupture. In an attempt to avoid this problem, the inexperienced surgeon will consider emulsifying the last remaining nuclear fragments, operating closer to the cornea, a procedure that will create endothelial cell loss.

If the surgeon suspects clinically significant zonular weakness, a condition frequently observed in these cases, he or she should use a capsular tension ring (CTR). There has been a lot of debate regarding the most suitable timing for this particular maneuver; some surgeons believe that the tension ring should be inserted as soon as any degree of weakness is observed, usually prior to the phacoemulsification procedure, while others feel that it should be inserted prior to irrigation/aspiration or before the IOL is implanted (the most popular solution). However, some surgeons do not recommend the application of the tension rings as they feel that with time, an extremely weakened bag could result in luxation of the IOL-tension ring-capsular bag into the posterior chamber, a situation that is difficult to manage when compared to the luxation of the IOL-capsular bag complex (refer to Chapter 15).

Phacoemulsification

When hydrodissection has been completed and the nucleus has been rotated, the surgeon can perform phacoemulsification. This procedure is more feasible and used more frequently due to the development of new phacoemulsification instruments and new surgical techniques (phaco chop, coaxial microincision cataract surgery [C-MICS]). Prior to emulsifying the nucleus, the surgeon should aspirate a small quantity of viscoelastic (positioned close to the lens surface) to avoid occluding the tip (wound burn) and to ensure better circulation of the BSS in the AC.

Regardless of the phacoemulsification technique the surgeon prefers, higher energy levels are required compared to the surgery for standard cataracts, with a potential increase in the risk of damaging the endothelium and rupturing the blood-ocular barrier.

These cataracts should only be operated by expert surgeons who should use the latest phacoemulsification equipment as these will allow modification of the parameters with a reduction in surgical times and the amount of energy used. In any case, compared to a standard cataract, phacoemulsification of this type of cataract requires considerably more time. When removing these nuclei, many surgeons still proceed with sculpting procedures. It is essential to create a space in the center of the nucleus, which will allow manipulation of the nuclear fragments and the phaco tip. This space is essential because the higher phaco power and more viscoelastic usage increase the risk of a wound burn. The maneuvers must be very delicate to avoid affecting the capsule and the zonules. A 45-degree phaco tip is usually used for these maneuvers, however, a 30-degree tip will permit better occlusion in the successive stages of phacoemulsification.

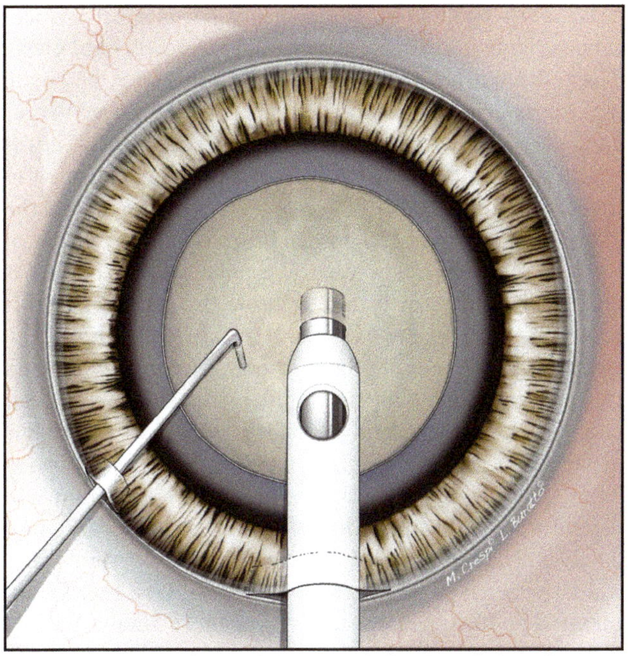

Figure 7-2. A step of coaxial phacoemulsification of a large brunescent cataract nucleus performed using the chop technique.

During sculpting, in our opinion, phaco power, flow rate, and the vacuum must be quite high (80%, 25 cc per minute, and 140 mm Hg, respectively), and this slightly increases the operative risks of capsular rupture, capsular-zonular damage, and contact between hard fragments and the corneal endothelium. Next, the surgeon can choose one of the techniques suitable for this type of nucleus (eg, Fine's "crack and flick" technique, Shepherd's "in situ" fracture, Gimbel's "divide and conquer" nuclear fracture technique, among others); these techniques involve fragmenting the nucleus into small pieces with external separation. However, each of these techniques creates capsule-zonular stress.[3-5]

There are other techniques (eg, "phaco chop" described by Nagahara[6] and the "stop and chop" technique described by Koch[7]) that reduce the capsular and zonular stress, an extremely important factor in these eyes.

The "quick chop" technique is a variation of the "phaco chop" with a reduction in the amount of ultrasound used and manual fragmentation required. This allows reduction of energy with a reduction in the risk of wound burn, shortened operating times, and a reduction in the amount of stress to the zonules (Figure 7-2). This technique is particularly suitable for the management of most brunescent nuclei (with the exception of the extremely hard ones). The technique involves the use of high vacuum (to create maximum grip) and a chopper; the phaco tip is used to create a deep groove in the center of the nucleus, using ultrasound pulses. The phaco tip is therefore used as a pivot point to fracture the nucleus into pieces, moving them toward the chopper, which has been pushed from top down in front of the phaco aperture. The vertical element of the chopper is pushed vertically downward to create the crack. With this technique, the chopper will always remain inside the rhexis, clearly visible and under the surgeon's full control. To avoid the risk of zonulolysis or capsular rupture, the vertical chopper does not extend beyond the edges of the rhexis as far as the equator, as is the case for the classical phaco chop technique. The movement of lateral separation will extend the crack across the nucleus and will separate the 2 halves. The same procedure is then repeated several times until the nucleus is gradually split into 4 or more fragments. The 15-degree phaco tip is the most suitable for this technique. With very hard nuclei the surgeon may wish to impale the nucleus in an off-center position, instead of the central position preferred during the removal of a standard cataract, to initiate the crack. If the surgeon does not set adequately high levels of vacuum (resulting in inadequate holding power), the chopper will dislocate the fragments away from the phaco tip, and it will be much more difficult to remove the larger fragments from the bag. With these unusually dense nuclei, the surgeon should create an anterior central groove to allow the phaco tip to impale the very compact nucleus in a deep and peripheral position (this would prove much more difficult if a groove is not created). For optimal impaling of the nucleus, with luxation, the surgeon should retract the irrigation sleeve and expose more of the phaco tip.

Regardless of the technique preferred by the modern surgeon (divide and conquer, stop and chop, chop), the basic principle is the same—the creation of multiple, small-size fragments that are larger and much denser than those of other types of nucleus. Subsequently, the fragments are split into even smaller pieces and pulled by the chopper close to the tip and delicately guided into it. As with a standard cataract, the pieces are successively emulsified and aspirated; in this case, however, the vacuum is much higher and occasional short bursts of ultrasound (20% to 40%) will be required. During this step, the movements of the surgeon's nondominant hand are fundamental.

In the past, blockage of the tubing by rigid nuclear fragments was a frequent problem, though this has been largely resolved. These pieces may occlude the phaco tip resulting in poor followability, resulting in excessive turbulence inside the AC with trauma to the endothelium. Today, modern phacoemulsification machines considerably reduce the amount of energy and heat produced with increased followability associated with reduced vibration of the fragments inside the phaco tip. This technology is called hyperpulsated and was introduced by WhiteStar Technology with the AMO (Abbott Park Laboratories) Sovereign phaco. At the time of this writing, it is also supplied by other companies (eg, Alcon). By modulating ultrasound power supplied by the Ozil torsional system (Alcon) and by the Ellipse transversal system (AMO), the axial pulses are replaced by nonlongitudinal movements of the phaco tip.[8,9] Along with the development of the hyperpulsated technology, these innovations significantly reduce the vibration and repulsion of brunescent particles at the phaco tip. Signs that the surgeon must recognize when the phaco tip is partially or completely occluded are sudden appearance of emulsified milky material in front of the ultrasound tip and suddenly decreased followability.

There are numerous advantages associated with the C-MICS technique with new phacoemulsification equipment. In addition to greater maneuverability of the instruments, better maintenance of the AC, reduction in induced astigmatism, less surgical trauma, with a hypermature cataract, the new technologies lead to a reduction in the intraocular flow, greater efficiency, a reduction in ultrasound, and easier execution of the chop technique (the finer instruments facilitate the cleaving of the nucleus).

During phacoemulsification, repeated injections of a dispersive or pseudo-adaptive (if used correctly) VES into the anterior and posterior chambers creates space, protects the endothelium, leads to better positioning of the nucleus for emulsification, and emulsifies at a safe distance from the posterior capsule. Because of the prolonged surgical times, these viscoelastics are indicated because of the better retention as opposed to cohesive viscoelastics (ie, they persist longer intraocularly).

In particular, given that the posterior capsule is frequently thinner and stretched by the large volume of the lens, it will be weak and flaccid with folds and laxity and will tend to be aspirated into the phaco tip with a major risk of rupture. This potential complication is exacerbated by the fact that this type of cataract is characterized by an absence or reduced amount of an epinucleus that protects the posterior capsule, forcing the surgeon to work closer to the posterior capsule and the equatorial periphery, particularly when a deep central groove has been created.

Consequently, it is advisable for several small injections of a dispersive or pseudo-adaptive VES behind the nucleus during phacoemulsification, injecting it into various areas to create a thin yet uniform layer of VES between the nucleus and the posterior capsule, creating an artificial epinucleus that separates the posterior capsule from the operating plane. Because of its intrinsic properties, it is not easily aspirated by the phaco tip, and this facilitates the safe emulsification of the fragments.

Small nuclear fragments are occasionally trapped in the secondary incision or beneath the iris, particularly if dispersive VESs are used. The surgeon must look for these fragments and be particularly diligent when removing the VES.

In order to reduce the risk of wound burn, given that a greater amount of ultrasound is required to fracture a dense nucleus compared to a standard cataract, the corneal tunnel constructed should be wider and shorter to allow the escape of fluid that will cool the phaco tip. This complication due to technological improvements, specifically designs of phaco tips, is not as common as in the past, with bound needles, double sleeve, and "aspiration bypass hole." At any rate, if the incision is created in clear cornea, at the end of phacoemulsification, the surgeon may see moderate edema of the corneal stroma due to the increased energy delivered.

Successive Steps

Once the nucleus has been completely removed, the remainder of the surgery is exactly the same as for the standard cataract: aspiration of the cortex, implantation of the IOL into the bag, and hydration of the tunnel (usually creating a self-sealing valve, not requiring sutures at the end of the procedure). However, at the end of the procedure, if the capsular bag appears to be compromised to such a degree as it will not support the IOL over time, the surgeon may opt to implant a posterior chamber IOL with trans-scleral or iris fixation or an AC-IOL.

Postoperative

Edema of the corneal stroma is frequently seen the day after phacoemulsification for a brunescent cataract. It is usually very mild and is the result of endothelial cell loss or trauma induced by turbulence of the hard nuclear fragments chafing the corneal endothelium, creating edema. However, this usually disappears within the space of a few days.

Conclusion

The removal of a brunescent cataract requires careful preoperative planning and must be performed by an experienced surgeon. We believe that topical anesthesia is the elective choice for removing this type of cataract with phacoemulsification. Using aids to minimize difficulties associated with this type of cataract (visualization of the anterior capsule with dyes, the use of pseudo-adaptive VESs, protection of the weakened zonules and the posterior capsule, phaco, etc), the use of the latest generation of phacoemulsification devices and surgical techniques associated with low levels of trauma in recent years means that the removal of the brunescent cataract has become a surgical operation that is performed more frequently and enjoys good success.

References

1. Hou P, Hu YJ. Phacoemulsification of hard nucleus cataracts. *J Cataract Refract Surg.* 2010;36(5):872-873.
2. Miyata K, Nagamoto T, Maruoka S, Tanabe T, Nakahara M, Amano S. Efficacy and safety of the soft-shell technique in cases with a hard lens nucleus. *J Cataract Refract Surg.* 2002;28(9):1546-1550.
3. Kim HK. Decrease and conquer: phacoemulsification technique for hard nucleus cataracts. *J Cataract Refract Surg.* 2009;35(10):1665-1670.
4. Park JH, Lee SM, Kwon JW, et al. Ultrasound energy in phacoemulsification: a comparative analysis of phaco-chop and stop-and-chop techniques according to the degree of nuclear density. *Ophthalmic Surg Lasers Imaging.* 2010;41(2):236-241.
5. Kamoi K, Mochizuki M. Phaco forward-chop technique for managing posterior nuclear plate of hard cataract. *J Cataract Refract Surg.* 2010;36(1):9-12.
6. Nagahara K. Video presentation. In: *ASCRS Film Festival*; 1993; Seattle, WA.
7. Koch PS, Katzen LE. Stop and chop phacoemulsification. *J Cataract Refract Surg.* 1994;20(5)566-570.
8. Zeng M, Liu X, Liu Y, et al. Torsional ultrasound modality for hard nucleus phacoemulsification cataract extraction. *Br J Ophthalmol.* 2008;92(8):1092-1096.
9. Fakhry MA, El Shazly MI. Torsional ultrasound mode versus combined torsional and conventional ultrasound mode phacoemulsification for eyes with hard cataract. *Clin Ophthalmology.* 2011;5:973-978.

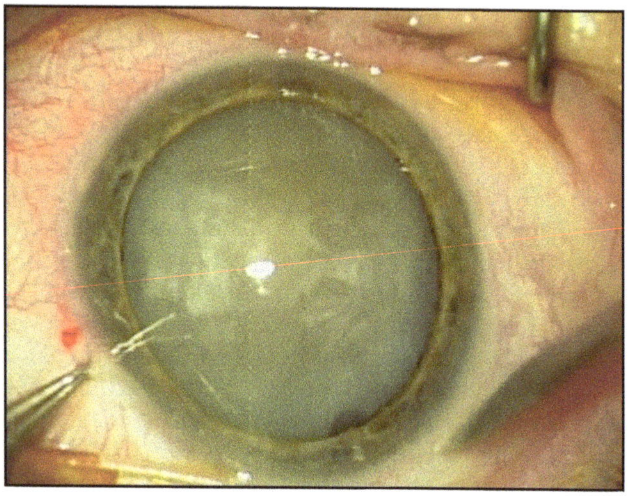

E-1. Complications in brunescent, intumescent cataract.

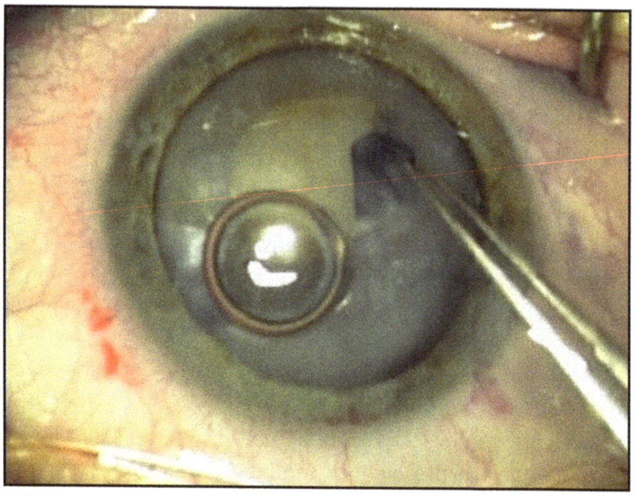

E-2. Trypan blue on the anterior capsule; the rhexis is escaping.

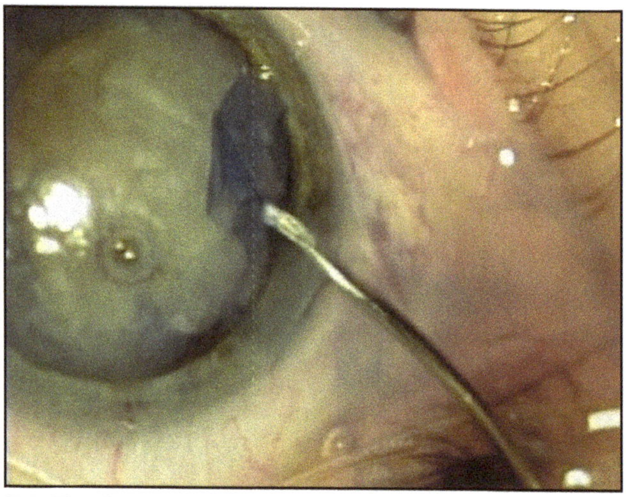

E-3. The rhexis has escaped the surgeon's control at 2 different points.

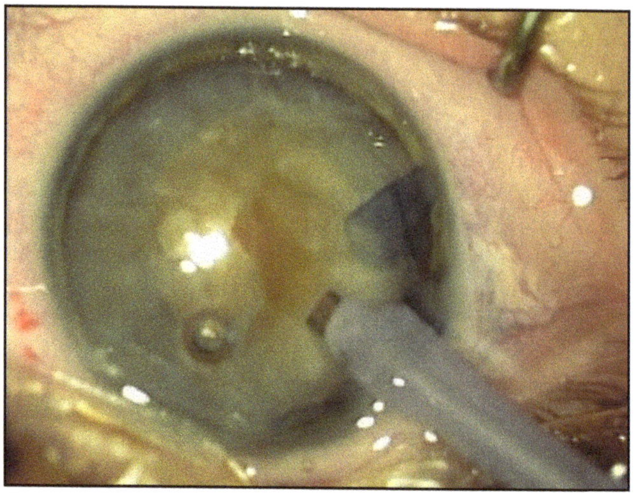

E-4. During phaco, the vitreous shifted forward.

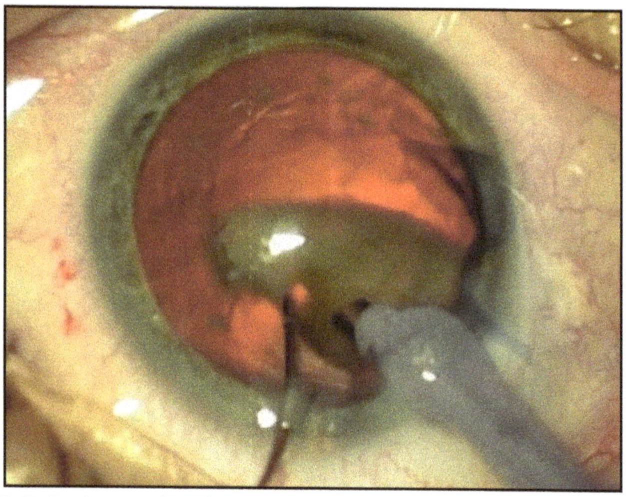

E-5. A mixture of nucleus and vitreous.

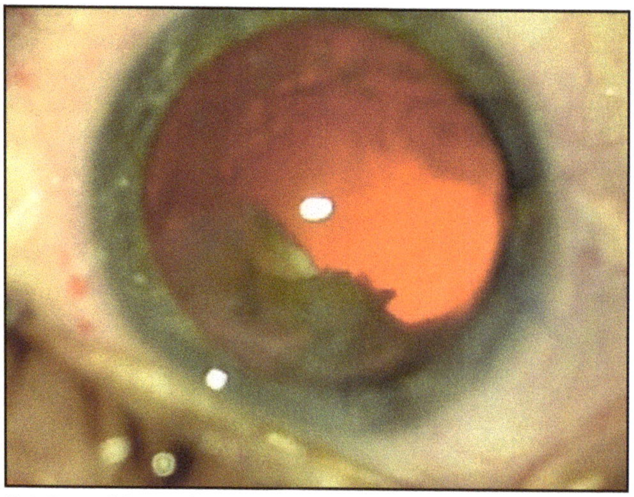

E-6. Part of the nucleus is in the vitreous. Posterior vitrectomy is necessary and scleral fixated IOL implantation.

8

Cataract in High Myopia

Cataract surgery in eyes with high myopia can be very challenging. Myopic eyes have an axial length in excess of 25.5 to 26.0 mm, with refraction usually greater than -8 diopters (D). This is associated with alterations of the sclera, choroid, retina, and vitreous, with differing degrees of severity.

In these eyes, one should prepare for a number of pre-, intra-, and postoperative difficulties. Preoperatively, problems begin with the initial examination, the examination of the fundus, treatment of rhegmatogenus lesions, calculation of power, and choice of the intraocular lens (IOL). Intraoperative difficulties include the type of anesthesia, reduced resistance or thinning of some tissues, vitreous degeneration, and fragility of the capsular-zonular complex. Finally, postoperatively, it is important to maintain the integrity and transparency of the posterior capsule to prevent vitreoretinal complications and maintain ability of examining the fundus in fine detail.

Anatomical-Surgical Considerations

There are several anatomical differences between myopic and emmetropic eyes. The ocular parameters, as observed by François and Goes,[1] showed the depth of the anterior chamber (AC) is greater in the myopic eye compared to the emmetropic eye. This difference is greater in young patients, less than 25 with myopia greater than – 15 D (AC equal or greater to 3.63 mm). Regarding lens power, the literature reports a wide range from + 10 to + 25.22 D; however, no significant differences in the thickness have been observed. The most obvious difference is the length of the posterior chamber. In myopia greater than 15 D, the difference in length is approximately 0.37 mm for each diopter.

The structure of the ciliary body is different because it has to work much less in the myopic eye than in emmetropic or hyperopic eyes. In the ciliary muscle of myopes, longitudinal fibers dominate over circular ones, which are almost totally absent, leading to reduction of accommodation.

This gives the muscle a tapered shape with the greatest thickness posteriorly with respect to the emmetropic eye.

The zonular fibers appear to be weaker due to the low levels of movement and stretching deriving from increased fiber diameter; this may result in increased weakness and greater incidence of subluxation of the lens, compared to emmetropic eyes.

The sclera can be variably thinner and weaker. This may lead to the formation of staphylomas that frequently develop in the posterior sclera; they may also occur at the equator, in particular in the superotemporal quadrant.

The choroid is distended, thinned, and atrophic, and Bruch's membrane may have breaks that allow neovascularization to invade the subretinal macular space with serious visual consequences.

These eyes have a greater tendency to acute intraoperative subchoroidal hemorrhage. A study by Hoffmann and Waubke[2] many years ago reported an incidence of 14.9% in severe myopic eyes undergoing intracapsular extraction technique, as compared to 0.77% of emmetropic eyes. More recently,[3] severe myopia is considered to be one of the major causes of subchoroidal hemorrhage (along with glaucoma and diabetes). The frequency shows no statistically significant differences between intra- and extracapsular cataract extraction (ICCE, ECCE, respectively). With phacoemulsification, this has become very rare.

In the high myope, great attention must be paid to the vitreoretinal complex. The vitreous undergoes early syneresis. This change of the vitreous, combined with zonular laxity, offers less resistance to the positive pressure from the infusion during surgery. There will be subsequent deepening of the AC and undesired traction forces on the zonules. According to a study by Coppè and Lapucci,[4] during phacoemulsification, 3 different mechanisms are activated, and these may be responsible for posterior vitreous detachment (PVD)—anterior shift of the vitreous, fluctuation and intracameral turbulence with destabilization of the vitreous and retinal traction, and finally, intra- or postoperative rupture of the posterior capsule. These causes of PVD may be responsible for postoperative detachment of the retina,

Buratto L, Brint SF, Caretti L.
Cataract Surgery in Complicated Cases (pp 105-110).

with or without peripheral retinal degeneration detected prior to surgery.

There may be central and peripheral retinal defects of the severely myopic patient, in proportion to the severity of the myopia; the surgeon must identify any peripheral rhegmatogenic degeneration. These may lead to retinal detachment from a previous rhegmatogenic lesion, particularly if the integrity of the posterior capsule has been compromised (intra- or postoperatively following ytrrium-aluminum-garnet [YAG] laser capsulotomy).

Cataract surgery is responsible for a 40-fold increase[5] in the risk of retinal detachment in severely myopic patients compared to emmetropic eyes. Even postoperative YAG laser capsulotomy increases the risk of retinal detachment, approximately 3.9 times greater in myopic eyes than in emmetropic eyes, according to some.[6] Capsulotomy destabilizes the matrix of the hyaluronic acid, destroys the anterior hyaloid, and reduces the concentration of hyaluronic acid. This can lead to posterior detachment of the vitreous and subsequently to detachment of the retina. The incidence of retinal detachment following YAG laser capsulotomy is less than 1% in emmetropic eyes. This figure rises to 10% in some studies of high myopes.[7] In a study by Ranta et al,[8] the risk of postcapsulotomy retinal detachment is 2%, and this figures rises to 5.8% in cases without prophylactic treatment. Moreover, the risk is greater if the axial length is greater than 25 mm.

In another recent study, Alimanovic[9] reports a similar risk of retinal detachment (2.5%), with an increase in frequency over time and is correlated to the size of the capsulotomy. To reduce the risk of this complication, the surgeon should create a capsulotomy diameter of 4 mm or smaller.

High Myopia and Cataracts

It is well known that cataracts in highly myopic patients appear more frequently in middle age, and the most frequent type is the posterior cortical cataract. Young patients with high myopia will experience a combination of lens opacity and deterioration in vision. These young patients will normally request surgery earlier than the emmetropic patient, as the patient's visual needs are very important

Surgery eliminates the visual problem caused by the lens opacity and will simultaneously correct the myopic refractive error. Some surgeons think clear lens extraction should be considered. There are enormous advantages, but it also increases the risk of postoperative detachment of the vitreous and the retina. Retinal detachment is the most frequent complication with this type of surgery and is highly debated.

There are also associations of cataract surgery in high myopia and progression of neovascular maculopathy. Some studies suggest that phacoemulsification induces a 12.5% increased risk of developing choroidal neovascularization.[10]

Surgically, ICCE is obsolete and has been abandoned for a number of reasons (eg, it induces an unacceptable increase in the frequency of postoperative retinal detachment, between 0.4% and 5.74%). ECCE is still a valid option as it maintains an intact posterior capsule, but reduces intraoperative control and increases astigmatism and slows postoperative recovery, thus it is rarely used in high myopia. By limiting the anterior movement of the vitreous, the intact posterior capsule reduces the incidence of anterior hyaloid rupture, vitreous traction, and loss of hyaluronic acid with a lower frequency of posterior detachment of the vitreous and possible retinal detachment. In the general population, the vitreoretinal complications are considerably lower for ECCE (with an intact capsule, with or without the implantation of an IOL) compared to ICCE, 1.5% (range 0% to 3.7%), increasing post YAG.

Phacoemulsification is preferred for the myopic eye because of intraoperative stability of the AC, a high level of control, insertion of the IOL in the bag, and the micro-incision. There is a vast amount of literature describing the correlation between phacoemulsification and retinal detachment. This complication is usually observed in 4.4% of cases (range 0% to 8%), following phacoemulsification with or without implantation of an IOL. A recent paper[11] reports the risk of retinal detachment is 1.17%; this risk rises to 5.17% in patients under 50 years of age. Another study, on a series of 2175 eyes with phacoemulsification and the implantation of the IOL in the bag, reported a 4.6% risk of retinal detachment.[12]

The risk of retinal detachment increases considerably if the posterior capsule is ruptured during surgery, as confirmed by a recent study by Jakobsson et al.[13] Another study,[14] on 9388 eyes with a follow-up of 4 years, reported that the cumulative risk of retinal detachment in high myopia following cataract extraction and implantation of an IOL increases over time, resulting in a late-onset increase of this serious complication.

Preoperative Evaluation

Prior to cataract surgery in a patient with high myopia, the surgeon should pay attention to the external evaluation, the anterior segment, and particularly the posterior segment. If the opacity of the lens permits, it is essential to evaluate the macula and periphery of the retina using modern diagnostic equipment. The condition of the posterior pole predicts the patient's postoperative visual recovery; precise biometry is required. The surgeon must also evaluate the ability of the pupil to dilate, the chamber depth, and particularly the stability of the lens.

Selection of Postoperative Refraction

In planning the surgery the situation of the other eye must also be taken into consideration. The surgeon may aim to reduce the overall discomfort in binocular vision of the highly myopic patient. Surgery aims to restore sharp vision, with or without the use of spectacles or contact lenses. With surgery, routine activities can be greatly improved with appropriate postoperative refraction, or quality of life may deteriorate, particularly if hyperopia has been induced.

The decision to aim for emmetropia or myopia is based on the patient's age and visual requirements. Normally, in a patient of middle-to-older age, particularly in patients who treasure their near vision, the surgeon should induce moderate myopia (1 to 4 D); this will allow good near vision with no need for optical correction. The patient will be able to perform routine functions (eg, reading and writing) with no need for spectacles or contact lenses. In nonpresbyopic patients, the surgeon should aim for emmetropia, using a contact lens for distance vision in the fellow eye and spectacles for near vision in the operated eye. In the younger patient with moderate presbyopia, the objective of surgery should be slight myopia in the operated eye and emmetropia with a contact lens in the nonoperated eye to achieve monovision.

When planning the postoperative refraction, the surgeon must consider the following:

- Hyperopia is to be avoided; this condition would require the patient to use spectacles for both near and distance vision. Hyperopia completely changes the refractive situation, interfering with everyday routine activities.
- One should avoid anisometropia. Normally patients will tolerate differences between the 2 eyes less than 3 D; greater differences will lead to binocular discomfort, anisiconia, and asthenopia.
- The situation of the contralateral eye must always be taken into consideration; the refractive plan will be more straightforward if both eyes require surgery.

If only one eye requires surgery, there are a number of different options: postoperative refraction of approximately -3 to 4 D or correction of the contralateral eye with a contact lens to create compatible refraction; in this case, the patient will have good binocular balance, good near vision, and will require contact lenses for distance vision. If the patient does not tolerate contact lenses, the myopia may be treated using excimer laser corneal correction.

Extraction of the contralateral lens is indicated if the lens has an early cataract; however, if the lens is completely clear, the surgeon should opt for a pure refractive solution.

Intraocular Lens

One of the final frontiers in ophthalmology lies with precise selection of the power of the IOL to be used. The calculation of the appropriate IOL power for eyes with high myopia is complicated by 2 factors: the measurement of axial length and the calculation formula used.

The presence of a posterior staphyloma, more frequent with an increased axial length, often causes an axial length error, with a subsequent IOL power miscalculation. The staphyloma will displace and tilt the macula with respect to the optical axis,[15,16] thus giving different measurements from repeated biometric readings. To reduce the margin of error in these cases, one can use B-scan immersion echography in an attempt to visualize the macula inside the staphyloma; the reference point is the optic nerve and the surgeon attempts to identify the macula on the temporal side of the insertion point. The use of biometry (IOL Master [Carl Zeiss Meditec, Dublin, CA]) can further improve the accuracy of the axial length measurement by using a precise point of retinal fixation inside the staphyloma.[17]

The second factor of difficulty lies with the choice of the formula. Two types of formulas have been developed over the years:

1. Theoretical optic formulas (laws of geometric optics applied to schematic eyes)
2. Regression formulas by SRK (analysis of mathematical regression of clinical findings obtained by Sanders, Retzlaff, and Kraff)[18]

Initially, theoretical formulas proved to be inadequate for the correction of myopic eyes.

The standard regression formulas, which work well for emmetropic eyes, are inadequate for very long or very short eyes.

Linear regression formulas were introduced with an A that is different for eyes with an axial length greater than 24.5 mm or alternatively polymodal analysis regression formulas, derived from the same group of myopic patients. The problem with these formulas is that they are all based on the axial length and the central corneal power to predict the postoperative position of the implant. Moreover, they are based on mathematical factors that often make the formulas inaccurate on a wide range of axial lengths. The Holladay 2 is considered to be better, because it uses the AC depth and a number of other variables, such as the thickness of the lens and the corneal diameter, to predict the final position of the IOL.[19-22]

Both types of formulas have been adapted to moderately myopic eyes with an axial length of between 22 and 24.5 mm.[23] According to Terzi et al[24] and Haigis,[25] optimization of the constants for the IOLs improves the accuracy of the power calculation. In a study, Petermeier et al[26] concluded that with optimized constants, the SRK-T, Haigis, Hoffer-Q, and Holladay 2 formulas only produce a small variation of the postoperative refraction with respect to the refractive target. Currently, Hoffer considers the SRK-T formula to be the most reliable for globes longer than 26 mm and is probably the most commonly used today; for eyes between 24.5 and 26 mm, the Holladay 2 is indicated, and below this length, the Hoffer Q is the most reliable[15,16] (Table 8-1).

Presently, another option is the light-adjustable IOL, produced by Calhoun Vision (Pasadena, CA) and now

Table 8-1.

Most Popular Formulas Used Depending on the Refraction

EMMETROPIA	SRK-T
MYOPIA	
Mild (axial length < 24.5 mm)	Hoffer-Q
Mild-moderate (axial length 24.5 to 26 mm)	Holladay-2
Severe (axial length > 26 mm)	SRK-T
HYPEROPIA	
Haigis (axial length< 22mm)	Hoffer-Q, Holladay-2
If anterior segment is reduced	SRK-II

commercially available outside the United States; the lens allows correction of residual myopic error of up to −2 D.[27]

For myopic eyes, it is preferable to implant acrylic lenses as they lead to less posterior capsule opacity than silicone and particularly their polymethylmethacrylate counterparts; these latter lenses require enlarging the main incision, losing one of the most important advantages of phacoemulsification. Acrylic IOLs possess chemical-physical characteristics that limit cell proliferation, and particularly IOLs with a square edge lead to a lower percentage of postoperative posterior capsule opacity.[28] Acrylic lenses are available with low or negative powers and can be implanted with injectors through microincisions. Moreover, with potential vitreoretinal surgery, acrylic IOLs are not associated with the problems of silicone oil interaction.

Surgical Procedures

Anesthesia

For phaco in high myopes, topical anesthesia is recommended, frequently combined with intracameral anesthesia. As mentioned previously, the myopic eye is longer and larger than the standard eye; moreover, the sclera is thinner with numerous staphylomas. Using topical anesthesia avoids serious risks associated with retrobulbar anesthesia, such as the accidental perforation of the eye, retinal complications secondary to compression required to diffuse the anesthetic (retinal detachment, retinal artery or vein occlusion), and retrobulbar hemorrhage that would require abortion of surgery. Other more infrequent complications of retrobulbar anesthesia are pain associated with the introduction of the needle and the anesthetic, a certain degree of respiratory and central nervous system depression, and the possibility of contralateral amaurosis.

In these myopic eyes, peribulbar anesthesia is preferable to retrobulbar as it is safer, more straightforward, easier, and less painful. It also avoids the complications and the discomfort associated with the retrobulbar and facial nerve block. The anesthetic agent is not injected into the muscular cone; anesthesia is achieved by diffusion and requires a greater quantity of anesthetic (8 to 10 mL) compared to retrobulbar (3 to 5 mL).

Surgical Technique

In terms of the corneal incisions, it should be remembered that in the myopic eye, due to the deepening of the AC associated with positive pressure from infusion, not counterbalanced by posterior vitreous pressure, frequently the phaco tip and the other instruments must be used more vertically than normal (Figure 8-1). The tunnel created is therefore slightly shorter to avoid corneal distortion that may occur when the tunnel is excessively long.

It is not appropriate to suggest a specific type of viscoelastic substance (VES). The choice must be based on each individual case; for example, with an extremely dense nucleus that requires more ultrasound energy, dispersive or pseudoadaptive VES is recommended to provide better protection of the corneal endothelium.

We recommend that the capsulorrhexis is always performed using forceps to allow tangential traction forces on the circular profile of the capsulotomy, avoiding centrifugal traction that is more damaging for the zonules. The surgeon should create small tears using tangential traction, frequently moving the forceps to grasp the edge of the rhexis at its insertion point with the capsule. Our recommendation is that the rhexis should be just slightly smaller than the diameter of the IOL so that the edge of the rhexis covers the edge of the IOL, with less creasing and less opacification of the posterior capsule. In cases with significant anterior-posterior fluctuations of the nucleus, a large anterior capsulorrhexis allows the surgeon the opportunity to luxate the nucleus into the AC and then proceed with its removal.

Hydrodissection must be completed perfectly, with the cleavage plane between the capsule and the cortex. This will minimize tension on the capsular bag and zonules during the maneuvers to rotate and remove the nucleus. Presently, with nucleofracture and the new instruments available, phacoaspiration is the most frequently used maneuver, with low ultrasound and high vacuum values. The main difference between phacoemulsification in these and normal eyes is that when the ultrasound tip is inserted, because of the positive infusion pressure, the chamber deepens; this is caused by a number of factors including zonular fragility, sclera thinning, and partial vitreous liquefaction. It may be responsible for undesired zonular traction, and the surgeon must try to maintain an appropriate chamber depth. Thus, the infusion bottle should be lowered; the surgeon can adjust the height case by case based on the AC depth (with infusion active). A lower flow rate in the AC will also result in lower intracameral turbulence with less stimulus of the iris thus less miosis, adding more difficulty.

No specific technique to deal with the cataract in the highly myopic patient is advocated; the surgeon must ensure that all movements are cautious and gentle, ensuring that the integrity of the posterior capsule and the zonules are preserved. All of the parameters are reduced: ultrasound power, aspiration flow rate, vacuum, and infusion. In young patients with very soft cataracts, the phaco roll technique may prove useful. In the case of harder nuclei in more elderly myopic patients, the technique that we would recommend is the quick chop, an endocapsular technique that normally uses high vacuum (140 to 160 mm Hg) and a chop hook used inside the margin of the rhexis, clearly visible to the surgeon.

If the surgeon is still faced with an excessively deep AC or with partial zonular disinsertion, the supracapsular phaco chop can be considered. This technique causes less zonular stress and the surgeon will not have to tilt the instruments as much. However, for this technique, the surgeon must perform a larger capsulorrhexis to allow the nucleus to be easily luxated in the supracapsular space, in front of the anterior rhexis.

A critical consideration is traction on the vitreous base induced at various stages during surgery. In particular, collapse of the AC is unwanted and may occur immediately following removal of the phaco tip or irrigation/aspiration cannula from the eye. When the AC collapses because of a lack of infusion, the posterior capsule and the vitreous move forward and this movement can be significant and sudden.

This phenomenon can be reduced by delicately removing the instruments from the AC or by filling the AC with cohesive VES injected through the paracentesis, prior to removing the phaco tip or the irrigation/aspiration cannula.

Once phacoemulsification has been completed, the surgeon proceeds with aspiration of the cortex, a maneuver facilitated by good hydrodissection. Meticulous removal of the cortex will be easier and safer, reducing posterior capsule opacity. The surgeon should use a low flow rate and a low vacuum, for complete removal of the material while reducing tension on the zonules. The common coaxial systems are ideal for removing a large part of the cortex; difficulties may appear with subincisional cortex particularly if the tunnel is excessively long or if the rhexis is small or decentered inferiorly. Buratto's bimanual system consists of 2 separate handpieces (one for irrigation and the other for aspiration) that are inserted through 2 separate paracentesis incisions. The aspiration cannula pulls the fragments toward the center; the irrigation cannula maintains bag distension.

The surgeon must use a low flow rate and low vacuum to reduce tension forces on the zonules. Inappropriate zonular stress can occur when the surgeon enters the AC with irrigation on and a chamber filled with VES.

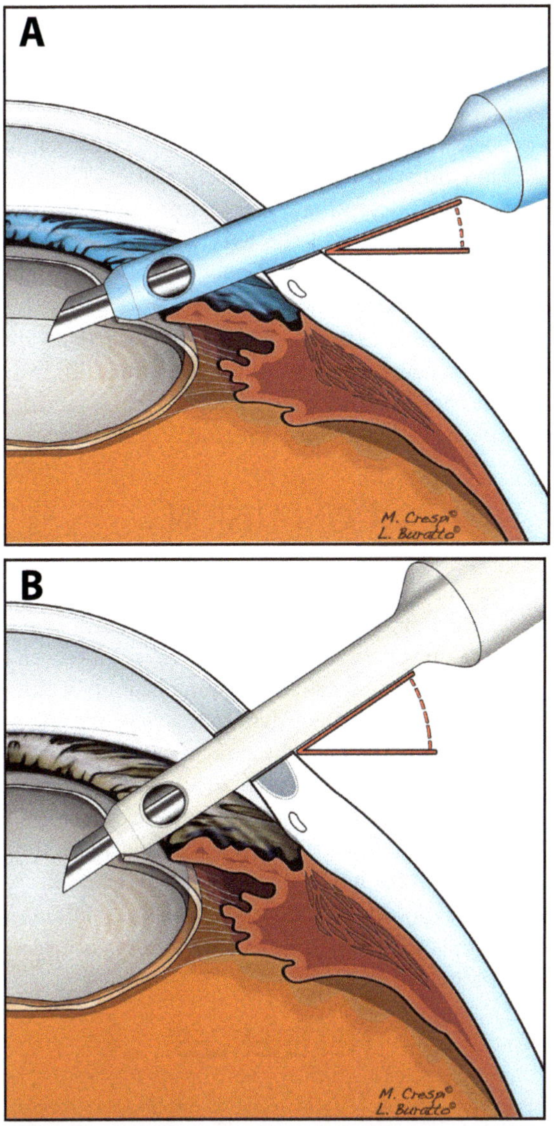

Figure 8-1. (A) The inclination of the instrument in the emmetropic eye and (B) the myopic eye in which the inclination is greater.

Bimanual cannulas also allow careful cleaning of the posterior capsule and the anterior subcapsular epithelium, if necessary.

There has been some debate about the use of capsular tension rings (CTRs) in severely myopic eyes (see Chapter 2). We feel that these devices are appropriate only with serious zonular weakness. Moreover, the timing for insertion is also a subject of discussion. Some surgeons feel that the CTR should be inserted as soon as laxity is observed (ie, prior to phacoemulsification), others believe that it should be prior to irrigation/aspiration, and others are of the opinion it should be inserted before the implantation of the IOL (the most popular solution). Others do not advocate CTRs because, in their opinion, in the long-term, an extremely weakened bag can result in the luxation of the IOL-tension ring-capsular bag complex into the vitreous, a situation that is much more difficult to manage as opposed to the luxation of the IOL-capsular bag complex alone (also refer to the chapter on traumatic cataract and on the congenital subluxation of the lens). In a recent article,[29] it was reported that in severe myopes, the implantation of the tension ring did not significantly matter. The authors concluded that implanting a ring did not cause significant change in the position of the IOL; consequently, the surgeon did not need to modify the power of the IOL, with or without a tension ring.

The IOL implantation, preferably acrylic, is no different from standard cataract surgery; an injector through a microincision induces minimal or no astigmatism. The completion of the procedure is performed as normal.

Conclusion

The myopic cataract patient usually has a high degree of satisfaction, improving quality of life, greatly reducing dependence on spectacles or contact lenses. Moreover, retinal detachment—the most serious complication of this surgery—is much less frequent than in the past. Opacification of the posterior capsule has been greatly reduced thanks to the use of acrylic IOLs. Future developments may include the possibility of instruments (such as Perfect Capsule [Milvella Ltd, Epping, Australia]) or substances to inject into the capsular bag or coat the IOL and block cell proliferation.

In the not-too-distant future, clear lens extraction in the highly myopic patient will be much more readily accepted by the ophthalmic community.

References

1. François J, Goes F. Oculometry of progressive myopia. *Bibl Ophthalmol.* 1975;(83):277-282.
2. Hoffmann DH, Waubke T. Results of cataract extraction with and without enzymatic zonulolysis. *Klin Monbl Augenheilkd Augenarztl Fortbild.* 1961;139:527-533.
3. Obuchowska I, Mariak Z. Risk factors of massive suprachoroidal hemorrhage during extracapsular cataract extraction surgery. *Eur J Ophthalmol.* 2005;15(6):712-717.
4. Coppè AM, Lapucci G. Posterior vitreous detachment and retinal detachment following cataract extraction. *Curr Opin Ophthalmol.* 2008;19(3):234-242.
5. Colin J, Robinet A. Clear lensectomy and implantation of low-power posterior chamber intraocular lens for correction of high myopia: a four-year follow-up. *Ophthalmology.* 1997;104(1):73-77.
6. Javitt JC, Tielsch J, Canner JK, Jolb MM, Sommer A, Steinberg EP. National outcomes of cataract extraction. Increased risk of retinal complications associated with Nd:YAG laser capsulotomy. The Cataract Patients Outcomes Research Team. *Ophthalmology.* 1996;103(10):1537-1545.
7. Koch DD, Liu JF, Gill EP, Parke DW. Axial myopia increases the risk of retinal complications after neodymium-YAG laser posterior capsulotomy. *Arch Ophthalmol.* 1989;107(7):986-990.
8. Ranta P, Tommila P, Kivelä T. Retinal breaks and detachment after neodymium: YAG laser posterior capsulotomy: five-year incidence in a prospective cohort. *J Cataract Refract Surg.* 2004:30(1):58-66.
9. Alimanovic HE. Correlation between eye aperture diameter and complications in the posterior eye segment after Nd-YAG capsulotomy. *Bosn J Basic Med Sci.* 2008;8(2):106-109.
10. Hayashi K, Ohno-Matsui K, Futagami S, Ohno S, Tokoro T, Mochizuki M. Choroidal neovascularization in highly myopic eyes after cataract surgery. *Jpn J Ophthalmol.* 2006;50(4):345-348.
11. Russell M, Gaskin B, Russell D, Polkinghorne PJ. Pseudophakic retinal detachment after phacoemulsification cataract surgery: ten-year retrospective review. *J Cataract Refract Surg.* 2006;32(3):442-445.
12. Grand MG. The risk of a new retinal break or detachment following cataract surgery in eyes that had undergone repair of phakic break or detachment: a hypothesis of a causal relationship to cataract surgery. *Trans Am Ophthalmol Soc.* 2003;101:335-369.
13. Jakobsson G, Montan P, Zetterberg M, Stenevi U, Behndig A, Lundström M. Capsule complication during cataract surgery: retinal detachment after cataract surgery with capsule complication: Swedish Capsule Rupture Study Group report 4. *J Cataract Refract Surg.* 2009;35(10):1699-1705.
14. Sheu SJ, Ger LP, Ho WL. Late increased risk of retinal detachment after cataract extraction. *Am J Ophthalmol.* 2010;149(1):113-119.
15. Update on IOL power calculations formulas. In: Garg A, Hoyos JE, Dementiev J, eds. *Mastering Techniques of IOL Power Calculations.* New Delhi, India: Jaypee Brothers; 2005:16-22.
16. Kohnen S, Brauweiler P. First results of cataract surgery and implantation of negative power intraocular lenses in highly myopic eyes. *J Cataract Refract Surg.* 1996;22:416-420.
17. MacLaren RE, Sagoo MS, Restore M, Allan BD. Biometry accuracy using zero-and negative-powered intraocular lenses. *J Cataract Refract Surg.* 2005;31:280-290.
18. Olsen T. Calculation of intraocular lens power: a review. *Acta Ophthalmol Scand.* 2007;85:427-485.
19. Holladay JT, Prager TC. Accurate ultrasonic biometry in pseudophakia. *Am J Ophthalmol.* 1989;107:189-190.
20. Smith LF, Stevens JD, Larkin F, Restori M. Errors leading to unexpected pseudophakic ametropia. *Eye.* 2001;15:728-732.
21. Kora Y, Koike M, Suzuki Y, Inatomi M, Fukado Y, Ozawa T. Errors in IOL power calculations for axial high myopia. *Ophthalmic Surg.* 1991;22:78-81.
22. Duffey RJ, Leaming D. US trends in refractive surgery: 2002 ISRS survey. *J Refract Surg.* 2003;19:357-363.
23. Hill WE, Byrne SF. Complex axial length measurements and unusual IOL power calculations. In: Points F, ed. *Clinical Modules for Ophthalmologists.* San Francisco, CA: American Academy of Ophthalmology; 2004.
24. Terzi E, Wang L, Kohnen T. Accuracy of modern intraocular lens power calculation formulas in refractive lens exchange for high myopia and high hyperopia. *J Cataract Refract Surg.* 2009;35:1181-1189.
25. Haigis W. Intraocular lens calculation in extreme myopia. *J Cataract Refract Surg.* 2009;35:906-911.
26. Petermeier K, Gekeler F, Messias A, Spitzer MS, Haigis W, Szurman P. Intraocular lens power calculation and optimized constants for highly myopic eyes. *J Cataract Refract Surg.* 2009;35:1575-1581.
27. Hengere FH, Hutz WW, Dick HB, Conrad-Heneger I. Combined correction of sphere and astigmatism using the light-adjustable intraocular lens in eyes with axial myopia. *J Cataract Refract Surg.* 2011;37(2):317-323.
28. Hayashi K, Yoshida M, Hayashi H. Posterior capsule opacification in myopic eyes. *J Cataract Refract Surg.* 2006;32(4):634-638.
29. Schild AM, Rosentreter A, Hellmich M, Lappas A, Dislage S, Dietlein TS. Effect of a capsular tension ring on refractive outcomes in eyes with high myopia. *J Cataract Refract Surg.* 2010;36(12):2087-2093.

9

Cataract in Severe Hyperopia

Hyperopia is usually considered to be a refractive error providing good distance vision and poor near vision. Eyes with severe hyperopia, greater than 3 to 4 diopters (D), have a number of different anatomical, pathological, and surgical features. Depending on the degree of hyperopia, young patients usually have good uncorrected vision for a long period of time, eventually losing accommodation and becoming dependent on optical correction. With severe hyperopia, optical correction is necessary for most of the patient's life.

Hyperopia may be due to a shorter axial length than normal due to a growth defect (axial hyperopia), a reduction in the refractive index of the cornea and/or the lens, an excessive distance between the lens and the cornea (the anterior chamber [AC] is deeper), or total absence of the lens (aphakia).

Severely hyperopic eyes are more prone to closed-angle glaucoma, particularly in elderly patients. This is due to a smaller-than-usual anterior segment, with a shallow AC and narrow angle.

Surgery in severely hyperopic patients may be quite challenging. Difficulties involve measuring the axial length, calculating the intraocular lens (IOL) power, and even obtaining commercially available IOLs. Intraoperative difficulties of these small eyes are associated with the diminished space in the anterior segment, greater risk of the suprachoroidal hemorrhage fluid misdirection syndrome, expulsive hemorrhage, and the frequent occurrence of poor mydriasis or even miosis. Intractable miosis, frequently seen in these patients, is often associated with prolonged use of miotic eyedrops that may be associated with the formation of posterior synechiae and/or pupillary membranes and alterations of the lens. Extremely difficult are those patients in which severe hyperopia is associated with microphthalmos. However, with improvements in biometry, phacoemulsification, and piggyback implantation techniques when necessary, it is possible to achieve highly satisfactory results even in these difficult patients.

Determination of the Axial Length and Power of the Intraocular Lens

Accurate axial length measurements and determining the correct power of the IOL are the most important steps to achieving a precise refractive result in severely hyperopic patients. For extremely precise measurements of axial length, partial coherence interferometry biometry is available, which also accurately calculates the corneal curvature and depth of the AC. The IOL Master (Carl Zeiss Meditec, Dublin, CA) was the first commercially available noncontact biometry device. It can provide extremely accurate measurements, without discomfort for the patient, and it is currently the most popular system used in calculation of the IOL power for cataract surgery, according to a recent consensus held in Padua, Italy, in early of 2011 (unpublished proceedings).

Contact ultrasound biometry devices, on the other hand, are normally calibrated at a moderate speed for eyes of normal dimensions. They can be sources of error when used in eyes that are excessively short, as with severe hyperopic patients, and may induce corneal indentation during applanation. Therefore, we prefer immersion biometry for the measurement of axial length, as this method avoids corneal applanation and allows an extremely accurate measurement.

AC depth and thickness of the lens must be measured extremely accurately, as the postoperative effective position of the IOL, and therefore its effective power in pseudophakia, depends on it. Also, along with slit-lamp observation, biometry is used to determine whether or not a hyperopic eye has a normal or short anterior segment; this may prove useful when scheduling and performing the surgery. It is

Buratto L, Brint SF, Caretti L.
Cataract Surgery in Complicated Cases (pp 111-116).

important to remember that neither very short nor very long eyes adapt perfectly to static IOL formulas, despite numerous modifications in existence. Consequently, in hyperopia, for the most part, the eyes are undercorrected (see the Intraocular Lens section in this chapter).

Surgical Anatomy of the Severely Hyperopic Eye

Accurate evaluation of the surgical anatomy of the hyperopic eye is fundamentally important when implementing a successful surgical strategy with a reduced risk of complications.

Hyperopic eyes can be divided into 2 categories: those with a short anterior segment and those with a normal anterior segment.[1,2] Some characteristics are present in all severely hyperopic or microphthalmic eyes. Other characteristics are found in just a portion of them.

Hyperopic Eyes With a Short Anterior Segment

Only a small amount of hyperopic eyes have a short anterior segment (17% according to an older study by Holladay[1]). The characteristic-reduced dimensions of the anterior segment are proportionate to the axial length (almost always less than 22 mm), associated with a crystalline lens of more-or-less normal dimensions, which tends to push the iris forward, reducing the AC depth. The cornea has a small diameter but normal thickness, the iris is often dark and thick, and the angle is very narrow (0 to 2 according to Shaffer's scale). As a result, these eyes are predisposed to acute glaucoma (which is not always associated with severe hyperopia). This condition may appear in young patients (ie, younger than 40 years of age). Frequently, this type of eye will require cataract surgery following a long-standing history of narrow- or closed-angle glaucoma, frequently post-yttrium-aluminum-garnet (YAG) laser iridotomy with a very small pupil that cannot be dilated well due to prolonged miotic therapy. Descemet's membrane adheres less firmly to the corneal stroma as opposed to normal eyes, and small areas of stripping near the incision due to the shallow AC should be closely monitored. The endothelial cell count is often reduced, an important consideration as the cataract nucleus is frequently hard and the surgeon has to work near the endothelium. Normally, the zonules are fairly strong, with the exception of some cases of microphthalmos in which they may be very weak. The sclera and the choroid are normally thick; the vitreous has a normal consistency with no breaks or detachments typical of severe myopia. During the cataract operation, vitreous pressure often occurs and may be associated with choroidal effusion.

Hyperopic Eyes With a Normal Anterior Segment

The majority of cases with severe hyperopia or microphthalmos are included in this group (83% according to the study by Holladay[1]). The characteristic features are an anterior segment of normal size not proportionate to the shortened axial length. The dimensions of the cornea and the AC depth are normal; the angle is open with no risk of closure. The reduced axial length is often unexpected and is apparent only with biometry. In these eyes, hyperopia is considered to be a refractive error for which the patient will often request early refractive surgery. The zonules are often weak and sometimes associated with subluxation of the lens. Similarly, the sclera and the choroid are thick, and the vitreous has a normal consistency.

Surgical Technique: Difficulties and Management (Eyes With a Small Anterior Segment)

When severely hyperopic eyes are operated, even experienced surgeons encounter difficulties when the anterior segment is reduced. (There will be postoperative refractive problems if the anterior segment is normal.) As usual, topical anesthesia is recommended, which will allow surgery to be safely performed and reduce the risk of vitreous pressure.

Incisions between 2 to 2.2 mm in clear cornea are preferable, sized for the fine micro-coaxial phacoemulsification tips. The advantage with a clear corneal incision of a severely hyperopic patient is basically a more direct approach to the cataract in eyes that frequently have a shallow AC depth. The phaco tip can be easily moved toward the lens with no significant distortion. On the other hand, with a sclerocorneal incision, as the surgeon will be working "upwards," he or she will be inclined to distort the incision to correctly orient the phaco tip toward the lens. Considering that the AC may have a depth of less than 2 mm (particularly if there is closed-angle glaucoma), the corneal tunnel must be slightly longer and narrower to reduce the risk of iris prolapse and to allow the AC to be deepened, thanks to better wound closure.

With a small, correct incision, maintaining AC depth, there is a reduction in the incidence of iris prolapse and endothelial damage. The use of microincision techniques greatly facilitates maneuvers of instruments in hypothalamic eyes, as AC depth is maintained.

Very high molecular weight adhesive or pseudoadaptive viscoelastic substances (VESs) should be used as these flatten the anterior curve of the lens, with decreased tendency toward the escape of the rhexis. This should be closely monitored. AC depth will also be increased. Initially, the VES will also dilate the pupil slightly, which may be small, stabilizes the iris and persists for a longer period of time inside the AC, and finally, reduces the chance for miosis.

A good option is the soft-shell technique by Arshinoff.[3] A dispersive viscoelastic is injected first and forms a meniscus in contact with the endothelium. A cohesive VES is then injected in contact with the anterior surface of the lens; this greatly reduces the incidence of iris prolapse and provides excellent protection of the endothelium. It will also decrease trapping of lens fragments by the dispersive VES itself, if used alone. However, the surgeon should never hesitate to add additional dispersive VES if there are difficulties or if necessary. During capsulorrhexis, the surgeon should avoid distortion of the corneal incision to prevent the escape of VES with consequent shallowing of the AC and the possibility of extension of the rhexis. If this occurs, additional VES should immediately be injected, prior to completing the capsulorrhexis. In these cases, some surgeons perform the rhexis through a side-port incision with coaxial microforceps, creating the main incision only once the rhexis has been completed.

In severely hyperopic eyes with a reduced anterior segment, the pupil will often be small, and this must be managed appropriately. As mentioned earlier, miosis is often caused by prolonged miotic therapy, possibly resulting in a fibrotic pupillary ring that can be removed using capsulorrhexis forceps or crocodile forceps for vitreoretinal surgery. This maneuver may allow modest dilation of the pupil.

Pupil stretching or sphincterotomies that include no more than approximately 1 mm of iris tissue are maneuvers that are recommended only with very marked miosis. Before surgery, the inexperienced surgeon may use excessive mydriatic drugs; however, this will not resolve the miosis and may also be responsible for an increase in arterial pressure with consequent choroidal congestion and intraoperative vitreous pressure. During phacoemulsification, poor visibility associated with extreme miosis may facilitate rupture or disinsertion of the capsule with consequent prolapse of the vitreous.

Hydrodissection must be performed by injecting fluid more carefully and more slowly as opposed to standard cases to avoid a sudden increase in the intraocular pressure (IOP) and iris prolapse.

There is no particular phacoemulsification technique that is considered to be more advantageous than the other. It stands to reason that supracapsular approaches are not recommended; neither is phaco flip because of the limited space inside the AC. In our opinion, the quick chop technique, a variation of the phaco chop, is preferable. This technique allows the chopper to work inside the area of the rhexis and for the surgeon to limit the energy. High levels of vacuum and a chopper are used; using ultrasound, the surgeon creates a deep central grove. The phaco tip will act as a pivot point to split the nucleus into pieces, working against the chopper that has been pushed from above downward in front of the opening of the phaco. The high level of vacuum is used to remove the fragments of the nucleus with short ultrasound pulses.

Given that less energy is used, it is suitable for the management of the majority of nuclei associated with severe hypothalamia, thus requiring the surgeon to work with the phaco tip in a position closer to the corneal endothelium. Low endothelial cell counts should also be taken into account.

Intraocular movements must be very well controlled. Another useful suggestion is to set the flow rate correctly. The surgeon can modify the flow rate to increase pressure and deepen the AC. This is achieved by modifying the parameters on the panel (infusion) and increasing the height of the balanced salt solution (BSS). The potential for miosis and iris prolapse must be taken into account. The coaxial microincisional cataract surgery (C-MICS) technique provides excellent maintenance of the AC during all steps of the operation, with the added advantages of sealed incisions with an increase in infusion pressure.

Another intraoperative problem is the vitreous pressure, which sometimes occurs in severely hyperopic eyes, in particular with microphthalmos (with an axial length of less than 20 mm) and narrow-angle glaucoma. When it occurs, posterior vitreous pressure usually begins shortly after commencing surgery and will often be even more evident toward the end of irrigation/aspiration. If this problem occurs and the surgeon feels that he or she cannot complete the operation without complications, stop, close the wound, and complete the operation a few hours later or the following day, when the pressure has resolved—a great advantage of phaco over extracapsular surgery.

Contributing factors to the development of posterior vitreous pressure are periretrobulbar anesthesia, excessive use of mydriatic drugs, and preoperative firm eye. Choroidal effusion is initially vessel dilation with no wall rupture or choroidal hemorrhage, seen rapidly with capsular rupture and with a vitrectomy that creates space inside the vitreous cavity.

Management of more serious cases of microphthalmic eyes with severe hyperopia may include a posterior pars plana mini-vitrectomy, which should be performed initially, to increase the space in the AC with a corresponding reduction in the posterior chamber. Currently, this approach is much less traumatic for the eye than in the past, thanks to the microincision-vitrectomy-surgery technique, in particular, the 25-gauge systems. The surgeon introduces a 25-gauge trocar into the vitreous chamber 4 mm from the limbus (at 10 o'clock for right-handed surgeons and at 2 o'clock for left-handed surgeons). The vitrectomy probe is inserted into the vitreous chamber immediately behind the lens, and the surgeon performs a dry vitrectomy lasting just a few seconds, which will shift the lens backwards with deepening of the AC. The surgeon must pay maximum attention during this maneuver to avoid complications because of possible and sometimes significant weakness of the zonules in eyes with microphthalmos. The recommended parameters for the vitrectomy are 5000 cuts, 400 aspiration, and 40 infusion. The phacoemulsification procedure can now be managed under conditions of greater safety.

In hyperopic eyes with a normal anterior segment, possible intraoperative difficulties are similar to routine cataract operations. One problem that may occur in these eyes is the weakness or laxity of the zonules, which will lead to an

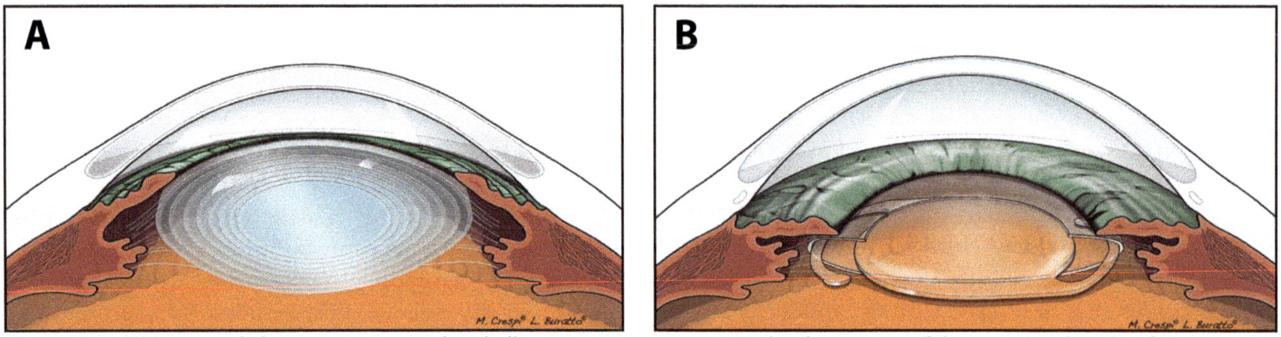

Figure 9-1. (A) In severely hyperopic eyes with a shallow anterior segment, (B) the deepening of the anterior chamber following the removal of the cataract or clear lens eliminates the risk of closed-angle glaucoma.

increase in the AC depth during phacoemulsification with the possibility of inducing zonular disinsertion; the surgeon may have to bring the instruments into a more vertical position due to the deeper position in the bag. The surgeon should lower the infusion bottle of BSS and reduce the parameters of aspiration to avoid collapse of the AC. Capsular weakness can be countered with the insertion of a tension ring; however, this will be difficult if not impossible to insert with miosis, possibly because of the vitreous pressure.

Refractive Lensectomy

Over the years, there have been many reasons why surgeons have considered removing the clear crystalline lens and implanting an IOL for refractive purposes, especially in hyperopic patients. As they age, severe hyperopes without correction have blurred vision for both near and distant vision, and also develop presbyopia, requiring addition of greater positive power to the already strong lenses they use. They do not tolerate contact lenses and even find it difficult to insert these lenses without the assistance of spectacles.

Consequently, severely hyperopic patients have a greater need for refractive surgery than the severely myopic patient; however, there are fewer surgical options available. Presently, corneal surgery cannot be used in these patients to correct errors greater than of 4 D. Phakic IOLs are not indicated for implantation in eyes with a shallow anterior segment; the risk of retinal detachment from phacoemulsification is lower as opposed to the severe myope. Lensectomy has a positive effect in the potential prevention of narrow-/closed-angle glaucoma (Figure 9-1).[4,5]

The removal of the clear lens, possibly associated with the implantation of a multifocal IOL, is a surgical option that should be considered.

Intraocular Lens

Following removal of the nucleus and cortex, the IOL is implanted in the capsular bag if the lens of appropriate dioptric power is available. The lens required is usually a high power. There are 2 reasons why the power of the IOL is high: the reduced axial length and the extreme posterior position of the IOL with respect to the corneal apex. In small eyes even with miosis, one-piece foldable acrylic lenses can be inserted fairly easily using an injector. If the surgeon decides to use an injector to implant a 3-piece acrylic lens, the insertion process may be possible in a single maneuver, however, it may prove difficult to position the polymethylmethacrylate (PMMA) loops (initially positioned in the sulcus) inside the bag.

It should be remembered that the lenses currently available rarely exceed 34 D because above this level the optical characteristics associated with the greater anterior curvature produce mediocre optical qualities. There is a basic difference between eyes with a shortened anterior segment and those with a normal one: the former require lenses of around 30 D, while the latter may require lenses of 40 D or more.

Regarding formulas, in our opinion the SRK-II is suitable only for hyperopic eyes with a small anterior segment. In a recent article,[6] the authors concluded that the Hoffer Q formula is more accurate than the SRK-T in eyes with an axial length of less than 22 mm, without customized constants of AC depth being used. An article published in 2007[7] reports findings on the largest group of severely hyperopic cataract patients. It evaluated biometry and accuracy of the formulas; according to the authors, the Haigis appears to be the most accurate. The same study highlighted an important difference between open-loop and plate-haptic IOLs, suggesting that the design of the loops can influence the effective position of the IOLs in very small eyes.

The older optical formulas (such as Binkhorst's formula with the AC depth constant varying in relation to the eye) have recently been joined by other formulas that provide more precise refractive results in eyes with severe ametropia in an attempt to reduce the approximations necessary with the static or older optic formulas. All of these formulas consider all possible variables—corneal diameter, keratometry, AC depth, lens thickness, and axial length. The most suitable optical formula is the Holladay 2; despite not being perfect, because of the anterior position of the IOL,[8] this has shown its superiority in hyperopic eyes that require implantation of an IOL of power greater than 30 D.

Piggyback

In cases that require implantation of a lens of 34 D or more to achieve emmetropia, the surgeon may decide to implant 2 IOLs (piggyback IOLs) normally used for a single implant (Figure 9-2). This is required by the power limitations of commercially available IOLs and the better optical quality supplied by aligned implants as opposed to a single implant of dioptric power close to 40 D. The first polypseudophakic implant dates back to 1993 and was used in 2 cases of microphthalmos.[9] It was rapidly adopted as a method for replacing the lens in severe hyperopia (primary piggyback) and for correction of unacceptable residual errors (myopic or hyperopic) in pseudophakic patients (secondary piggyback). When piggyback IOLs were first used, both lenses were implanted in the capsular bag; this technique was later abandoned because of possible complications, such as a late hyperopic shift that was partly linked to the dislocation of both IOLs,[10] intralenticular fibrotic membranes that were difficult to treat, and reduced visual acuity. It is no longer advisable to implant the 2 IOLs in the capsular bag; the optimal situation is to implant the posterior lens in the bag and the anterior one in the sulcus, even though this technique has resulted in a higher percentage of decentration of the anterior IOL, as reported by Baumeister and Kohnen in their studies with the Scheimpflug camera.[10]

There are 2 systems for splitting the dioptric power of the IOLs:

1. The anterior and posterior IOLs have equal power (Gills' method)[11]
2. The posterior IOL has the highest possible corrective power

We prefer the second option for 2 reasons. First, it reduces the optic distortion that may appear if the anterior IOL is decentered. Second, in the event it is necessary to replace the anterior IOL with a lens of greater power, there are more options available.

When 2 IOLs are implanted, they will be in contact at the apex, and the resulting dioptric power will be the sum of the power of the individual lenses (as long as the second lens, positioned in the sulcus, does not compress the lens implanted in the bag). The contact zone between the 2 lenses may be reduced to points when the 2 surfaces are convex and the optic is PMMA. In the case of foldable acrylic lenses, the contact may be circular and of variable size depending on the type of IOL and the dioptric power. This contact area can cause a slight reduction in visual acuity and lead to the appearance of phenomena of multifocality, recorded for the first time by Findl et al.[12]

Regarding dioptric power, the Holladay 2 formula is extremely useful because it allows the accurate calculation of the lens power based on both IOLs positioned in the bag or on one of the lenses implanted in the sulcus. In the event of residual refractive error, the anterior IOL can be replaced as soon as the day after surgery. However, this procedure does not always produce a precise refractive result as tractional forces on the capsular bag over the first month post-surgery can still modify the position of the lens optic and influence the refractive state.

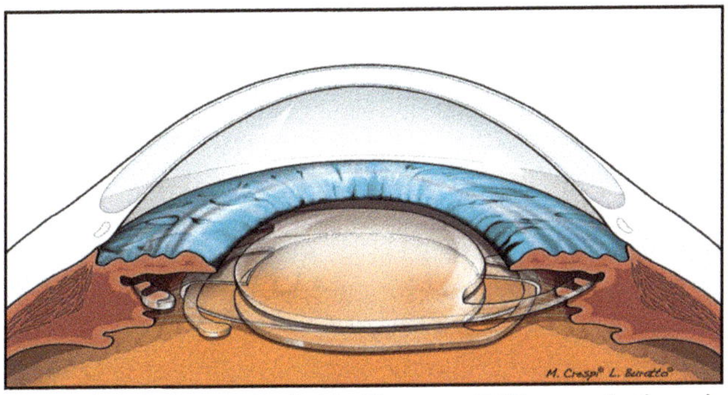
Figure 9-2. Polypseudophakia. There are 2 IOLs, one in the sulcus and one in the capsular bag.

Multifocal IOLs[13] and silicone IOLs[14] have also been used in the technique of multiple implants with good results as shown fairly recently. The authors of both papers reported findings with a group of patients implanted with a multifocal IOL in the bag and a monofocal IOL in the sulcus.

As mentioned earlier, problems can arise in eyes that have a piggyback implant both placed in the bag (not seen with lenses in PMMA); specifically, whitish matter may form between 2 foldable acrylic lenses, and this will reduce visual acuity. This phenomenon is probably due to an accumulation of VES; however, a histopathological study by Werner et al[15] suggested that the formation of this matter was linked to proliferation of cortical material from Soemmering's ring into the interlenticular space. This observation had been previously presented by Gayton,[9] who suggested meticulous removal of the cortex to prevent the formation of the opaque substance.

Another potential drawback is proliferation of Elschnig pearls between the 2 lenses, which will be responsible for a reduction in visual acuity associated with a late increase in hyperopia, as reported for the first time by Shugar and Schwartz in 1999.[16] Both of these complications are difficult to treat with the neodymium:YAG (Nd:YAG) laser and they necessitate regular and extremely complex surgery with a frequently unsatisfactory outcome. Consequently, double implantation in the bag of acrylic lenses is strongly discouraged.

The literature includes a number of cases of glaucoma associated with implantation of piggyback IOLs caused by a number of factors: pupillary block,[17] closed angle,[18] and particularly, pigment dispersion. Usually, the anterior IOL is responsible for the mechanical chafing of the iris with consequent development of glaucoma secondary to pigment dispersion.[19-21]

Another valid option is the light-adjustable IOL, available from Calhoun Vision (Pasadena, CA). These lenses allow the correction of residual hyperopic error within the range of +0.25 and +2.00 D, without jeopardizing visual acuity.

If the surgeon has to treat a primary cataract in a severely hyperopic patient or has to correct a residual refractive error in a pseudophakic patient, he or she may choose to implant the STAAR (Monrovia, CA) Collamer phakic IOL in the posterior chamber. This lens is easy to insert and remove if necessary. However, the literature reported a hyperopic shift in 2 cases of implantation in the capsular bag due to dislocation (backward movement of the IOL implanted).[22]

Yet another alternative to fine tune procedures is hyperopic laser-assisted in situ keratomileusis (LASIK), which should be performed some months following phacoemulsification to correct residual hyperopia or astigmatism.

If the capsule ruptures during surgery and the damage prevents positioning of the IOL in the bag or in the sulcus, the implant must be fixed to the sclera or the iris, as long as the appropriate lens is available and clinical conditions permit. Preferably, this implant should be performed at a later stage; it should be remembered that scleral fixation of the IOL may also be accompanied by hemorrhage in eyes with microphthalmos.

Regarding the implantation of the iris-fixated IOL, it should be remembered that the smaller dimensions of microphthalmic eyes frequently do not permit implantation of a lens in the AC.

Removal of Viscoelastic

Adequate removal of the VES injected during surgery is important to prevent onset of transient increased IOP postoperatively. If the IOP is elevated immediately postoperatively, it is not difficult to manage because the IOP can be reduced by decompressing the AC under slit-lamp control. The VES is allowed to escape through the side-port incision that has been depressed using a blunt 30-gauge cannula needle.

Conclusion

With the advent of phacoemulsification, cataract surgery in patients with severe hyperopia is possible without any major complications as compared to the past. Preoperatively, maximum attention must be given to accurate measurement of the axial length and the calculation of the IOL power, 2 components that are often imprecise. Currently, surgery is often performed earlier to allow either refractive correction or avoid angle-closure; however, the procedures may prove difficult because of anatomical conditions, partially controllable with appropriate VES, methods of pupil dilation and endothelial protection, and with low-energy phacoemulsification techniques. In addition to anatomical difficulties, these eyes also pose problems with the calculation of the IOLs and the availability of suitable IOL dioptric powers.

Piggyback IOL implantation is an option that will allow these patients to reach emmetropia with excellent vision quality. In the near future, femtosecond laser technology will allow us to further improve the already-satisfactory outcome of cataract surgery in patients affected by severe hyperopia.

References

1. Holladay JR. Achieving emmetropia in extremely short eyes. Presented at: the 1996 Annual Meeting of American Academy of Ophthalmology; 1996; Chicago, IL.
2. Gills JP, Cherchio M. Phacoemulsification in high hyperopic cataract patients. In: Lu LW, Fine IH. *Phacoemulsification in difficult and challenging cases.* New York, NY: Thieme; 1999:21-31.
3. Arshinoff SA. Dispersive-cohesive viscoelastic soft shell technique. *J Cataract Refract Surg.* 1999;25(2):167-173.
4. Greve EL. Primary angle-closure glaucoma: extracapsular cataract extraction or filtering procedure? *Int Ophthalmol.* 1988;12(3):157-162.
5. Gunning FP, Greve EL. Lens extraction for uncontrolled angle-closure glaucoma: long-term follow-up. *J Cataract Refract Surg.* 1998;24(10):1347-1356.
6. Gavin EA, Hammond CJ. Intraocular lens power calculation in short eyes. *Eye (Lond).* 2008;22(7):935-938.
7. MacLaren RE, Natkunarajah M, Riaz Y, Bourne RR, Restori M, Allan BD. Biometry and formula accuracy with intraocular lenses used for cataract surgery in extreme hyperopia. *Am J Ophthalmology.* 2007;143(6):920-931.
8. Fenzl RE, Gills JP, Cherchio M. Refractive and visual outcome of hyperopic cataract cases operated on before and after implementation of the Holladay II formula. *Ophthalmology.* 1998;105(9):1759-1764.
9. Gayton JL, Sanders VN. Implanting two posterior chamber intraocular lenses in a case of microphthalmos. *J Cataract Refract Surg.* 1993;19(6):776-777.
10. Baumeister M, Kohnen T. Scheimpflug measurement of intraocular lens position after piggyback implantation of foldable intraocular lenses in eyes with high hyperopia. *J Cataract Refract Surg.* 2006;32(12):2098-2104.
11. Gills JP, Fenzl RE. Piggyback intraocular lens implantation. *Dev Ophthalmol.* 2002;34:209-216.
12. Findl O, Menapace R, Georgopoulos M, Kiss B, Petternel V, Rainer G. Morphological appearance and size of contact zones of piggyback intraocular lenses. *J Cataract Refract Surg.* 2001;27(2):219-223.
13. Akaishi L, Tzelikis PF. Primary piggyback implantation using the ReSTOR intraocular lens: case series. *J Cataract Refract Surg.* 2007;33(5):791-795.
14. Akaishi L, Tzelikis PF, Gondim J, Vaz R. Primary piggyback implantation using the Tecnis ZM900 multifocal intraocular lens: case series. *J Cataract Refract Surg.* 2007;33(12):2067-2071.
15. Werner L, Mamalis N, Stevens S, Hunter B, Chew JJ, Vargas LG. Interlenticular opacification: dual-optic versus piggyback intraocular lenses. *J Cataract Refract Surg.* 2006;32(4):655-661.
16. Shugar JK, Schwartz T. Interpseudophakos Elschnig pearls associated with late hyperopic shift: a complication of piggyback posterior chamber intraocular lens implantation. *J Cataract Refract Surg.* 1999;25(6):863-867.
17. Kim SK, Lanciano RC Jr, Sulewski ME. Pupillary block glaucoma associated with a secondary piggyback intraocular lens. *J Cataract Refract Surg.* 2007;33(10):1813-1814.
18. García-Feijo J, Saenz-Frances F, Martinez-De-La-Casa JM, et al. Angle-closure glaucoma after piggyback intraocular lens implantation. *Eur J Ophthalmol.* 2008;18(5):822-826.
19. Chang SH, Lim G. Secondary pigmentary glaucoma associated with piggyback intraocular lens implantation. *J Cataract Refract Surg.* 2004;30(10):2219-2222.
20. Iwase T, Tanaka N. Elevated intraocular pressure in secondary piggyback intraocular lens implantation. *J Cataract Refract Surg.* 2005;31(9):1821-1823.
21. Chang WH, Werner L, Fry LL, Johnson JT, Kamae K, Mamalis N. Pigmentary dispersion syndrome with a secondary piggyback 3-piece hydrophobic acrylic lens. Case report with clinicopathological correlation. *J Cataract Refract Surg.* 2007;33(6):1106-1109.
22. Ozturk F, Snyder ME, Osher RH, Bishop JR 3rd. Hyperopic shift with posterior bowing of a Collamer posterior chamber intraocular lens. *J Cataract Refract Surg.* 2007;33(1):159-161.

10

Cataract in Retinitis Pigmentosa

Retinitis pigmentosa (RP) is a group of hereditary disorders affecting the photoreceptors and retinal pigment epithelium (RPE) that gradually causes night blindness and progressive contraction of the visual field. It is the most common retinal degeneration worldwide with an incidence of approximately 1 in 4000.[1] It normally appears during the first 4 decades of life, and the incidence decreases in the subsequent 2 to 3 decades.

The group of pathologies included in RP is phenotypically similar but genetically extremely heterogeneous, including more than 50 genes (identifiable in 60% of patients). Because of the genetic and functional differences of the various proteins involved in the pathogenesis, it is not completely clear what mechanisms are responsible for the various forms of RP. It is assumed that mutation of the gene causes a structural abnormality of a protein that in some ways is involved in visual function. This abnormality causes degeneration of the photoreceptors, and the disease begins. In all of the experimental animal models of RP and in humans apoptosis is the final cause of photoreceptor degeneration, and the apoptotic pathway involved has been recently identified.[2] Apoptosis predominantly affects the rods; the genetic defects affect the cones and RPE less frequently.[3]

More than 25% of patients affected by RP will eventually become legally blind in both eyes. However, they will rarely lose their sight completely. More than half of the patients with RP have a visual acuity of 5/10 in at least one eye.[4]

RP generally only affects one eye, but rarely it may be associated with other systemic conditions. There is a difference between primary RP, characterized by involvement of the eye alone, and secondary RP, associated with extraocular conditions (involving the ear in particular).

The hereditary patterns of primary RP may be autosomal dominant, autosomal recessive, X-linked, or isolated (most frequent). X-linked PR may be recessive, largely affecting males, or it may be dominant that affects both sexes, even though females are always affected to a lesser degree. Some of the dysgenic and mitochondrial forms have also been described.[5] Normally, patients do not have any family history of RP.

The age of onset and severity of the disease depends on the hereditary pattern (the autosomal dominant having the mildest expression). RP may have very different degrees of severity; some patients have only a sectional loss of visual field, others have severe loss of the peripheral visual field associated with variable loss of central macular function.

Visual deterioration in RP is particularly due to a loss of photoreceptors. This causes damage to the RPE and the other layers of retinal neuroepithelium[6]; the process progresses posteriorly and can cause loss of vision due to involvement of the macula and a contraction of the visual field.

The clinical signs of RP on fundus exam are attenuation of retinal vessels initially and fibrotic generation in the late stages (Figure 10-1). In almost all cases, there is waxy pallor of the optic disc, arteriolar constriction, and hyalinization. Pigmentary changes can generally be seen; however, they can be absent or mild at the onset of the disease. They include characteristic bone spicules, widespread granulation, or pigment clumps. These are due to degeneration of the photoreceptors, atrophy of the external retina and the RPE, and the intraretinal migration of the RPE.

Diagnosis of RP is based on the visual field and electroretinogram documentation of the progressive loss of photoreceptor functions. This examination picks up the damage, generally many years prior to the onset of symptoms. Genetic consulting facilitates an accurate diagnosis and determines the hereditary factor in each family, via the molecular genetic test (available for some of the genes involved); this information may be useful in preventing the disease.

Buratto L, Brint SF, Caretti L.
Cataract Surgery in Complicated Cases (pp 117-120).

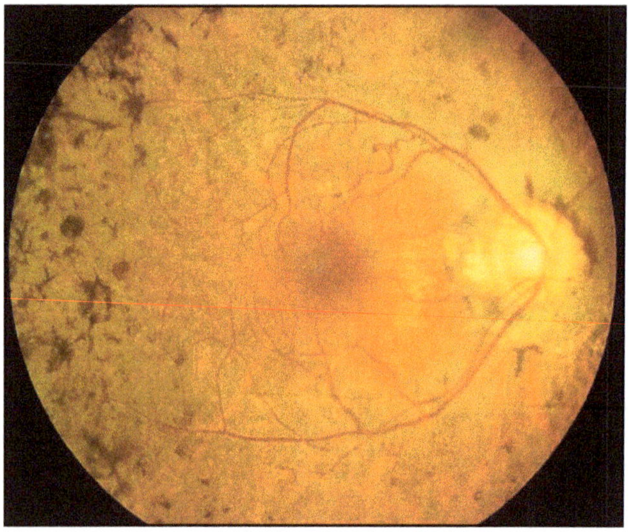

Figure 10-1. Retinogram in an RP patient with significant contraction of the temporal retinal blood vessels and pigmentary changes.

The progression of RP is extremely variable; however, the disease is always progressive and debilitating. As mentioned before, visual loss in RP is due, in some cases, to progressive retinal degeneration, but can also occur with the onset of cystoid macular edema (CME) or cataract.

CME occurs in approximately 10% to 15% of patients,[7,8] even though an incidence of up to 70% of ME detected by angiography has been reported.[9] The pathogenesis of CME is not known; a low-grade chronic ocular inflammation has been suggested as being responsible by the rupture of the blood-retinal barrier and therefore ME.

Cataract is present in approximately 50% of patients and would also appear to be caused by low-grade inflammation. Other possible ocular associations are myopia (above all), astigmatism, high-order aberrations, floaters (due to cells in the vitreous, clumps, and posterior detachment of the vitreous), retinal detachment (the incidence is identical to that in the myopic population), glaucoma, and ectopia lentis.[10,11]

Posterior dislocation of the lens in RP was described for the first time in 2002 by Sato et al.[11] A case of anterior bilateral lens dislocation following acute ocular hypertension was reported recently.[12] According to the authors, the anterior bilateral dislocation following an acute attack of glaucoma is caused by moderate mydriasis associated with weakening of the iris and the ciliary body.

There is no medical treatment for RP, even though progression of the disease can be slowed by daily administration of 15,000 IU of vitamin A. Research in possible treatments is ongoing; future treatments may include retinal transplant, implantation of retinal chips, gene therapy, stem cells, nutritional supplements, and/or therapy with drugs or growth factors.

Cataract Associated With Retinitis Pigmentosa

Cataract is a recognized complication of all types of RP. Patients with RP develop lens opacities when they are still fairly young.[13-15] Typically, these patients develop both a posterior cortical or posterior subcapsular cataract. When this is associated with constriction of the visual field, it can cause further visual loss, even when the lens opacity is mild. It should be emphasized that with RP even relatively mild degrees of lens opacity can cause significant vision loss Most patients complain of glare, requiring surgery when they are fairly young. The scientific literature reports an average of 47 to 58 years of age requiring surgery.[16-21]

In reference to cataract surgery, in addition to the general risks associated with surgery, with RP, there are additional factors that can cause poor postoperative results. They include the following:

- Atrophy of the peripheral retina in the late stages of RP.
- CME is common with RP. It is reasonable to assume that ME will be increased after surgery: the frequency reported in the literature is approximately 15%,[21] unexpectedly low considering the use of the extracapsular cataract extraction (ECCE) in some of the cases.
- The threshold of phototoxcity, a risk that also exists in patients without RP,[22] is probably lower in RP.
- Posterior capsule opacification (PCO) and contraction of the anterior capsule are more frequent, early and aggressive with RP.[16-29] The reason for increased capsular cell proliferation in retinal dystrophy is not known; however, the mediator released in the retinal neuroepithelium can modify the growth and differentiation of the lens fibers.[25] It has been suggested that the retinal pathology induces capsular cell proliferation, and the characteristic posterior cataract in RP[20,26,28,29]; it can therefore be assumed that this also occurs following cataract surgery. A similar stimulus could also be responsible for the phimosis of the anterior capsule that develops in RP patients more frequently than in non-RP patients and can cause tilting or dislocation of the IOL in the anterior or posterior chamber.[22-24,30] Like ectopia lentis, the dislocation of the IOL is probably due to weakness of the zonular fibers and the degeneration of the anterior vitreous.[11,23,31] In a Korean patient with RP, the IOL dislocated in the anterior chamber 6 years following phacoemulsification in the left eye and 8 years after ECCE in the right eye.[32] Hayashi et al[31] documented possible predisposing factors for late dislocation of the IOL inside and outside the capsular bag following cataract surgery with bag implantation of an IOL: it is reported that RP is associated with an increased incidence of dislocation of the IOL-capsular bag complex.

Severe capsular contractions, anterior vitreous degeneration and zonule weakness may cause possible IOL dislocation in patients with RP. Another recent study described a patient with RP who developed posterior dislocation of the IOL one year after a neodymium: yttrium-aluminum-garnet (Nd:YAG) capsulotomy.[33]

Surgical Tips and Functional Results

When the surgeon is planning phacoemulsification in RP patients, in light of these considerations, he or she should create a large capsulorrhexis (approximately 6 mm) to minimize contraction of the anterior capsule. It is important to preserve the integrity of the zonules and minimize risk of posterior capsule rupture. The chop phacoemulsification technique is preferred in order to reduce the stress on the zonules. Likewise, hydrodissection must be extremely delicate. Consider using a 3-piece IOL, tension rings, or performing relaxing radial incisions of the anterior capsule to minimize the risk of capsular phimosis and the associated consequences.[34]

Considering that the opacification of the lens acts as a natural filter, and the threshold of phototoxicity is probably lower in these patients, the extraction of the lens theoretically causes more toxicity potential, so the surgeon should consider the use of a filtering IOL to reduce the incidence of phototoxicity. As coaxial light is used in the microscope; the light intensity should be reduced to a minimum, the surgeon should reduce light during implantation of the IOL and try to perform the surgery as quickly as possible

Despite the potentially poor visual results, it is important to consider early surgery in RP patients. The patients should have realistic expectations and understand possible complications.[16,21] The benefits are realized early postoperatively, especially glare reduction.

Benefits of surgery in patients with poor preoperative vision in the more advanced stages of the disease will be less obvious, because of pre-existing macular pathology, even though postoperative ME is less frequent than would be expected.[21]

Conclusion

RP patients often benefit from cataract surgery, frequently performed at an early age, with significant improvement in the visual capacity and symptoms. It should be performed with a technique that preserves the zonules and attempts to reduce the incidence of post-operative complications. These RP patients are at a greater risk of PCO and CME.

Even though posterior dislocation of the IOL does not occur very often, it is a complication that must be discussed prior to surgery, as this is difficult to manage in these delicate eyes.

References

1. Boughman JA, Conneally PM, Nance WE. Population genetic studies of retinitis pigmentosa. *Am J Hum Genet.* 1980;32(2)223-235.
2. Marigo V. Programmed cell death in retinal degeneration: targeting apoptosis in photoreceptors as potential therapy for retinal degeneration. *Cell Cycle.* 2007;6(6)652-655.
3. Cottet S, Schorderet DF. Mechanisms of apoptosis in retinitis pigmentosa. *Curr Mol Med.* 2009;9(3):375-383.
4. Grover S, Fishman GA, Anderson RJ, et al. Visual acuity impairment in patients with retinitis pigmentosa at age 45 years or older. *Ophthalmology.* 1999;106(9):1780-1785.
5. Fahim AT, Bowne SJ, Sullivan LS, et al. Allelic Heterogeneity and genetic modifier loci contribute to clinical variation in males with X-linked retinitis pigmentosa due to RPGR mutations. *PLoS One.* 2011;6(8):e23021.
6. Humayun MS, Prince M, de Juan E Jr, et al. Morphometric analysis of the extramacular retina from postmortem eyes with retinitis pigmentosa. *Invest Ophthalmol Vis Sci.* 1999;40(1)143-148.
7. Fishman GA, Gilbert LD, Fiscella RG, Kimura AE, Jampol LM. Acetazolamide for treatment of chronic macular edema in retinitis pigmentosa. *Arch Ophthalmol.* 1989;107(10):1445-1452.
8. Spalton DJ, Bird AC, Cleary PE. Retinitis pigmentosa and retinal oedema. *Br J Ophthalmol.* 1978;62(3):174-182.
9. Newsome DA. Retinal fluorescein leakage in retinitis pigmentosa. *Am J Ophthalmol.* 1986;101(3):354-360.
10. Berson EL, Rosner B, Sandberg MA, Weigel-DiFranco C, Dryja TP. Ocular findings in patients with autosomal dominant retinitis pigmentosa and rhodopsin, proline-347-leucine. *Am J Ophthalmol.* 1991;111(5):614-623.
11. Sato H, Wada Y, Abe T, Kawamura M, Wakusawa R, Tamai M. Retinitis pigmentosa associated with ectopia lentis. *Arch Ophthalmol.* 2002;120(6):852-854.
12. Kwon YA, Bae SH, Sohn YH. Bilateral spontaneous anterior lens dislocation in a retinitis pigmentosa patient. *Korean J Ophthalmol.* 2007;21(2):124-126.
13. Pruett RC. Retinitis pigmentosa: clinical observations and correlations. *Trans Am Ophthalmol Soc.* 1983;81:693-735.
14. Fishman GA, Anderson RJ, Lourenco P. Prevalence of posterior subcapsular lens opacities in patients with retinitis pigmentosa. *Br J Ophthalmol.* 1985;69(4):263-266.
15. Heckenlively J. The frequency of posterior subcapsular cataract in the hereditary retinal degenerations. *Am J Ophthalmol.* 1982;93(6):733-738.
16. Auffarth GU, Tetz MR, Krastel H, Blankenagel A, Völcker HE. Indikationen und Erfolgsaussichten der Kataraktoperation bei Patienten mit Retinitis pigmentosa. *Ophthalmologe.* 1996;93(2):168-176.
17. Bastek JV, Heckenlively JR, Straatsma BR. Cataract surgery in retinitis pigmentosa patients. Ophthalmology. 1982;89(8):880-884.
18. Reccia R, Scala A, Bosone G. Posterior chamber intraocular lens implantation in patients with retinitis pigmentosa. *Doc Ophthalmol.* 1989;72(2):115-118.
19. Newsome DA, Stark WJ Jr, Maumenee IH. Cataract extraction and intraocular lens implantation in patients with retinitis pigmentosa or Usher's syndrome. *Arch Ophthalmol.* 1986;104(6):852-854.
20. Fagerholm PP, Philipson BT. Cataract in retinitis pigmentosa. An analysis of cataract surgery results and pathological lens changes. *Acta Ophthalmol (Copenh).* 1985;63(1):50-58.

21. Jackson H, Garway-Heath D, Rosen P, Bird AC, Tuft SJ. Outcome of cataract surgery in patients with retinitis pigmentosa. *Br J Ophthalmol.* 2001;85(8):936-938.
22. Lee BL, Sternberg JP. Microscope light toxicity. *Sem Ophthalmol.* 1993;8:151-155.
23. Hayashi K, Hayashi H, Matsuo K, Nakao F, Hayashi F. Anterior capsule contraction and intraocular lens dislocation after implant surgery in eyes with retinitis pigmentosa. *Ophthalmology.* 1998;105(7):1239-1243.
24. Nishi O, Nishi K. Intraocular lens encapsulation by shrinkage of the capsulorhexis opening. *J Cataract Refract Surg.* 1993;19(4):544-545.
25. Nishi O, Nishi K, Fujiwara T, Shirasawa E, Ohmoto Y. Effects of the cytokines on the proliferation of and collagen synthesis by human cataract lens epithelial cells. *Br J Ophthalmol.* 1996;80(1):63-68.
26. Eshaghian J, Rafferty NS, Goossens W. Ultrastructure of human cataract in retinitis pigmentosa. *Arch Ophthalmol.* 1980;98(12):2227-2230.
27. Auffarth GU, Nimsgern C, Tetz MR, Krastel H, Völcker HE. Erhöhte Nachstarrate und Besonderheiten der Nd:YAG-Laserkapsulotomie bei Retinitis pigmentosa. *Ophthalmologe.* 1997;94(11):791-795.
28. Streeten BW, Eshaghian J. Human posterior subcapsular cataract. A gross and flat preparation study. *Arch Ophthalmol.* 1978;96(9):1653-1658.
29. Al-ghoul KJ, Novak LA, Kuszak JR. The structure of posterior subcapsular cataracts in the Royal College of Surgeons (RCS) rats. *Exp Eye Res.* 1998;67(2):163-177.
30. Najjar DM, Igbre AO, Tsai FF Late capsular bag contraction and intraocular lens subluxation in retinitis pigmentosa: a case report. *J Med Case Reports.* 2011;5:65.
31. Hayashi K, Hirata A, Hayashi H. Possible predisposing factors for in-the-bag and out-of-the-bag intraocular lens dislocation and outcomes of intraocular lens exchange surgery. *Ophthalmology.* 2007;114(5):969-975.
32. Lee HJ, Min SH, Kim TY. Bilateral spontaneous dislocation of intraocular lenses within the capsular bag in a retinitis pigmentosa patient. *Korean J Ophthalmol.* 2004;18(1):52-57.
33. Smith M, Pappas G, Evans N. Intraocular lens migration following posterior capsulotomy in retinitis pigmentosa. *Eye (Lond).* 2007;21(6):867-869.
34. Nikpoor N, Stone DU. Rapid capsular phimosis in retinitis pigmentosa. *Ophthalmic Surg Lasers Imaging.* 2010;29:41.

11

Cataract Surgery in Patients With Uveitis

Cataracts are the greatest cause of vision loss in uveitis patients. The incidence of cataract reported depends primarily on the type of uveitis. The incidence varies between 50% in patients with juvenile rheumatoid arthritis (JRA) and other forms of posterior uveitis and 75% of cases with chronic anterior uveitis.[1-8] It commonly appears in all forms of anterior and intermediate uveitis,[9-11] due to chronic inflammation and the chronic use of corticosteroid drugs.

Generally speaking, posterior uveitis per se does not have specific cataractogenic effects compared to other forms of inflammation; however, the cataract may be induced by systemic steroid therapy. Actually, the development of a cataract depends on the type of uveitis and the duration, intensity, and treatment of the inflammation (dose, duration, type, and drug administration method).[12]

This cataract is not associated with old age (senile cataract); the cataract associated with uveitis develops in the early years of life and affects children and young adults.

This type of cataract has a number of characteristics that require a different therapy/surgical approach compared to the senile cataract.[11] Preoperative anti-inflammatory drug regimes are essential and must be accurately planned for each individual patient, being different from the routine surgical regime.

Postoperative follow-up must both control the inflammation and monitor the higher incidence of complications, such as posterior capsule opacification (PCO), glaucoma, relapsed episodes of iritis, and macular edema (ME). Consequently, cataract surgery in this type of eye is more difficult in technical terms and is much more complicated for the surgeon due to the onset or increase in intraocular inflammation.[4,13-16]

Recently, improvements in surgical techniques, intraocular lens (IOL) design, and basic pre- and postoperative control of the inflammation have allowed surgeons to operate on the cataract earlier, with better results in adults and, to a lesser degree, in children.[14]

It is essential to determine the basic pathology as this will allow the surgeon to formulate a correct prognosis and determine precise therapeutic strategy.

Physiopathology, Signs, and Symptoms

The physiopathology of cataract formation in patients with uveitis is not clear. Multiple factors have been advanced, most importantly free radicals of oxygen, lysosomal enzymes, immunocomplex deposits on the posterior capsule, hypoxia, and an altered or abnormal flow of aqueous humor.[11] Posterior synechiae to the anterior lens capsule or posterior subcapsular cataract may have been caused by chronic inflammation of the ciliary body or the use of corticosteroids. An increased incidence of nuclear cataract has also been reported.

Symptoms correlated to the cataract will be related to the patient's age, the type of uveitis, and the type of cataract.

Uveitic patients typically complain of deterioration in visual acuity, similar to patients with other forms of cataract. Near vision can be affected with subcapsular cataracts, and glare is frequently the main problem.[17]

If the doctor makes an incorrect diagnosis of cataract in young patients affected by active uveitis or JRA, severe amblyopia may occur. With treatment (amblyopic surgery), it is possible to maintain the visual acuity of most children better than 20/40.

Buratto L, Brint SF, Caretti L.
Cataract Surgery in Complicated Cases (pp 121-129).

Timing of Surgery

There are 2 main indications for cataract surgery in patients with uveitis. The first is a cataract that causes a significant deterioration in vision with reasonably good prognosis for improved vision following the cataract operation. The second indication is a cataract that prevents examination of the fundus.

First, the decision to operate must be taken on a case-by-case basis. Techniques to predict postoperative visual acuity can be used in patients in which standard estimation of visual acuity is not sufficient and the condition of the macula cannot be determined. Measurement of the potential visual acuity and laser interferometry are techniques that can be used and reassure us of useful vision. In patients with good visual acuity but severe glare with posterior subcapsular opacities, cataract surgery is essential.

Second, the operation aims to improve visualization of the posterior pole. Occasionally, the cataract will prevent the surgeon from recognizing specific diseases of the posterior segment (eg, posterior uveitis, vasculitis, or ME) and can also prevent proper treatment (eg, corticosteroid or immunosuppressive therapy).

The cataract may prevent diagnostic techniques, such as retinal angiography and optical coherence tomography, and interfere with some therapeutic techniques, such as argon laser photocoagulation or cryotherapy.

To achieve clear vision of the ocular fundus, cataract surgery may be necessary. Generally it should be performed only when the eyes are quiescent. There is one obvious exception—where iritis is induced by the lens, such as in the case of phacolytic glaucoma.

Perioperative Treatment (Anti-Inflammatory and Immunosuppressive Therapy)

It is essential to try to achieve total (or almost total) control of the inflammation for 3 months prior to surgery. This is not easy; however, with a progressive approach to therapy, complete control of the inflammation is possible in the majority of patients.

The most important indication of inflammation is the presence (or absence) of inflammatory cells in the anterior chamber (AC) or in the vitreous.[11] Aqueous flare, on the other hand, in chronic anterior uveitis simply indicates a vascular "incompetence" of the iris and the ciliary body, resulting from vascular damage caused by recurrent uveitis. Consequently, flare should not be routinely used as a parameter to evaluate the amount of inflammation. Recognizing inflammatory cells in the vitreous in the presence of an advanced cataract may prove to be extremely difficult. Thus, the surgeon must do everything in his or her power to eliminate or reduce inflammation prior to surgery. Inflammatory cells in the vitreous disappear much more slowly than in the AC; consequently, their presence does not necessarily indicate active disease.

When inflammation cannot be evaluated, the eye can be treated prophylactically for a few days, as though it were affected by an active inflammation.[18] However, in patients with Vogt-Koyanagi-Harada syndrome, vitreous inflammation is not associated with cataract development, as reported by Moorthy et al.[19]

When uveitis is part of a systemic disease, treatment with oral anti-inflammatory drugs may be necessary, and medical control may necessitate a multidisciplinary approach.[11]

The surgeon should be aware that surgery could also aggravate the underlying inflammatory process due to the release of lens material, in addition to the surgical trauma itself. It is therefore essential that the surgery be performed in a quiet eye. It is worth repeating that the inflammation must be kept under control for at least the 3-month period prior to surgery.

A correct therapeutic approach considers splitting the patients into 2 groups: complicated cases and noncomplicated cases.[15] Noncomplicated patients are affected by uveitis, controlled with topical steroids, and routine surgery is simply anticipated. The therapeutic approach begins 1 week prior to surgery; one drop of a topical corticosteroid (1% prednisolone acetate or 0.5% dexamethasone) is administered 4 times a day.

Complicated patients necessitate systemic and periocular therapy to maintain the uveitis in a quiescent state, or they may be patients in which the surgeons expect surgery to be technically difficult. All patients classified as complicated should undergo topical therapy and oral prednisolone (1 mg/kg/day). Some authors recommend intravenous administration of the drug. Some authors also suggest treating high-risk patients (ie, patients with a previous history of ME or patients who had a poor result in the first eye operated due to postoperative uveitis or ME).

Due to possible side effects of corticosteroids, some authors suggest the administration of immunomodulating drugs and antimetabolites to control the ocular inflammation, even though universal guidelines are still not available.

In the past, some authors recommended the use of biodegradable slow-release inserts of dexamethasone to the AC to control the inflammation; however, this is no longer advocated.

Surgical Technique: Phacoemulsification

Precise phacoemulsification is recommended for uveitic patients. Issues that must be considered are miotic pupil, pupil membrane, posterior synechiae, and band keratopathy.

Phacoemulsification utilizes a small wound, causing minimal trauma, minimizing postoperative inflammation. It is useful for young patients and for those treated with high doses of corticosteroids. General anesthesia is not required, and most surgeons prefer topical anesthesia or local anesthesia with a retrobulbar or peribulbar block. Occasionally patients are very young and may be uncooperative, so general anesthesia may be necessary.

A clear cornea (preferable) or scleral tunnel may be used. The advantages of clear cornea compared to sclera include absence of postoperative redness, the absence of filtering blebs, and the fact that cauterization is unnecessary.

When a rigid polymethylmethacrylate (PMMA) lens is implanted, a limbal approach with a short scleral tunnel is preferred.

The surgeon should be cautious as the corneal endothelium and iris tissue are often compromised.

Viscoelastic substances are used routinely to break adhesions and increase mydriasis. A combination of hyaluronic acid and chondroitin sulfate (Healon Endocoat [Abbott Laboratories, Abbott Park, IL]) is preferred or high-viscosity viscoelastic substances (eg, Healon GV [Abbott Laboratories] and Amvisc Plus [Bausch & Lomb, Rochester, NY]) can be used. Many patients with uveitis will have sclerosis of the dilatory muscle of the pupil or extensive posterior synechiae. Posterior synechiae, causing miosis, can be broken by visco separation (with the help of viscoelastic substances, synechiolysis can be performed with an iris spatula) or cut with scissors.

Two-handed pupil stretching maneuvers can be performed once the synechiae have been broken. If further mydriasis is required, the surgeon can use 4 De Juan iris retractor hooks applied in each quadrant through 4 small paracenteses. Multiple sphincterotomies may be necessary.

When the entire pupil edge is involved, occasionally a fibrotic membrane can be dissected or removed 360 degrees to produce a completely free pupil edge. There is marked pupillary dilation after this maneuver of peripupillary membranectomy.

The continuous circular capsulorrhexis should be as large as possible (5.5 mm) given that there is a tendency for iridocapsular adhesions to form postoperatively. The rhexis can also be enlarged at later stages during surgery.

Minimum phaco time should be used. The majority of cataracts are removed following hydrodissection and hydroexpression into the AC, or the nucleus may be removed with the chop technique.

The subcapsular cortex can be removed with a 1- or 2-handed irrigation/aspiration technique. The bimanual or 2-handed technique is safer and better for cleaning of the posterior capsule and the aspiration of the residual epithelial cells from the anterior capsule. In some cases, hydro cleaning of the posterior capsule is a safe, useful technique (Blumenthal, personal communication).

Iris atrophy, sclerosis of the pupil sphincter, cyclitic membranes, posterior synechiae, anterior capsular sclerosis, band keratopathy, neovascularization of the angle, and possible iris hemorrhage (as often happens in cases of Fuchs heterochromic cyclitis) are all factors that can increase the difficulty of the surgery.

Some authors suggest a small iridectomy in cases with uveitis, given that pupillary block has been reported postoperatively.

Finally, in cases of noninfective uveitis, the surgeon should consider the injection of intravitreal, sub-Tenon's, or periocular steroids at the end of surgery. Recent literature suggests, despite being off label, 4 mg of intravitreal triamcinolone for controlling inflammation and postoperative ME.[20-23] The intraoperative use of this drug is safe and extremely useful, allowing the surgeon to avoid using systemic corticosteroids. The sub-Tenon's administration of 40 mg of triamcinolone also proved to be helpful, equal to the use of 1% prednisolone eyedrops postoperatively[24] or periocular administration (inferior, adjacent to the orbit floor).[25]

One topic that is still debatable is whether the posterior capsule should be left intact during cataract surgery with uveitis. Posterior capsulorrhexis can avoid frequent PCO and provide access to the anterior vitreous to remove the inflammatory elements it contains. Vice versa, leaving the posterior capsule intact has the advantage of reducing the anterior diffusion of the inflammation. In our opinion, in eyes with extensive membrane formation, the surgeon should consider an automated anterior vitrectomy following a central posterior capsulorrhexis.

If extensive fibrosis and exudate formation is seen in the vitreous, a pars plana vitrectomy may be indicated (see the Vitrectomy section in this chapter).

An intracapsular operation should be reserved for situations where a significant, phaco-induced complication occurred in the patient's other eye.

If the patient has also developed chronic ME, the surgery should include both an anterior and a posterior approach. The majority of surgeons opt for a conventional pars plana vitrectomy technique.

Intraocular Lenses

Until a few years ago, the majority of surgeons considered chronic uveitis as a relative contraindication to the implantation of an IOL: implantation in the sulcus or in the AC was always contraindicated and even placing an IOL in the capsular bag was controversial. Currently, a number of studies have suggested that in selected cases in conjunction with appropriate perioperative anti-inflammatory therapy, the implantation of a posterior chamber IOL (PC-IOL) in the capsular bag is not associated with additional risks.[1-8,11-14,18-29]

There is a large amount of information regarding small incision phacoemulsification with implantation of a foldable IOL in patients with chronic uveitis; these articles compared the implantation of a foldable IOL through a 3.2-mm incision and the implantation of a PMMA IOL with an incision of 5.5 mm or larger. Postoperative inflammation was significantly lower with the smaller incisions.

In patients with severe uveitis, in-the-bag implantation is important, not simply to prevent irritation of the uvea that can lead to prolonged breakdown of the blood-aqueous barrier and a more serious inflammatory response, but also to ensure that the IOL is well centered and stable.

Regarding IOL materials, in the past, PMMA was the most widely used for IOLs. This material is inert and stable. Subsequently, silicone and hydrogel lenses were introduced and were rapidly adopted, partly because of the popularity of phacoemulsification.

The interest in these materials was based on their ability to be inserted through small incisions. The use of silicone IOLs in patients with uveitis resulted in a greater inflammatory reaction than IOLs of other materials (PMMA, heparin-modified, hydrogel, and/or hydrophobic acrylic). A greater number of complications have been described following phacoemulsification, such as intense inflammatory reactions in the AC, total contraction of the anterior capsule, subluxation of the IOL, and (mild) increase in PCO compared to PMMA implants.[30-34]

We do not recommend the use of silicone lenses in patients in which the blood-aqueous barrier is compromised, such as patients with uveitis, and this has also been validated in the literature.[12] Surgeons should remember that silicone IOLs will tend to adhere to silicone oil[35]; consequently, this material is generally not suitable for implantation in uveitic patients.

Several years ago, IOLs with a modified surface (eg, by the addition of heparin) were introduced. Heparin-coated lenses theoretically reduce the number and the severity of deposits on the surface of the IOL[27,36]; however, they have fallen out of favor as they are not associated with any real benefit for the patient.[37]

Doubts relative to the implantation of the IOLs following the extraction of cataract in eyes with uveitis are a key problem in these patients.

A uveitic eye is unique regarding different types of pathology, preoperative inflammation and its treatment, postoperative inflammation, and specific complications. Presently, with modern PC-IOLs, the implantation of IOLs is less problematic. These IOLs are well tolerated in most patients, particularly when implanted in the capsular bag as we mentioned earlier

The long-term prognosis of the eye with uveitis in relation to the biocompatibility of the IOL and inflammation is now better understood. A number of studies have been published recently on IOLs in uveitic eyes[14,28,38,39]: some of these articles[28,38] suggest that hydrophilic IOLs have good uveal biocompatibility, but poor capsular biocompatibility compared to hydrophobic lenses; nevertheless, long-term results indicate that all of the acrylic lenses (hydrophobic and hydrophilic) with squared edges produce good functional results[38] (see the Follow-Up and Results of Surgery section in this chapter).

Consequently, the implantation of IOLs in these eyes is safe and effective in adults; there is still some controversy regarding the use of IOLs in children's eyes, even though recent literature advocates implantation of IOLs as long as the degree of inflammation present is carefully controlled prior to surgery (see Chapter 1).[39]

Combined Surgery: Glaucoma

The combination of glaucoma with uveitis is one of the most serious problems of intraocular inflammation. This condition exists in various syndromes and can be difficult to treat. Many patients have a very poor response to this surgery. The surgeon must determine the severity of the inflammation and, if possible, the associated syndrome. One should treat the underlying inflammation and the glaucoma itself.

A number of mechanisms can produce secondary glaucoma, and it is important to diagnose them to define appropriate therapy. With acute or chronic intraocular inflammation, the role of corticosteroids as a treatment and as the cause of the high intraocular pressure (IOP) must be determined.

Pharmacological therapy is the first step in the treatment of glaucoma associated with uveitis; steroids, acetazolamide, beta-blockers, cycloplegics, among others are used.

When medical treatment fails to control high IOP, a surgical approach is indicated. A number of surgical procedures are available for the treatment of glaucoma associated with uveitis.[40,41] The surgeon is free to perform the type of procedure best indicated.

Generally speaking, control of glaucoma in patients with uveitis is not as easy as in patients without uveitis. Trabeculectomy in patients with glaucoma and uveitis is generally successful, but not as high as with the general population because of wound scarring and loss of the trabeculectomy (particularly when the operation is combined with phacoemulsification)[42,43]; however, some authors suggest that pre-existing uveitis should not be considered to be a risk factor in the failure of filtering surgery.[44]

Aggressive anti-inflammatory therapy should be administered to patients with glaucoma before and after the trabeculectomy.

Antimetabolites have been used in association with trabeculectomy for at least 20 years. In the past, 5-fluorouracil has been replaced by mitomycin C to retard wound healing following trabeculectomy.[42,43,45] Good results have been reported for mitomycin C used in traumatic aphakic and pseudophakic glaucoma. A sponge is soaked in mitomycin C at a concentration of 0.02 mg/mL, and this is placed on the bed covered by the scleral flap. The sponge is left in position for 2 minutes, removed, and then the flap is sutured.

Nevertheless, the use of this drug is not free from side effects. Greater success of filtration is actually associated with an increased risk of hypotony, loss of the bleb, and late-onset endophthalmitis associated with the bleb.[46,47]

An alternative to trabeculectomy could be a deep sclerectomy. This may produce IOP control equivalent to that of the trabeculectomy procedure, with less postoperative inflammation; however, postoperative management is more complex (the patient must have more frequent clinical checks therapeutic corrective procedures).[48]

The use of drainage systems offers an additional surgical strategy when the surgeon is faced with refractory glaucoma secondary to uveitis. The most commonly used device is the Molteno (Dunedin, New Zealand) implant.[40,41] This technique has been exclusively developed for eyes with inflammatory glaucoma; it functions simply because the artificial material of the stent cannot form scar tissue. The surface of this plate allows the formation of a fibrotic area that is suitable for the absorption of the aqueous. These devices are reserved for refractory glaucomatous patients with uveitis after medical treatment has failed and when recurrent inflammation is the cause of failure of the standard filtering procedure.

Cyclitic Membrane

Some patients with a long history of chronic uveitis will develop a cyclitic membrane. This membrane extends from the ciliary body above the posterior surface of the lens and can be observed directly or can be diagnosed with ultrasound technology. It stretches the ciliary body and can cause it to detach, resulting in hypotony and phthisis of the globe.

In the past, when cataract surgery procedures required a large incision, the membrane was excised with scissors in the pupillary area. With modern surgical techniques, it can be completely excised along with the cataract and the anterior vitreous. In aphakic eyes, some cyclitic membranes can be cut successfully with the neodymium:yttrium-aluminum-garnet (Nd:YAG) laser.

Inflammatory or fibrotic membranes above the surface of the lens are common after anterior segment surgery in patients with uveitis. These membranes can grow across the iris and obstruct the pupillary area. They can be removed with a Nd:YAG laser or with surgery. Some bleeding is common; however, it is normally free from serious consequences.

Recombinant tissue plasminogen activator is commonly used in patients following myocardial infarction. A number of years ago, the intraocular use of this substance was also suggested to dissolve postoperative fibrin. For the treatment of persistent fibrin in the anterior segment, a single dose of 25 mcg was injected into the AC through a paracentesis. The membrane retracts and dissolves rapidly. Even though there is a small incidence of fibrin reformation and a minor risk of bleeding, neither of these complications is serious. This intracameral procedure should be considered in children having cataract surgery to prevent the frequent severe postoperative inflammatory reaction.[49]

The use of heparin to prevent intraocular postoperative formation of clots of fibrin following eye surgery has been evaluated.[50-54] A single injection into the AC, the addition of heparin to the infusion solution, and a single intravenous injection produce a statistically significant reduction in the amount of postoperative intraocular fibrin. There are no reports of postoperative ocular bleeding in the literature.

Vitrectomy

There is increasing evidence showing that pars plana vitrectomy in some uveitic syndromes brings therapeutic benefit with elimination of inflammatory debris, the risk of fibrinous bands, chronic opacification of the vitreous, and reduction of ME (believed to be correlated to the inflammation of the vitreous and retina). In our experience, phacoemulsification and pars plana vitrectomy have demonstrated significant advantages as opposed to other techniques.[55-60]

The small sealed incision used in cataract surgery provides the perfect closure following the implantation of the IOL for subsequent vitrectomy, a procedure that can now be performed with 23- and 25-gauge techniques that do not require sutures.

Postoperative Treatment

The surgeon should implement a strategy to prevent postoperative inflammation and avoid potential ocular complications. Postoperatively, severe inflammatory phenomena are a possibility, particularly in children.

The use of topical steroids is the standard treatment protocol. These drugs reduce the morbidity associated with ocular inflammation, prevent structural damage to the eye, and reduce discomfort for the patient.[61]

Currently, prednisolone or dexamethazone eye drops are administered 4 times a day starting the first day postoperative. The dosage will be gradually reduced over the next 4 to 8 weeks.

Even though topical steroids are usually the most common anti-inflammatory agents used following cataract extraction, their potential side effects limit their use in some situations. This is particularly true for steroids that tend to increase IOP. Consequently, anti-inflammatory agents that control postoperative inflammation with little or no effect on IOP would be a useful therapeutic addition. One of the current strategies in the development of new steroid drugs is the identification of substances that have a marked anti-inflammatory activity associated with a low tendency to increase IOP or induce other side effects. There are no strict guidelines in an emergency when there is pre-existing uveitis in the eye. The surgeon should expect a severe postoperative exacerbation of the existing inflammation.

The following guidelines can be applied to all intraocular procedures in eyes with uveitis:

- Depending on the severity of the case, topical or systemic corticosteroids should be administered 1 week prior to surgery.
- At surgery, subconjunctival corticosteroids should be injected as far as possible from any surgical wound. The authors prefer intravitreal, sub-Tenon's, or inferior periocular sites.
- Postoperatively, topical and systemic corticosteroids can be used in a dosage proportional to the severity of the inflammation.
- In more severe cases, moderate or high doses of oral prednisolone should be administered (between 1 and 1.5 mg/kg/day) and aggressive doses of topical corticosteroids every hour prior to surgery, then tapering the doses progressively in the 4 to 8 weeks postoperatively.

In cases of glaucoma induced by steroids, the treatment can be extremely difficult. In these cases, the surgeon should consider temporary immunosuppressive therapy as an alternative to cortisone to control the inflammation.

Efficacy of nonsteroidal anti-inflammatory drugs in the treatment of intraocular inflammation is important. Some currently used nonsteroidal anti-inflammatory drugs inhibit the enzyme cyclooxygenase. They reduce the formation of prostaglandin, a substance that plays an important role in ocular inflammation, producing a break in the blood-aqueous barrier. Diclofenac or ketorolac reduces inflammation following argon laser trabeculoplasty and following cataract surgery.[62-64] The role of these drugs in postoperative inflammation is accepted given that they are not linked to any increase in IOP.

Follow-Up and Results of Surgery

Generally speaking, severe inflammatory reaction is seen following implantation of IOLs in patients with chronic anterior uveitis (34% to 53%), particularly in children, even when pre- and postoperative anti-inflammatory measures are taken. The complications that arise following surgery are fairly frequent and are generally much more severe in children[1-8,12-14,26-29,39,40]; they include the following:

- PCO (high incidence: 38% to 62%). In some groups of patients, this complication occurs in 50% of cases,[29] in other groups the percentage was slightly lower,[12] and in others slightly higher.[2,3,5] Some articles reported a rate of onset of PCO required an Nd:YAG laser capsulotomy was greater in patients under 55 years of age and in patients with a hydrogel IOL as opposed to silicone or PMMA. The increased percentage of Nd:YAG laser capsulotomies in patients following a hydrogel IOL was reported for cases with[12,28] and those without uveitis.[16,65] The problem was attributed to the high water content of these lenses (18% to 30%), in contrast to the low water content of hydrophobic acrylic IOLs (<2%) and silicone or PMMA (both containing less than 1% water).[66,67] In some clinical trials, including a fairly recent randomized study,[15] hydrophobic acrylic IOLs implanted in the eyes of patients were associated with a lower incidence of postoperative inflammation and PCO. In another relatively recent study,[12] it was demonstrated for the first time that prophylactic steroid treatment reduces the incidence of PCO; this effect may be linked to the inhibitory action on the proliferation of lens epithelial cells, as shown in in vitro studies,[68,69] or it may be linked to an indirect effect associated with the inhibition of the uveal inflammatory response.[70]
- Fibrinous membranes (more frequent in pars planitis). These are frequently very dense and are not always broken by the Nd:YAG laser even when high energy levels are used. These also tend to reform; they can be localized behind the IOL (retrolenticular membranes) and are associated with dislocation of the lens and retinal detachment.
- Reduced visual acuity. The greatest causes of reduction in visual acuity in these patients are cystoid ME (CME; 2% to 56%), epiretinal membranes (approximately 15%), glaucomatous damage of the optic nerve, and vitreous inflammations, all resulting from postoperative inflammatory complications. In children particularly, there is frequent development of fibrinous-type inflammatory reactions, in varying degrees of severity, and these may be responsible for these important complications. In pediatric cases, high IOP may be caused by several basic mechanisms in patients with or without JRA. In children with JRA, AC inflammation tends to be more severe, resulting in the formation of pupillary membranes, anterior synechiae, goniosynechiae, pupillary block, and successively closed-angle glaucoma. However, in young patients without JRA, the degree of inflammation in the AC is associated with a smaller increase in IOP.

The prevalence of all of the previously mentioned complications was higher in older studies of extracapsular cataract extraction as opposed to phacoemulsification. It has been confirmed that smaller incisions and reduced uveal trauma resulting from phacoemulsification reduce the degree of early-onset postoperative inflammation and induce less damage to the blood-aqueous barrier,[13,16] both considered to be contributing factors in ME.[3,71] These observations suggest that intense pre- and postoperative topical antinflammatory therapy should always be used in high-risk patients and in patients who develop inflammatory signs for adequate control of the inflammatory response and consequently the ME.

Moreover, improvements in cortex removal and the use of better IOL materials with better biocompatibility have led to a considerable reduction in the incidence of PCO following phacoemulsification.[28-35,38]

Useful visual acuity can be achieved in the majority of patients with uveitis as reported in the more important trials.[4-6,12,15,72-76] Cataract surgery is associated with a significant increase in visual acuity both short- and long-term; best-corrected visual acuity of 20/40 with an increase in 2 or more Snellen lines compared to preoperative has been reported in 20% to 93% of patients.[4-6,12,15,72-76]

Currently, cataract surgery in uveitic patients can be considered to be a safe, efficacious procedure in adults; controversy still surrounds the functional results from surgery in children. Important steps are precise diagnosis and careful classification of cases that are at a high risk of a poor functional result following cataract surgery. In particular, the outcome in eyes with preoperative evidence of macular pathology (and/or also of the optic nerve) will probably be unsatisfactory, because in these patients, there is often a reduction of vision long-term.

According to some but not all authors, negative predictive factors for a poor postoperative result are the origins of the uveitis, such as the patient's sex, the patient's age at the time of surgery (younger than 30 years), and pathologies of the anterior segment such as anterior synechiae.

Regarding the feasibility of implanting an IOL in a pediatric cataract patient with uveitis, it should be noted that a number of clinical studies pointed out that children who have become unilaterally aphakic will not tolerate contact lenses for long periods of time for a number of reasons (eg, corneal pathology and band keratopathy).[76] Severe amblyopia and strabismus follows in small children with JRA, and they will have a more aggressive uveitis (eg, worse postoperative vision, more dangerous surgery, greater incidence of complications) as opposed to children without JRA.[77] Moreover, if a secondary IOL implant is required, a real possibility during the patient's life to correct the severe anisometropia, this will be associated with more complex surgery and a greater incidence of complications. As a result, contemporaneous implantation of an IOL allowing immediate correction of the refractive error associated with aphakia is the best option and preferred over the use of contact lenses.[77,78] Several years ago, Lundvall and Zetterstrom[79] suggested the implantation of a heparin-modified PMMA IOL to correct aphakia in pediatric patients with uveitis including uveitis associated with JRA.

In both adults and children, chronic inflammation, even low grade, can permanently damage the optic nerve, the retina, the angle of the AC, and other ocular structures. This can jeopardize our efforts to achieve good visual rehabilitation following cataract surgery. Aggressive therapy and early surgery prior to the appearance of permanent structural damage to the eye may prove useful in the future.

Conclusion

Cataracts are frequently observed in uveitic patients. These patients will be destined for surgery. The surgical approach must be personalized based on the patient's symptoms and the origins of the uveitis; the treatment administered must keep the eye in a quiescent state anticipating the difficulties from the surgical procedure. Perioperative control of the inflammation, excellent understanding of the available literature, and a meticulous modern surgical technique must be combined to provide the patient with uveitis undergoing cataract surgery with the best possibilities of success. The degree of success from the surgery has increased significantly from the not-too-distant past.

References

1. Foster RE, Lowder CY, Meisler DM, et al. Extracapsular cataract extraction and posterior chamber intraocular lens implantation in uveitis patients. *Ophthalmology.* 1992;99:1234-1241.
2. Krishna R, Meisler DM, Lowder CY, et al. Long term follow-up of extracapsular cataract extraction and posterior chamber intraocular lens implantation in patients with uveitis. *Ophthalmology.* 1998;105:1765-1769.
3. Okhravi N, Lightman SL, Towler HM. Assessment of visual outcome after cataract surgery in patients with uveitis. *Ophthalmology.* 1999;106:710-722.
4. Rauz S, Stavrou P, Murray PI. Evaluation of foldable intraocular lenses in patients with uveitis. *Ophthalmology.* 2000;107:909-919.
5. Estafanous MF, Lowder CY, Meisler DM, et al. Phacoemulsification cataract extraction and posterior chamber lens implantation in patients with uveitis. *Am J Ophthalmol.* 2001;131:620-625.
6. Suresh PS, Jones NP. Phacoemulsification with intraocular lens implantation in patients with uveitis. *Eye.* 2001;15:621-628.
7. Meacock WR, Spalton DJ, Bender L, et al. Steroid prophylaxis in eyes with uveitis undergoing phacoemulsification. *Br J Ophthalmol.* 2004;88:1122-1124.
8. Heger H, Drolsum L, Haaskjold E. Cataract surgery with implantation of IOL in patients with uveitis. *Acta Ophthalmol.* 1994;72:478-482.
9. Kanski JJ, Shun-Shin GA. Systemic uveitis syndromes in childhood: an analysis of 340 cases. *Ophthalmology.* 1984;91(10):1247-1252.
10. Michelson JB, Friedlaender MH, Nozik RA. Lens implant surgery in pars planitis. *Ophthalmology.* 1990;97(8):1023-1026.
11. Hooper PL, Rao NA, Smith RE. Cataract extraction in uveitis patients. *Surv Ophthalmol.* 1990;35(2):120-144.
12. Elgohary MA, McCluskey PJ, Towler HM, et al. Outcome of phacoemulsification in patients with uveitis. *Br J Ophthalmol.* 2007;91(7):916-921.
13. Chee SP, Ti SE, Sivakumar M, et al. Postoperative inflammation: extracapsular cataract extraction versus phacoemulsification. *J Cataract Refract Surg.* 1999;25:1280-1285.

14. Roesel M, Heinz C, Koch JM, Heiligenhaus A. Cataract surgery in uveitis. *Ophthalmology.* 2008;115(8):1431.
15. Alio JL, Chipont E, BenEzra D, et al. Comparative performance of intraocular lenses in eyes with cataract and uveitis. *J Cataract Refract Surg.* 2002;28:2096-2108.
16. Hollick EJ, Spalton DJ, Ursell PG, et al. Posterior capsular opacification with hydrogel, polymethylmethacrylate, and silicone intraocular lenses: two-year results of a randomized prospective trial. *Am J Ophthalmol.* 2000;129:577-584.
17. Ram J, Jain S, Pandav SS, Gupta A, Mangat GS. Postoperative complications of intraocular lens implantation in patients with Fuchs' heterochromic cyclitis. *J Cataract Refract Surg.* 1995;21(5):548-551.
18. Foster CS, Barrett F. Cataract development and cataract surgery in patients with juvenile rheumatoid arthritis-associated iridocyclitis. *Ophthalmology.* 1993;100(6):809-817.
19. Moorthy RS, Rajeev B, Smith RE, Rao NA. Incidence and management of cataracts in Vogt-Koyanagi-Harada syndrome. *Am J Ophthalmol.* 1994;118(2):197-204.
20. Alkawas AA, Hamdy AM, Shahien EA. Intraoperative intravitreal injection of triamcinolone acetonide for cataract extraction in patients with uveitis. *Ocul Immunol Inflamm.* 2010;18(5):402-407.
21. Okhravi N, Morris A, Kok HS, et al. Intraoperative use of intravitreal triamcinolone in uveitic eyes having cataract surgery: pilot study. *J Cataract Refract Surg.* 2007;33(7):1278-1283.
22. Dada T, Dhawan M, Garg S, Nair S, Mandal S. Safety and efficacy of intraoperative intravitreal injection of triamcinolone acetonide injection after phacoemulsification in cases of uveitic cataract. *J Cataract Refract Surg.* 2007;33(9):1613-1618.
23. Li J, Heinz C, Zurek-Imhoff B, Heiligenhaus A. Intraoperative intraocular triamcinolone injection prophylaxis for post-cataract surgery fibrin formation in uveitis associated with juvenile idiopathic arthritis. *J Cataract Refract Surg.* 2006;32(9):1535-1539.
24. Paganelli F, Cardillo JA, Melo LA Jr, Oliveira AG, Skaf M, Costa RA; Brazilian Ocular Pharmacology and Pharmaceutical Technology Research Group. A single intraoperative sub-Tenon's capsule triamcinolone acetonide injection for the treatment of post-cataract surgery inflammation. *Ophthalmology.* 2004;111(11):2102-2108.
25. Roesel M, Heinz C, Koch JM, Heiligenhaus A. Comparison of orbital floor triamcinolone acetonide and oral prednisolone for cataract surgery management in patients with non-infectious uveitis. *Graefes Arch Clin Exp Ophthalmol.* 2010;248(5):715-720.
26. Alió JL, Sayans JA, Chipont E. Flare-cell meter measurement of inflammation after uneventful cataract surgery with intraocular lens implantation. *J Cataract Refract Surg.* 1997;23(6):935-939.
27. Terrada C, Julian K, Cassoux N, et al. Cataract surgery with primary intraocular lens implantation in children with uveitis: long-term outcomes. *J Cataract Refract Surg.* 2011;37(11):1977-1983.
28. Abela-Formanek C, Amon M, Schauersberger J, et al. Results of hydrophilic acrylic, hydrophobic acrylic, and silicone intraocular lenses in uveitic eyes with cataract: comparison to a control group. *J Cataract Refract Surg.* 2002;28:1141-1152.
29. Akova YA, Foster CS Cataract surgery in patients with sarcoidosis-associated uveitis. *Ophthalmology.* 1994;101(3):473-479.
30. Martínez Toldos JJ, Artola Roig A, Chipont Benabent E. Total anterior capsule closure after silicone intraocular lens implantation. *J Cataract Refract Surg.* 1996;22(2):269-271.
31. Davison JA. Capsule contraction syndrome. *J Cataract Refract Surg.* 1993;19:582-589.
32. Tuft SJ, Talks SJ. Delayed dislocation of foldable plate-haptic silicone lenses after Nd:YAG laser anterior capsulotomy. *Am J Ophthalmol.* 1998;126:586-588.
33. Mamalis N, Davis B, Nilson CD, et al. Complications of foldable intraocular lenses requiring explantation or secondary intervention-2003 survey update. *J Cataract Refract Surg.* 2004;30: 2209-2218.
34. Oner FH, Saatci OA, Sarioglu S, et al. Interaction of intraocular lenses with various concentrations of silicone oil: an experimental study. *Ophthalmologica.* 2003;217:124-128.
35. Apple DJ, Federman JL, Krolicki TJ, et al. Irreversible silicone oil adhesion to silicone intraocular lenses. A clinicopathologic analysis. *Ophthalmology.* 1996;103:1555-1561.
36. Percival SP, Pai V Heparin-modified lenses for eyes at risk for breakdown of the blood-aqueous barrier during cataract surgery. *J Cataract Refract Surg.* 1993;19(6):760-765.
37. Lardenoye CW, van der Lelij A, Berendschot TT, Rothova A. A retrospective analysis of heparin-surface-modified intraocular lenses versus regular polymethylmethacrylate intraocular lenses in patients with uveitis. *Doc Ophthalmol.* 1996-1997;92(1):41-50.
38. Abela-Formanek C, Amon M, Kahraman G, Schauersberger J, Dunavoelgyi R. Biocompatibility of hydrophilic acrylic, hydrophobic acrylic, and silicone intraocular lenses in eyes with uveitis having cataract surgery: long-term follow-up. *J Cataract Refract Surg.* 2011;37(1):104-112.
39. Hug D. Intraocular lens use in challenging pediatric cases. *Curr Opin Ophthalmol.* 2010;21(5):345-349.
40. Hill RA, Nguyen QH, Baerveldt G, et al. Trabeculectomy and Molteno implantation for glaucomas associated with uveitis. *Ophthalmology.* 1993;100(6):903-908.
41. Gedde SJ, Heuer DK, Parrish RK 2nd; Tube Versus Trabeculectomy Study Group. Review of results from the Tube Versus Trabeculectomy Study. *Curr Opin Ophthalmol.* 2010;21(2):123-128.
42. Park UC, Ahn JK, Park KH, Yu HG. Phacotrabeculectomy with mitomycin C in patients with uveitis. *Am J Ophthalmol.* 2006;142(6):1005-1112.
43. Carreño E, Villarón S, Portero A, Herreras JM, Maquet JA, Calonge M. Surgical outcomes of uveitic glaucoma. *J Ophthalmic Inflamm Infect.* 2011;1(2):43-53.
44. Kaburaki T, Koshino T, Kawashima H, et al. Initial trabeculectomy with mitomycin C in eyes with uveitic glaucoma with inactive uveitis. *Eye (Lond).* 2009;23(7):1509-1517.
45. Palmer SS. Mitomycin as adjunct chemotherapy with trabeculectomy. *Ophthalmology.* 1991;98(3):317-321.
46. Wolner B, Liebmann JM, Sassani JW, Ritch R, Speaker M, Marmor M. Late bleb-related endophthalmitis after trabeculectomy with adjunctive 5-fluorouracil. *Ophthalmology.* 1991;98(7):1053-1060.
47. Song A, Scott IU, Flynn HW Jr, Budenz DL. Delayed-onset bleb-associated endophthalmitis: clinical features and visual acuity outcomes. *Ophthalmology.* 2002;109(5):985-991.
48. Dupas B, Fardeau C, Cassoux N, Bodaghi B, LeHoang P Deep sclerectomy and trabeculectomy in uveitic glaucoma. *Eye (Lond).* 2010;24(2):310-314.
49. Klais CM, Hattenbach LO, Steinkamp GW, Zubcov AA, Kohnen T. Intraocular recombinant tissue-plasminogen activator fibrinolysis of fibrin formation after cataract surgery in children. *J Cataract Refract Surg.* 1999;25:357-362.
50. Johnson RN, Balyeat E, Stern WH. Heparin prophylaxis for intraocular fibrin. *Ophthalmology.* 1987;94(6):597-601.
51. Ozkurt YB, Taşkiran A, Erdogan N, Kandemir B, Doğan OK. Effect of heparin in the intraocular irrigating solution on postoperative inflammation in the pediatric cataract surgery. *Clin Ophthalmol.* 2009;3:363-365.
52. Kruger A, Amon M, Abela-Formanek C, Schild G, Kolodjaschna J, Schauersberger J. Effect of heparin in the irrigation solution on postoperative inflammation and cellular reaction on the intraocular lens surface. *J Cataract Refract Surg.* 2002;28(1):87-92.
53. Terrada C, Julian K, Cassoux N, et al. Cataract surgery with primary intraocular lens implantation in children with uveitis: long-term outcomes. *J Cataract Refract Surg.* 2011;37(11):1977-1983.
54. Zarei R, Azimi R, Moghimi S, et al. Inhibition of intraocular fibrin formation after infusion of low-molecular-weight heparin during combined phacoemulsification-trabeculectomy surgery. *J Cataract Refract Surg.* 2006;32(11):1921-1925.

55. Svozilkova P, Heissigerova J, Brichova M, Kalvodova B, Dvorak J, Rihova E. The role of pars plana vitrectomy in the diagnosis and treatment of uveitis. *Eur J Ophthalmol.* 2011;21(1):89-97.
56. Margolis R, Brasil OF, Lowder CY, et al. Vitrectomy for the diagnosis and management of uveitis of unknown cause. *Ophthalmology.* 2007;114(10):1893-1897.
57. Androudi S, Ahmed M, Fiore T, Brazitikos P, Foster CS. Combined pars plana vitrectomy and phacoemulsification to restore visual acuity in patients with chronic uveitis. *J Cataract Refract Surg.* 2005;31(3):472-478.
58. Soheilian M, Mirdehghan SA, Peyman GA. Sutureless combined 25-gauge vitrectomy, phacoemulsification, and posterior chamber intraocular lens implantation for management of uveitic cataract associated with posterior segment disease. *Retina.* 2008;28(7):941-946.
59. Giuliari GP, Chang PY, Thakuria P, Hinkle DM, Foster CS. Pars plana vitrectomy in the management of paediatric uveitis: the Massachusetts Eye Research and Surgery Institution experience. *Eye (Lond).* 2010;24(1):7-13.
60. Margolis R. Diagnostic vitrectomy for the diagnosis and management of posterior uveitis of unknown etiology. *Curr Opin Ophthalmol.* 2008;19(3):218-224.
61. Jaanus SD. Anti-inflammatory drugs. In: Bartlett JD, Jaanus SD, eds. *Clinical Ocular Pharmacology.* Boston, MA: Butterworth Publishers; 1989:163-197.
62. Herbort CP, Mermoud A, Schnyder C, Pittet N. Anti-inflammatory effect of diclofenac drops after argon laser trabeculoplasty. *Arch Ophthalmol.* 1993;111(4):481-483.
63. Bodaghi B, Weber ME, Arnoux YV, Jaulerry SD, Le Hoang P, Colin J. Comparison of the efficacy and safety of two formulations of diclofenac sodium 0.1% eyedrops in controlling postoperative inflammation after cataract surgery. *Eur J Ophthalmol.* 2005;15(6):702-711.
64. Maca SM, Amon M, Findl O, Kahraman G, Barisani-Asenbauer T. Efficacy and tolerability of preservative-free and preserved diclofenac and preserved ketorolac eyedrops after cataract surgery. *Am J Ophthalmol.* 2010;149(5):777-784.
65. Javdani SM, Huygens MM, Callebaut F. Neodymium: YAG capsulotomy rates after phacoemulsification with hydrophobic and hydrophilic acrylic intraocular lenses. *Bull Soc Belge Ophtalmol.* 2002;(283):13-17.
66. Doan KT, Olson RJ, Mamalis N. Survey of intraocular lens material and design. *Curr Opin Ophthalmol.* 2002;13:24-29.
67. Tehrani M, Dick HB, Wolters B, et al. Material properties of various intraocular lenses in an experimental study. *Ophthalmologica.* 2004;218:57-63.
68. McDonnell PJ, Krause W, Glaser BM. In vitro inhibition of lens epithelial cell proliferation and migration. *Ophthalmic Surg.* 1988;19:25-30.
69. Cortina P, Gomez-Lechon MJ, Navea A, et al. Diclofenac sodium and cyclosporin A inhibit human lens epithelial cell proliferation in culture. *Graefes Arch Clin Exp Ophthalmol.* 1997;235:180-185.
70. Oshika T, Yoshimura K, Miyata N. Postsurgical inflammation after phacoemulsification and extracapsular extraction with soft or conventional intraocular lens implantation. *J Cataract Refract Surg.* 1992;18:356-361.
71. Ursell PG, Spalton DJ, Whitcup SM, Nussenblatt RB. Cystoid macular edema after phacoemulsification: relationship to blood-aqueous barrier damage and visual acuity. *J Cataract Refract Surg.* 1999;25(11):1492-1497.
72. Yoeruek E, Deuter C, Gieselmann S, et al. Long-term visual acuity and its predictors after cataract surgery in patients with uveitis. *Eur J Ophthalmol.* 2010;20(4):694-701.
73. Jancevski M, Foster CS. Cataracts and uveitis. *Curr Opin Ophthalmol.* 2010;21(1):10-14.
74. Ram J, Gupta A, Kumar S, Kaushik S, Gupta N, Severia S. Phacoemulsification with intraocular lens implantation in patients with uveitis. *J Cataract Refract Surg.* 2010;36(8):1283-1288.
75. Van Gelder RN, Leveque TK. Cataract surgery in the setting of uveitis. *Curr Opin Ophthalmol.* 2009;20(1):42-45.
76. Nemet AY, Raz J, Sachs D, et al. Primary intraocular lens implantation in pediatric uveitis: a comparison of 2 populations. *Arch Ophthalmol.* 2007;125(3):354-360.
77. BenEzra D, Cohen E. Cataract surgery in children with chronic uveitis. *Ophthalmology.* 2000;107:1255-1260.
78. Quiñones K, Cervantes-Castañeda RA, Hynes AY, Daoud YJ, Foster CS. Outcomes of cataract surgery in children with chronic uveitis. *J Cataract Refract Surg.* 2009;35(4):725-731.
79. Lundvall A, Zetterstrom C. Cataract extraction and intraocular lens implantation in children with uveitis. *Br J Ophthalmol.* 2000;84:791-793.

12

Floppy Iris Syndrome

In 2005, Chang and Campbell described a new clinical entity called intraoperative floppy iris syndrome (IFIS)[1] characterized by a triad of intraoperative signs:

- A lax iris stroma with a tendency to flap or wave (floppy iris syndrome) in normal intraocular fluids
- A tendency for the floppy iris to prolapse in the corneal incisions
- Progressive intraoperative miosis

This syndrome is not always bilateral and does not have the same severity in all cases. There is a grading or classification for the syndrome: mild, moderate,[2-4] severe, or complete (with all elements of the triad present).[1,5,6] An analysis of one of the large case studies on IFIS published (167 cases)[7] showed that the severe form is most common (in 43% of cases), followed by the moderate form (30%), and lastly, the mild form (17%).

IFIS is a relatively rare syndrome seen in approximately 2% of cataract surgeries. The appearance of this syndrome is predominantly linked to the use of tamsulosin, a drug that blocks the α-1 receptors and is used in the treatment of benign prostate hyperplasia (BPH); however, as will be explained in this chapter, it can also be caused by other factors. In the first and in subsequent papers, a higher incidence of complications was observed during cataract surgery in these patients, including iris trauma (pupillary deformation, iris transillumination, and iridodialysis), hyphema, rupture of the posterior capsule, and herniation of the vitreous into the anterior chamber (AC). Preoperatively, the surgeon must identify the risk factors, note any prostate-related drug usage, and refer the patient to an experienced surgeon who is able to manage the floppy iris.

Etiology and Pathogenesis

According to a recent White Paper of the American Society of Cataract and Refractive Surgery (ASCRS),[7] the onset of IFIS is largely due to the use of systemic α-1 adrenergic antagonist drugs, such as tamsulosin.[1-13] According to some trials, this drug can cause IFIS in 94% of cases (with a range of 43% to 94% observed in different groups).[14]

The first paper by Chang and Campbell[1] described the syndrome and consisted of 2 studies: a retrospective study that examined 511 patients (706 eyes) to identify those being treated with tamsulosin and a prospective study that examined 741 patients (900 eyes) with analysis of the frequency of IFIS.

In the first series, the surgeons identified 16 patients using tamsulosin, and 10 of these had IFIS (63%). It should be pointed out that, from the entire series, these were the only eyes that showed IFIS (2%, 10/511). In the second series, IFIS was seen in 16 patients (2.2%, 16/741), and of these, 15 were being treated with tamsulosin (the remaining patient was diabetic).

Because α-1 antagonist drugs act by relaxing the smooth muscle of the prostate, they increase the flow in the lower urinary tract. Tamsulosin is the only one that is truly selective for the receptors of the receptor subtype α-1A, present in the prostate and in the smooth dilator muscle of the iris.[7,13-17] Tamsulosin is the most uroselective drug (with an affinity for the α-1A receptor that is 20 times greater than the affinity of the α-1B receptor) and therefore used more frequently in BPH; however, it is also more to blame for the onset of IFIS. In the United States, approximately 3% of all patients undergoing cataract surgery use this drug.

Buratto L, Brint SF, Caretti L.
Cataract Surgery in Complicated Cases (pp 131-140).

The real mechanism behind the development of IFIS is not known.

Molecular biology studies have demonstrated that these α-1A receptors are present in mouse iris and are those mostly responsible for mydriasis in that species.[18]

No similar studies have been performed on humans; however, it is probable that the situation is similar.[18,19] According to the most credible theory, by blocking the α-1A receptors consistently and for a prolonged period, tamsulosin induces a reduction in the tone of the iris dilator muscle and causes irreversible atrophy (from lack of use) of the muscle itself (explaining the poor mydriasis and the floppy iris). These phenomena may persist for years after the use of the drug has been discontinued.

Also recent tests on experimental models (rabbits[18,19]) suggested the role of another hypothetical receptor, in addition to the known α-1A receptor, in the contraction of the iris dilatory muscle and consequently in the pathogenesis of IFIS. This hypothetical receptor could have an extremely high affinity for tamsulosin.

In a recent study,[20] a postmortem examination under the optical microscope, the smooth dilatory muscle and the stroma of the iris in patients treated with tamsulosin were compared with human iris control eyes. The authors demonstrated a statistically significant reduction of the mean thickness of the iris dilatory muscle (a reduction of 23.2%) and the iris stroma in a group of patients who used tamsulosin. This reduction was not dose dependent. Moreover, under the electron microscope, the iris stroma contained myofibrils and vacuoles; however, these are not always associated with muscular atrophy.

A similar result was documented in a recent study by Prata et al[21]; using spectral-domain optical coherence tomography (OCT), researchers performed an in vivo comparison of the ultrastructure in humans and iris thickness in patients treated with nonselective α-1 antagonist drugs compared to controls. In patients (63% of the total) undergoing treatment or previously treated with this class of drugs, tamsulosin in particular, the researchers observed a dose-dependent thinning of the middle peripheral iris and a smaller pupil diameter. These findings confirm previous observations on animals.[22,23] The effect was dose dependent (duration of the treatment). This was in contrast with the results from the study by Santaella et al,[20] with the observations reported by Palea et al[24] on tamsulosin and with the clinical findings of Chang et al[7] that demonstrated cases of IFIS even in patients undergoing a short period of treatment with tamsulosin or patients who had stopped treatment several years previously (even 3 to 5 years).

The thinning of the iris stroma may be secondary to increased pupillary miosis and stretching of the stromal tissue and will give an explanation for the intraoperative behavior of the iris during IFIS.

Some authors[20] believe that the documented thinning of the iris dilatory muscle supports the theory of its atrophy because of a lack of adrenergic stimulation caused by the receptor inhibition of tamsulosin. Again, according to this study, the thinning and the atrophy of the dilatory muscle could explain the intraoperative behavior of the iris in IFIS. Given that the iris stroma is formed by dense fibrocollagenous tissue crossed by blood vessels, melanocytes, and fibroblasts, it is possible that the dilatory muscle makes a significant contribution to the structural rigidity of the iris to counteract the hydrostatic forces present in the AC during phacoemulsification. All of these permanent anatomical modifications can explain why IFIS is still present months and sometimes years after tamsulosin use is discontinued.[7,25]

Nevertheless, given that normally 50% to 55% of patients who use tamsulosin do not develop IFIS, the use of the drug does not necessarily predict the onset of IFIS. The fact that IFIS does not appear in all patients treated with tamsulosin is probably due to other factors.

In addition to its appearance following treatment with tamsulosin, IFIS can develop in some patients treated with nonselective α-1 antagonist drugs that inhibit all of the subtypes of α-1 receptors—alfuzosin, doxazosin, terazosin, prazonsin, naptopidil, and indoramin—even though in these cases the associated IFIS is less frequent (2% to 19% of cases) and generally less severe than in patients treated with selective α-1 antagonist drugs, as reported in numerous publications.[2,5,8,11,13-17,24,26] The retrospective studies by Palea et al[24] showed a much higher percentage of IFIS in patients treated with tamsulosin (86.4%) compared to those treated with alfuzosin (15.4%).

The difference in the incidence of IFIS could be (as mentioned earlier) that compared to the nonselective α-1 antagonist drugs, tamsulosin has a significantly higher affinity for the α-1A receptor subtype. Moreover, Michel et al[27] studied the effects of the different α-1 agonist and antagonist drugs in rabbits and reported that the α-1 antagonists were associated with a dose-dependent, reversible inhibition of the mydriasis induced by phenylephrine, and when the dose was increased, it induces reversible miosis. Another trial examined the effects of tamsulosin and alfuzosin on the pupil diameter in humans: following treatment with tamsulosin, the pupillary diameter decreases with the presence of mesopic and scotopic light; following treatment with alfuzosin it decreases only with scotopic light.[28] Oshika et al[5] made another interesting observation—the non-selective α-1 antagonist drugs induce IFIS only if administered systemically and not when administered topically.

As these are drugs used in female patients for the treatment of urinary retention and high blood pressure, IFIS can also be observed in women, though this is rare.[1,9]

IFIS has also been noted following the use of a number of drugs that can influence the tone of the iris dilatory muscle, examples include labetalol (α- and β-blocker), finasteride (a drug that inhibits 5-α reductase and indicated for BPH), mianserin (an antidepressant), zuclopenthixol and risperidone (antipsychotics with an α-blocker mechanism), and chlorpromazine and donepezil (α-blockers).[7,11,15,29,30] There is a report in the literature that documents the appearance of IFIS following the use of saw palmetto, an herbal remedy used in the treatment of BPH that has documented muscarinic and α-1 adrenergic activity (the latter also seen in men).[31]

Schwinn and Afshari[13] suggested a series of cofactors that are responsible for IFIS, such as high blood pressure, diabetes mellitus, and heart failure, even though a recent meta-analysis of the risk factors of IFIS in the literature[30] reported a link between high blood pressure and IFIS, though the same was not reported for diabetes mellitus. The authors concluded that multiple factors are involved in the onset of this complex syndrome.

Moreover, given that a significant percentage of cases appear without any clearly identifiable risk factors, it is plausible that the combination of different drugs and pathological states can cause IFIS not associated with the use of α-1 antagonist drugs[32]: saw palmetto, antagonists of angiotensin, cholinergic agonists and antagonists, myorelaxants, and nitric oxide do not appear to cause IFIS on their own; however, the combination of these drugs and pathologies for which they are indicated (high blood pressure, etc) may contribute to the appearance of IFIS. The complexity of the iris physiology, the drug dose and duration of treatment, individual sensitivity to the drugs, pharmacokinetics, and coexistence of systemic and ocular factors all probably play a role in the appearance of this complex syndrome. The reason why the use of α-blocker drugs (such as tamsulosin) does not predict the onset of IFIS can probably be explained by this. A topic that is the subject of ongoing discussion and still with no conclusion is the minimum preoperative length of treatment with α-antagonist drugs that can cause the onset of the syndrome. According to Chang et al,[14] the syndrome can appear after just 2 weeks of treatment; however, Shah et al[33] reported its appearance after just 2 days. This is an additional factor that would explain why not all patients treated with the drugs develop IFIS.

In routine clinical practice, the surgeon will deal with cases of IFIS that cannot be traced back to any specific cause.

Grading

As mentioned previously, the range of severity of IFIS is extremely variable; it varies between patients, even between the 2 eyes of the same patient.[9,11-14,34] The condition can be classified by the following:

- Mild: signs of iris laxity (without prolapse or miosis), good preoperative mydriasis
- Moderate: a tendency to iris prolapse and progressive miosis is observed, moderate preoperative mydriasis is observed
- Severe: classical triad of symptoms, often accompanied by poor preoperative mydriasis.

In the various study groups, the severe and moderate forms are more frequent than the mild forms. It should be pointed out that some of the evaluation criteria, such as iris laxity, are subjective, and this can lead to a variable definition or diagnosis between different observers.

Unfortunately, the onset and severity of IFIS cannot be predicted with certainty, even though poor preoperative mydriasis (< 6.5 mm according to some authors, < 7 mm according to others) generally precedes severe IFIS. With IFIS, during surgery many pupils constrict even when preoperative pupil dilation is sometimes excellent.[12,14]

No correlation has been demonstrated between the severities of IFIS, the color of the eyes, the patient's age, or the length of time the patient has been treated with α-1 antagonists. However, many researchers agree that the use of tamsulosin is associated with more severe IFIS[12,14] than other α-1 antagonist drugs.

The study by Prata et al,[21] which used spectral domain OCT, showed ultrastructural alterations of the iris that may predict the onset of IFIS.

Intraoperatively, iris flopping during the initial fluid injections into the AC indicates imminent onset of IFIS.

Management Strategies

A number or approaches have been proposed to manage the behavior of the iris during IFIS. These include the following:

- Numerous pharmacological strategies
- The use of a high viscosity or viscoadaptive viscoelastic substances (VES), combined with low flow parameters of phacoemulsification
- The insertion of mechanical pupil-dilating devices

With IFIS, the surgeon must always respect some general surgical principles. For example, the corneal incisions should always be constructed very carefully; the incisions should start in an anterior position at the root of the iris to reduce the incidence of iris prolapse. The corneal tunnel should be longer, again to reduce the risk of prolapse. Modern techniques of phacoemulsification—coaxial and bimanual microincisional cataract surgery (C-MICS and B-MICS, respectively)—using smaller, tighter incisions will reduce the risk of iris prolapse, but cannot prevent this happening in the case of severe IFIS.

Hydrodissection must be performed very slowly to avoid the risk of iris prolapse. The surgeon should reduce the flow of irrigation and aspiration and orient the direction of the irrigation flow away from the pupil edge to reduce mechanical stimulation that could cause further miosis. Phacoemulsification using central nucleofracture (modified

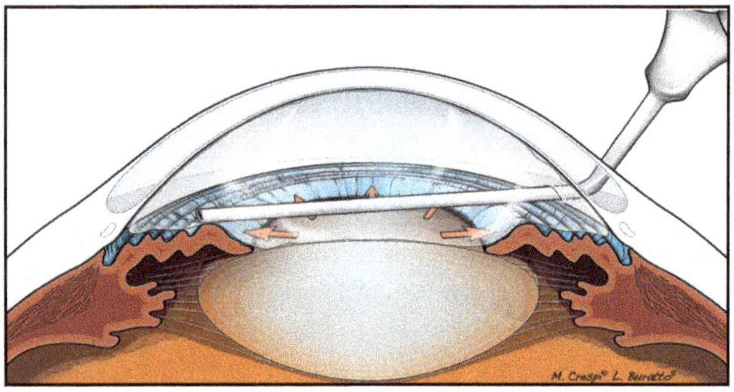

Figure 12-1. Viscomydriasis achieved with Healon 5.

phaco chop), which allows the surgeon to perform all of the movements of the instrument within the reduced pupillary diameter with constant visualization of the tip, is the elective technique in this type of eye as it reduces engaging the iris with the phaco tip. Other techniques (such as the cross), apart from requiring the surgeon to move the phaco tip into a blind peripheral area (behind a poorly dilated iris), increase the risk of accidental iris capture by the phaco or irrigation/aspiration tip with additional miotic stimulus.

An injector should be used to implant the intraocular lens (IOL), eliminating the need to enlarge the tunnel, thus reducing the possibility of the iris prolapse while providing better control of the intraocular maneuvers. Some suggest inserting the injector cartridge in the bevel-up position and injecting the IOL without rotation in the bevel-down position; most surgeons would consider this system to be unusual, however, by introducing and removing the injector from the eye like a shoe-horn, there will be a reduction in the incidence of iris prolapse into the tunnel and the cartridge.

Finally, the surgeon should avoid partial sphincterotomies and mechanical pupil stretching. In addition to not being helpful, they can exacerbate iris floppiness.

Considering that IFIS can also be unilateral, the surgeon should remember the syndrome may affect the other eye of patients scheduled for cataract surgery using all types of α-antagonists, even when there has been no evidence of IFIS in the first eye operated.

Pharmacological Strategies

Some authors have suggested that stopping use of tamsulosin (that has a plasma half-life of just 48 to 72 hours) prior to cataract surgery could reduce the risk of the syndrome developing.[1,7,9,13,14,34] Like others, we believe that in the absence of objective scientific evidence, the drug treatment should not be stopped, because the syndrome may appear years after discontinuation of the drugs.[7,9,21,25,34] The suspension of the drug was tested in 2 important clinical trials[14,35]: in both cases, the authors concluded that stopping treatment did not prevent IFIS nor did it reduce the severity.

An intracameral injection of α-1 agonists, underneath the iris, was suggested to directly stimulate the iris dilatory muscles.[4,36-42] In some cases, an intracameral injection of phenylephrine was efficacious in the management of IFIS; others suggested intracameral epinephrine. To balance the acid pH, avoid solutions containing preservatives and use diluted solutions (eg, 1:1000 epinephrine [without bisulfites] associated with 1:3 [or 1:4] balanced salt solution [BSS] Plus or plain BSS).[39] An intracameral injection of phenylephrine or epinephrine can increase the dilation of the pupil in some cases of IFIS, but not all of them. According to some authors,[36] the intracameral injection of epinephrine does not change the incidence of IFIS, but can prevent the onset of intraoperative miosis. Moreover, both agents often increase iris rigidity, increasing the tone of the iris muscle, greatly reducing the tendency of the iris to flop or prolapse. However, there have been reports of risk of acute hypertension following the intracameral injection of α-1 agonists, though to date, the link has not been definitively confirmed.[42]

The use of Mydriacyl (tropicamide), indicated in theory for cases of IFIS, has nothing to support the claims of its efficacy.

Masket and Belani[40] were the first to suggest the use of atropine eye drops to maximize cycloplegia in eyes at risk of IFIS. As this approach is not useful in all cases of IFIS, 1% atropine (3 times a day for 1 to 2 days prior to surgery), is a reliable method to counteract miosis in IFIS.[25,39,40] It generally leads to a larger preoperative pupil diameter; however, for general management of the pupil, other devices are often required such as iris retractors. The results from a small clinical trial demonstrated the success of a combination of topical atropine and intracameral epinephrine,[40] suggesting a synergism of the 2 drugs.

Nevertheless, when atropine is used, patients with BPH should not stop treatment with α-blocker drugs to avoid risking acute urinary retention.

Viscoelastics

As described in the literature,[14] Healon 5 (2.3% sodium hyaluronate) is an extremely cohesive VES with enormous viscomydriatic capacity. It should be injected close to the pupil margin and successively in segments around the pupil (Figure 12-1).

Because of its high viscosity, this substance enlarges the pupil (facilitating the creation of the capsulorrhexis); it has a unique property of blocking the tendency of iris prolapse in the corneal incisions.

Nevertheless, during phacoemulsification, the surgeon should reduce aspiration flow and vacuum settings (<25 cc/min, <200 to 250 mm Hg, respectively) to prolong the presence of the VES in the AC. If progressive miosis is seen during phacoemulsification, additional Healon 5 can be injected.

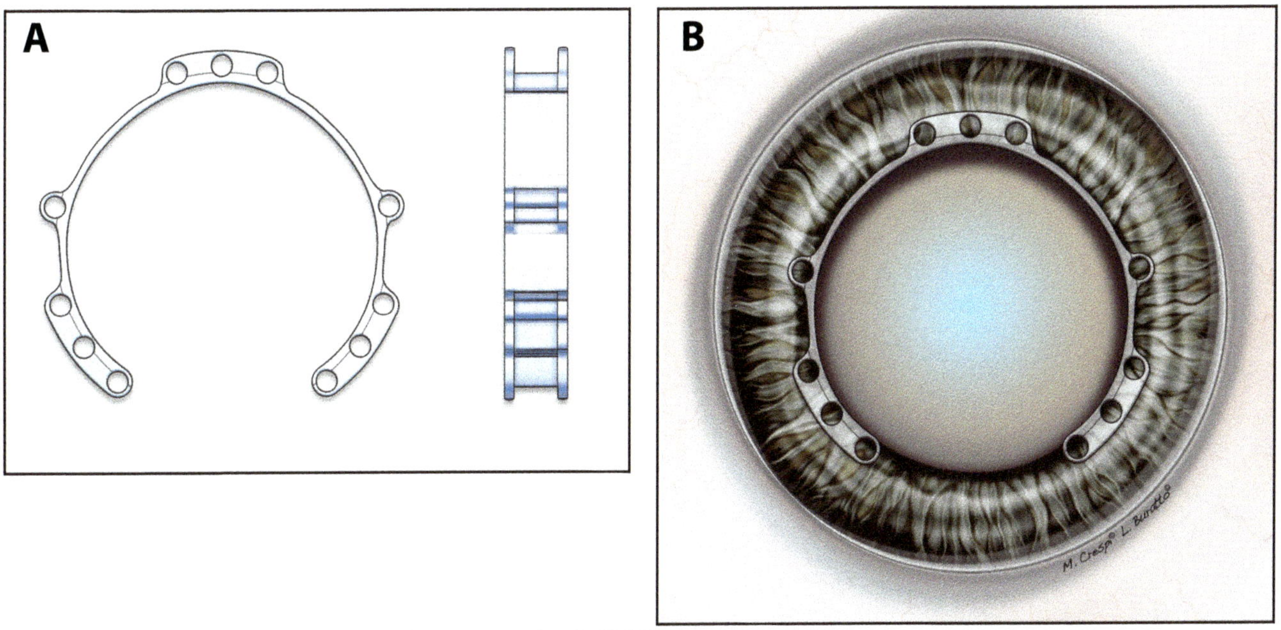

Figure 12-2. (A and B) A Morcher 5S pupil expansion ring in PMMA.

When compared to the devices for mechanical expansion, Healon 5 depends more on appropriate phacoemulsification technique and correct settings of the parameters. Clearly, this strategy is not indicated when high vacuum levels are required, as in the case of very dense nuclei or if the surgeon is not comfortable using this setting.

With the aspiration of Healon 5, the pupil can constrict rapidly and the floppy iris will be more evident when the cortex is being removed or following the insertion of the IOL (VES must be completely removed from below the IOL). With these maneuvers, the surgeon should keep the bottle at a moderate height (not excessively high) and perform the surgical procedures precisely and delicately to avoid problems.

Other VESs can be used as an alternative to, or in association with, Healon 5. Arshinoff[43] suggested injecting a dispersive substance such as Viscoat (3% sodium hyaluronate-4% chondroitin sulfate) into the peripheral area of the AC, followed by an injection of Healon 5 centrally to create what he described as the "soft-shell technique to resolve IFIS."

Modi et al[44] demonstrated that DisCoVisc (1.6% hyaluronic acid-4% chondroitin sulfate) lasts longer inside the eye and is a better VES than Healon 5 when high flow and vacuum parameters are used.

Devices for the Mechanical Expansion of the Pupil

Iris retractors and pupil expansion rings produce stable mechanical pupillary dilation. They prevent miosis and avoid iris prolapse[45-49] (refer to Chapter 5).

The rings can be complete or incomplete; some are manufactured in solid polymethylmethacrylate (PMMA), while others are produced in silicone or expandable hydrogel (ie, Morcher, Perfect Pupil, Graether, Siepser).

Both the 5S pupillary ring (Morcher Gmbh, Stuttgart, Germany) and the Perfect Pupil (Milvella, Savage, MN) are disposable plastic rings that are positioned at the margin of the pupil with a sterilizable metal injector[47] (Figure 12-2). These rings have an opening that allows the passage of the phaco tip.

The Graether pupillary expansion ring in silicone (Eagle Vision, Memphis, TN) is inserted with a preloaded disposable plastic injector.[48]

When dehydrated, the Siepser ring has an irregular oval shape and is easily inserted through a 3-mm opening. Once hydrated inside the AC, it expands into a circular shape and is positioned across the pupil margin with a positioning hook; in this way, the feet engage the iris and expand it (Figure 12-3).

All of these devices are difficult to insert with pupils of diameter less than 4 mm or with small eyes.

Recently, Malyugin developed an expansion device that is squared, foldable, and disposable (Micro Surgical Technology, Redmond, WA) (Figure 12-4)[45]: in 5-0 polypropylene, this flexible device is inserted into the AC with a disposable injector. Its 4 circular spirals engage the pupil edge and expand it to 6 to 7 mm for the duration of surgery. This pupil expansion device is the easiest to insert and remove. The main advantage of this device is its straightforward, nontraumatic engagement of the iris edge and the well-controlled pupil stretching it produces.

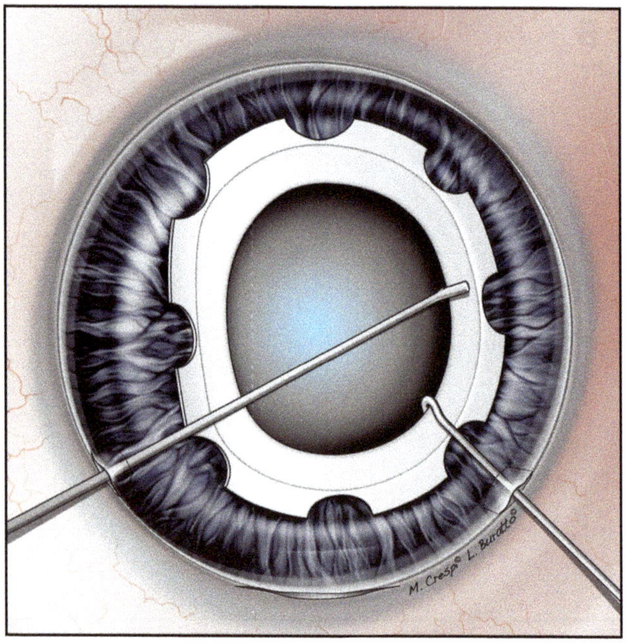

Figure 12-3. Positioning of the Siepser pupil expansion ring.

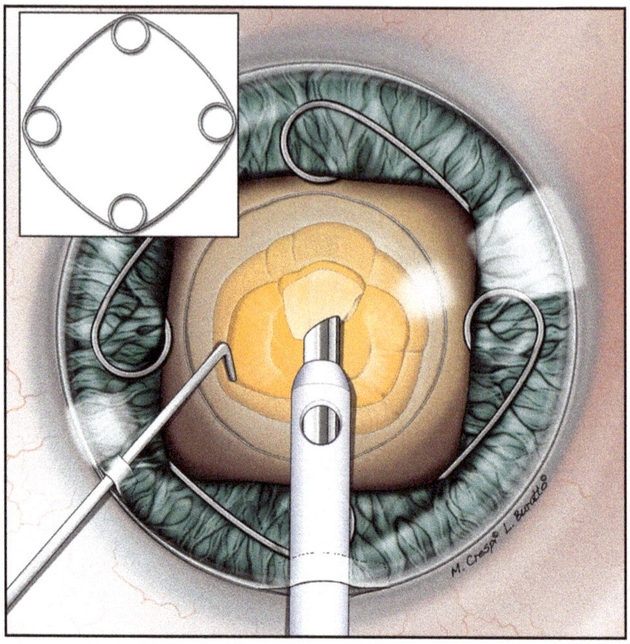

Figure 12-4. Malyugin's pupil expander.

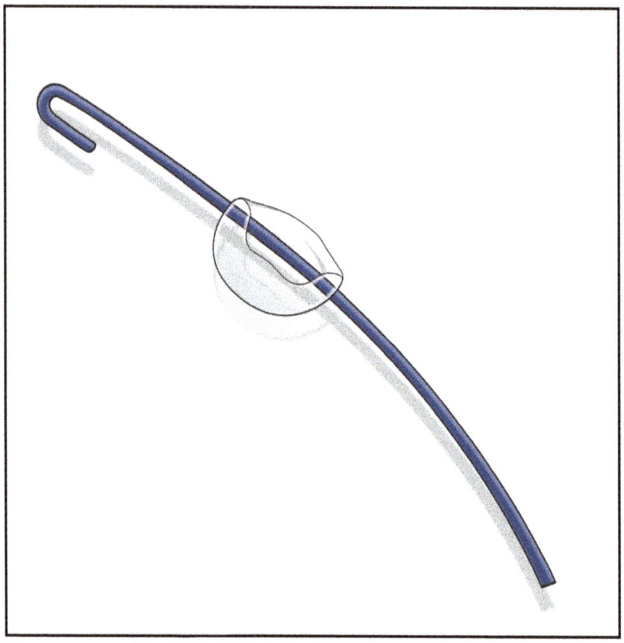

Figure 12-5. Iris retractors: a Grieshaber disposable hook.

Iris retractors are the most commonly used mechanical strategy for pupil expansion during IFIS (Figure 12-5).[9,14,35] Disposable retractors are produced in 6-0 nylon (Alcon Laboratories, Fort Worth, TX); ones that can be sterilized are produced in 4-0 polypropylene (Katena Products, Denville, NJ). Having the same size and stiffness as the haptics of the IOL, the reusable retractors are easy to manage, and the fact that they can be sterilized in the autoclave means that they have an excellent cost-benefit ratio.

Oetting and Omphroy[49] were the first to suggest that positioning the retractors to form a diamond-shaped pupil was associated with a number of advantages (see Chapter 5). The retractors are introduced into the AC through 4 paracenteses, created just at the clear cornea; the position is important for the functional and safe diamond-shape pupil expansion. The subincisional retractor is inserted through a different paracentesis than the main incision. Thus, the iris is retracted posteriorly and underneath the main incision; consequently, exposure of the iris to the phaco tip is minimized (Figure 12-6). The retractor positioned close to the side-port incision facilitates the movements of the chopper.

In a relatively recent study,[50] a new and interesting method was proposed to manage iris prolapse: the prolapsed iris is reposited and a single subincisional iris retractor is inserted to manage the iris prolapse of IFIS.

Some authors suggest inserting the retractors and the expansion rings following the capsulotomy and hydrodissection procedures. In this case, the pupil edge can be stretched using a positioning hook or with VES to avoid tearing the edge of the capsulorrhexis with the retractor. It should be remembered that if the pupil is fibrotic (due to the chronic use of miotic agents or due to posterior synechiae), excessive stretching with retractors may cause bleeding, rupture of the sphincter, and permanent mydriasis. This normally does not happen with IFIS, a syndrome in which the pupil is so elastic that it will rapidly return to its physiological size even if it has been stretched to a maximum.[1]

Both of these devices, indicated with severe IFIS, despite prolonging the surgical time allow surgery to proceed

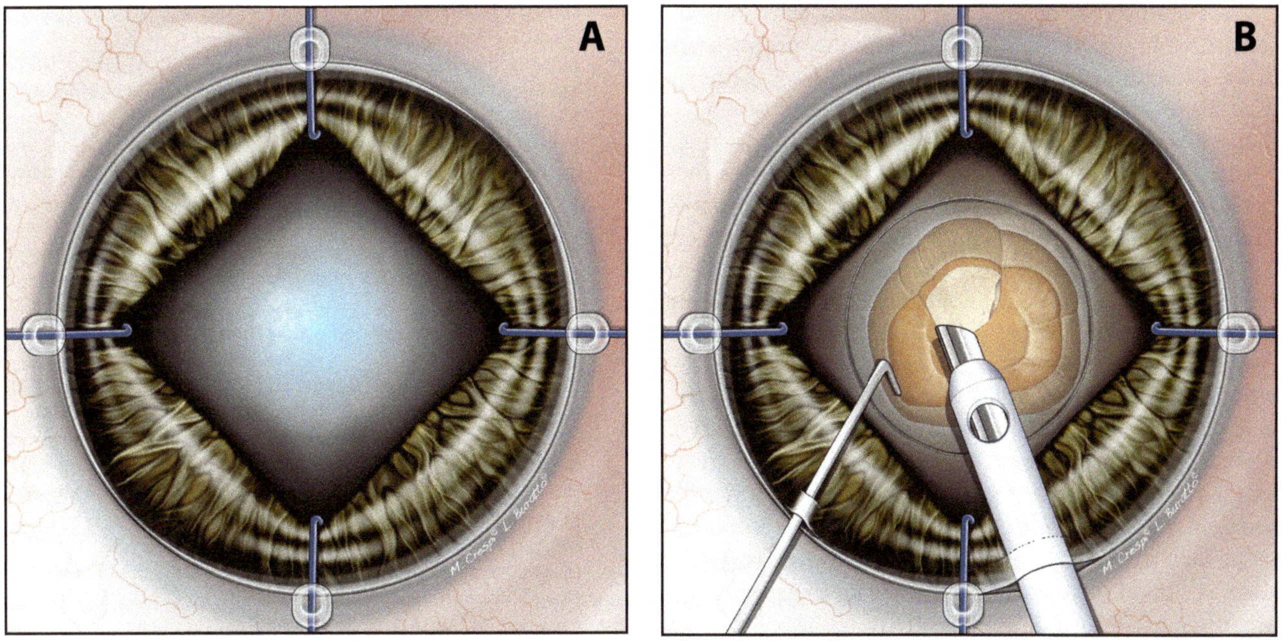

Figure 12-6. Iris retractors in 4-0 polypropylene. (A) Diamond-shaped pupil achieved by positioning 4 iris retractors. (B) Positioning a subincisional iris retractor inserted through a paracentesis close to the main incision.

under conditions of maximum safety and the creation of stable mydriasis.

Combined Strategies

Given the enormous variation in the severity of IFIS, determining the best single technique for managing the problem is difficult in the absence of a randomized prospective trial.

According to a study by the ASCRS,[35] in decreasing order, the most frequently used management strategies are as follows:

- Intracameral α-agonist (38%)
- Iris retractors (23%)
- Preoperative administration of atropine (19%)
- Healon 5 VES (15%)
- Pupillary expansion rings (4%)

Because of the varied severity of the IFIS syndrome, an approach that involves several steps can be used in these eyes.[41] All of the previously described strategies can be successfully combined, and one-third of the eye-surgeons interviewed during the ASCRS study preferred this approach.[35]

In cases of mild or moderate IFIS, pharmacological strategies alone may be sufficient. The intracameral injection of α-1 agonists will dilate the pupil and prevent or reduce iris flopping and prolapse through increased tone of the dilating muscle.

If the diameter of the pupil is inadequate for surgery, a viscoadaptive VES can be injected.

Finally, with severe IFIS or other surgical difficulties (eg, dense nucleus, pseudoexfoliation, relaxed zonules), iris retractors and devices to expand the pupil are extremely useful and are also indicated in cases of less experienced surgeons or phaco techniques performed with high levels of vacuum.

The surgeon must remember that it is extremely difficult to compare the efficacy of the various strategies given the enormous variability in the degree of severity of IFIS and its unpredictability from patient to patient.[51]

Surgical Risks

Before this syndrome was well described, cataract surgery in patients treated with α-1 antagonist drugs was associated with an increase in surgical complications. Due to unexpected iris prolapse and miosis, problems seen with IFIS—iris defects (pupil deformation, iris transillumination, and iris dialysis), accidental aspiration of the iris by the phaco or irrigation/aspiration tip, hyphema, and capsule rupture or loss of vitreous—were observed in 0% and 22% of cases. The percentage is higher for beginning surgeons and lower in more recent publications.[1,8,14,27,52-65]

Cases of IFIS with iris prolapse have been reported during trabeculectomy.[66,67] An interesting case report of choroidal detachment in a patient using tamsulosin would suggest that this drug might also inhibit the α-1 receptors of the choroid.[68]

In a multicenter prospective study[14] to determine the incidence of surgical complications, with the surgeon aware of the patient's history of use of α-blocker drugs, he or she used his or her discretion to select one of the 4 systems to manage the pupil: iris retractors, pupil expansion rings, Healon 5 with a low aspiration rate, or preoperative topical atropine (intracameral epinephrine was not included in the study). The surgeon could employ a second strategy in the event the first is not successful. The study demonstrated that Healon 5 was the most common first-line strategy (60%), followed by iris retractors (31%), preoperative atropine (5%), and pupil extension rings (4%). The most common complication was a mild or moderate iris defect (asymptomatic), usually caused by iris prolapse and observed in 16% of cases. Capsule rupture and vitreous loss were observed in just 0.6% of cases (a much lower figure than the 12% to 15% seen in other studies[1,15]).

In the trial by ASCRS,[35] the most frequent complications were damage to the iris and posterior capsule rupture; according to 53% and 23%, respectively, of the ophthalmologists surveyed, these percentages were significantly higher than those observed in eyes not affected by IFIS.

Finally, several reports have been published that analyze large numbers of patients having cataract surgery in association with IFIS. Even though there are numerous operating difficulties and problematic management with these eyes, patients operated by expert surgeons reported excellent functional outcomes and no complications were observed.

Conclusion

Preoperative recognition of the potential presence of IFIS is extremely important in modern cataract surgery. Poor mydriasis (<6.5 mm) is an important risk factor that increases the degree of operating difficulty and requires careful surgical planning. When the experienced surgeon is fully aware of the risk of IFIS in a patient, appropriate operative strategies to reduce the incidence of complications and achieve an excellent outcome can be used. The patient must also be informed on the possible problems that face the surgeon and that the surgery may proceed differently from routine cataract surgery, with associated complications. It should be remembered that not all patients using anti-α-1 adrenergic drugs develop IFIS and that this syndrome may manifest with differing degrees of severity, even between the 2 eyes of the same patient.

References

1. Chang DF, Campbell JR. Intraoperative floppy iris syndrome associated with tamsulosin. *J Cataract Refract Surg.* 2005;31:664-673.
2. Dhingra N, Rajkumar KN, Kumar V. Intraoperative floppy iris syndrome with doxazosin [letter]. *Eye (Lond).* 2007;21:678-679.
3. Bidaguren A, Irigoyen C, Mendicute J, et al. Floppy-iris syndrome associated with tamsulosin: a prospective case-control stud. *Arch Soc Esp Oftalmol.* 2007;82:349-354.
4. Keklikci U, Isen K, Unlu K, et al. Incidence, clinical findings and management of intraoperative floppy iris syndrome associated with tamsulosin. *Acta Ophthalmol.* 2009;87:306-309.
5. Oshika T, Ohashi Y, Inamura M, et al. Incidence of intraoperative floppy iris syndrome in patients on either systemic or topical alpha(1)-adrenoceptor antagonist. *Am J Ophthalmol.* 2007;143:150-151.
6. Mazal Z. Intraoperative floppy iris syndrome. *Cesk Slov Oftalmol.* 2007;63:91-94.
7. Chang DF, Braga-Mele R, Mamalis N, Masket S, Miller KM, Nichamin LD, Packard RB, Packer M; ASCRS Cataract Clinical Committee. ASCRS White Paper: clinical review of intraoperative floppy-iris syndrome. *J Cataract Refract Surg.* 2008;34(12):2153-2162.
8. Herd MK. Intraoperative floppy-iris syndrome with doxazosin. *J Cataract Refract Surg.* 2007;33(4):562.
9. Nguyen DQ, Sebastian RT, Kyle G. Surgeon's experiences of the intraoperative floppy iris syndrome in the United Kingdom. *Eye (Lond).* 2007;21(3):443-444.
10. Cheung CM, Awan MA, Sandramouli S. Prevalence and clinical findings of tamsulosin-associated intraoperative floppy-iris syndrome. *J Cataract Refract Surg.* 2006;32:1336-1339.
11. Chadha V, Borooah S, Tey A, et al. Floppy iris behaviour during cataract surgery: associations and variations. *Br J Ophthalmol.* 2006;91:40-42.
12. Parssinen O, Leppanen E, Keski-Rahkonen P, et al. Influence of tamsulosin on the iris and its implications for cataract surgery. *Invest Ophthalmol Vis Sci.* 2006;47:3766-3771.
13. Schwinn DA, Afshari NA. Alpha1-adrenergic antagonists and floppy iris syndrome: tip of the iceberg? *Ophthalmology.* 2005;112:2059-2060.
14. Chang DF, Osher RH, Wang L, Koch DD. Prospective multicenter evaluation of cataract surgery in patients taking tamsulosin (Flomax). *Ophthalmology.* 2007;114(5):957-964.
15. El-Ghatit AM. Association of IFIS and vasodepressor medication [letter]. *J Cataract Refract Surg.* 2006;32:546-547.
16. Settas G, Fitt AW. Intraoperative floppy iris syndrome in a patient taking alfuzosin for benign prostatic hypertrophy [letter]. *Eye.* 2006;20:1431-1432.
17. Muqit MM, Menage MJ. Intraoperative floppy iris syndrome [letter]. *Ophthalmology.* 2006;113:1885-1886.
18. Nakaura S, Taniguchi T, Suzuki F, et al. Evaluation of α1-adrenoreceptors in the rabbit iris: pharmacological characterization and expression of mRNA. *Br J Pharmacol.* 1999;127:1367-1374.
19. Ishikawa H, Miller DD, Patil PN. Comparison of post-junctional alpha-adrenoceptors in iris dilator muscle of humans, and albino and pigmented rabbits. *Naunyn Schmiedebergs Arch Pharmacol.* 1996;354(6):765-772.
20. Santaella RM, Destafeno JJ, Stinnett SS, Proia AD, Chang DF, Kim T. The effect of alpha1-adrenergic receptor antagonist tamsulosin (Flomax) on iris dilator smooth muscle anatomy. *Ophthalmology.* 2010;117(9):1743-1749.
21. Prata TS, Palmiero PM, Angelilli A, Sbeity Z, De Moraes CG, Liebmann JM, Ritch R. Iris morphologic changes related to alpha(1)-adrenergic receptor antagonists implications for intraoperative floppy iris syndrome. *Ophthalmology.* 2009;116(5):877-881.
22. Wikberg-Matsson A, Uhlén S, Wikberg JE. Characterization of alpha(1)-adrenoceptor subtypes in the eye. *Exp Eye Res.* 2000;70(1):51-60.
23. Yu Y, Koss MC. Alpha(1A)-adrenoceptors mediate sympathetically evoked pupillary dilation in rats. *J Pharmacol Exp Ther.* 2002;300(2):521-525.

24. Palea S, Chang D, Rekik M, et al. Comparative effect of alfuzosin and tamsulosin on the contractile response of isolated rabbit prostatic and iris dilator smooth muscles: possible model for intraoperative floppy-iris syndrome. *J Cataract Refract Surg.* 2008;34:489-496.
25. Bendel RE, Phillips MB. Preoperative use of atropine to prevent intraoperative floppy-iris syndrome in patients taking tamsulosin. *J Cataract Refract Surg.* 2006;32:1603-1605.
26. Blouin MC, Blouin J, Perreault S, Lapointe A, Dragomir A. Intraoperative floppy-iris syndrome associated with alpha1-adrenoreceptors: comparison of tamsulosin and alfuzosin. *J Cataract Refract Surg.* 2007;33(7):1227-1234.
27. Michel M, Okutsu H, Noguchi Y, et al. In vivo studies on the effects of alpha1-adrenoceptor antagonists on pupil diameter and urethral tone in rabbits. *Naunyn Schmiedebergs Arch Pharmacol.* 2006;372:346-353.
28. Altan-Yaycioglu R, Yaycioglu O, Gul U, et al. The effects of two systemic alpha1-adrenergic blockers on pupil diameter: a prospective randomized single-blind study. *Naunyn Schmiedebergs Arch Pharmacol.* 2007;375:199-203.
29. Issa SA, Dagres EJ. Intraoperative floppy-iris syndrome and finasteride intake. J Cataract Refract Surg. 2007;33(12):2142-2143.
30. Yeu E, Grostern R. Saw palmetto and intraoperative floppy-iris syndrome. *J Cataract Refract Surg.* 2007;33(5):927-928.
31. Chatziralli IP, Sergentanis TN. Risk factors for intraoperative floppy iris syndrome: a meta-analysis. *Ophthalmology.* 2011;118(4):730-735.
32. Neff KD, Sandoval HP, Fernández de Castro LE, Nowacki AS, Vroman DT, Solomon KD. Factors associated with intraoperative floppy iris syndrome. *Ophthalmology.* 2009;116(4):658-663.
33. Shah N, Tendulkar M, Brown R. Should we anticipate intraoperative floppy iris syndrome (IFIS) even with very short history of tamsulosin? *Eye (Lond).* 2009;23(3):740.
34. Osher RH. Association between IFIS and Flomax. *J Cataract Refract Surg.* 2006;32(4):547.
35. Chang DF, Braga-Mele R, Mamalis N, Masket S, Miller KM, Nichamin LD, Packard RB, Packer M; ASCRS Cataract Clinical Committee. Clinical experience with intraoperative floppy-iris syndrome. Results of the 2008 ASCRS member survey. *J Cataract Refract Surg.* 2008;34(7):1201-1209.
36. Takmaz T, Can I. Clinical features, complications, and incidence of intraoperative floppy iris syndrome in patients taking tamsulosin. *Eur J Ophthalmol.* 2007;17(6):909-913.
37. Williams GP, Tsaloumas MD. The use of intracameral phenylephrine in the management of intraoperative floppy-iris syndrome with doxazosin. *Eye (Lond).* 2008;22(8):1094.
38. Gurbaxani A, Packard R. Intracameral phenylephrine to prevent floppy iris syndrome during cataract surgery in patients on tamsulosin. *Eye (Lond).* 2007;21(3):331-332.
39. Shugar JK. Prophylaxis for IFIS. *J Cataract Refract Surg.* 2007;33(6):942-943.
40. Masket S, Belani S. Combined preoperative topical atropine sulfate 1% and intracameral nonpreserved epinephrine hydrochloride 1:4000 [corrected] for management of intraoperative floppy-iris syndrome. *J Cataract Refract Surg.* 2007;33(4):580-582.
41. Manvikar S, Allen D. Cataract surgery management in patients taking tamsulosin staged approach. *J Cataract Refract Surg.* 2006;32(10):1611-1614.
42. Lee KJ, Figueira EC, Sharma NS, et al. Iris prolapse and the floppy-iris syndrome. *J Cataract Refract Surg.* 2007;33(5):757-758.
43. Arshinoff SA. Modified SST-USST for tamsulosin-associated intraoperative [corrected] floppy-iris syndrome. *J Cataract Refract Surg.* 2006;32(4):559-561.
44. Modi SS, Davison JA, Walters T. Safety, efficacy, and intraoperative characteristics of DisCoVisc and Healon ophthalmic viscosurgical devices for cataract surgery. *Clin Ophthalmol.* 2011;5:1381-1389.
45. Chang DF. Use of Malyugin pupil expansion device for intraoperative floppy-iris syndrome: results in 30 consecutive cases. *J Cataract Refract Surg.* 2008;34(5):835-841.
46. Akman A, Yilmaz G, Oto S, Akova YA. Comparison of various pupil dilatation methods for phacoemulsification in eyes with a small pupil secondary to pseudoexfoliation. *Ophthalmology.* 2004;111(9):1693-1698.
47. Kershner RM. Management of the small pupil for clear corneal cataract surgery. *J Cataract Refract Surg.* 2002;28(10):1826-1831.
48. Graether JM.Graether pupil expander for managing the small pupil during surgery. *J Cataract Refract Surg.* 1996;22(5):530-535.
49. Oetting TA, Omphroy LC. Modified technique using flexible iris retractors in clear corneal cataract surgery. *J Cataract Refract Surg.* 2002;28(4):596-598.
50. Tint NL, Yeung AM, Alexander P. Management of intraoperative floppy-iris syndrome-associated iris prolapse using a single iris retractor. *J Cataract Refract Surg.* 2009;35(11):1849-1852.
51. Flach AJ. Intraoperative floppy iris syndrome: pathophysiology, prevention, and treatment. *Trans Am Ophthalmol Soc.* 2009;107:234-239.
52. Mamalis N. Intraoperative floppy-iris syndrome. *J Cataract Refract Surg.* 2006;32(10):1589-1590.
53. Chitkara DK, Smerdon DL. Risk factors, complications, and results in extracapsular cataract extraction. *J Cataract Refract Surg.* 1997;23:570-574.
54. Corey RP, Olson RJ. Surgical outcomes of cataract extractions performed by residents using phacoemulsification. *J Cataract Refract Surg.* 1998;24:66-72.
55. Desai P, Minassian DC, Reidy A. National cataract surgery survey 1997-98: a report of the results of the clinical outcomes. *Br J Ophthalmol.* 1999;83:1336-1340.
56. Martin KR, Burton RL. The phacoemulsification learning curve: per-operative complications in the first 3000 cases of an experienced surgeon. *Eye.* 2000;14:190-195.
57. Lundstrom M, Barry P, Leite E, et al. 1998 European Cataract Outcome Study: report from the European Cataract Outcome Study Group. *J Cataract Refract Surg.* 2001;27:1176-1184.
58. Ionides A, Minassian D, Tuft S. Visual outcome following posterior capsule rupture during cataract surgery. *Br J Ophthalmol.* 2001;85:222-224.
59. Gimbel HV, Sun R, Ferensowicz M, et al. Intraoperative management of posterior capsule tears in phacoemulsification and intraocular lens implantation. *Ophthalmology.* 2001;108:2186-2189.
60. Blomquist PH, Rugwani RM. Visual outcomes after vitreous loss during cataract surgery performed by residents. *J Cataract Refract* Surg. 2002;28:847-852.
61. Tan JH, Karwatowski WS. Phacoemulsification cataract surgery and unplanned anterior vitrectomyis it bad news? *Eye.* 2002;16:117-120.
62. Chan FM, Mathur R, Ku JJ, et al. Short-term outcomes in eyes with posterior capsule rupture during cataract surgery. *J Cataract Refract Surg.* 2003;29:537-541.
63. Androudi S, Brazitikos PD, Papadopoulos NT, et al. Posterior capsule rupture and vitreous loss during phacoemulsification with or without the use of an anterior chamber maintainer. *J Cataract Refract Surg.* 2004;30:449-452.
64. Hyams M, Mathalone N, Herskovitz M, et al. Intraoperative complications of phacoemulsification in eyes with and without pseudoexfoliation. *J Cataract Refract Surg.* 2005;31:1002-1005.

65. Ang GS, Whyte IF. Effect and outcomes of posterior capsule rupture in a district general hospital setting. *J Cataract Refract Surg.* 2006;32:623-627.
66. Au L, Wechsler D, Fenerty C. Alpha antagonists and intraoperative floppy iris syndrome (IFIS) during trabeculectomy. *Eye (Lond).* 2007;21(5):671-672.
67. Norris JH, Mall S, Burnett CA.Floppy Iris Syndrome Hull Hooks (FISH Hooks): a new technique for managing IFIS in trabeculectomy surgery. *Eye (Lond).* 2009;23(3):743-744.
68. Shapiro BL, Petrovic V, Lee SE, Flach A, McCaffery S, O'Brien JM. Choroidal detachment following the use of tamsulosin (Flomax). *Am J Ophthalmol.* 2007;143(2):351-353.

13

Management of Cataract in Diabetic Patients

Epidemiological data suggest that there has been an increased incidence of diabetes mellitus (DM) in industrialized countries.[1,2] In 2010, it was estimated that more than 220 million people suffered from DM and that number will have increased to 300 million by 2025. DM affects approximately 69% of the White population with a higher frequency in Blacks, American Indians, and Hispanic populations.[1,2]

Type 1 diabetes is characterized by reduced secretion of insulin caused by destruction of beta cells in the islets of Langerhans. Diabetes type 2, on the other hand, is caused by a resistance to insulin, rather than reduced secretion, and typically develops later in life.

Monitoring type 1 and type 2 patients with good glycemic control and equal duration of the disease shows greater similarities than differences between the 2 forms of the disease.

Type 2 diabetes is increasing because of poor dietary habits and obesity; however, retinal complications and cardiovascular diseases can be significantly reduced by maintaining strict glycemic control, as described in the Diabetes Control and Complications Trial.[3] Blood glucose values ideally should be between 80 and 120 mg/dL and glycosylated hemoglobin (Hb1AC) should have a value of below 6.5.[3]

Cataract is more common in diabetic than in nondiabetic patients.[4] Poor glycemic control increases the incidence of cataracts and accelerates their evolution.

Two-thirds of patients with type 2 diabetes develop cataracts[5] and 20.8% of those with diabetes type 1 undergo cataract surgery after 25 years of disease.[6]

Cataract is the second most common ocular complication in DM.[7] In the UK, about 20% of cataract surgeries were performed on patients with diabetes.[8]

Cataract surgery in diabetic patients has 2 objectives: to improve visual acuity and allow better classification and treatment of retinopathy.[9] This second objective is pursued mainly in industrialized countries[10]; diabetic patients in developing countries undergo surgery when the cataract is mature or hypermature.[11,12]

Cataract surgery can often be responsible for rapid progression of diabetic retinopathy (DR) and may be associated with a poor functional outcome after surgery,[4,7,13] but this was prior to widespread use of phacoemulsification, implantation of intraocular lenses (IOLs) in the bag, fluorescein angiography, focal photocoagulation, panretinal photocoagulation, and vitrectomy, and it was prevalent when strict glycemic control was not considered essential. DR progression ranged from 15% to 70%, with reduction in the degree of progression due to improvements in surgical techniques.

Between the late 1970s and early 1990s, the literature showed rapid progression of DR (diabetic retinopathy and maculopathy) following cataract surgery performed with intracapsular (ICCE) and extracapsular (ECCE) cataract extraction techniques.[14-17]

DR after cataract surgery with phacoemulsification has not produced a consensus,[18,19] especially as there have been very few studies that included nonoperated eyes as controls.[20-23] Several studies documented a rate of progression of DR after phacoemulsification of between 21% and 32% 12 months after surgery[17,18,24-28] or 25% after 6 months.[29]

The rate of progression of DR in eyes with phacoemulsification is lower than the rate associated with older types of cataract surgery. Jaffe et al[15] and Pollack et al[30] reported a progression of DR of 37% and 38.2% 12 to 18 months after cataract extraction (ECCE), compared to progression of 30% or less reported for phacoemulsification. Only 4 studies[20-23] compared operated and nonoperated eyes to assess progression of DR after phacoemulsification; in all these studies, there were no statistically significant differences in progression of DR between operated and nonoperated

Buratto L, Brint SF, Caretti L.
Cataract Surgery in Complicated Cases (pp 141-147).

eyes, although the progression was slightly higher in operated eyes.

A recent review by Saha and Chen[31] shows phacoemulsification did not accelerate development of retinopathy and macular edema (ME) in all patients with diabetes.

There is no doubt that the use of increasingly smaller incisions and reduced surgical times associated with phacoemulsification decrease postoperative inflammation and may induce less blood-ocular barrier breakdown. Higher levels of vascular endothelial growth factor (VEGF) and other angiogenic factors have been detected in operated eyes, on the day immediately after phacoemulsification. The levels tend to drop a month after surgery. Elevated levels of these angiogenic factors may be responsible for subclinical or clinical progression of DR and ME.

There is no doubt that the degree of severity of DR contributes to increased risk of postoperative progression. Studies have shown that in diabetic patients without retinopathy or with mild retinopathy, the results of cataract surgery are excellent and reflect those obtained in nondiabetic patients.[32]

Patients with nonproliferative diabetic retinopathy ([non-PDR] moderate to medium) without ME show functional results that are close to those of nondiabetic subjects, although there may be increased macular retinal thickness by optical coherence tomography that is often not clinically significant.[33]

It has been shown that in the later stages of DR, phacoemulsification may be associated with a risk of visual deterioration secondary to DR progression[18,19,34,35]; however, it would appear that only a minority of patients with advanced DR (with ME and history of previous laser treatments) were worse after cataract surgery.[32]

Several studies also suggest that poor metabolic control contributes to progression of DR after surgery.[36,37]

At least one study completed a few years ago has shown that cystoid ME (CME) resolved spontaneously without treatment.[38] Thus, laser or early injection treatment is not indicated; waiting up to 6 months before any intervention is more appropriate.

The belief that cataract surgery leads to poorer results in patients with preoperative CME or neovascularization is still true when results are compared to those of nondiabetics. This has been partly contradicted by an important long-term study that demonstrated stable visual function 5 years after cataract surgery in the majority of patients with diabetes.[39]

If the fundus can be examined, new blood vessels and ME should be treated by photocoagulation or with anti-VEGF drugs before cataract surgery, even if not clinically significant.[3,29,40] It is accepted that ME is a frequent cause of poor functional outcome following cataract surgery, although it is sometimes difficult to distinguish diabetic maculopathy from pseudophakic CME (Irvine-Gass syndrome). The progression of pre-existing ME after cataract surgery is a situation that surgeons dread, and may appear even up to 1 year after surgery. Therefore, whenever possible, the surgeon should attempt to eliminate ME and neovascularization prior to cataract surgery.

With rubeosis, iridis, immediate retinal panphotocoagulation, or anti-VEGF drug treatment is essential. However, if neovascular glaucoma has already occurred, medical therapy alone will normally not be sufficient. Topical pressure-lowering drugs, cycloplegics, and topical steroids may reduce the intraocular pressure (IOP) and associated inflammation but will not resolve the problem. Anti-VEGF drugs lead to a rapid regression of neovascularization and reduction in IOP, at least for a short period of time. In the presence of active iris neovascularization, the risk of intra- and postoperative complications is high, so for patients with both cataracts and active iris neovascularization, the following approach should be employed: intravitreal or intracameral injection of anti-VEGF (that can cause temporary regression of neovascularization), cataract surgery, and subsequent immediate panretinal photocoagulation.

Focal treatment should be performed with CME, as recommended by the Early Treatment Diabetic Retinopathy Study (ETDRS); it should be considered when retinal thickening, fluorescein leakage, or exudates are seen in the posterior pole.[41]

Although the indication for panretinal photocoagulation requires the presence of characteristic high-risk lesions, according to ETDRS standards, many retinal specialists tend to recommend panphotocoagulation with any type of neovascularization if cataract surgery is planned. ETDRS has demonstrated that early panphotocoagulation may limit visual impairment.[40] If vision through a contact lens is not sufficiently clear to allow photocoagulation, the surgeon can sometimes perform panphotocoagulation with indirect ophthalmoscopy.

The role of VEGF in the development of new vessels in PDR is well known.[42] VEGF is also known to be associated with an increase in vascular permeability in patients with non-PDR. Increased perimacular capillary permeability is considered to be the most likely factor in the onset of ME in patients with diabetes.

Panphotocoagulation can also have beneficial effects on ME as well as on new vessels, thus the surgeon usually waits 3 months after panphotocoagulation before considering other forms of treatment for ME. Fluorescein angiography is useful for identifying significant leakage sites and determining need for any focal treatments. Panphotocoagulation should be repeated until all active neovascularization has disappeared.

If opacity of the lens prevents photocoagulation, laser treatment should be performed as soon as possible after cataract removal. Full cooperation between the cataract surgeon and the retinal specialist is essential to avoid delays and minimize risk of complications.

If ME cannot be controlled prior to cataract surgery and the surgeon opts to proceed, at the end of surgery, intravitreal injection of agents that will reduce ME should be given. There is abundant literature on this topic[43-52]; it reports on use of triamcinolone acetonide (4 mg) and bevacizumab; (Avastin; 1.25 mg). Both can attenuate progression of ME, although follow-up of these studies is short, just 6 months. As reported in one of these studies,[52] 6 months after surgery there may be no difference in terms of visual acuity and foveal retinal thickness between patients having this type of treatment and patients having cataract surgery only.

In summary, the progression of DR can be affected by the following variables: severity of DR (and ME), duration of DM, metabolic and blood pressure control, and surgical technique used for cataract surgery.

Thus, it is important that prior to surgery, the surgeon assesses the status of the DR, the impact cataract surgery may have on DR, and the treatment of ME. Close monitoring should be continued for at least 6 months after surgery.

Generally speaking, visual prognosis after cataract surgery in diabetic patients is good.

General Considerations on Cataract Surgery in Diabetic Patients

In the past, IOL implantation was discouraged in diabetic patients, but presently phacoemulsification and implantation of posterior chamber IOLs (PC-IOLs) are now considered proper and safe surgical procedures even in diabetic patients (see the Management of Cataract in Patients Requiring Vitrectomy section in this chapter).

The surgical technique does not differ substantially from standard cataract surgery, although in these cases some factors that can affect visual outcome must be considered. It is essential to perform a relatively large capsulorrhexis and remove as much of the cortex and subcapsular epithelial cells (for better visualization of the fundus and in anticipation of subsequent laser treatment for DR). Anterior capsular phimosis is more common in diabetic patients than in nondiabetics,[53] so the capsulorrhexis should be slightly larger and cleaner than in standard cases.

The surgeon should also avoid prolonged surgical time and not rupture the posterior capsule as there is an association in progression of DR and reduction in visual acuity.[54] It is essential to minimize surgical trauma in diabetic patients.

There is evidence[55] suggesting that diabetic patients may be more susceptible to phototoxic stress during surgery and the surgeon should take this into consideration.

One should minimize corneal endothelial damage as this could make subsequent laser photocoagulation more difficult. The endothelial cell count is lower in diabetic patients and there is an increased disruption of cell morphology[56-58]; it is subjected to major metabolic stress following phacoemulsification and has a lower functional reserve compared to the endothelium in nondiabetic patients.

The iris in diabetics is more fragile and surgically induced (intraoperative) miosis occurs more frequently than nondiabetic patients. Therefore, this surgery should only be performed by experienced surgeons[59,60]; consider using a viscoadaptive viscoelastic substance (VES) such as Healon 5 (Abbott Laboratories, Abbott Park, IL). The pigmented iris epithelium often contains vacuoles due to accumulation of glycogen (probably of ischemic origin), and frequently there is loss of pigment following trauma or surgery.

Diabetic patients should avoid silicone IOLs because, in later stages of the disease, vitrectomy may be required, which involves use of a silicone oil tamponade.[61] Theoretically, an IOL with a flat large optic (>6 mm) facilitates visualization and eventual treatment of the peripheral retina (eg, a 6.5-mm IOL provides an optic zone that is 39.7% larger than that with a 5.5-mm IOL).

Posterior capsule opacification (PCO) develops more frequently in diabetics than nondiabetics, even if reports in the literature are not consistent. PCO appears to be affected by the edge of the optic and to a lesser extent by the junction between the optic and haptics and the IOL material. A square edge appears to inhibit proliferation of lens epithelial cells and may therefore prevent formation of PCO, as reported recently by Cochrane.[62] In this paper, given the highly significant difference between the rounded edge and the square edge of the optic, surgeons should choose a square edged optic to reduce the incidence of PCO in diabetic patients.

Many studies have compared biocompatibility of IOL materials in diabetic patients (eg, hydrophobic acrylic IOLs are associated with increased AC flare immediately postoperatively postoperative period). However, this develops less frequently with silicone PC-IOLs. Cochrane reported[62] that no major difference in the rate of PCO was seen with various IOL materials.

Another important factor in PCO appears to be the degree of postoperative inflammation, higher in diabetics than nondiabetics. Postoperative anti-inflammatory treatment does not seem to influence the frequency with which this occurs.

The level of phosphorus in the blood serum and in the aqueous of diabetic patients, particularly those with PDR, is significantly higher than in normal individuals. This may give rise to another type of complication: opacification of hydrophilic acrylic IOLs. There are increased reports of progressive calcified opacification in hydrophilic acrylic IOLs used in diabetic patients.[63,64]

Finally, there is controversy associated with the use of multifocal or accommodative IOLs in diabetic patients.

Regarding IOL implantation, the preferred site is the capsular bag.[53-64] Here the IOL acts as a barrier between the anterior and posterior segments, while the AC-IOL (including the iris claw) or sulcus fixed should not be used, as they are associated with increased risk of iris neovascularization.

The incidence of postoperative endophthalmitis is higher in diabetics,[65,66] and the surgeon should be extra cautious. Moreover, in diabetic patients, the corneal epithelium is not firmly adhered and any adhesions heal more slowly.[67,68] Confocal microscopy shows a reduced baseline cell count in patients with diabetes (this may be due to reduced nerve density in the sub-basal nerve plexus), alterations of the basement membrane, increased basal epithelial cell turnover, and reduced cell count of the middle corneal stroma. In addition to the modified density of sub-basal nerve plexus, the nerve plexus of the corneal stroma is also changed; nerve disorders are more frequent than in diabetic patients without DR. This explains the epitheliopathies often seen after cataract surgery.

Following cataract surgery, progression of ME is possible. Treatment with nonsteroidal anti-inflammatory drugs (NSAIDs) is recommended. Numerous studies have shown that when treatment with NSAIDs is started before surgery and prolonged postoperatively for at least 4 weeks, it is effective in reducing this complication.[69-71] By blocking the inflammatory cascade with NSAIDs, possibly in association with anti-VEGF drugs, the surgeon can reduce the risk of DR progression.

Finally, it should be remembered that these eyes may develop fibrous uveal reactions postoperatively (reported in up to 13.7% of cases) and unexpected bleeding in the AC in a higher percentage than in nondiabetic patients.

After cataract surgery, the fundus of all patients with non-PDR should be carefully examined within 3 months after surgery; patients with PDR or in those patients where it was not possible to determine the condition of the retina prior to surgery should be reassessed after a shorter interval.

Management of Cataract in Patients Requiring Vitrectomy

Combining lens and vitreous removal is associated with an increased incidence of postoperative neovascular glaucoma; however, this combination prevents fibrovascular proliferation of the anterior vitreous cortex (retrolenticular neovascularization, and neovascularization of the anterior hyaloid).

The vitreous cortex and lens act as barriers against diffusion of VEGF into the anterior segment, and their presence limits the incidence of neovascular glaucoma.

If the lens is preserved during vitrectomy, the surgeon should also attempt to leave the anterior vitreous cortex intact.

In diabetic patients, endocapsular lensectomy can be performed to preserve the anterior capsule, with sulcus implantation of a PC-IOL.

IOL implantation after endocapsular lensectomy or after phacoemulsification tends to keep the capsule (anterior for endocapsular lensectomy, posterior for phaco) and anterior hyaloid intact, reducing the risk of neovascular glaucoma.

Even today, some authors believe that endocapsular lensectomy with ultrasound fragmentation via pars plana with a 20-gauge tip is preferable to a combined phacoemulsification-vitrectomy procedure.

Before surgery, the surgeon should decide whether the cataract interferes with his or her view of the surgical field. He or she must then plan combined endocapsular lensectomy (standard, limbal, or cornea procedure) or phaco.

In all cases with active iris or retinal neovascularization, the surgeon must perform panretinal endophotocoagulation during the vitrectomy.

Phacoemulsification Combined With Vitrectomy (Combined Surgery) and Phacoemulsification Before or After Vitrectomy (Sequential Surgery)

Many surgeons now perform phacoemulsification to remove a clinically significant cataract. However, if the surgery involves the joint expertise of an anterior segment surgeon and a vitreoretinal surgeon (combined phaco-vitrectomy surgery, possibly associated with a posterior capsulectomy), the patient will benefit from greater and more rapid functional recovery[72-76] compared to sequential treatment, avoiding the need for a second operation. Many clinical studies show that, with careful patient selection, combined surgery leads to significant anatomical and functional improvement in most cases, especially considering the role of the vitreoretinal interface in the development of clinically significant ME appearing after laser photocoagulation.

As previously mentioned, patient selection is critical; patients over 60 years of age tend to develop cataracts following vitrectomy. The presentation of vitreous membranes for dissection is greatly facilitated if the cataract is removed at the same time. Another indication is an opacity that has progressed slowly over the previous 2 years.

Conversely, patients with severe vitreous-retinal traction, widespread retinal ischemia, or active rubeosis iridis or young patients with minor lens opacities can be managed more efficiently without simultaneous removal of the lens.

The disadvantage of the combined procedure is primarily the fact that surgical time is prolonged. Moreover, phaco and vitrectomy performed simultaneously may cause miosis, retention of viscoelastic substances in the AC, corneal edema, striate keratopathy, and mobilization of pigment into the AC. A study compares combined surgery of vitrectomy with phacoemulsification with vitrectomy combined with ECCE.[77] Both methods are effective, but when phacoemulsification is combined with vitrectomy, visual acuity is better, astigmatism is reduced, and there are fewer complications.

Today, thanks to technological progress, even complex cases can be treated safely with combined surgery of vitrectomy with cataract and using a minimal invasive technique (23 or 25 gauge).[78,79]

The percentage of PCO is lower in patients undergoing combined phaco-vitrectomy surgery than those having the sequential procedure.[80]

If iris clips or traction sutures are required during vitrectomy because of miosis caused by phaco, there will be greater postoperative inflammation, response time will be longer, and costs will be higher—the technique has not enjoyed widespread success.

Finally, if vitrectomy is performed prior to phaco, visibility of the vitreous will be compromised. Moreover, the patient will experience slower visual recovery prior to the second surgery for cataract removal[75] (see Chapter 14).

Endocapsular Lensectomy Combined With Vitrectomy

The endocapsular lensectomy technique was developed to preserve the anterior capsule (Blankenship[81] and Kokame et al[82]) and avoid damaging the iris. Some surgeons prefer endocapsular lensectomy with anterior capsule preservation to combination surgery with phaco. The PC-IOL is implanted at the end of the vitrectomy procedure.

Indications for Endocapsular Lensectomy Without Intraocular Lens Implantation

In some cases, endocapsular lensectomy with removal of the entire capsular bag without IOL implantation is preferable to phacoemulsification with implantation of an IOL. Aphakic eyes allow better visibility of the fundus, convenient access to the anterior cortical vitreous and peripheral vitreous, and smoother gas-fluid exchange. Removal of the lens and entire capsule without IOL implantation eliminates the substrate that leads to formation of cyclitic membranes and fibrovascular proliferation of the anterior cortical vitreous (retrolenticular neovascularization, and fibrovascular proliferation of the anterior hyaloid) unless a fibrinous syndrome develops. An eye with a single compartment will lead to more rapid escape of cells, proteins, fibrin, fibronectin, blood, and VEGF.

Contact lenses for correction of aphakia should be used with caution in diabetic patients because of reduced corneal sensitivity, while correction with spectacles is usually well tolerated, especially after panretinal photocoagulation restricting the peripheral visual field.

If the lens is clear, it should not be removed; with vitrectomy for PDR due to increased risk of neovascular glaucoma, unless there is a fibrinous syndrome underway, there is a high risk of postoperative bleeding or if the surgeon uses silicone oil as a tamponade for large retinal breaks or retinotomies. It is a general opinion that the anterior cortical vitreous and lens act as barriers against diffusion of VEGF into the anterior segment; this is the beginning of neovascularization of the iris and the trabeculum. In vitrectomies performed on diabetics in which the lens is left in position, the surgeon should also preserve the anterior cortical vitreous, unless it is opaque or a source of tension.

References

1. Kokiwar PR, Gupta S, Durge PM. Prevalence of diabetes in a rural area of central India. *Int J Diab Dev Ctries.* 2007;27:8-10.
2. Klein R, Moss S. A comparison of the study populations in the Diabetes Control and Complications Trial and the Wisconsin Epidemiologic Study of Diabetic Retinopathy. *Arch Intern Med.* 1995;155(7):745-754.
3. Absence of a glycemic threshold for the development of long term complications: the perspective of the Diabetes Control and Complications Trial. *Diabetes.* 1996;45:1289-1298.
4. Raman R, Pal SS, Adams JS, Rani PK, Vaitheeswaran K, Sharma T. Prevalence and risk factors for cataract in diabetes: Sankara Nethralaya Diabetic Retinopathy Epidemiology and Molecular Genetics Study. Report number 17. *Invest Ophthalmol Vis Sci.* 2010;51(12):6253-6261.
5. Grauslund J, Green A, Sjølie AK. Cataract surgery in a population-based cohort of patients with type 1 diabetes: long-term incidence and risk factors. *Acta Ophthalmol.* 2011;89(1):25-29.
6. Mechini U, Cappelli S, Virgili G. Cataract surgery and diabetic retinopathy. *Semin Ophthalmol.* 2003;18:103-108.
7. Ivancic D, Mandic Z, Barac C, Kopic M. Cataract surgery and post operative complication in diabetic patients. *Coll Antropol.* 2005;29:55-58.
8. Hamilton AMP, Ulbig MW, Polkinghorne P. *Management of Diabetic Retinopathy.* London, England: BMJ Publishing Group; 1996.
9. Cunliffe IA, Flanagan DW, George NDL, Aggarwaal RJ, Moore AT. Extracapsular cataract surgery with lens implantation in diabetics with or without proliferative retinopathy. *Br J Ophthalmol.* 1991;75:9-12.
10. Gabric N, Henc-Petrinovic L, Dekaris I, Busic M, Ptrinovic-Doresic J. Timing of cataract surgery in diabetics. *Acta Med Croatia.* 1996;50:25-28.

11. Yorston D, Wood M, Cichuli S, Foster A. Does monitoring improve cataract surgery outcomes in Africa? *Br J Ophthalmol.* 2002;86:543-547.
12. Salman A, Parmar P, Vanila CG, Thomas PA, Nelsen Jesudasan CA. Is ultrasonography essential before surgery in eyes with advanced cataract? *J Postgrad Med.* 2006;52:19-22.
13. Dowler JG, Hykin PG, Lightman SL, Hamilton AM. Visual acuity following extracapsular cataract extraction in diabetics: a meta-analysis. *Eye.* 1995;9:313-317.
14. Benson WE, Brown GC, Tasman W, et al. Extracapsular cataract extraction with placement of a posterior chamber lens in patients with diabetic retinopathy. *Ophthalmology.* 1993;100:730-738.
15. Jaffe GJ, Burton TC, Kuhn E, et al. Progression of nonproliferative diabetic retinopathy and visual outcome after extracapsular cataract extraction and intraocular lens implantation. *Am J Ophthalmol.* 1992;114:448-456.
16. Hykin PG, Gregson RM, Stevens JD, Hamilton PA. Extracapsular cataract extraction in proliferative diabetic retinopathy. *Ophthalmology.* 1993;100:394-399.
17. Zaczek A, Olivestedt G, Zetterstrom C. Visual outcome after phacoemulsification and IOL implantation in diabetic patients. *Br J Ophthalmol.* 1999;83:1036-1041.
18. Mittra RA, Borrillo JL, Dev S, et al. Retinopathy progression and visual outcomes after phacoemulsification in patients with diabetes mellitus. *Arch Ophthalmol.* 2000;118:912-917.
19. Liu Y, Luo L, He M, Liu X. Disorders of the blood-aqueous barrier after phacoemulsification in diabetic patients. *Eye.* 2004;18:900-904.
20. Krepler K, Biowski R, Schrey S, et al. Cataract surgery in patients with diabetic retinopathy: visual outcome, progression of diabetic retinopathy, and incidence of diabetic macular oedema. *Graefes Arch Clin Exp Ophthalmol.* 2002;240:735-738.
21. Squirrell D, Bhola R, Bush J, et al. A prospective, case controlled study of the natural history of diabetic retinopathy and maculopathy after uncomplicated phacoemulsification cataract surgery in patients with type 2 diabetes. *Br J Ophthalmol.* 2002;86:565-571.
22. Liao SB, Ku WC. Progression of diabetic retinopathy after phacoemulsification in diabetic patients: a three-year analysis. *Chang Gung Med J.* 2003;26:829-834.
23. Hong T, Mitchell P, de Loryn T, et al. Development and progression of diabetic retinopathy 12 months after phacoemulsification cataract surgery. *Ophthalmology.* 2009;116:1510-1514.
24. Kato S, Fukada Y, Hori S, et al. Influence of phacoemulsification and intraocular lens implantation on the course of diabetic retinopathy. *J Cataract Refract Surg.* 1999;25:788-793.
25. Kim SJ, Equi R, Bressler NM. Analysis of macular edema after cataract surgery in patients with diabetes using optical coherence tomography. *Ophthalmology.* 2007;114(5):881-889.
26. Hayashi K, Igarashi C, Hirata A, Hayashi H. Changes in diabetic macular oedema after phacoemulsification surgery. *Eye (Lond).* 2009;23(2):389-396.
27. Rashid S, Young LH. Progression of diabetic retinopathy and maculopathy after phacoemulsification surgery. *Int Ophthalmol Clin.* 2010;50(1):155-166.
28. Hartnett ME, Tinkham N, Paynter L, et al. Aqueous vascular endothelial growth factor as a predictor of macular thickening following cataract surgery in patients with diabetes mellitus. *Am J Ophthalmol.* 2009;148(6):895-901.
29. Borrillo JL, Mittra RA, Dev S, et al. Retinopathy progression and visual outcomes after phacoemulsification in patients with diabetes mellitus. *Trans Am Ophthalmol Soc.* 1999;97:435-445.
30. Pollack A, Dotan S, Oliver M. Progression of diabetic retinopathy after cataract extraction. *Br J Ophthalmol.* 1991;75:547-551.
31. Shah AS, Chen SH. Cataract surgery and diabetes. *Curr Opin Ophthalmol.* 2010;21(1):4-9.
32. Murtha T, Cavallerano J. The management of diabetic eye disease in the setting of cataract surgery. *Curr Opin Ophthalmol.* 2007;18(1):13-18.
33. Eriksson U, Alm A, Bjärnhall G, Granstam E, Matsson AW. Macular edema and visual outcome following cataract surgery in patients with diabetic retinopathy and controls. *Graefes Arch Clin Exp Ophthalmol.* 2011;249(3):349-359.
34. Mozaffarieh M, Heinzl H, Sacu S, Wedrich A. Clinical outcomes of phacoemulsification cataract surgery in diabetes patients: visual function (VF-14), visual acuity and patient satisfaction. *Acta Ophthalmol Scand.* 2005;83:176-183.
35. Stein JD, Grossman DS, Mundy KM, Sugar A, Sloan FA. Severe adverse events after cataract surgery among Medicare beneficiaries. *Ophthalmology.* 2011; 118(9):1716-1723.
36. Hauser D, Katz H, Pokroy R, et al. Occurrence and progression of diabetic retinopathy after phacoemulsification cataract surgery. *J Cataract Refract Surg.* 2004;30:428-432.
37. Henricsson M, Heijl A, Janzon L. Diabetic retinopathy before and after cataract surgery. *Br J Ophthalmol.* 1996;80:789-793.
38. Dowler JG, Sehmi KS, Hykin PG, Hamilton AM. The natural history of macular edema after cataract surgery in diabetes. *Ophthalmology.* 1999;106(4):663-668.
39. Lundqvist B, Mönestam E. Longitudinal changes in subjective and objective visual function in diabetics 5 years after cataract surgery. *Acta Ophthalmol.* 2012;90(3):215-220.
40. Suto C, Kitano S, Hori S. Optimal timing of cataract surgery and panretinal photocoagulation for diabetic retinopathy. *Diabetes Care.* 2011;34(7):e123.
41. Early Treatment Diabetic Retinopathy Study research group. Photocoagulation for diabetic macular edema. Early Treatment Diabetic Retinopathy Study. Report number 1. *Arch Ophthalmol.* 1985;103(12):1796-1806.
42. Aiello LP, Avery RL, Arrigg PG, et al. Vascular endothelial growth factor in ocular fluid of patients with diabetic retinopathy and other retinal disorders. *N Engl J Med.* 1994;331(22):1480-1487.
43. Takata C, Messias A, Folgosa MS, et al. Intravitreal injection versus subtenoninfusion of triamcinolone acetonide during cataract surgery in patients with refractory diabetic macular edema. *Retina.* 2010;30(4):562-569.
44. Kim SY, Yang J, Lee YC, Park YH. Effect of a single intraoperative sub-Tenoninjection of triamcinolone acetonide on the progression of diabetic retinopathy and visual outcomes after cataract surgery. *Cataract Refract Surg.* 2008;34(5):823-826.
45. Habib MS, Cannon PS, Steel DH. The combination of intravitreal triamcinolone and phacoemulsification surgery in patients with diabeticfoveal oedema and cataract. *BMC Ophthalmol.* 2005;5:15.
46. Wahab S, Ahmed J. Management of cataract with macular oedema due to diabetes mellitus type-II and hypertension with grid laser prior to surgery and intra-vitreal bevacizumab (Avastin) peroperatively. *J Pak Med Assoc.* 2010;60(10):836-839.
47. Akinci A, Batman C, Ozkilic E, Altinsoy A. Phacoemulsification with intravitreal bevacizumab injection in diabetic patients with macular edema and cataract. *Retina.* 2009;29(10):1432-1435.
48. Takamura Y, Kubo E, Akagi Y. Analysis of the effect of intravitreal bevacizumab injection on diabetic macular edema after cataract surgery. *Ophthalmology.* 2009;116(6):1151-1157.
49. Lanzagorta-Aresti A, Palacios-Pozo E, Menezo Rozalen JL, Navea-Tejerina A. Prevention of vision loss after cataract surgery in diabetic macular edema with intravitreal bevacizumab: a pilot study. *Retina.* 2009;29(4):530-535.
50. Chen CH, Liu YC, Wu PC. The combination of intravitreal bevacizumab and phacoemulsification surgery in patients with cataract and coexisting diabetic macular edema. *J Ocul Pharmacol Ther.* 2009;25(1):83-89.
51. Cheema RA, Al-Mubarak MM, Amin YM, Cheema MA. Role of combined cataract surgery and intravitreal bevacizumab injection in preventing progression of diabetic retinopathy: prospective randomized study. *J Cataract Refract Surg.* 2009;35(1):18-25.

52. Fard MA, Yazdanei Abyane A, Malihi M. Prophylactic intravitreal bevacizumab for diabetic macular edema (thickening) after cataract surgery: prospective randomized study. *Eur J Ophthalmol.* 2011;21(3):276-281.
53. Ebihara Y, Kato S, Oshika T, Yoshizaki M, Sugita G. Posterior capsule opacification after cataract surgery in patients with diabetes mellitus. *J Cataract Refract Surg.* 2006;32(7):1184-1187.
54. Mittra RA, Borrillo JL, Dev S, Miller WF, Koenig B. Retinopathy progression and visual outcomes after phacoemulsification in patients with diabetes mellitus. *Arch Ophthalmol.* 2000;118:912-917.
55. Altug C, Gursel Y, Aydin A. Photic retinopathy after cataract surgery in diabetic patients. *Retina.* 2006;26:1021-1028.
56. Mathew PT, David S, Thomas N. Endothelial cell loss and central corneal thickness in patients with and without diabetes after manual small incision cataract surgery. *Cornea.* 2011;30(4):424-428.
57. Tsai CC, Kao SC, Kau HC, Isenberg SJ. Risk factors for corneal endothelial injury during small-incision cataract surgery in patients with diabetes mellitis. *Arch Ophthalmol.* 2005;123(7):1020-1021; author reply, 1021.
58. Morikubo S, Takamura Y, Kubo E, Tsuzuki S, Akagi Y. Corneal changes after small-incision cataract surgery in patients with diabetes mellitus. *Arch Ophthalmol.* 2004;122(7):966-969.
59. Zaczek A, Zetterström C. Cataract surgery and pupil size in patients with diabetes mellitus. *Acta Ophthalmol Scand.* 1997;75(4):429-432.
60. Mirza SA, Alexandridou A, Marshall T, Stavrou P. Surgically induced miosis during phacoemulsification in patients with diabetes mellitus. *Eye (Lond).* 2003;17(2):194-199.
61. Khawly JA, Lambert RJ, Jaffe GJ. Intraocular lens changes after short- and long-term exposure to intraocular silicone oil. An in vivo study. *Ophthalmology.* 1998;105(7):1227-1233.
62. Javadi MA, Zarei-Ghanavati S. Cataracts in diabetic patients: a review article. *J Ophthalmic Vis Res.* 2008; 3(1):52-65.
63. Kim CJ, Choi SK. Analysis of aqueous humor calcium and phosphate from cataract eyes with and without diabetes mellitus. *Korean J Ophthalmol.* 2007;21:90-94.
64. Lee DH, Seo Y, Joo CK. Progressive opacification of hydrophilic acrylic intraocular lenses in diabetic patients. *J Cataract Refr Surg.* 2002;28:1271-1275.
65. Doft BH, Wisniewski SR, Kelsey SF, Groer-Fitzgerald S; Endophthalmitis Vitrectomy Study Group. Diabetes and post-cataract extraction endophthalmitis. *Curr Opin Ophthalmol.* 2002;13(3):147-151.
66. Doft BH, Wisniewski SR, Kelsey SF, Fitzgerald SG; Endophthalmitis Vitrectomy Study Group. Diabetes and postoperative endophthalmitis in the endophthalmitis vitrectomy study. *Arch Ophthalmol.* 2001;119(5):650-656.
67. Tabatabay CA, Bumbacher M, Baumgartner B, Leuenberger PM. Reduced number of hemidesmosomes in the corneal epithelium of diabetics with proliferative vitreoretinopathy. *Graefes Arch Clin Exp Ophthalmol.* 1988;226(4):389-392.
68. Tsubota K, Chiba K, Shimazaki J. Corneal epithelium in diabetic patients. *Cornea.* 1991;10(2):156-160.
69. Endo N, Kato S, Haruyama K, Shoji M, Kitano S. Efficacy of bromfenac sodium ophthalmic solution in preventing cystoid macular oedema after cataract surgery in patients with diabetes. *Acta Ophthalmol.* 2010;88(8):896-900.
70. Hariprasad SM, Akduman L, Clever JA, Ober M, Recchia FM, Mieler WF. Treatment of cystoid macular edema with the new-generation NSAID nepafenac 0.1%. *Clin Ophthalmol.* 2009;3:147-154.
71. Wittpenn JR, Silverstein S, Heier J, Kenyon KR, Hunkeler JD, Earl M; Acular LS for Cystoid Macular Edema (ACME) Study Group. A randomized, masked comparison of topical ketorolac 0.4% plus steroid vs steroid alone in low-risk cataract surgery patients. *Am J Ophthalmol.* 2008;146(4):554-560.
72. Diolaiuti S, Senn P, Schmid MK, Job O, Maloca P, Schipper I. Combined pars plana vitrectomy and phacoemulsification with intraocular lens implantation in severe proliferative diabetic retinopathy. *Ophthalmic Surg Lasers Imaging.* 2006;37(6):468-474.
73. Lahey JM, Francis RR, Kearney J. Combining phacoemulsification with pars plana vitrectomy in patients with proliferative diabetic retinopathy: a series of 223 cases. *Ophthalmology.* 2003;110(7):1335-1339.
74. Kim SH, Chung JW, Chung H, Yu HG. Phacoemulsification and foldable intraocular lens implantation combined with vitrectomy and silicone oil tamponade for severe proliferative diabetic retinopathy. *J Cataract Refract Surg.* 2004;30(8):1721-1726.
75. Lahey JM, Francis RR, Kearney JJ, Cheung M. Combining phacoemulsification and vitrectomy in patients with proliferative diabetic retinopathy. *Curr Opin Ophthalmol.* 2004;15(3):192-196.
76. Rivas-Aguiño P, García-Amaris RA, Berrocal MH, Sánchez JG, Rivas A, Arévalo JF. Pars plana vitrectomy, phacoemulsification and intraocular lens implantation for the management of cataract and proliferative diabetic retinopathy: comparison of a combined versus two-step surgical approach. *Arch Soc Esp Oftalmol.* 2009;84(1):31-38.
77. Hsu SY, Wu WC. Comparison of phacoemulsification and planned extracapsular cataract extraction in combined pars plana vitrectomy and posterior chamber intraocular lens implantation. *Ophthalmic Surg Lasers Imaging.* 2005;36(2):108-113.
78. Lee DY, Jeong HS, Sohn HJ, Nam DH. Combined 23-gauge sutureless vitrectomy and clear corneal phacoemulsification in patients with proliferative diabetic retinopathy. *Retina.* 2011;31(9):1753-1758.
79. Altan T, Acar N, Kapran Z, Unver YB, Ozdogan S. Transconjunctival 25-gauge sutureless vitrectomy and silicone oil injection in diabetic tractional retinal detachment. *Retina.* 2008;28(9):1201-1206.
80. Roh JH, Sohn HJ, Lee DY, Shyn KH, Nam DH. Comparison of posterior capsular opacification between a combined procedure and a sequential procedure of pars plana vitrectomy and cataract surgery. *Ophthalmologica.* 2010;224(1):42-46.
81. Blankenship GW. The lens influence on diaetic vitrectomy results. Report of a prospective randomized study. *Arch Ophthalmol.* 1980;98(12)2196-2198.
82. Kokame G, Flynn HW, Blankenship GW. Posterior chamber intraocular lens implantation during diabetic pars plana vitrectomy. *Ophthalmology.* 1989;96(5):603-610.

14

Role of Vitreoretinal Surgery in Cataract Surgery

Widespread use of technology, improvements in surgical techniques, and increased indications for vitreoretinal surgery have led to an increased frequency of cataract surgery following vitreoretinal procedures. The same applies to combined cataract-vitreoretinal and vitreoretinal surgery in the management of complications associated with cataract extraction. This chapter will take an in-depth look at the first 2 topics.

Cataract Extraction Following Vitreoretinal Surgery

Cataract, in particular nuclear cataract, can be induced or accelerated following vitreoretinal surgery. This is well confirmed in the literature; prospective studies on eyes undergoing vitrectomy for macular pathologies have shown that the frequency of nuclear sclerosis was approximately 80% 1 year after surgery.[1-3]

Progressive nuclear cataract formation following vitrectomy can be slowly progressive and can obviate the improvements in macular function following vitrectomy. Frequently, posterior subcapsular lens opacities are seen in cases in which a tamponade substance is used at the end of vitreoretinal surgery. Episcleral surgery without vitrectomy differs from vitreous surgery in that it does not cause a significant increase in the frequency of cataract.

Why Does a Cataract Develop?

There are a number of reasons why cataracts develop following vitreoretinal surgery.[1-4] One is accidental contact between the lens and an intraocular surgical instrument; in these cases, there may be rupture of the posterior capsule that leads to hydration of the lens cortex.[4] Normally the cataract is self-limiting and localized and will not affect vision to any significant degree unless the posterior pole is involved; however, sometimes it may be extensive, necessitating an unplanned lensectomy or the removal of a cataract immediately after the vitrectomy.

Another reason for the development of nuclear sclerosis or posterior subcapsular lens opacity is the use of intraocular gas. The mechanism by which an intraocular gas causes lens opacity is unknown. The layered appearance of the posterior subcapsular lens is normally a reversible phenomenon associated with the crystallization of the anterior hyaloid and the posterior capsule. Even though many surgeons consider this layered appearance to be a precursor of progressive lens opacity, this has not been proven.

The third potential cause of cataract following vitreoretinal surgery is vitreous hemorrhage or inflammation. This may be an additional variable; however, many other pathological inflammatory processes have been associated with the formation of lens opacity.[1-4] Large numbers of patients undergoing vitrectomy for macular pucker have been examined for the onset of nuclear sclerosis. The duration of this surgery is relatively short, pre- and postoperative inflammation relatively minimal, and other variables, such as prolonged inflammation or presence of blood or gas, are minimal or absent.

The pathogenesis of cataracts in patients undergoing vitrectomy include the chemical composition of the infusion fluids, and despite the fact that new formulations of infusion fluids have been advanced in recent years, the frequency of nuclear sclerosis remains high.

Another suggestion is that the vitreous acts as a barrier or a tamponade, protecting the lens from cataract

Buratto L, Brint SF, Caretti L.
Cataract Surgery in Complicated Cases (pp 149-154).

formation, and its removal facilitates the onset of cataracts.[2] It has been suggested[2] that cataracts form because of exposure to non-neutralized free radicals generated by the posterior segment; normally, these are neutralized by the normal composition of the vitreous. This hypothesis corresponds to the higher frequency of cataract in older patients who have a more liquid vitreous. Hypothetically, surgical removal of the vitreous will rapidly simulate this process and accelerate cataract formation. For this reason, some surgeons opt for a minimal or core vitrectomy, as one of the theoretical advantages is a reduction in postoperative cataracts.

Preoperative Patient Evaluation

Preoperative patient evaluation is similar to the examination prior to cataract surgery; however, occasionally, additional tests may be necessary based on the type of lens opacity. An accurate anatomical evaluation is crucial, sometimes requiring a B-scan to determine the integrity of the posterior segment and consequently, predict the visual prognosis.

Special attention must be paid to the calculation of the intraocular lens (IOL) power. It is helpful to perform biometry on patients scheduled for vitreoretinal surgery, even if the surgeon does not plan a contemporaneous phaco. This avoids the potential problems with measuring the axial length in an extremely dense lens. Moreover, if silicone oil has been used to tamponade the eye with vitrectomy, the calculations for the IOL must be adjusted if the oil is removed immediately or later. Another consideration is that a patient with a cataract in a vitrectomized eye may develop another one more slowly in the contralateral eye; consequently, the patient may have a prolonged period of unilateral pseudophakia. This should be taken into account in selecting the power of the IOL.

Some additional testing may be necessary preoperatively (eg, macular optical coherence tomography, angiography, potential acuity test, and electroretinographic tests).

Surgical Technique

Extracapsular techniques with a large incision and nuclear expression are more difficult in postvitrectomy patients. There is an increase in frequency of complications caused by zonular and capsular fragility.[5-8]

Currently, phacoemulsification is the standard cataract procedure following vitrectomy and in almost all cases can be performed under topical anesthesia.[9]

A prospective study by Misra and Burton[10] examined the incidence of intraoperative complications on 117 vitrectomized eyes. The authors reported that in expert hands, in spite of potential intraoperative difficulties associated with these eyes, the incidence of posterior capsule rupture was 1.7%, similar to that for the standard procedure.

Potential problems involve zonular and capsular weakness. As discussed in Chapter 8, there are some common maneuvers that may prove useful in postvitrectomy eyes, even though a study published by Cochrane in 2008 demonstrated that there are no randomized trial results available that can be used for the definition of the guidelines for this type of patient.[11]

Hydrodissection should be complete and should be cortical cleaving to minimize tension between the capsule, and consequently the zonules, during nuclear rotation and extraction.

The primary difference in phacoemulsification in these eyes compared to standard eyes is that when the ultrasound tip is introduced into the anterior chamber (AC), the depth of the AC and mydriasis increase with positive infusion pressure, due to lack of support from the vitreous, leading to undesired zonular traction. Thus, the infusion bottle should be lowered prior to introducing the tip into the AC. The bottle height can be adjusted on the basis of the chamber depth (with infusion). Another option is to allow some viscoelastic substance (VES) to escape prior to introducing the ultrasound tip into the AC. As with highly myopic eyes, the instruments are typically more vertically oriented.

For posterior capsule instability due to a lack of vitreous support, the removal of the cortex may be extremely difficult and the posterior lens capsule may rupture unexpectedly.

There may also be loss of zonular support in vitrectomized eyes, possibly due to the lens floating on a bubble. The surgeon should choose techniques that do not subject the zonules to additional stress (quick chop technique).[12]

With extreme laxity, instead of implanting the IOL in the capsular bag, the surgeon can consider placing the IOL in the ciliary sulcus. The implantation of an AC-IOL should be avoided when there is any risk that the pathology of the posterior segment can be reactivated; however, implantation is acceptable in selected cases and iris enclavation is recommended.

Another problem that may occur in vitrectomized eyes is the presence of a posterior capsular plate, often difficult to cleave and remove. In eyes with a previous vitrectomy and serious postoperative inflammation, there may be preoperative miosis or posterior synechiae; consequently, pupil stretching or use of iris retractor hooks may be necessary.

Cataract removal in the presence of silicone oil is now a safe procedure. In these cases, the following elegant and minimally invasive approach can be taken. Phacoemulsification is performed as described above; the surgeon proceeds with a central posterior capsulorrhexis, and the silicone oil is removed through the limbus. The surgeon introduces an aspiration system (held in the dominant hand and introduced through the primary incision) and a continuous balanced salt solution (BSS) infusion cannula (held in the nondominant hand and introduced through a paracentesis), positioning both instruments behind the posterior capsulorrhexis. The surgeon then begins the slow and complete removal of the silicone oil. As the oil is lighter than water, it will escape more easily with the flow of intraocular fluids. The IOL is implanted in the sulcus; in these cases, a 3-piece hydrophobic acrylic lens with a 6-mm optic is used (overall diameter 13 mm). Prior to the implantation, the surgeon injects a small quantity of dispersive VES, some into the AC but for the most part between the posterior face of the iris and the anterior capsule, to create an opening for the implant. Implantation of the IOL is performed with an injector and is a 2-step process. The distal loop and the optic are positioned using the injector; the proximal loop is maneuvered into its final position in the sulcus using tying forceps. Finally, the surgeon aspirates the VES from the AC with the bottle of BSS in a very low position. Acetylcholine is then injected.

The surgical techniques in patients following previous episcleral operations are no different from standard cases.

The majority of patients having cataract surgery following vitreoretinal or episcleral surgery achieve good visual acuity; vision is influenced only by retinal comorbidity. Moreover, the percentage of intra- and postoperative complications reported is not significantly greater than in routine cataract surgery.[13]

Following cataract surgery a very low incidence of recurrent retinal detachment was reported. With a scleral band, the eye was elongated by an average of 2 diopters (D). Consequently, the determination of the axial length and the calculation of the power of the IOL should reflect this structural modification.

Cataract Removal Combined With Vitreoretinal Surgery

Clinical Situations and Surgical Indications

Cataract surgery combined with vitrectomy (20-, 23-, and 25-gauge) is a procedure that has been performed recently with different vitreoretinal pathologies—macular pathologies, vitreous hemorrhage, rhegmatogenous retinal detachment, proliferative retinopathy, and proliferative diabetic retinopathy.[14,15]

In vitreoretinal surgery, surgeons believe that a lensectomy allows better access to the vitreous base and improves intraoperative visualization in cases with diseases of the posterior segment such as proliferative retinopathy or proliferative diabetic retinopathy. On the other hand, with less serious pathologies of the posterior segment (such as epiretinal membranes, macular holes, or limited trauma), combined surgery is performed only if the simultaneous objective of rehabilitating the patient's vision is required. Combined surgery is indicated when the cataract is clinically significant, assuming that intraoperative visualization of the posterior segment during vitrectomy is poor. Combined surgery is typically performed if the patient is over 60 years of age, even when the cataract is not highly significant because, as previously mentioned, vitrectomy and the use of tamponades can accelerate cataract development.

Normally, an IOL is implanted during the vitrectomy procedure. In more serious cases, however, a lensectomy with removal of residual lens material will be performed without IOL implantation to avoid compromising success of the primary vitreoretinal objectives (ie, complete removal of the vitreous base); however, total vitrectomy is still considered to be ideal.

There are a number of advantages associated with a combined approach: better intraoperative visualization of the retina, better access to the vitreous base, rapid visual rehabilitation, lower risks associated with anesthesia (if the surgeon decides to perform the subsequent cataract operation under local anesthesia), economic convenience, and benefits with a single operation.[16] There is a single period of convalescence and a shorter visual rehabilitation interval.

Combined procedures are also associated with potential drawbacks; it may jeopardize the outcome of the vitreoretinal surgery by increasing the level of difficulty of the surgery and its duration. This may be the cause of greater postoperative inflammation.

Chung et al reported that in 13.5% of cases, fibrinous exudate was seen in the AC following combined cataract and 20-gauge vitrectomy, a percentage greater than in the group of sequential surgery.[17]

Also postoperative inflammation may be responsible for secondary posterior capsule opacification (PCO), a fairly frequent occurrence according to Sood et al. In all of the cases of combined surgery in which PCO developed, gas had been used as a tamponade.[14]

Technological improvement in vitreoretinal surgery advocates routine use of 23- and 25-gauge microincision vitrectomy surgery (MIVS) systems, resulting in lower postoperative inflammation and less surgically induced astigmatism, compared to traditional 20-gauge systems[18,19] (Figure 14-1).

In a recent publication,[20] a significantly higher occurrence of choroidal effusion was reported in patients having a combined operation compared to the group of patients with vitrectomy alone for proliferative diabetic retinopathy. Choroidal effusion causes shallowing of the angle, reduction of AC depth, and inflammatory complications.

Another potential drawback in the case of vitreous hemorrhage is that the absence of a red reflex or a poor red reflex may make visualization of the capsulorrhexis more difficult with subsequent complications.[17,21]

A technique was described recently[22,23] to help this problem; by using light supplied by a 23-gauge illuminated infusion cannula, the red reflex can be increased, producing better visualization of the lens structures and the

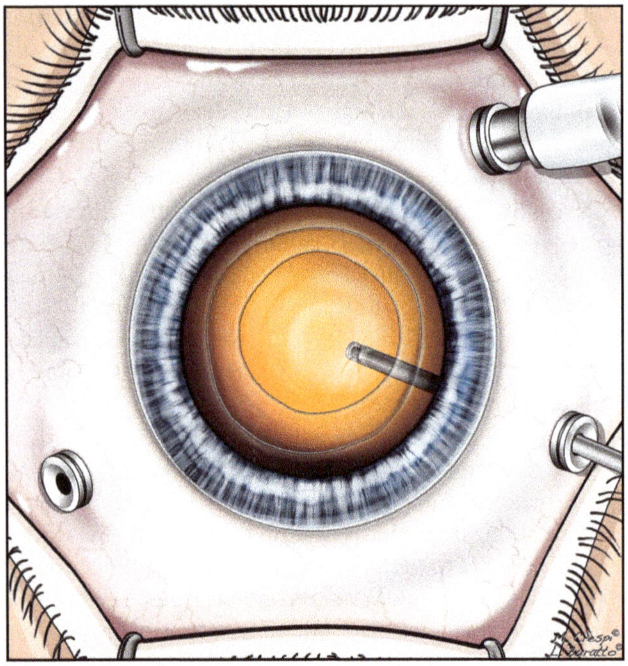

Figure 14-1. Image of the anterior segment with 3 23-gauge trocars in position, prior to the start of phacoemulsification.

posterior capsule, facilitating the capsulorrhexis, assisting phacoemulsification, and cleaning of the posterior capsule.

The surgeon should be cautious recommending combined cataract and vitreoretinal surgery, as the influence of the cataract on visual acuity may be overestimated, particularly when there is blood in the vitreous that eliminates the red reflex.

Surgical Options

There are various options with combined surgery. The first is phacoemulsification and implantation of an IOL, followed by a vitrectomy. The majority of surgeons prefer to insert the 3 MIVS trocars first (an infusion cannula and the other 2 capped temporarily); the surgeon then proceeds with cataract surgery with implantation of an IOL followed by the vitrectomy. The advantages are good visualization of the posterior segment, easier access to the vitreous base, and a better tamponade effect permitting more complete removal of the vitreous. The main problem may be leakage into the AC during the indentation steps with possible luxation of the IOL. Corneal edema, Descemet's folds, and miosis may also occur.

Some surgeons prefer the sequence of vitrectomy, phacoemulsification, and implantation of the IOL. Here the IOL will be stable during vitrectomy; however, there are some drawbacks: poor visibility because of the cataract, difficult access to the vitreous base with possible iatrogenic damage to the PC, and a phaco procedure performed without vitreous support (see the previous paragraphs).

Another surgical variation is phaco, vitrectomy, and IOL implantation. The disadvantage is that during vitrectomy, the PC may oscillate as it is not distended and stabilized by the IOL. This can be reduced by the injection of a VES into the capsule or by insertion of a tension ring.

Yet another option is pars plana lensectomy with preservation of the anterior lens capsule, followed by vitrectomy and concluded with implantation of a posterior chamber IOL in the sulcus on the residual anterior capsule (see also Chapter 13). It is essential to perform a large anterior capsulotomy given that subsequent opacification will also lead to a contraction of the capsular opening. This approach offers excellent visibility during the vitrectomy and is not associated with the risk of reopening the cataract incision created during the vitrectomy.

Functional Results

Functional results appear to be similar with both combined procedures and 2 separate surgeries. In a previous nonrandomized study on 32 eyes with an epiretinal membrane,[24] 15 eyes were treated with simultaneous procedures of cataract extraction, IOL implantation, and vitrectomy; the remaining 17 eyes were treated with vitrectomy alone. In the vitrectomy alone group, 65% of the eyes developed a cataract and required cataract surgery approximately 2 years later. In both groups, postsurgical visual results were similar; however after 2 years, the vitrectomy only group reported a decrease in vision due to progressive nuclear sclerosis. The authors concluded that simultaneous or combined surgery achieved more rapid rehabilitation with reduced costs and greater benefit for the patient.

These initial observations have been confirmed with comparative studies on combined and sequential surgery that included patients with epiretinal membranes and macular holes.[25,26]

Moreover, there are a number of surgeons who recommend combined surgery in other types of vitreoretinal pathology, involving even more complex operations.[27-31]

The power of the IOL for patients with combined phacovitrectomy surgery deserves some consideration: in a recent study,[32] a slight myopic shift was reported (approximately 0.4 D) in patients undergoing macular surgery. The shift was seen more frequently in patients with macular pucker as opposed to those with macular holes, thus with combined surgery, the authors suggest implanting a lens with a slight hyperopic correction to achieve emmetropia.

Conclusion

Currently, the problem associated with potential cataracts is increasingly taken into consideration during vitreoretinal surgery. As there are new therapeutic options available for the various vitreoretinal diseases that were deemed untreatable in the past, the frequency of cataract surgery in the postvitrectomy patient is constantly increasing. The phacoemulsification surgeon is now much more confident when approaching this type of surgery.

The mini-incisional combined technique of phaco-vitrectomy is a treatment option of enormous interest and benefit for the patient.

Coordinated treatment strategies between surgeons, expert in the anterior and posterior segments, as summarized in this chapter, can maximize the final visual outcome.

REFERENCES

1. Michels RG. Vitrectomy for macular pucker. *Ophthalmology.* 1984;91:134-138.
2. Thompson JT, Glaser BM, Sjaarda RN, Murphy RP. Progression of nuclear sclerosis and long-term visual results of vitrectomy with transforming growth factor beta-2 for macular holes. *Am J Ophthalmol.* 1995;119:48-54.
3. FreemanWR, Stanley PA, Kim JW, El-Haig W, et al. Vitrectomy for the treatment of full-thickness stage 3 or 4 macular holes. *Arch Ophthalmol.* 1997;115:11-21.
4. Edelhauser HF, Gonnering R, Van Horn DL. Intraocular irrigating solutions: a comparative study of BSS plus and lactated Ringer's solution. *Arch Ophthalmol.* 1984;102:1077-1078.
5. Siegelman J, Ketover BP, Coleman DJ. Spontaneous lens rupture follow pars plana vitrectomy. *Ann Ophthalmol.* 1978;10:65-71.
6. Cohen SB, Peyman GA, DeCorral LR. Extracapsular cataract extraction after silicone oil injection [letter]. *Ophthalmic Surg.* 1985;16:660.
7. Smiddy WE, Stark WJ, Micels RG. Cataract extraction after vitrectomy. *Ophthalmology.* 1987;94:483-487.
8. Biró Z, Kovacs B. Results of cataract surgery in previously vitrectomized eyes. *J Cataract Refract Surg.* 2002;28(6):1003-1006.
9. Zaheer I, Taylor SR, Pearson RV. Phacoemulsification in vitrectomized eyes under topical anesthesia. *Eur J Ophthalmol.* 2007;17(3):336-340.
10. Misra A, Burton RL. Incidence of intra-operative complications during phacoemulsification in vitrectomized and non-vitrectomized eyes: prospective study. *J Cataract Refract Surg.* 2005;31(5):1011-1014.
11. Do DV, Hawkins B, Gichuhi S, Vedula SS. Surgery for post-vitrectomy cataract. *Cochrane Database Syst Rev.* 2008;(3):CD006366.
12. Sachdev N, Brar GS, Sukhija J, Gupta V, Ram J. Phacoemulsification in vitrectomized eyes: results using a "phaco chop" technique. *Acta Ophthalmol.* 2009;87(4):382-385.
13. Chang MA, Parides MK, Chang S, Braunstein RE. Outcome of phacoemulsification after pars plana vitrectomy. *Ophthalmology.* 2002;109(5):948-954.
14. Sood V, Rahman R, Denniston AK. Phacoemulsification and foldable intraocular lens implantation combined with 23-gauge transconjunctival sutureless vitrectomy. *J Cataract Refract Surg.* 2009;35:1380-1384.
15. Kim MJ, Park KH, Hwang JM, Yu HG, Yu SK, Chung H. The safety and efficacy of transconjunctival sutureless 23-gauge vitrectomy. *Korean J Ophthalmol.* 2007;21:201-207.
16. Kim SH, Chung JW, Chung H, Yo HG. Phacoemulsification and foldable intraocular lens implantation combined with vitrectomy and silicone oil tamponade for severe proliferative diabetic retinopathy. *J Cataract Refract Surg.* 2004;30:1721-1726.
17. Chung TY, Chung H, Lee JH. Combined surgery and sequential surgery comprising phacoemulsification, pars plana vitrectomy, and intraocular lens implantation: comparison of clinical outcomes. *J Cataract Refract Surg.* 2002;28:2001-2005.
18. Scharwey K, Pavlovic S, Jacobi KW. Combined clear corneal phacoemulsification, vitreoretinal surgery, and intraocular lens implantation. *J Cataract Refract Surg.* 1999;25:693-698.
19. Jang SY, Choi KS, Lee SJ. Chandelier retroillumination-assisted cataract extraction in eyes with vitreous hemorrhage. *Arch Ophthalmol.* 2010;128(7):911-914.
20. Kim KH, Sohn HJ, Song HJ, Lee DY, Nam DH. Surgeon-controlled-endoillumination-guided irrigation and aspiration during combined 23-gauge sutureless vitrectomy and cataract surgery in eyes with poor fundus reflex. *J Cataract Refract Surg.* 2010;36(12):2028-2031.
21. Chang CJ, Chang YH, Chiang SY, Lin LT. Comparison of clear corneal phacoemulsification combined with 25-gauge transconjunctival sutureless vitrectomy and standard 20-gauge vitrectomy for patients with cataract and vitreoretinal diseases. *J Cataract Refract Surg.* 2005;31(6):1198-1207.
22. Park DH, Shin JP, Kim SY. Surgically induced astigmatism in combined phacoemulsification and vitrectomy; 23-gauge transconjunctival sutureless vitrectomy versus 20-gauge standard vitrectomy. *Graefes Arch Clin Exp Ophthalmol.* 2009;247(10):1331-1337.
23. Park SP, Ahn JK, Lee GH. Morphologic changes in the anterior segment after phaco-vitrectomy for proliferative diabetic retinopathy. *J Cataract Refract Surg.* 2009;35(5):868-873.
24. Ando A, Nishimura T, Uyama M. Surgical outcome on combined procedures of lens extraction, intraocular lens implantation, and vitrectomy during removal of epiretinal membrane. *Ophthalmic Surg Lasers.* 1998;29:974-979.
25. Dugas B, Ouled-Moussa R, Lafontaine PO, et al. Idiopathic epiretinal macular membrane and cataract extraction: combined versus consecutive surgery. *Am J Ophthalmol.* 2010;149(2):302-306.
26. Muselier A, Dugas B, Burelle X, et al. Macular hole surgery and cataract extraction: combined vs. consecutive surgery. *Am J Ophthalmol.* 2010;150(3):387-391.
27. Sisk RA, Murray TG. Combined phacoemulsification and sutureless 23-gauge pars plana vitrectomy for complex vitreoretinal diseases. *Br J Ophthalmol.* 2010;94(8):1028-1032.
28. Wensheng L, Wu R, Wang X, Xu M, Sun G, Sun C.Clinical complications of combined phacoemulsification and vitrectomy for eyes with coexisting cataract and vitreoretinal diseases. *Eur J Ophthalmol.* 2009;19(1):37-45.
29. Li W, Sun G, Wu R, Wang X, Xu M, Sun C. Long term results after phaco-vitrectomy and foldable intraocular lens implantation. *Acta Ophthalmol.* 2009;87(8):896-900.
30. Treumer F, Bunse A, Rudolf M, Roider J. Pars plana vitrectomy, phacoemulsification and intraocular lens implantation. Comparison of clinical complications in a combined versus two-step surgical approach. *Graefes Arch Clin Exp Ophthalmol.* 2006;244(7):808-815.
31. Lahey JM, Francis RR, Kearney JJ, Cheung M. Combining phacoemulsification and vitrectomy in patients with proliferative diabetic retinopathy. *Curr Opin Ophthalmol.* 2004;15(3):192-196.
32. Falkner-Radler CI, Benesch T, Binder S. Accuracy of pre-operative biometry in vitrectomy combined with cataract surgery for patients with epiretinal membranes and macular holes: results of a prospective controlled clinical trial. *J Cataract Refract Surg.* 2008;34(10):1754-1760.

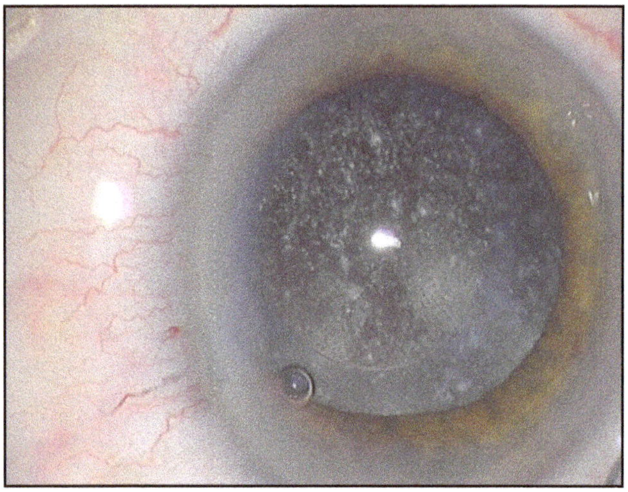

F-1. Phaco in asteroid degeneration of the vitreous.

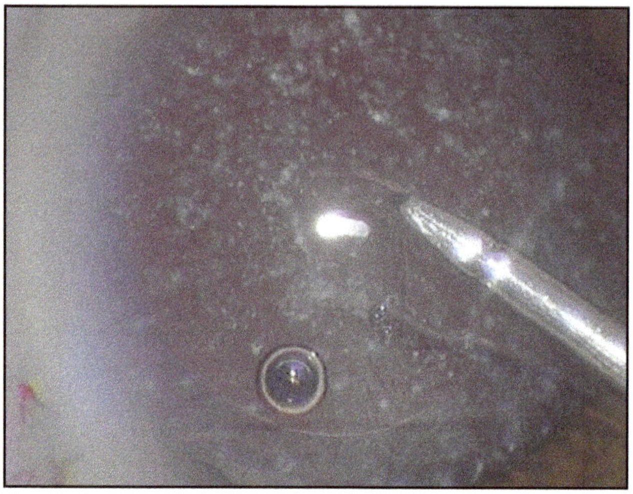

F-2. With asteroid degeneration of the vitreous at the end of phaco, the surgeon can perform the posterior rhexis.

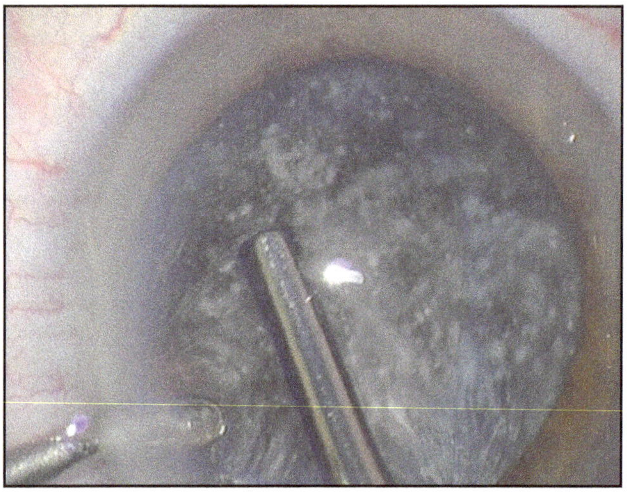

F-3. The surgeon can perform a vitrectomy through the rhexis.

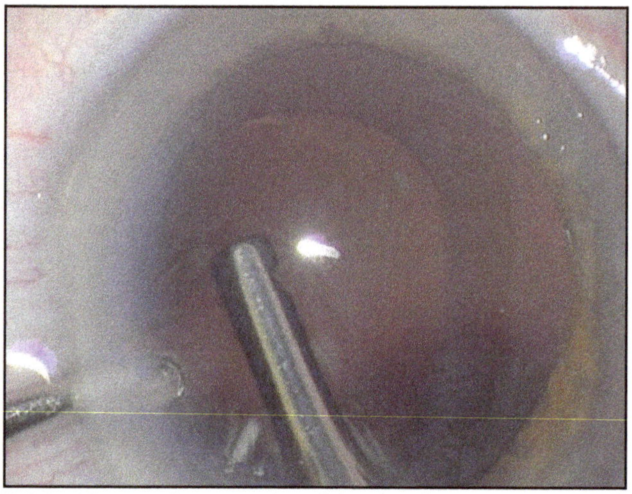

F-4. In this way, a large portion of the vitreal opacity is removed; IOL implantation in the bag follows.

15

Traumatic Cataract

Cataract surgery in traumatized eyes is one of the most difficult clinical situations an anterior segment surgeon is likely to encounter. There are many causes of traumatic cataract, including penetration, perforation, or contusive trauma. Subsequent traumatic wounds can be variable, and the extent of the damage may be difficult to evaluate. Two possible scenarios of lenticular ocular trauma are dislocation and loss of lens transparency; these can be complicated by fragmentation or swelling of the lens. Cataracts may develop early or late and may be caused by mechanical or nonmechanical (eg, lightning) factors.

The concomitant presence of posterior segment disruption may necessitate vitreoretinal surgery that can be performed before, after, or during cataract surgery. This requires careful planning and a close working relationship with a posterior segment surgeon.

As with all surgery, and particularly with trauma, the surgeon must prepare for any expected or unexpected intraoperative situation, as this will maximize surgical confidence. With traumatic cataracts, normally acute, the patient complains of sudden loss of visual acuity, usually expecting to return to pretrauma acuity. It is essential that the surgeon fully explain that the outcome of this surgery is unpredictable. The surgeon should advise a reasonable visual prognosis because the possible trauma is difficult to assess.

With the introduction of the Birmingham Terminology System, the examination and definition of ocular trauma has been standardized.[1] As a result, it is possible to study the postoperative visual outcome in the traumatic cataract and estimate visual predictability, with special reference to the Birmingham Terminology System.

The literature reports functional results of traumatic cataracts, often grouped together, isolated clinical cases, and small clinical numbers.[2,3]

This chapter will provide an attentive and systematic approach to traumatic cataract surgery, describing various surgical techniques.

Clinical Evaluation

A careful preoperative evaluation of the patient with a traumatic cataract is essential to fully understand the altered ocular anatomy and allow the surgeon to plan accordingly. This preoperatively evaluates the degree of damage to the eye and formulates a plan for surgery, choosing instruments, equipment, sutures, and implants that may be necessary during the operation. Careful preoperative planning reduces unexpected intraoperative events, resulting in a better visual outcome for the patient.

Clinical History

The patient's clinical history differentiates acute or previous trauma. In emergency cases, the preoperative examination must determine how the trauma occurred and the force of impact, as it may provide indications of the existence of a hidden perforating wound or an intraocular foreign body. Possible concomitant lesions in the posterior segment should be evaluated.

Trauma resulting from metallic impacts should lead the surgeon to suspect the presence of a metallic intraocular foreign body. In the event of an obvious perforation, the surgeon should assess how the injury occurred, considering possible infection.

In some cases, a traumatic cataract may appear months or even years after the injury. Sometimes the patient cannot remember how the trauma occurred and may even have

Buratto L, Brint SF, Caretti L.
Cataract Surgery in Complicated Cases (pp 155-168).

forgotten all about it. Probing questions from the surgeon may facilitate remembering.

Objective Examination

The visit should always begin with an examination of the best-corrected visual acuity. When hand motion or light perception vision is detected, maintenance or loss of the patient's ability to recognize the color of a lighted object can provide some prognostic information on central vision. The response to Purkinje's phenomenon can provide an indirect indication on the presence of a detached retina or existence of glaucomatous damage, or more rarely, a range of neurological complications.

Slit-lamp biomicroscopy can provide interesting information for the planned surgery. First, the surgeon should examine the anterior chamber (AC) for signs of vitreous prolapse or intraocular foreign bodies. The surgeon will be able to evaluate the damage and presenting vitreous.

The lens must be examined very carefully. It may be possible to confirm the traumatic origin of the cataract by very careful observation: a space between the pupil margin and the lens surface or dislocation of the Y-suture with respect to the pupil. The presence and extent of phacodonesis and decentration of the lens zonular disinsertion must be recorded. If the anterior capsule appears to be damaged, the amount and course of the capsular laceration must be recorded; a wrinkled capsular surface may indicate discontinuity of the capsule itself or the zonules. It should be remembered that the integrity of the capsule may be compromised even with contusive (not penetrating) trauma.[4,5] With capsular laceration, the surgeon should try to plan a rhexis that will circumvent the tear. Remember that the laceration will tend to extend as the lens swells; consequently, if the laceration is near the edge of what could be the largest capsulorrhexis possible, surgery should be performed as quickly as possible.

Similarly, the posterior capsule may be lacerated following penetrating or contusive trauma[6]; however, in this case, it is unlikely that this will be seen with the clinical examination as the cataract will limit visibility.

Sometimes it is possible to examine the fundus depending on the opacity of the media, and its examination should include identification of holes, retinal lacerations, or retinal edema. The presence of subretinal or suprachoroidal hemorrhage should lead to greater prognostic caution, as any degree of suprachoroidal hemorrhage would cause posterior pressure during surgery.

Special Tests

If the cataract is particularly dense, planning the surgery should include the B-scan. This can document the state of the posterior segment and also provide crucial information on the state of the posterior capsule.

In the case of a mature cataract resulting from a penetrating wound, the B-scan can provide information on the posterior capsule (eg, it can highlight a decentered rupture of the posterior capsule).

The results of the B-scan may modify the surgeon's approach to the cataract surgery itself.

When a suprachoroidal hemorrhage is detected, the surgeon should consider a pars plana vitrectomy. If possible, surgery should be postponed until the hemorrhage has been reabsorbed. If the hemorrhage is large, a vitreoretinal surgeon must be consulted; evacuation of the hemorrhage may be required and while this is technically a simple procedure, it is associated with an increased risk of retinal detachment.

A computed tomography (CT) scan of the orbit is indicated if the surgeon suspects the presence of an intraocular or intraorbital foreign body. Acutely, a CT scan can provide information useful for formulating the diagnosis of traumatic cataract; a slight change in the lens may indicate the presence or imminent development of a visually important cataract. The CT scan may indicate an intumescent cataract, misleading to the diagnosis of traumatic aphakia.[7]

A preoperative evaluation of potential vision with traumatic cataracts, especially if opaque, is very difficult, thus a B-scan, CT scan, and electroretinogram can be very helpful. The age of the patient and preoperative visual acuity are important predictive factors for visual function. Normally, satisfactory visual acuity following traumatic blunt related cataract surgery is achieved more frequently, as compared to penetrating or perforating trauma, because of the lower incidence of postoperative complications.

Objective Examination With an Open Globe

In the emergency room, Snellen visual acuity is usually impossible to obtain; however, it is possible to document light perception, hand motion or finger-counting, facial recognition, or even reading the print on the informed consent. With penetrating trauma, measurement of visual acuity can underestimate the real visual potential. Family or patient recollection of the trauma can be helpful in determining potential. Light response may be extremely useful in the formulation of the prognosis, if possible, with an open globe. As traumatic mydriasis, miosis, lacerations, or incarceration of the iris can limit pupil motility in the traumatized eye, one should remember that to determine the presence of an afferent pupillary defect, only one pupil needs to be examined. The surgeon should not force the eyelids open if the patient is squeezing.

With an open corneal scleral laceration, it is probable that a good slit-lamp examination will be unlikely or even impossible, making surgical planning even more critical. Some recommend removal of the cataract when the globe is being repaired (primary cataract removal),[8,9] though a deferred approach may prove to be more advantageous (secondary removal of the cataract).[10]

The advantages of deferred removal of the cataract include better visibility inside the eye, stabilization of the blood-eye barrier, more precise determination of the intraocular lens (IOL), and the possibility for better reconstruction of the anterior segment. In many cases, poor corneal transparency, clots, or anatomical changes can prevent examination of the anterior segment, leading to unexpected complications. Following initial surgical, additional examination and evaluation can lead to better surgical planning. Moreover, with an open globe, keratometry and biometry are almost impossible, and patient cooperation will be poor. This may be the source of significant ametropia when the visual result could otherwise be excellent.

On initial examination, the damage to the lens can sometimes appear to be more significant than it actually is; it may not even be necessary to remove the cataract. This may occur with a corneal laceration that penetrates the anterior capsule. Here, the cornea is sutured without removing the cataract; the lens capsule may close autonomously, leaving just a tiny point of opacity in the lens. With a small peripheral perforation, the lens may remain essentially clear following the careful removal of the intraocular foreign body.[11] Inert foreign bodies (such as glass) are well tolerated even when left in situ; however, a foreign body of a ferrous nature must be removed, as it could lead to ocular siderosis with iron deposits in the eye and potentially devastating visual consequences.[12]

One of the major advantages of primary cataract surgery is that the surgeon can inspect the posterior segment. If the traumatic cataract prevents adequate exploration impeding the removal of an identified foreign body, the lens must be removed, particularly if the surgeon suspects that the foreign body may contain biological matter or other contaminating substances.

If the foreign body is located in the posterior segment, the anterior segment surgeon should collaborate with the vitreoretinal surgeon.

The traumatic cataract should ideally be removed through an anterior approach; a pars plana vitrectomy usually ends up with aphakia or requiring a scleral fixated IOL. If the vitreoretinal surgeon feels a pars plana vitrectomy is necessary, he or she should try to preserve as much of the capsular diaphragm as possible to provide support for the IOL.

Generally, primary removal of the cataract is recommended if the lens is fragmented, swollen, or if it induces pupillary block.

Moreover, some patients may have medical conditions, making it more feasible to perform a single surgery under general anesthesia. We prefer to postpone the cataract surgery whenever possible to allow local anesthesia. The patient should be well informed preoperatively regarding his or her prognosis.

Surgical Planning and Technique

The preliminary evaluation should decide primary or secondary cataract removal, and good preoperative planning is essential.

The first decision in every surgery is the choice of anesthesia; with traumatic cataracts, there are usually 2 options: local or general anesthesia. If the globe is open, general anesthesia usually gives the surgeon greater operating safety. If the globe is closed, the choice depends largely on the patient's cooperation and the expected duration of the surgery.

Topical anesthesia should be used only in the most straightforward cases of traumatic cataract.

If the surgeon expects to see significant posterior pressure, mannitol may be used to reduce intraocular pressure prior to transferring the patient to the operating room.

Some have suggested a possible association between intravenous mannitol and suprachoroidal hemorrhage; however, no studies have ever identified mannitol as an independent risk factor, whereas ocular trauma is a risk factor that has been extensively documented.[13-17]

Determining the Incision Location

Once the surgeon has selected the anesthesia, he or she must decide on the position for the scleral or conjunctival incision. This incision should be placed in an area of the anterior segment that has been least damaged; an incision performed near zonular dialysis will make insertion of a Cionni modified capsular tension ring (MCTR [Morcher, Stuttgart, Germany]) or IOL for scleral fixation unnecessarily difficult. Moreover, the surgeon will be working in an area of anterior hyaloid exposure, with greater risk of vitreous loss.

Sometimes a prominent brow will dictate a temporal approach; however, if the wound crosses temporally, the surgeon may consider an inferior incision.

If the above are not factors, the position can be placed depending on the astigmatism. The surgeon should also be comfortable.

Conjunctiva

Although the conjunctival incision is by no means a critical step of the surgery, the surgeon should carefully determine the position and the extension of the peritomy. Opening the conjunctiva must allow straightforward access to the tunnel leaving room for a pars plana sclerotomy, suturing of an IOL with scleral fixation, or insertion of a Cionni MCTR. As much conjuntiva as possible

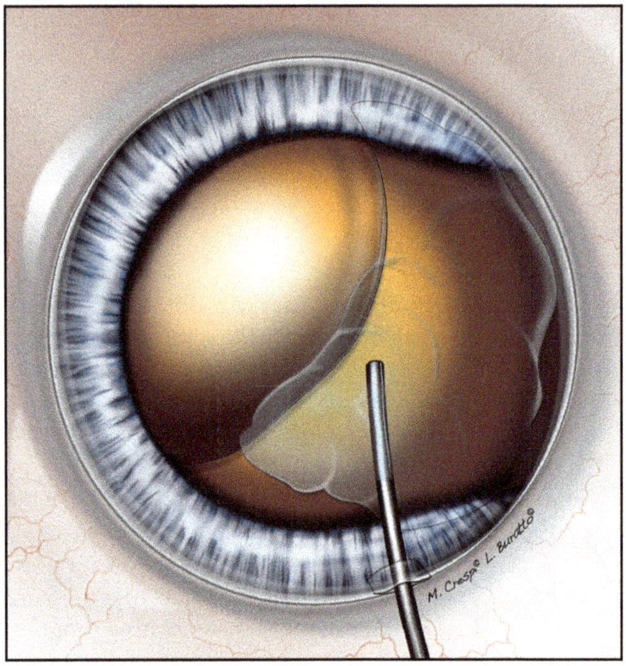

Figure 15-1. Use of a dispersive VES to create a plug to protect the exposed vitreous face.

should be spared, as many cases of traumatic cataract may eventually require glaucoma surgery.

Choice of Viscoelastic Substance

In traumatic cataracts, the choice of viscoelastic substance (VES) depends on a number of factors, and in some cases, more than one VES may prove useful. If the anterior hyaloid is partly exposed, a dispersive VES, such as Viscoat (Alcon Laboratories, Fort Worth, TX) or Healon Endocoat or Healon 5 (Abbott Laboratories, Abbott Park, IL), can tamponade the vitreous[18] (Figure 15-1). This type of VES will also provide excellent protection for the endothelium, as endothelial cell density has been reduced by the trauma.[19]

The ability to maintain spaces and ease of removal of a highly cohesive VES such as Healon GV (Abbott Laboratories) or Biolon (SIFI, Catania, Italy) make these substances ideal for IOL implantation.

In some cases, the surgeon may opt for Arshinoff's "soft shell" technique; it combines the superior endothelial protection of a dispersive VES with the ability to maintain spaces and ease of removal and transparency typical of cohesive agents.[20] The soft shell is created by partially filling the anterior AC with a dispersive VES and subsequently injecting a cohesive VES directly in front of the lens. This pushes the dispersive agent against the endothelium, creating a thin protective layer. This approach is not useful if the goal is to protect the vitreous face.

When the surgeon has planned to dry aspirate the lens material located below the VES, a moderately cohesive VES should be used, such as Healon or Provisc (sodium hyaluronate [Alcon]). A highly cohesive VES such as Healon GV will tend to obstruct the cannula used in the techniques of manual aspiration.

Capsulotomy and Hydrodissection

The anterior capsulotomy often determines the success of the remainder of the surgery. If the trauma has caused a lens perforation, the surgeon should attempt to convert the perforation into an anterior capsulorrhexis.

A continuous circular capsulorrhexis provides much greater mechanical resistance than a partial capsulorrhexis or one created using the old "can-opener" technique[21,22]; it also facilitates the rest of the surgery.

Occasionally, the anterior capsular opening can be performed using a vitrectomy probe; however, this type of capsulotomy, despite being structurally more stable than the can-opener technique, is still not as safe as a continuous circular capsulorrhexis.[23,24] The vitrectorhexis technique may be more difficult in practice than in theory as the capsule is not always easily aspirated. Moreover, when the capsule is grasped by the probe, zonular integrity may be compromised. With a traumatic cataract, visualization of the capsule may be particularly difficult, especially if the capsule is torn or the cortex is opaque. A number of dyes have been suggested to improve visibility: indocyanine green (ICG), trypan blue, methylene blue, gentian violet, and fluorescein.

Clinically, ICG is extremely good and has an acceptable safety profile, as does trypan blue.[25] Initial usage of ICG recommended injection under air; however, Lenni Buratto found that if the capsule is still intact, one could simply spread a drop of dye over the anterior capsule, below the VES. This can also outline the edges of a capsular perforation.

Gimbel and Willerscheidt[26] proposed a decompression technique for the capsular bag in white cataracts—the aspiration of the whitish liquefied cortical material through a small central opening created in the capsule to decompress the intumescent capsular bag. This can reduce the risk of rhexis extension and reduce the pressure inside the bag.

The surgeon must be especially careful when creating the rhexis in a traumatized lens; the chosen surgical technique must be perfect. The zonular barrier may not always be uniform, and consequently, the tearing technique used may be different from the usual one. The surgeon must attempt to keep the leading edge of the flap folded to ensure a more predictable progression of the tear.

In order to avoid traction on the zonules, it is often necessary to use a technique that tears in a direction tangential to the circular profile of the capsulotomy, avoiding centrifugal forces that carry greater risk of damage to the damaged zonules. The maneuver is much more controlled if the surgeon creates small segments with tangential traction, regrasping frequently.

Dyes

Trypan blue has some potential advantages: it is useful for "finding" the edge of a capsulorrhexis that was "lost" as it was being created.[27,28] Tangential illumination of the anterior capsule with a sterile endo-illuminator can also improve visibility with a white lens. It has been shown that staining with trypan blue modifies biomechanical properties of the human lens capsule and induces a significant reduction in elasticity, increasing rigidity,[29,30] the same effect achieved with ICG. There have been recent reports of toxicity induced by this dye, one of the most popular used during capsulorrhexis.[31,32] In a recent study, its effects on the lens epithelial cells and on the capsule by optical microscopy, electron microscopy, and immune-histochemistry[29] concluded that trypan blue induced lens epithelial cell death, supporting the theory that a 0.1% solution of this dye can reduce the incidence of posterior capsule opacification.

In another recent paper,[33] several different vital dyes were compared (ie, the triarylmethanes [methylene blue and aniline blue] with patent blue and trypan blue). The researchers examined their capsular staining capacity and cytotoxicity in cultures of human corneal endothelial cells. The authors observed that high concentrations of trypan blue and aniline blue were significantly cytotoxic to cultures of human corneal endothelial cells compared to patent blue and methylene blue, which caused less damage. All of the dyes tested stained the lens capsule adequately for capsulorrhexis.

In had been felt that methylene blue and gentian violet were extremely cytotoxic. However, some years ago, safe exposure times and dosages were determined for a number of dyes[34]: 1 minute of exposure for 0.25% ICG, 0.20% methylene blue, 0.40% trypan blue, 0.01% gentian violet, and 10% fluorescein do not appear to have cytotoxic effects on cell cultures. Moreover, concentrations have been determined for optimal staining of the anterior capsule[35]: 0.25% ICG, 0.10% methylene blue, 0.10% trypan blue, 0.01% gentian violet, and 1.25% sodium fluorescein.

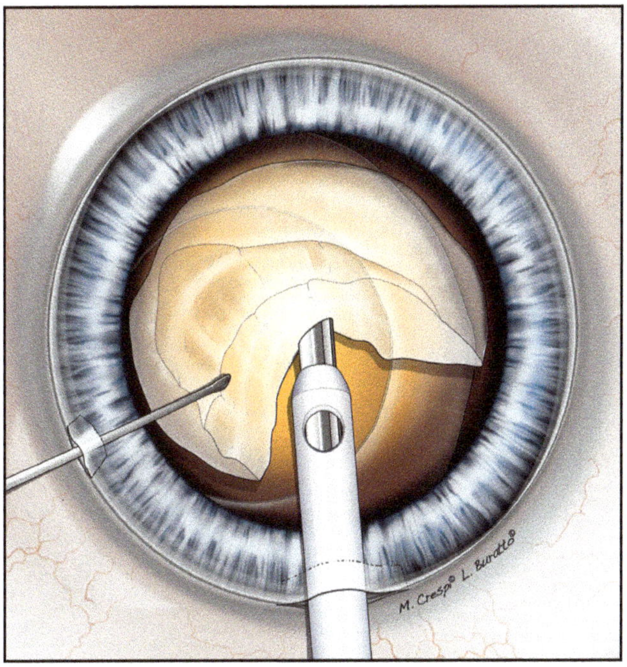

Figure 15-2. Phacoemulsification in the AC following expression of the nucleus outside of the capsule.

When there is loss or extensive weakness of the zonules, the surgeon may find it necessary to start by cutting the anterior capsule with a cystotome, a sharp 15-degree blade, or a diamond knife. Once this first opening has been created, the surgeon may sometimes encounter difficulty with the rhexis, associated with lack of resistance by the zonules.

We recommend a large capsulorrhexis measuring 5.5 to 6.0 mm, as this will facilitate the manipulation of the nucleus. In children with traumatic cataracts, the rhexis may prove to be even more challenging than in adults, given that the young anterior capsule is stronger and much more elastic. For these patients, it may be much easier to create a small rhexis initially enlarging it at a later stage as these capsules have a greater tendency to rhexis extension.

If there is marked zonular instability, the surgeon can use a fixation instrument inserted through a side incision to stabilize the nucleus during capsulorrhexis.

Hydrodissection should be performed slowly and carefully to completely free the nucleus and reduce zonular stress during its manipulation. If the nucleus is soft, as it usually is, complete hydrodissection of the nucleus and its subluxation into the AC will greatly simplify the removal of the nucleus, virtually eliminating zonular stress[36] (Figure 15-2).

Hydrodelineation is recommended. The surgeon should rotate the nucleus with great care and attention, performing minimal or no rotation of the nucleus to avoid inducing stress on the residual zonular fibers. Rather than rotating the nucleus, the surgeon should rotate the aspiration port to limit stress on residual zonular fibers.

Removal of the Nucleus

Removal of the nucleus can be performed with several techniques, each with advantages and disadvantages depending on the specific case. The nucleus in a young eye will normally be soft, with a choice of techniques to choose from. If the capsulorrhexis is intact, phaco-aspiration of the nucleus is generally safe and rapid. If there is rupture of the anterior or posterior capsule, manual aspiration with a Simcoe cannula (Katalyst Surgical, Chesterfield, MO), or similar cannula, will afford better control, while dry

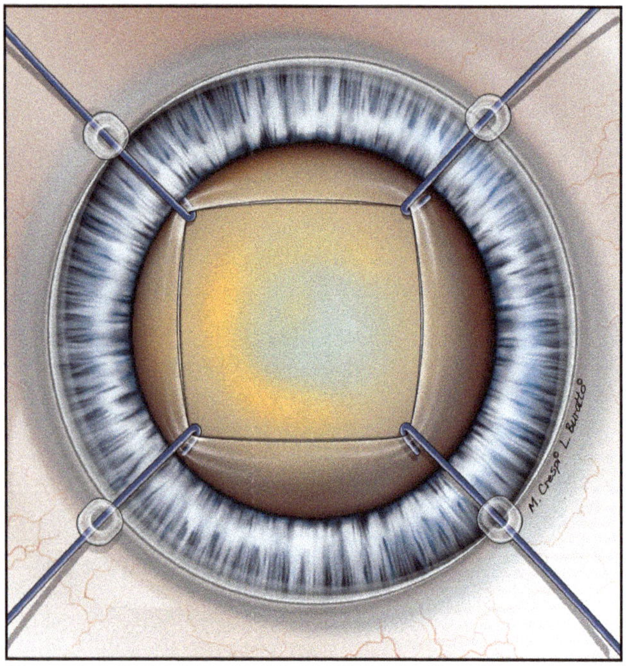

Figure 15-3. Four iris hooks used to stabilize the subluxated capsular bag.

aspiration of the soft nucleus under VES ensures excellent control, particularly in the more complex cases.[18]

As the density of the nucleus is greater in older patients, removal becomes more difficult. Improvements with small incisions and working in a closed system (coaxial MICS) help greatly in these weakened zonule cases. As traumatized eyes are associated with an increased risk of suprachoroidal hemorrhage, the closed system minimizes the risk of expulsive hemorrhage. Also, if the posterior capsule has ruptured or if there is zonular dehiscence, tamponading the vitreous with VES will be more successful in a closed system.

Conversely, manual extracapsular extraction requires an open wound, greatly compromising the surgeon's control. Some basic nuclear manipulation principles must be considered in traumatic cases. The techniques of phaco flip and chip and flip are not recommended as these can exert dangerous traction forces on the remaining zonules. Many variations of delicate divide and conquer and particularly phaco chop techniques can be adapted to the principles of slow-motion phaco.

Phacoemulsification With Compromised Zonules

In some patients with extremely weak zonules, creation of the groove for a divide and conquer phaco or other endocapsular manipulations can add extra stress to the already compromised capsular support. A relatively large capsulorrhexis will facilitate viscoexpression of the nucleus in the AC.

A better alternative would be a delicate chopping procedure that would protect the remaining zonular fibers as all of the force would be absorbed by the chopper, the nucleus, and the force against the phaco handpiece.

Phacoemulsification should proceed with lower vacuum and aspiration, and the bottle is kept as low as possible (Osher's "slow motion phaco").[37] These modifications will allow reduced pressure in the AC with lower traction on the fragile and already partially absent zonules; there will be less chance of vitreous disruption stabilization of the lens and less turbulence in the AC. Initially, the ultrasound tip should enter with the bottle very low to prevent excessive deepening of the anterior segment that has already been filled with VES. As soon as part of the VES has been removed, the bottle can be raised slightly.

If the surgeon is operating at the 12 o'clock position, another useful maneuver to limit stress on the zonular fibers is to rotate the bevel of the phaco tip and orient it toward the nasal or temporal segments, without rotating the nucleus.

Some feel the aspiration must always be centrifugal relative to the area of weakness. It depends on the position of the zonular weakness; if not extensive, forces must be directed toward the weakened area.

With significant zonular damage, a CTR can be used to stabilize the nucleus prior to starting phaco. To facilitate the introduction of the ring into the bag, the surgeon should perform a delicate viscodissection of the cortex to create space for the insertion of the ring. If the zonular damage involves more than 4 hours (90 degrees), suturing a Cionni MCTR can strengthen the area of greater zonular weakness.[38] This improves the stability of the lens during all of the successive steps of the operation.

If the nucleus is particularly large and dense, the introduction of the ring can be difficult or even impossible prior to phaco. In these cases, the surgeon can enhance zonular support with flexible nylon iris retractors, introduced through a limbal incision. These hook to the edge of the capsulorrhexis (Figure 15-3). The retractor can be introduced easily through a paracentesis. After emulsification of the nucleus, the CTR can be introduced and positioned much more easily.

Theoretically, it is also possible to introduce the CTR following posterior capsule rupture, if an anterior and a posterior rhexis have been performed. Otherwise, the use of this device should be avoided. If the capsule ruptures or tears after the ring has already been positioned, the surgeon must remove it immediately, as its stability is no longer guaranteed.

Cortical Removal

The capsular bag must be inspected very carefully following nuclear removal, to rule out capsular rupture. Isolated rupture of the posterior capsule has been described as the result of contusive trauma.[39-41]

If the bag and the zonules are intact, the cortex can be aspirated as usual; however, if the zonules are damaged, extreme care is required to remove the cortex. If the cortex has been separated from the bag using hydrodissection at the beginning of the operation, this is much easier. However, if the hydrodissection is incomplete or has not been performed, viscodissection can be performed using dispersive or pseudoadaptive VES to separate the cortex from the bag (Figure 15-4). Moreover, cortical viscodissection will limit stress on the remaining zonules during the aspiration of the cortex.

It may be difficult for the surgeon to aspirate the cortex due to a lack of resistance by the zonular fibers and he or she may increase zonular dialysis. If the surgeon uses automated irrigation/aspiration, one should remove pieces of cortex with a tangential (as opposed to a radial) movement.

Irrigation/aspiration instruments can cause hydration of the vitreous, positive pressure, and vitreous prolapse. The Buratto bimanual cannulas (Ophthalmic Surgical Instruments, Como, Italy) are recommended as they will provide better control than coaxial techniques.

The same principle of tangential movement applies to manual aspiration with Simcoe-type cannulas (Beaver-Visitec International, Inc, Waltham, MA), which offer better control inside a stable chamber.

If there is posterior capsular rupture, once the intact anterior hyaloid has been covered with VES, the surgeon can complete the removal of the cortex. This procedure should be performed as a manual dry aspiration using a 25- or 27-gauge cannula attached to a 3-mL syringe, the chamber filled with VES, and without allowing vitreous escape. It is a long, tedious procedure; nevertheless, control is excellent.[42]

Removal of the Lens Material in the Event of Vitreous Presentation

The loss of vitreous from the anterior segment, with VES mixed with lens material, may lead to the onset of complications involving the posterior segment. If the object that caused the penetrating wound is removed, vitreous may infiltrate the lacerated lens and even cross it to reach the AC. The surgeon must always avoid aspirating vitreous given the tenacious adhesion of the VES to the base of the vitreous. Any traction exerted on the anterior vitreous can create retinal tears and eventually lead to retinal detachment.

If there is extensive zonular disinsertion and the residual fragments of the capsule are severely torn, the best approach may be a pars plana lensectomy with an anterior vitrectomy.

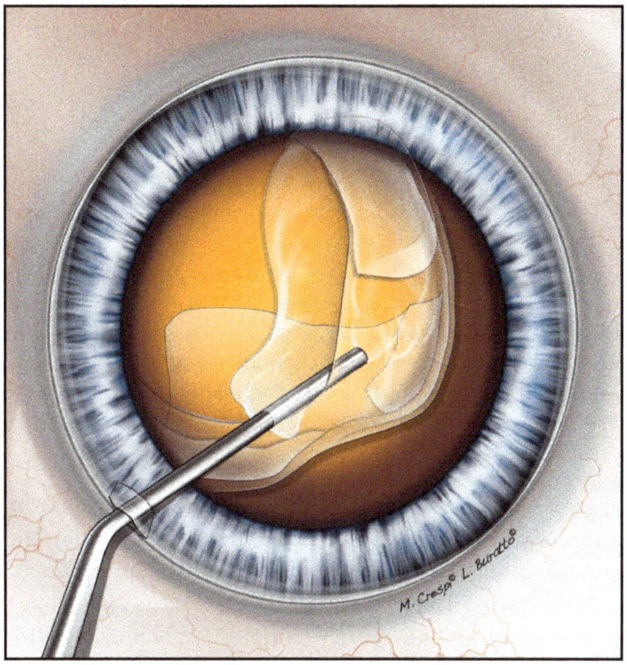

Figure 15-4. Viscodissection.

When the surgeon first detects vitreous mixed with lens material, with lens support and the peripheral areas of the lens intact, he or she should develop a specific approach. First, protruding vitreous must be removed by vitrectomy. It may be possible to perform a dry vitrectomy by placing the mouth of the vitrectomy probe at the corneal opening; this will allow good removal of all of the external vitreous without exerting traction. The parameters must be set with low flow rate, low aspiration, and a high cut rate. We suggest the dual linear method: the surgeon has an infusion foot control positioned at a preset height (on-off) that can regulate the level of aspiration linearly, until moving the foot pedal laterally to the cutting position, then again linear. Thus, during aspiration, the surgeon can select the cut desired at that particular instance.

Subsequently, the vitrectomy can be introduced into the AC. The surgeon can perform a delicate vitrectomy using the parameters indicated previously to remove the vitreous from the anterior segment, removing all of the incarcerated tissue from the wounds and incisions. Even low values of coaxial infusion introduced through the handpiece of the vitrectomy handpiece will tend to repulse the vitreous from the mouth of the instrument, causing unnecessary turbulence in the AC. Consequently, separate or 2-handed infusion through an accessory paracentesis is preferable, using a 21-gauge butterfly needle or a blunt cannula to ensure good control of the irrigation flow direction.

Once the vitreous has been completely removed from the AC, the surgeon should then concentrate on the lens material. If this material is soft, it can be aspirated using the vitrectomy probe. This instrument affords greater levels

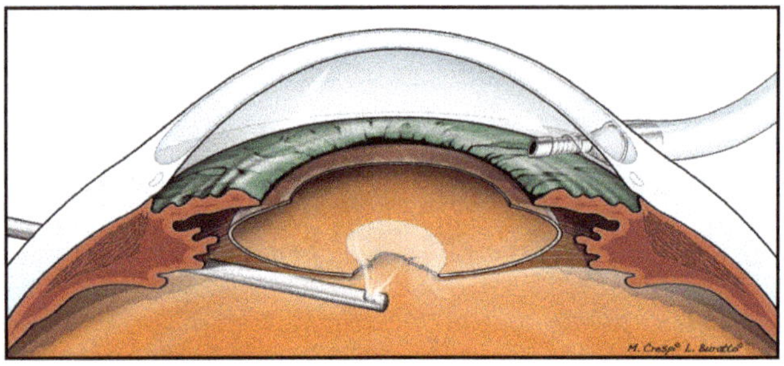

Figure 15-5. During the pars plana anterior vitrectomy, the irrigation liquid is infused through a 21-gauge butterfly needle inserted through a corneal paracentesis. The prolapsed vitreous is removed anteriorly by drawing it posteriorly with a vitrectomy device inserted through a sclerotomy.

of safety to the procedure in the event the lens material is mixed with vitreous. If some of the vitreous is caught in the aspiration hole, it is possible to start cutting immediately, thus releasing vitreous traction.

With zonular damage, a dry aspiration is possible with a chamber filled with VES. A moderately cohesive VES can be injected to deepen the chamber, taking care to inject it first in the wound site without overfilling the chamber. If excessive VES is injected, the associated increase in intraocular pressure can result in prolapse of the vitreous during injection. Aspiration efficacy is maximized if a 25- or 27-gauge cannula is introduced into the soft lens material as far away as possible from the capsular laceration. The lens material can therefore be aspirated by starting at a point distant from the laceration. If the vitreous is aspirated by the cannula, it should be released, and the surgeon should continue with additional vitrectomy.

Dense Nucleus and the Presence of a Lacerated Posterior Capsule

If the cataractous material is dense, phacoemulsification may be necessary. If the surgeon has managed to completely clean the anterior segment of vitreous, he or she can cautiously perform a phaco in the AC on a bed of dispersive VES or simply on a Sheets glide (BD Medical, Franklin Lakes, NJ). It may prove useful to introduce an instrument to support the lens material through an accessory corneal incision. The technique for the introduction of the Sheets glide (that may be a more complicated procedure) with a pseudo-posterior capsular function must be done with extreme care as to avowing any additional tearing of the capsule.

If the tear of the posterior capsule is extensive or there is widespread zonular weakness, the lens material may be supported from behind using a second instrument introduced pars plana, as described by Dr. Charles Kelman.[43] The surgeon must always avoid vitreous being aspirated by the phaco.

Cleaning the Anterior Segment

Following the complete removal of the lens material, the surgeon must check carefully and ensure there is no additional vitreous in the anterior segment. If this is not the case, he or she must perform a second vitrectomy.

Once the media of the anterior segment allows a clear view, a pars plana vitrectomy must be performed, using separate (anterior) infusion. The tip of the vitrectomy probe is inserted through a sclerotomy created with a 20-gauge V-blade 3.5 mm behind the limbus following a conjunctival peritomy (Figure 15-5). Better still, the surgeon can use a 23- or 25-gauge trocar inserted through the conjunctiva with the biplanar angled (5 to 30 degrees) technique, following opening of the conjunctiva with respect to the sclera below.

The pars plana approach has a number of advantages over a limbal vitrectomy. First, the vitreous is aspirated from behind, opposite the wounds of the anterior segment, and drawn into the vitreous cavity, generating less traction and allowing better access to the vitreous surrounding the pupil.[44] Moreover, when the probe is introduced with an anterior approach, the corneal dome is likely to be distorted, obscuring the surgeon's view. With a pars plana approach, there is better visualization. After completing the vitrectomy, if a 20-gauge blade has been used, the sclerotomy should be cleaned from the outside and the incision closed with a 6-0 Vicryl suture.

Management of the Lacerated Capsule

Once the lens material and vitreous have been removed from the AC, the surgeon should evaluate zonular and capsular support. After having filled the anterior segment with VES, the iris should be retracted to inspect the capsule and zonules.

If the anterior rhexis is still intact, and there is only a small laceration of the posterior capsule, VES can be injected into the tear to push the vitreous backward and convert the tear into a circular posterior rhexis. This will allow sufficient capsular support to implant a posterior chamber (PC) lens in the bag.

When the posterior capsule tear cannot be safely converted into a rhexis, the haptics of the PC-IOL can be placed into the sulcus. If the rhexis is intact and has a diameter of 5 mm or less, the optic can be pushed posterior to the rhexis, with better fixation and centration. In this case, the power of the IOL remains as usual; however, if both the haptics and the optic are at the level of the ciliary sulcus, the surgeon must subtract half a diopter from the optic power calculated (unpublished data presented at the annual conference of the American Society of Cataract and Refractive Surgery, 1984).

If the capsular damage is extensive, the surgeon must decide whether there is sufficient support to allow implantation of a PC-IOL in the sulcus. Despite the fact that the capsule is lacerated, it still may be able to provide long-term support for the IOL; however, the surgeon must be able to implant the lens carefully without damaging what is left of the capsule. The surgeon must pay maximum attention to the inferior support as the force of gravity can gradually cause an initially well-positioned lens to decenter inferiorly. When the IOL has been inserted and appears to be well centered, fixation can be confirmed using Osher's "Bounce test." This involves delicately decentering the optic toward each one of the 2 haptics and then releasing it. The IOL should recenter spontaneously.

If there is inadequate capsular support, the surgeon may opt to suture one or both haptics of the PC-IOL to the sclera or the iris. (The techniques for this maneuver are covered in detail in Chapter 19.)

Choice of Intraocular Lens

Following successful removal of the cataract, the surgeon must then choose the most suitable IOL.

Regarding materials, it should be remembered that silicone lenses will increase the difficulty of a successive vitrectomy using silicone oil, thus they are not the best choice with posterior segment wounds.[45,46] Polymethylmethacrylate (PMMA) lenses and acrylic are well tolerated by the eye and are the elective choices of vitreoretinal surgeons.

As traumatic cataracts are often associated with a certain degree of traumatic mydriasis, the lens chosen should have a diameter of 6 mm or more. A large optic will also attenuate the effects of decentration that is more frequent in these cases.

With inadequate capsular support, the surgeon has a choice of several types of IOL: scleral fixation, iris suture fixation, AC-IOL (open loop), and iris enclavation. If scleral fixation is required, a rigid one-piece PMMA lens will provide greater stability and can be sutured to the sclera at 2 or 4 points, the latter reducing the risks associated with tilting.

An IOL with a fixation element at the tip of each haptic is preferable. Foldable 3-piece acrylic lenses can also be sutured in the ciliary sulcus, each haptic fixed with a single suture, resulting in just 2-point fixation.

The results of fixation ab externo or ab interno are similar and equally valid. Ab externo fixation has the advantage of not requiring sutures inside the globe; it reduces the time needed for surgical manipulation resulting in less ocular trauma[47] (see Chapter 19).

If the patient has glaucoma or there is a risk of glaucoma following trauma, respect for the conjunctiva is crucial for possible future surgery for glaucoma. An acrylic lens may be implanted in clear cornea either in the bag or sulcus as indicated (see the Positioning of the Lens section in this chapter).

PMMA IOLs are ideal for implantation in the sulcus, with minimal capsular support. Ranges of optic sizes are available (6.0, 6.5, and even 7.0 mm).

Some recommend AC-IOLs, particularly in the traumatized eye (see Chapter 19). Even if an implant with angle fixation has been perfectly positioned, it will be in contact with the delicate ciliary body, which may induce mild chronic cyclitis and cystoid macular edema. Moreover, proximity to the trabecular meshwork may aggravate traumatic glaucoma. A study published several years ago reported late-onset pupillary deformation in 58% of patients implanted with a Kelman-type AC-IOL,[48] possibly due to a chronic inflammatory response. Moreover, the optics of the AC-IOL may not be large enough, accentuating the risk of undesired visual phenomena (eg, haloes, rainbow-like distortions, and glare due to the edge of the lens).

This is another reason why the use of an iris-enclavated AC-IOL (AMO) is recommended in the event of inadequate capsular support. This lens is also used frequently in post-traumatic cases as it can be enclavated on the posterior surface of the iris.[49]

Some feel implanting an IOL in the AC is a relatively safe procedure.[50] In a comparative study between primary AC-IOL implantation and primary implantation of an IOL with scleral fixation in complicated cataract surgery, it was felt in the medium term (12 to 18 months), results with the implantation of the IOL in the AC were superior to those of the IOL with scleral fixation.

A review[51] published in 2004 supported these claims. The authors concluded that due to the improvements in design of the IOLs, the number of complications caused by AC-IOLs (with iris enclavation in particular) was lower than those associated with the use of an IOL for scleral fixation.[51]

The literature reports substantially equal efficacy between scleral fixation IOLs and PC-IOLs with iris fixation[52] and between AC-IOLs and the sutured PC-IOLs.[53]

A review published by the American Academy of Ophthalmology concurs in the safety and the efficacy of all of these approaches.[54]

With traumatic cataracts, plate haptic silicone implants should be avoided, as they are unforgiving of capsule or zonular problems, as well as not tolerated in the event of a vitrectomy requiring silicone oil.[55-60]

Positioning of the Lens

If the integrity of the capsular bag is maintained, the IOL should be implanted inside the bag. Even in the presence of zonular damage, there are several possibilities for maintaining capsular fixation. As described previously, tension rings can be inserted at any stage during surgery, as long as the anterior rhexis and the bag are intact. If a CTR is not available and the surgeon detects just a small area of zonular dehiscence, the haptic can be oriented along the axis of least resistance, as long as it is not obvious that the best centration can be achieved along a different axis.

Allowing a foldable lens, preferably acrylic, to unfold slowly will minimize the stress on the residual zonular fibers.

With a posterior capsular rupture or zonular dialysis, a PC-IOL can still be inserted in the ciliary sulcus. If the anterior rhexis is intact but there is a large rupture of the posterior capsule, the surgeon must position the haptics in the sulcus and attempt to trap the optic behind the rhexis. This maneuver affords the best support and reduces the risk of decentration.

If the rhexis is torn or is larger than the optic, a large-diameter IOL can be implanted in the sulcus. In the event there is inferior zonular lysis and it is not possible to trap the optic in the rhexis, the implanted lens can be stabilized with a suture.

Intraocular Lenses in Pediatric Cases

Even though many surgeons implant IOLs in children, correction of aphakia in very young patients is still an extremely controversial subject. Traumatic injuries are typically unilateral and in monocular aphakia, the use of contact lenses will often prove to be more uncomfortable than in patients with bilateral aphakia.

IOLs are well tolerated by most children, even when they are inserted under conditions of trauma.[61-64] The implantation of an IOL will be considerably easier if performed as part of cataract removal, compared to subsequent implantation; a secondary implant may be more difficult because of iridocapsular adhesions and fusion of anterior and posterior capsules. If the posterior capsule is intact, the presence of a lens will reduce the risk of developing PCO, the most frequent late-onset complication.[63] If a yttrium-aluminum-garnet (YAG) capsulotomy is required, the IOL will prevent vitreous in the AC. The IOL will also reduce the formation of posterior synechiae.[64,65]

PC-IOLs with scleral fixation have been used successfully in children. The question remains: Is 10-0 polypropylene suture stable enough to ensure scleral fixation of the IOL for the rest of the child's life? Late-onset dislocation of the IOL secondary to rupture of the polypropylene suture has been reported, particularly in young patients.[66-68] Asadi and Kheirkhah[69] recently reported late-onset dislocation of the IOL with scleral fixation in children. In the patients they observed, the late-onset dislocation due to the rupture of the polypropylene suture occurred 10 years from surgery in 6 of 25 eyes (24%). Theoretically, this suture has a fairly long mean lifespan. However, Cionni et al reported that approximately 10% of the sutures ruptured on average after 18 months.[70]

Scleral fixation of the IOL should not be abandoned in children, but other sutures should be considered. The best alternative is probably 9-0 polypropylene, which has the same characteristics as 10-0 polypropylene, but is more resistant to degradation over time. An 8-0 Gore-Tex suture (W. L. Gore & Associates, Flagstaff, AZ) has also been suggested.

With inadequate capsular support, surgeons recently have suggested the use of lenses with iris enclavation. These lenses provide a valid alternative for the correction of post-traumatic aphakia in children and seem to preserve the endothelial cell count[71,72] (see Chapter 19).

Even though the use of IOLs for pediatric cases is encouraged, each ophthalmologist must weigh the pros and cons of every option available on a case-by-case basis and discuss the alternatives with the parents or guardians when obtaining the informed consent.

Repair of the Iris and Restoration of the Pupil Opening

Unless damage to the iris is extensive and prevents access to the lens or interferes with surgical maneuvers, the surgeon can repair the iris following cataract removal and implantation of the IOL.

The artificial lens is considerably thinner than the intumescent cataract; consequently the AC will be deeper, facilitating the intraocular maneuvers.

Moreover, the long needles used to suture the iris may inadvertently tear the capsule, the cortex, or the vitreous if they are used early in the surgery. Delicate detachment of the iridocapsular adhesions can be performed early; however, if the zonules are damaged, these adhesions will provide greater support during capsulorrhexis and phacoemulsification.

Trauma can result in 5 types of iris lesions: perforations or holes, sphincter disruption, iridodialysis, traumatic mydriasis, and partial or total loss of the iris tissue.

Iris defects can be repaired by overlapping the tissue and using transchamber Prolene 10-0 sutures (Ethichon, Cornelia, GA). A paracentesis is created in a position and in a direction that will permit a long, curved suture needle to pass easily through the tissues in the direction of the defect. The needle is inserted slowly into the paracentesis with a slight lateral oscillation to avoid engaging the stromal corneal fibers. The tip of the needle is pushed through the iris near the proximal edge of the defect and successively pushed from below through the distal iris flap, then penetrating the peripheral cornea. A more elegant and less traumatic procedure is for the needle to enter the lumen of an insulin needle inserted into the AC through a paracentesis (Figure 15-6).

If the iris sphincter is lacerated, it is best to identify the 2 edges of the lesion and impale the suture in healthy iris tissue. The suture can be tied inside the AC with a slipknot created using the technique described by Siepser.[73] The correct orientation of the ends of the suture is essential

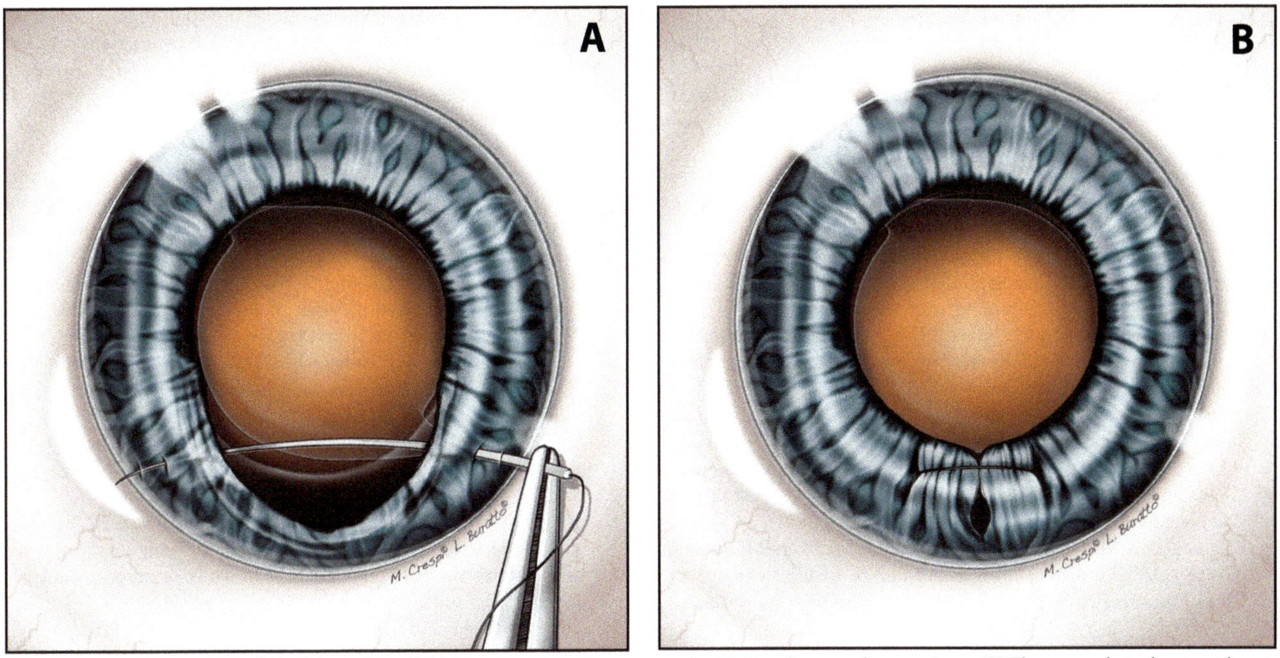

Figure 15-6. Correction of the iris defect. (A) The transchamber pass of a 10-0 polypropylene suture. (B) The completed suture knot.

because the suture is used to form a knot and is not just loosely tied.

The normal suture technique involves a double throw followed by a single one. This can be performed by the surgeon without an assistant. Once the suture has been passed through the tissue and the needle cut free, a hook or a push-pull forceps can be introduced into the AC to pull the 2 ends of the thread to the outside of the eye through the main corneal incision. The surgeon will tie a double throw outside; the 2 ends of the suture are grasped with suture forceps held in the nondominant hand, and with the assistance of an Osher hook (Asico, LLC, Westmont, IL) held in the dominant hand, the surgeon pushes the double knot in the AC to the desired position. He or she then proceeds with a single knot, which is tightened and positioned in the same way.

Iris dialysis can be repaired by impaling 2 needles with double 10-0 Prolene suture into the peripheral iris in the disinserted portion; these exit from the sclera close to the iris root.[74-76] The knot can be tied on the outside and then buried by rotation inside.

Post-traumatic mydriasis can lead to postoperative glare due to symptoms created by the pupillary edge. The surgeon is advised to create a restraining ring or cerclage to reduce the pupillary diameter.[77,78] Even though several techniques can be used to pass the suture through the iris tissue, every approach must have the objective of achieving a total or partial draw string contraction of the iris edge.

With significant loss of iris substance, the surgeon must consider the possibility of implanting a diaphragmed IOL (Morcher), a replacement diaphragm for the iris (Ophtec, Boca Raton, FL), intracapsular iris rings (Morcher), or occlusion segment rings (Morcher). The repair and the integration of the iris diaphragm is covered in greater detail in Chapter 16.

Membranous Cataract and Long-Standing Changes

Sometimes a patient will be referred to the ophthalmologist for the examination of a white or brunescent cataract many years after a penetrating wound. Sometimes a considerable amount of the lens matter will have already been reabsorbed, leaving minimal separation between the anterior and posterior capsules. The surgeon must be careful not to inadvertently enter the vitreous cavity. In some cases the capsule or residual lens is fibrotic or calcified and this may necessitate an incision with a blade or with scissors and removal of the hardened material with the vitrectomy probe. It is good for the surgeon to know that long-standing capsular lacerations do not tend to extend as rapidly as acute ruptures.

Conclusion

The traumatic cataract is extremely difficult to manage; every case is different. If the surgeon examines the eye carefully and chooses the appropriate surgical technique, he or she will be able to achieve excellent visual, functional, and esthetic results relative to the overall degree of trauma and damage to the eye.

References

1. Kuhn F, Morris R, Witherspoon CD, Mester V. The Birmingham Eye Trauma Terminology system (BETT). *J Fr Ophtalmol.* 2004;27:206-210.
2. Weinand F, Plag M, Pavlovic S. Primary implantation of posterior chamber lenses after traumatic cataract penetration. *Ophthalmology.* 2003;100:843-846.
3. Baykara M, Dogru M, Ozçetin H, Ertürk H. Primary repair and intraocular lens implantation after perforating eye injury. *J Cataract Refract Surg.* 2002;28:1832-1835.
4. Zabriskie NA, Hwang IP, Ramsey JF, Crandall AS. Anterior lens capsule rupture caused by air bag trauma. *Am J Ophthalmol.* 1997;123(6):832-833.
5. Saika S, Kin K, Ohmi S, Ohnishi Y. Posterior capsule rupture by blunt ocular trauma. *J Cataract Refract Surg.* 1997;23(1):139-140.
6. Angra SK, Vajpayee RB, Titiyal JS, Sharma YR, Sandramouli S, Kishore K. Types of posterior capsular breaks and their surgical implications. *Ophthalmic Surg.* 1991;22(7):388-391.
7. Almog Y, Reider-Groswasser I, Goldstein M, Lazar M, Segev Y, Geyer O. "The disappearing lens": failure of CT to image the lens in traumatic intumescent cataract. *J Comput Assist Tomogr.* 1999;23(3):354-356.
8. Rubsamen PE, Irvin WD, McCuen BW 2nd, Smiddy WE, Bowman CB. Primary intraocular lens implantation in the setting of penetrating ocular trauma. *Ophthalmology.* 1995;102(1):101-107.
9. Moisseiev J, Segev F, Harizman N, Arazi T, Rotenstreich Y, Assia EI. Primary cataract extraction and intraocular lens implantation in penetrating ocular trauma. *Ophthalmology.* 2001;108(6):1099-1103.
10. Agarwal A, Kumar DA, Nair V. Cataract surgery in the setting of trauma. *Curr Opin Ophthalmol.* 2010;21(1):65-70.
11. Pieramici DJ, Capone A Jr, Rubsamen PE, Roseman RL. Lens preservation after intraocular foreign body injuries. *Ophthalmology.* 1996;103(10):1563-1567.
12. O'Duffy D, Salmon JF. Siderosis bulbi resulting from an intralenticular foreign body. *Am J Ophthalmol.* 1999;127(2):218-219.
13. Speaker MG, Guerriero PN, Met JA, Coad CT, Berger A, Marmor M. A case-control study of risk factors for intraoperative suprachoroidal expulsive hemorrhage. Ophthalmology. 1991;98(2):202-209.
14. Arnold PN. Study of acute intraoperative suprachoroidal hemorrhage. *J Cataract Refract Surg.* 1992;18(5):489-494.
15. Beatty S, Lotery A, Kent D, et al. Acute intraoperative suprachoroidal haemorrhage in ocular surgery. *Eye (Lond).* 1998;2 (pt 5):815-820.
16. Ling R, Kamalarajah S, Cole M, James C, Shaw S. Suprachoroidal haemorrhage complicating cataract surgery in the UK: a case control study of risk factors. *Br J Ophthalmol.* 2004;88(4):474-477.
17. Moshfeghi DM, Kim BY, Kaiser PK, Sears JE, Smith SD. Appositional suprachoroidal hemorrhage: a case-control study. *Am J Ophthalmol.* 2004;138(6):959-963.
18. Osher RH, Cionni RJ. The torn posterior capsule: its intraoperative behavior, surgical management, and long-term consequences. *J Cataract Refract Surg.* 1990;16(4):490-494.
19. Fukagawa K, Tsubota K, Kimura C, et al. Corneal endothelial cell loss induced by air bags. *Ophthalmology.* 1993;100(12):1819-1823.
20. Arshinoff SA, Dispersive-cohesive viscoelastic soft shell technique. *J Cataract Refract Surg.* 1999;25(2):167-173.
21. Krag S, Thim K, Corydon L, Kyster B. Biomechanical aspects of the anterior capsulotomy. *J Cataract Refract Surg.* 1994;20(4):410-416.
22. David G, Humphrey JD. Finite element model of stresses in the anterior lens capsule of the eye. *Comput Methods Biomech Biomed Engin.* 2007;10(3):237-243.
23. Andreo LK, Wilson ME, Apple DJ. Elastic properties and scanning electron microscopic appearance of manual continuous curvilinear capsulorrhexis and vitrectorhexis in an animal model of pediatric cataract. *J Cataract Refract Surg.* 1999;25(4):534-539.
24. Comparison of anterior vitrectorhexis and continuous curvilinear capsulorrhexis in pediatric cataract and intraocular lens implantation surgery: a 10-year analysis. *J AAPOS.* 2007;11(5):443-446.
25. Ozturk F, Osher RH. Capsular staining: recent developments. *Curr Opin Ophthalmol.* 2006;17(1):42-44.
26. Gimbel HV, Willerscheidt AB. What to do with limited view: the intumescent cataract. *J Cataract Refract Surg.* 1993;19(5):657-661.
27. Melles GR, de Waard PW, Pameyer JH, Houdijn Beekhuis W. Trypan blue capsule staining to visualize the capsulorrhexis in cataract surgery. *J Cataract Refract Surg.* 1999;25(1):7-9.
28. de Waard PW, Budo CJ, Melles GR. Trypan blue capsular staining to "find" the leading edge of a "lost" capsulorrhexis. *Am J Ophthalmol.* 2002;134(2):271-272.
29. Dick HB, Aliyeva SE, Hengerer F. Effect of trypan blue on the elasticity of the human anterior lens capsule. *J Cataract Refract Surg.* 2008;34(8):1367-1373.
30. Wollensak G, Spörl E, Pham DT. Biomechanical changes in the anterior lens capsule after trypan blue staining. J *Cataract Refract Surg.* 2004;30(7):1526-1530.
31. Nanavaty MA, Johar K, Sivasankaran MA, Vasavada AR, Praveen MR, Zetterström C. Effect of trypan blue staining on the density and viability of lens epithelial cells in white cataract. *J Cataract Refract Surg.* 2006;32(9):1483-1488.
32. Portes AL, Almeida AC, Allodi S, Monteiro ML, Miguel NC. Trypan blue staining for capsulorrhexis: ultrastructural effect on lens epithelial cells and capsules. *J Cataract Refract Surg.* 2010;36(4):582-587.
33. Thaler S, Hofmann J, Bartz-Schmidt KU, Schuettauf F, Haritoglou C, Yoeruek E. Methyl blue and aniline blue versus patent blue and trypan blue as vital dyes in cataract surgery: Capsule staining properties and cytotoxicity to human cultured corneal endothelial cells. *J Cataract Refract Surg.* 2011;37(6):1147-1153.
34. Chang YS, Tseng SY, Tseng SH, Chen YT, Hsiao JH. Comparison of dyes for cataract surgery. Part 1: cytotoxicity to corneal endothelial cells in a rabbit model. *Cataract Refract Surg.* 2005;31(4):792-798.
35. Chang YS, Tseng SY, Tseng SH. Comparison of dyes for cataract surgery. Part 2: efficacy of capsule staining in a rabbit model. *J Cataract Refract Surg.* 2005;31(4):799-804.
36. Maloney WF. Supracapsular phaco: achieving greater efficacy with phaco outside of the capsular bag-a 3 years experience. Presented at: the American Society of Cataract and Refractive Surgery; April 1999; Seattle, WA.
37. Osher RH. Slow motion phacoemulsification approach. *J Cataract Refract Surg.* 1993;19(5):667.
38. Cionni RJ, Osher RH. Management of profound zonular dialysis or weakness with a new endocapsular ring designed for scleral fixation. *J Cataract Refract Surg.* 1998;24(10):1299-1306.
39. Campanella PC, Aminlari A, DeMaio R. Traumatic cataract and Wieger's ligament. *Ophthalmic Surg Lasers.* 1997;28(5):422-423.
40. Yasukawa T, Kita M, Honda Y. Traumatic cataract with a ruptured posterior capsule from a nonpenetrating ocular injury. *J Cataract Refract Surg.* 1998;24(6):868-869.
41. Thomas R. Posterior capsule rupture after blunt trauma. *J Cataract Refract Surg.* 1998;24(2):283-284.
42. Metz G. Lens induced glaucoma. Audiovisual *J Cataract Refrect Surg.* 1986;2(3).
43. Kelman C. Posterior capsular rupture. *Video J Cataract Refract Surg.* 1996;12(2).
44. Eller AW, Barad RF. Miyake analysis of anterior vitrectomy techniques. *J Cataract Refract Surg.* 1996;22(2):213-217.
45. Khawly JA, Lambert RJ, Jaffe GJ. Intraocular lens changes after short- and long-term exposure to intraocular silicone oil. An in vivo study. *Ophthalmology.* 1998;105(7):1227-1233.
46. Bartz-Schmidt KU, Kirchhof B, Heimann K. Condensation on IOLs during fluid-air exchange. *Ophthalmology.* 1996;103(2):199.

47. Kulkarni K, Zarbin M, Del Priore LV, Tezel TH. Ab externo technique for accurate haptic placement of transscleral sutured posterior chamber intraocular lenses. *Ophthalmic Surg Lasers Imaging.* 2007;38(1):72-75.
48. Sawada T, Kimura W, Kimura T, et al. Long-term follow-up of primary anterior chamber intraocular lens implantation. *J Cataract Refract Surg.* 1998;24(11):1515-1520.
49. Güell JL, Manero F. Artiflex (foldable iris claw IOL) secondary implantation for correction of aphakia after penetrating ocular injury. *J Refract Surg.* 2004;20(3):282-283.
50. Kwong YY, Yuen HK, Lam RF, Lee VY, Rao SK, Lam DS. Comparison of outcomes of primary scleral-fixated versus primary anterior chamber intraocular lens implantation in complicated cataract surgeries. *Ophthalmology.* 2007;114(1):80-85.
51. Güell JL, Barrera A, Manero F. A review of suturing techniques for posterior chamber lenses. *Curr Opin Ophthalmol.* 2004;15(1):44-50.
52. Michaeli A, Assia EI. Scleral and iris fixation of posterior chamber lenses in the absence of capsular support. *Curr Opin Ophthalmol.* 2005;16(1):57-60.
53. Donaldson KE, Gorscak JJ, Budenz DL, Feuer WJ, Benz MS, Forster RK. Anterior chamber and sutured posterior chamber intraocular lenses in eyes with poor capsular support. *J Cataract Refract Surg.* 2005;31(5):903-909.
54. Wagoner MD, Cox TA, Ariyasu RG, Jacobs DS, Karp CL; American Academy of Ophthalmology. Intraocular lens implantation in the absence of capsular support: a report by the American Academy of Ophthalmology. *Ophthalmology.* 2003;110(4):840-859.
55. Dick B, Schwenn O, Stoffelns B, Pfeiffer N. Late dislocation of a plate haptic silicone lens into the vitreous body after Nd:YAG capsulotomy. A case report. *Ophthalmology.* 1998; 95(3):181-185.
56. Petersen AM, Bluth LL, Campion M. Delayed posterior dislocation of silicone plate-haptic lenses after neodymium:yag capsulotomy. *J Cataract Refract Surg.* 2000;26(12):1827-1829.
57. Tuft SJ, Talks SJ. Delayed dislocation of foldable plate-haptic silicone lenses after Nd:YAG laser anterior capsulotomy. *Am J Ophthalmol.* 1998;126(4):586-588.
58. Johnson MW, Schneiderman TE. Surgical management of posteriorly dislocated silicone plate intraocular lenses. *Curr Opin Ophthalmol.* 1998;9(3):11-15.
59. Faucher A, Rootman DS. Dislocation of a plate-haptic silicone intraocular lens into the anterior chamber. *J Cataract Refract Surg.* 2001;27(1):169-171.
60. Agustin AL, Miller KM. Posterior dislocation of a plate-haptic silicone intraocular lens with large fixation holes. *J Cataract Refract Surg.* 2000;26(9):1428-1429.
61. Churchill AJ, Noble BA, Etchells DE, George NJ. Factors affecting visual outcome in children following uniocular traumatic cataract. *Eye (Lond).* 1995;9(pt 3):285-291.
62. BenEzra D, Cohen E, Rose L. Traumatic cataract in children: correction of aphakia by contact lens or intraocular lens. *Am J Ophthalmol.* 1997;123(6):773-782.
63. Ram J, Apple DJ, Peng Q, et al. Update on fixation of rigid and foldable posterior chamber intraocular lenses. Part II: choosing the correct haptic fixation and intraocular lens design to help eradicate posterior capsule opacification. *Ophthalmology.* 1999;106(5):891-900.
64. Holland GN, Van Horn SD, Margolis TP. Cataract surgery with ciliary sulcus fixation of intraocular lenses in patients with uveitis. *Am J Ophthalmol.* 1999;128(1):21-30.
65. Pandey SK, Ram J, Werner L, et al. Visual results and postoperative complications of capsular bag and ciliary sulcus fixation of posterior chamber intraocular lenses in children with traumatic cataracts. *J Cataract Refract Surg.* 1999;25(12):1576-1584.
66. Buckley EG. Hanging by a thread: the long-term efficacy and safety of transscleral sutured intraocular lenses in children (an American Ophthalmological Society thesis). *Trans Am Ophthalmol Soc.* 2007;105:294-311.
67. Vote BJ, Tranos P, Bunce C, Charteris DG, Da Cruz L. Long term outcome of combined pars plana vitrectomy and scleral fixated sutured posterior chamber intraocular lens implantation. *Am J Ophthalmol.* 2006;41:308-312.
68. Assia EI, Nemet A, Sachs D. Bilateral spontaneous subluxation of scleral fixated intraocular lenses. *J Cataract Refract Surg.* 2002;28:2214-2216.
69. Asadi R, Kheirkhah A. Long term results of scleral fixation of posterior chamber intraocular lenses in children. *Ophthalmology.* 2008;115:67-72.
70. Cionni RJ, Osher RH, Marques DM, et al. Modified capsular tension ring for patient with congenital loss of zonular support. *J Catract Refract Surg.* 2003;29:1668-1673.
71. Sminia ML, Odenthal MT, Wenniger-Prick LJ, Gortzak-Moorstein N, Völker-Dieben HJ. Traumatic pediatric cataract: a decade of follow-up after Artisan aphakia intraocular lens implantation. *J AAPOS.* 2007;11(6):555-558.
72. Odenthal MT, Sminia ML, Prick LJ, Gortzak-Moorstein N, Völker-Dieben HJ. Long-term follow-up of the corneal endothelium after artisan lens implantation for unilateral traumatic and unilateral congenital cataract in children: two case series. *Cornea.* 2006;25(10):1173-1177.
73. Siepser SB. The closed chamber slipping suture technique for iris repair. *Ann Ophthalmol.* 1994;26(3):71-72.
74. Wachler BB, Krueger RR. Double-armed McCannell suture for repair of traumatic iridodialysis. *Am J Ophthalmol.* 1996;122(1):109-110.
75. Erakgun T, Kaskaloglu M, Kayikcioglu O. A simple closed chamber technique for repair of traumatic iridodialysis in phakic eyes. *Ophthalmic Surg Lasers.* 2001;32(1):83-85.
76. Kaufman SC, Insler MS. Surgical repair of a traumatic iridodialysis. *Ophthalmic Surg Lasers.* 1996;27(11):963-966.
77. Osher RH. Consultation section. *J Cataract Refract Surg.* 1994;20:665-669.
78. Ogawa GS. The iris cerclage suture for permanent mydriasis: a running suture technique. *Ophthalmic Surg Lasers.* 1998;29: 1001-1009.

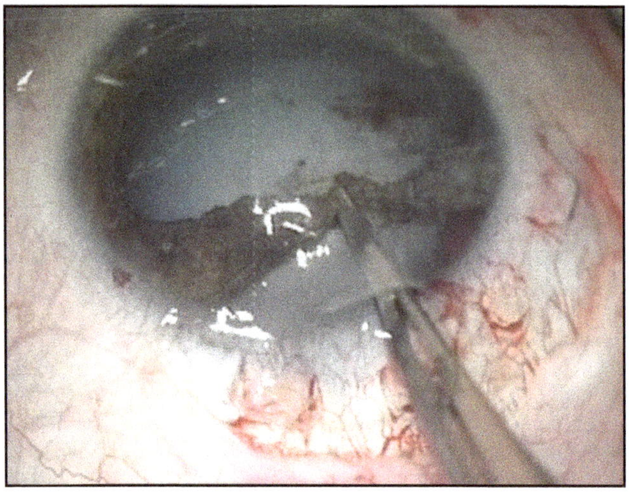

G-1. Traumatic cataract with iris disinsertion. (Reprinted with permission of Rudy Nuijts.)

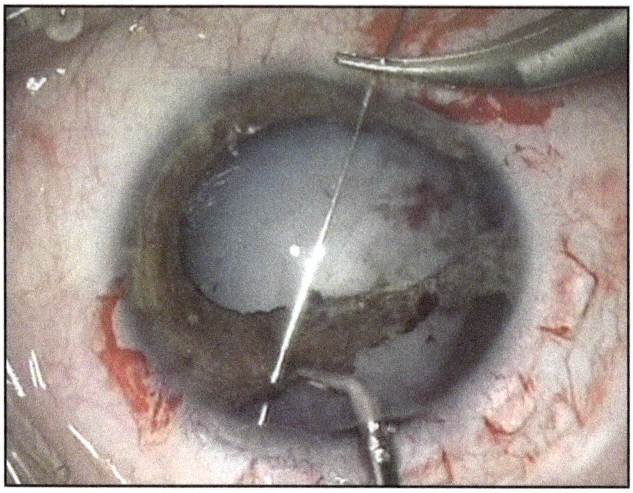

G-2. Iris suture. (Reprinted with permission of Rudy Nuijts.)

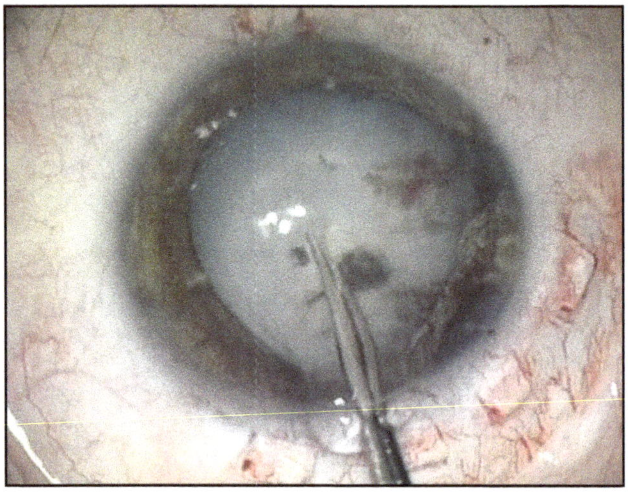

G-3. Anterior capsulotomy. (Reprinted with permission of Rudy Nuijts.)

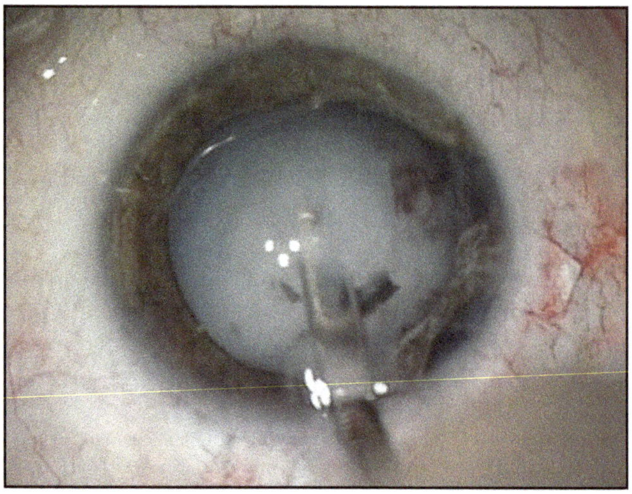

G-4. Phacoemulsification. (Reprinted with permission of Rudy Nuijts.)

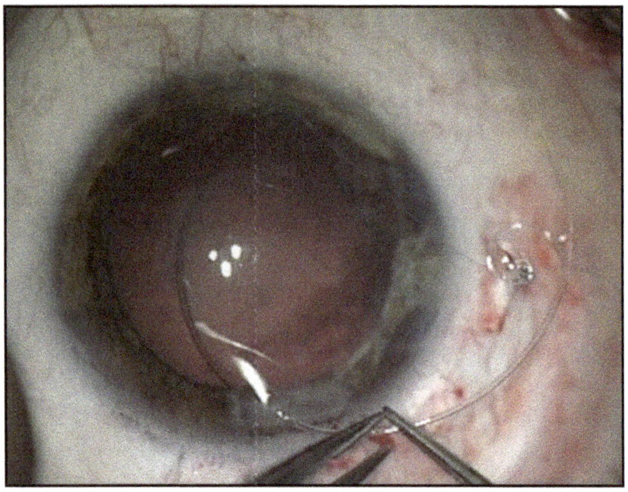

G-5. Insertion of a capsular ring and an IOL. (Reprinted with permission of Rudy Nuijts.)

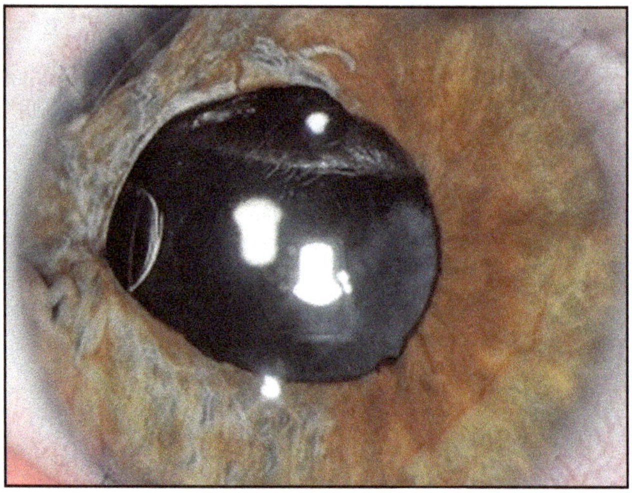

G-6. Results after 1 month. (Reprinted with permission of Rudy Nuijts.)

16

Cataract in Aniridic Eyes and Other Iris Defects

Iris defects are seen in different clinical conditions, such as congenital aniridia, coloboma, endothelial iridocorneal syndrome, Axenfeld-Rieger's syndrome, trauma (surgical and nonsurgical), uveitis, postoperative idiopathic mydriasis, and ocular albinism.

Aniridia is a rare congenital panocular disorder (predominantly profibrotic) that involves the cornea, the anterior chamber (AC), the iris, the crystalline lens, the retina, and the optic nerve. It is associated with a number of different syndromes, such as Wilms' tumor, bilateral sporadic aniridia, genital urinary abnormalities, and mental deficiencies. One of the frequently seen manifestations is cataract associated with capsular fragility. Glaucoma observed in these cases is associated with abnormalities of angle differentiation; however, it can also develop because of progressive angle-closure from synechiae.

Under all of the clinical conditions mentioned, implants that simulate the iris (artificial iris) can reduce glare, photophobia, and polyopia in the patient's eye and improve visual function.

Some of these devices can also eliminate optic aberrations present in the peripheral cornea and eliminate the visual competition between images that are in focus and images that are not.

Options Available to Repair Iris Defects

Given that each defect is individual to that particular patient, the surgical approach must be personalized to each eye. The primary repair of an iris defect with techniques such as iris sphincterectomy, synechiolysis, iris sutures, and restraining ring or cerclage may be adequate in some patients and should be evaluated before a prosthetic iris or other device is considered for implantation.

In reference to iris sutures,[1-6] the surgeon can use 1 or 2 iris sutures of 10-0 Prolene (a material that is practically inert) to correct the defect. The ideal needle should be very fine, short, and sharp because the iris is extremely mobile and tends to resist perforation. Once it has been perforated, it will move and follow the needle along its course and risks easy laceration. The most suitable needle in our opinion is the STC-6 Plus (Ethicon, Cornelia, GA); it has the rigidity and length necessary for the surgical maneuver, without inducing excessive lesions to the iris. This is introduced into the AC at the limbus, perforates the edges of the 2 iris flaps, and exits from the opposite limbus. The needle is then removed and the suture drawn and tied through a suitably positioned limbal incision. The needle is used in conjunction with an iris hook that will keep the iris stretched through counterpressure around the tip of the needle, facilitating penetration. Sometimes it may be necessary to curve the pass of the needle slightly in relation to the different shape of the anterior segment; alternately, the surgeon may use a curved needle and 10-0 Prolene (CIF-4 [Ethicon]). All of these maneuvers are performed inside the AC filled with high molecular weight viscoelastic substance (VES) that will isolate and stabilize the iris, maintain spaces, and minimize hemorrhage.

If the surgeon needs to suture the iris coloboma through a minimal opening in the cornea (eg, phaco in coaxial microincision cataract surgery [C-MICS]) or the sclera, a mixed technique can be used. A transcorneal maneuver is added to the intracameral step; the needle is passed to the outside as in the McCannel suture (Figure 16-1). In the modified McCannel suture method,

Buratto L, Brint SF, Caretti L.
Cataract Surgery in Complicated Cases (pp 169-175).

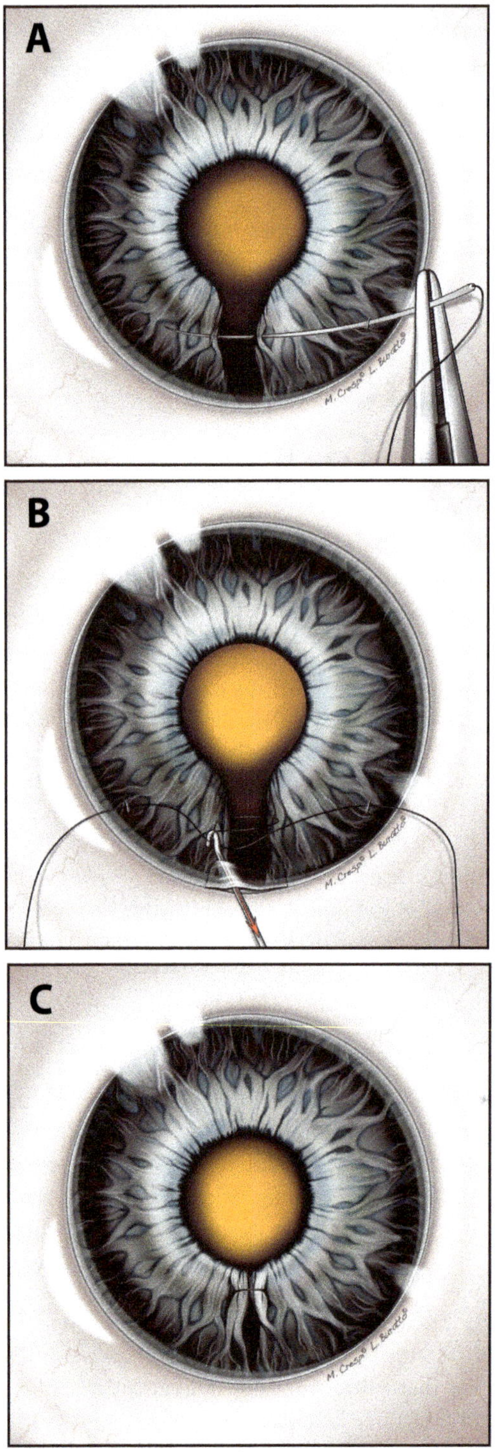

Figure 16-1. Suture of an iris coloboma using the McCannel transcorneal technique. (A) The needle passes through the cornea, the edges of the iris coloboma and again through the cornea. (B) Retrieval of one end of the suture thread. (C) Tying the knot.

proposed by Blackmon and Lambert,[4] a long, straight needle is used, with a slipknot tied on one side, using the Siepser technique.[7]

Unfortunately, it is not always possible to perform these techniques, and they may not be adequate for eyes with large iris defects. Iris defects up to 3 hours (or 90 degrees) can usually be well corrected with suture techniques. With larger defects, the surgeon should avoid excessively aggressive techniques, as the iris tissue in these cases is abnormal. There is considerable risk of iatrogenic iridodialysis, hemorrhage, and localized iris atrophy in the area adjacent to the tension pull of the suture. The speed and intensity of iris atrophy is proportionate to how tight the knot is pulled and how much traction is exerted by the suture on the tissue to bring the wound edges together. Once the suture has been positioned, the surgeon can create relaxing incisions along the lines of greater tension.

An alternative suture technique is iris cerclage, developed to correct permanent mydriasis (a condition that will respond to mydriatic agents but not to miotics) caused by widespread damage to the iris sphincter, a problem that may appear following cataract surgery.[8] In this technique, the surgeon creates a continuous suture around the iris; a long, curved needle (PC-7 [Alcon, Fort Worth, TX]) passes 10-0 polypropylene (Prolene) suture into and out of the AC through a limbal paracentesis, impaling the iris close to the pupillary margin to form a restraining ring or cerclage. With the AC filled with high molecular weight VES, the needle is inserted in the opening at 9 o'clock; a vitreoretinal crocodile clip is inserted at 1 o'clock to grasp the iris at 10 o'clock and pull it toward the center, allowing the needle to pass close to the pupil edge. This maneuver is repeated 3 to 4 times along the tempero-inferior sectors of the iris. The forceps are then removed. The tip of the needle is inserted in the channel of an irrigation cannula that penetrates the AC through a limbal incision at 5 o'clock. The iris suture maneuvers are repeated to create a long, continuous suture along the entire pupil edge. The ends of the suture are retrieved from the incision at 9 o'clock and tied allowing the size of the pupil to be adjusted by tightening the suture appropriately. The knot will lie in the AC. The technique minimizes stretching and the distortion of the iris and creates a fairly round iris of precise dimensions.

With extremely large iris defects (more than one quadrant of iris tissue missing or aniridia), colored contact lenses or corneal tattoos can be applied. Artificial iris implants are also available.[9-12]

Currently, a number of artificial iris implants are available and can be inserted at any stage during cataract surgery. They were introduced in 1994 and have functional benefits, such as an improvement in visual acuity and a reduction in visual discomfort. They also have cosmetic/esthetic advantages as they also restore the physiological appearance of the eye.[9,13-15] These devices can be implanted in the capsular bag in the ciliary sulcus or can be fixed to the sclera in the event of inadequate capsular support.

The coloboma ring with diaphragm (type 96C [Morcher GmbH, Stuttgart, Germany and Ophtec, Boca Raton, FL])

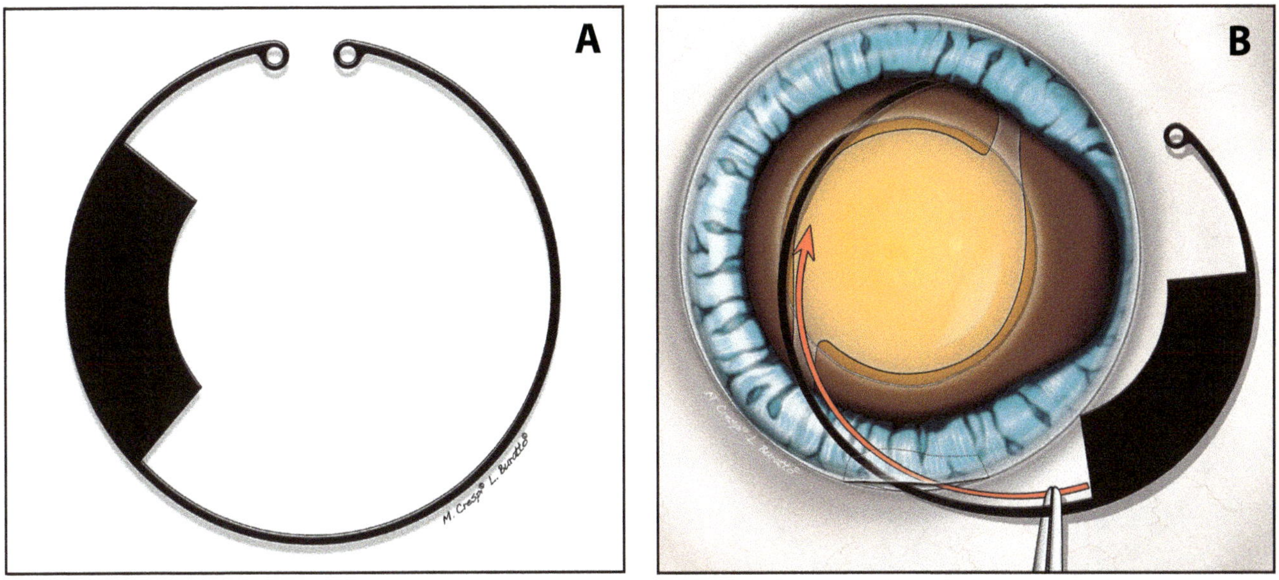

Figure 16-2. (A) CTR with coloboma diaphragm, model 96C (Morcher GmbH). (B) Intraocular insertion of the device.

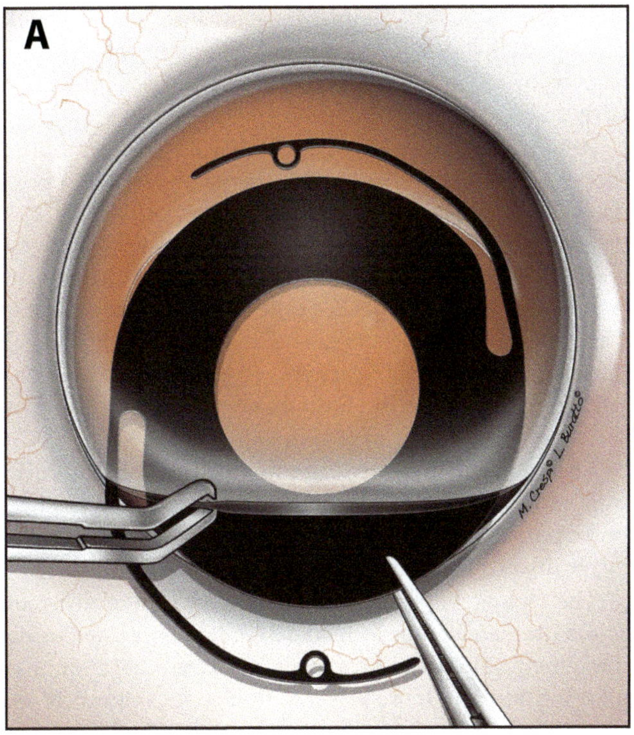

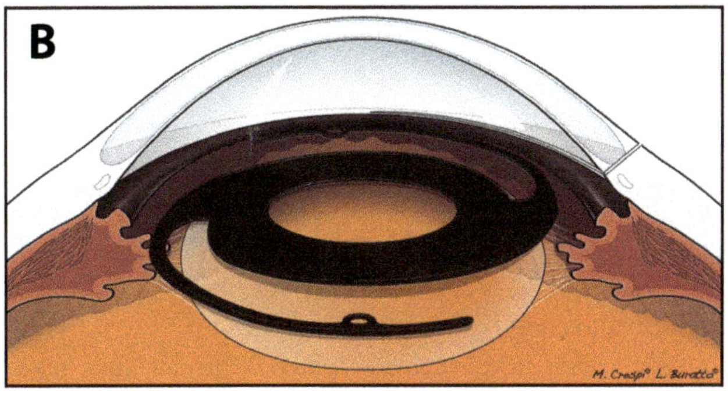

Figure 16-3. (A and B) Insertion of the diaphragm IOL.

is a device that Legler and Wischel[16] created by modifying the capsular tension ring ([CTR] described in Chapter 2). This device is made of polymethylmethacrylate (PMMA); it includes a single opaque segment of 2.5 mm and 90-degree extension, and its overall diameter is 11/13 mm (Figure 16-2). This device is used when there is a large peripheral iridectomy, an iris coloboma, or a localized post-traumatic iris defect; it will reduce discomfort from glare in patients with intense photophobia. Two or more rings can be used when the iris defects are larger. As this acts similar to a CTR, it will also correct any associated partial capsular bag instability.

In cases of complete aniridia (congenital or traumatic), a diaphragm intraocular lens (IOL) can be used. This device was presented in a publication by Sundmacher et al[15]; it is PMMA and consists of a transparent optic surrounded by a dark opaque circle that acts as the artificial iris diaphragm (types 67F and 67G [Morcher GmbH]). It is implanted in the sulcus and requires a very large incision as the device has an overall diameter of approximately 10 mm with optics in a range of dimensions (Figure 16-3). In the event of inadequate capsular support (eg, following trauma), it can be fixed by scleral suspension. This device provides good visual rehabilitation (reduction of glare, ghosting and other undesired images, and occasionally, the postoperative disappearance of nystagmus); however, postoperatively, it can cause serious inflammation, rise in intraocular pressure, high astigmatism (linked to the large corneal incision), hyperemia (bloodshot eyes), macular edema, corneal decompensation, and progression of any associated congenital epithelial disorders.[15,17-22] In a recent report[22] published in the literature, the long-term follow-up

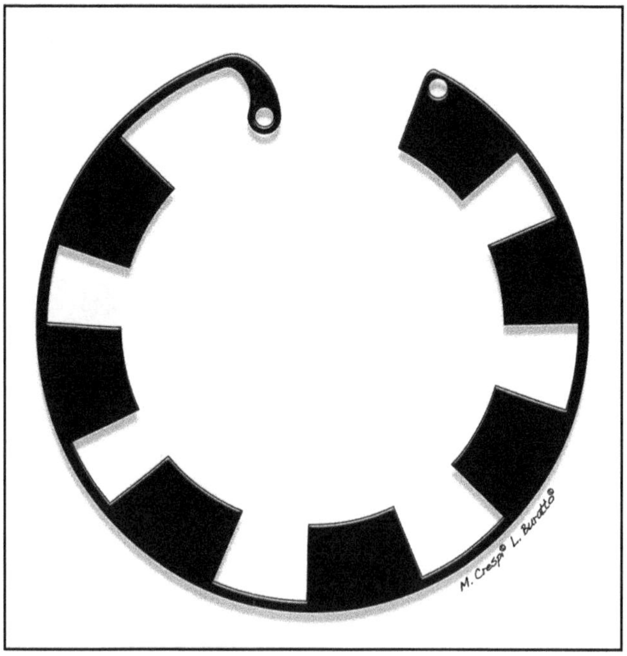

Figure 16-4. CTR with coloboma diaphragm, model 50C (Morcher GmbH).

of these diaphragm IOLs was analyzed following their use in the treatment of post-traumatic aniridia. The authors concluded that this device is safe and effective in the majority of cases. The 2 major complications observed long-term are glaucoma and corneal decompensation.[22]

Other companies, such as Ophtec B, produce one-piece diaphragm IOLs in a range of colors so that the final outcome will be as close as possible to the patient's natural iris, with significant esthetic advantages. The versions in blue, pale green, and brown are PMMA; the black diaphragm IOL is polycarbonate. The Ophtec model 311 requires a 9-mm corneal incision, and its feet are more resistant to manipulation compared to the lenses produced by Morcher. Other differences between the 2 brands are the pupillary opening (Ophtec 4 mm; Morcher 5 mm) and the arrangement of the edges of the optic (Ophtec model 311 has a rounded edge; the models from the Morcher Series 67 have a squared optic fused to the black segment).

Morcher recently produced model 30B, which has a diaphragm of clear PMMA and a colored opaque layer applied to the anterior surface, giving the IOL a multicolored dotted appearance.

An alternative to the diaphragm IOL is the CTR with an iris diaphragm (type 50C [Morcher]) that can be assembled with up to 7 black PMMA multiple fin segments (Figure 16-4). If 2 of these PMMA rings are implanted in the bag, one after the other, they can be rotated above each other and the fins will interlink to form a complete diaphragm (Figure 16-5). The surgeon must pay maximum attention when implanting these very delicate devices, as they are extremely susceptible to breakage. The use of multiple implants is not problematic even though the aspiration maneuver must be much slower and more delicate to avoid displacing them. The 50C rings can be implanted through a 3-mm corneal incision; these create an iris diaphragm with a pupil width of approximately 6 mm. They will reduce entrance diameter of light into the eye by 75% and will allow excellent postoperative observation of the fundus. If the surgeon wishes to achieve a smaller pupil diameter, he or she can use the new models 50D, 50E, and 50F—these will create pupils of 6.0, 3.5, and 4 mm, respectively. They can be implanted through 3-mm superior corneal incisions. The model 50F has been designed with less space between the fins, and this facilitates alignment of the 2 pieces. If a 50C ring is used, the optic size of the foldable IOL chosen should have a diameter of 6.5 mm to eliminate glare induced at the edge of the IOL. IOLs with a standard 6-mm optic are acceptable for the models 50D, 50E, and 50F. Ideally, the optic of the IOL in these cases should be positioned behind the rings. It is recommended to add 0.5 to 1 diopters (D) to the dioptric power of the IOL implanted to achieve emmetropia because of the optic's more posterior position due to its volume in the capsular bag. Following implantation, the artificial iris rings will be fairly stable.

Another endocapsular device that is similar to the Morcher 50 series is the Iris Prosthetic System (IPS) produced by Ophtec BV.[23] These modular multipiece IPS devices include bilobed elements; when assembled, these create an intact diaphragm and a CTR. They also have a system of closure that increases the stability of the implant. These devices can be implanted through 5-mm corneal incisions and maximum care and attention should be paid during the delicate procedures of assembly and locking of the components in the bag.

The Morcher implant is produced exclusively of fairly fragile black PMMA. Consequently, it should be implanted very carefully during implantation, to avoid excessive folding or distortion that may fracture the device.

The Ophtec implant is available in a range of different colors (the same range as model 311). It is implanted using the same technique as previously described; however, it is more flexible and more resistant to damage (Figure 16-6). The color will be chosen to match residual iris tissue. In order to protect the color and maintain the diameter of the rhexis, the surgeon should pay attention when aspirating the epithelial cells on the internal surface of the anterior capsule, to avoid fibrosis of the anterior capsule and consequent postoperative dislocation of the sectors secondary to contraction of the rhexis.

The clean empty capsular bag will therefore be ready to receive the sector(s) introduced using the same technique illustrated for the simple CTRs (see Chapter 2). Each sector will be positioned exactly in front of the zone it will cover. With total aniridia, the sectors should be arranged in the bag to create an artificial iris and pupil.

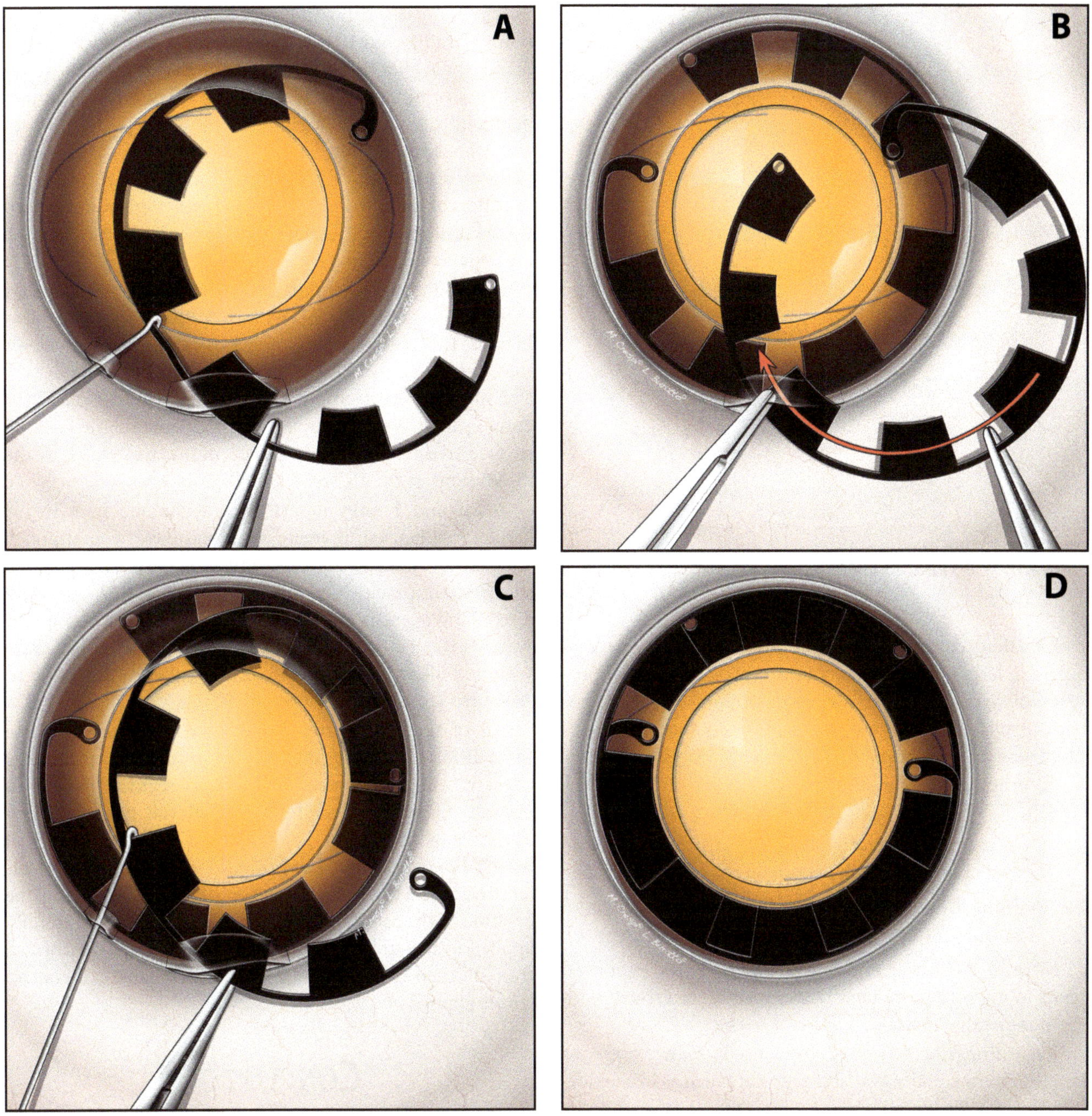

Figure 16-5. Implantation of 2 CTRs with coloboma diaphragm, model 50C (Morcher GmbH).

To prevent superimposition of the sectors, the ends of the rings are joined together with clips to create a complete and stable restraining ring/cerclage; the haptics of the lens will be positioned behind the iris sectors.

Currently, IPS can be implanted in eyes with extensive iris defects (aniridia, extensive deformations, or functional imperfections) that cannot be corrected with a simple repair technique.[23-28] They will reduce photophobia following cataract removal.

Some years ago, secondary implant with IPS was successfully presented for already pseudophakic patients affected by total post-traumatic aniridia.[28] In these patients, the traumatic event caused the total expulsion of the iris without affecting the IOL; because of intolerable glare, the patient's fibrotic capsular bag was reopened, and the artificial iris was implanted leaving the IOL in situ.

The IPS improves visual acuity and reduces glare and also allows the surgeon to create a pupil of predictable and repeatable diameter, with a relatively low incidence of complications (iritis, glaucoma, macular edema) that are easily managed.[14]

The ancient procedure of corneal tattoos was introduced by Claudius Galenus in AD 129 to hide the white

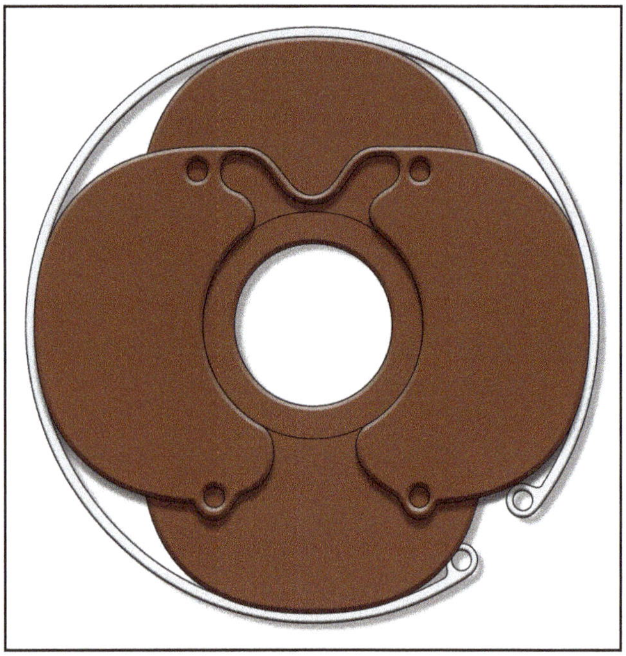

Figure 16-6. IPS with a PMMA ring.

leukomatous cornea.[29] These tattoos are currently used in aniridia, large iridectomies, and eccentric pupils and provide considerable visual comfort, particularly in patients with corneal leukomas and intolerant of contact lenses, and more generally for cosmetic reasons in inoperable eyes.

A corneal tattoo can be performed in one of 2 ways[30]:

1. Chemically: This involves a chemical reaction of precipitated pigments, typically metal salts (such as platinum or gold chloride), which deposit on the corneal surface
2. Staining: The dye is introduced directly (impregnation of carbon) into the depth of the cornea

Method 1 is easier and faster, but the tattoo produced tends to dissolve more rapidly than the tattoo created with the nonmetallic method.

Regarding the stains or dyes used, many surgeons employ commercially available pigments such as iron oxide, iron hydroxide, carbon black, titanium dioxide, and the Blue 15 pigment, even though the long-term safety and toxicity of these agents has not yet been demonstrated. Many authors recommend them for use in eyes that are severely visually impaired and for which less-invasive surgery is not an option.[30,31]

There are a number of dyes used for the impregnation of carbon. Indian ink is the most popular; however, Chinese ink, gold dust, organic pigments, uveal pigment, among others, are also available.

The most recent techniques of corneal tattoo involve the application of the dye directly into the corneal stroma. One of the techniques available was developed by Pfeiffer, in which the distal portion of a 3-sided spatulated needle (with a traditional 10-0 nylon suture) coated with a commercially available ink is used to create multiple sequential punctures in the corneal stroma.[31] There are a number of possible problems: a risk of full-depth perforation of the cornea, activation of the inflammation cascade and phagocytosis of the dye resulting in a reduction in the duration of the results, recurrent corneal erosions (caused by the multiple incisions across the Bowman membrane), and uneven pigmentation.

Another group of authors reported the use of a lamellar dissector (such as with INTACS [Addition Technology, Des Plaines, IL) for the creation of lamellar intrastromal canals that are then injected with commercially available dyes.[32] The limits of this technique include the fact that it is difficult to produce a uniform layer of pigment and the reduced surface area available to the effects of the dye created by the dimensions of the INTACS lamellar dissectors.

Islam and Franks described a technique in which a keratotome is used to create a corneal intrastromal pouch anterior to a peripheral iridectomy.[33] Filter paper soaked in sterile platinum chloride is then inserted in the pouch and a reducing agent is slowly added beneath the filter. In the patients treated, the authors achieved a reduction in glare with no bulbar inflammation or corneal erosions observed 2 months from surgery.

All of the previously mentioned techniques have the same limitations: it is difficult to accurately outline the edges of the tattoo resulting in an irregular border, an uneven distribution of the dye, and the nonpermanent duration of the tattoo. A number of authors have tried recently to overcome these limitations by creating a lamellar free cap with the femtosecond laser.[34] Following the creation of the cap, a commercially available dye is carefully applied to the stromal side of the lamellar cap; the corneal free cap then is repositioned on the stroma, and a contact lens is applied.

Conclusion

Surgeons nowadays have a number of different solutions available for treating patients affected by iris defects that create visual disturbances. These techniques include primary repair, corneal tattoos, and artificial iris implants.

The artificial iris implants can be positioned in the capsular bag; however, they necessitate a large capsulorrhexis and the hands of an extremely experienced surgeon due to the intraoperative difficulties that may occur. These devices or systems improve visual acuity and reduce visual discomfort for the patient. They are relatively safe though significant complications may develop, the most important being glaucoma.

References

1. Watt RH. Inferior congenital iris coloboma repair and IOL implantation. *J Cataract Refract Surg.* 1993;19:669-671.
2. McCannel MA. A retrievable suture idea for anterior uveal problems. *Ophthalmic Surg.* 1976;7:98-103.
3. Worst JGF, Los JRLI. Iris reconstruction by coloboma repair. *Ophthalmic Surg.* 1989;20:790-793.
4. Blackmon DM, Lambert SR. Congenital iris coloboma repair using a modified McCannel suture technique. *Am J Ophthalmol.* 2003;135:730-732.
5. Cionni RJ, Karatza EC, Osher RH, Shah M. Surgical technique for congenital iris coloboma repair. *J Cataract Refract Surg.* 2006;32(11):1913-1916.
6. Ogawa GS, O'Gawa GM. Single wound, in situ tying technique for iris repair. *Ophthalmic Surg Lasers.* 1998;29(11):943-948.
7. Chang DF. Siepser slipknot for McCannel iris-suture fixation of subluxated intraocular lenses. *J Cataract Refract Surg.* 2004;30:1170-1176.
8. Ogawa GS. The iris cerclage suture for permanent mydriasis: a running suture technique. *Ophthalmic Surg Lasers.* 1998;29(12):1001-1009.
9. Lee H, Khan R, O'Keefe M. Aniridia: current pathology and management. *Acta Ophthalmol.* 2008;86(7):708-715.
10. Alger LG. The cause and treatment of poor vision in aniridia. *Am J Ophthalmol.* 1945;28:730-735.
11. Choyce P. *Intraocular Lenses and Implants.* London, England: 1966; HK Lewis.
12. Burris TE, Holmes-Higgin DK, Silvestrini TA. Lamellar intrastromal corneal tattoo for treating iris defects (artificial iris). *Cornea.* 1998;17(2):169-173.
13. Menezo JL, Martínez-Costa R, Cisneros A, Desco MC. Implantation of iris devices in congenital and traumatic aniridias: surgery solutions and complications. *Eur J Ophthalmol.* 2005;15(4):451-457.
14. Neuhann IM, Neuhann TF. Cataract surgery and aniridia. *Curr Opin Ophthalmol.* 2010;21(1):60-64.
15. Sundmacher R, Reinhard T, Althaus C. Black-diaphragm intraocular lens for correction of aniridia. *Ophthalmic Surg.* 1994;25(3):180-185.
16. Legler U, Wischel B. The capsular tension ring, a new device for complicated cataract surgery. Presented at the American Society of Cataract and Refractive Surgery;May 1993; Seattle, WA.
17. Reinhard T, Engelhardt S, Sundmacher R. Black diaphragm aniridia intraocular lens for congenital aniridia: long-term follow-up. *J Cataract Refract Surg.* 2000;26(3):375-381.
18. Osher RH, Burk SE. Cataract surgery combined with implantation of an artificial iris. *J Cataract Refract Surg.* 1999;25(11):1540-1547.
19. Beltrame G, Salvetat ML, Chizzolini M, et al. Implantation of a black diaphragm intraocular lens in ten cases of post-traumatic aniridia. *Eur J Ophthalmol.* 2003;13(1):62-68.
20. Dong X, Yu B, Xie L. Black diaphragm intraocular lens implantation in aphakic eyes with traumatic aniridia and previous pars plana vitrectomy. *J Cataract Refract Surg.* 2003;29(11):2168-2173.
21. Aslam SA, Wong SC, Ficker LA, MacLaren RE. Implantation of the black diaphragm intraocular lens in congenital and traumatic aniridia. *Ophthalmology.* 2008;115(10):1705-1712.
22. Dong X, Xu H, Yu B, Ying L, Xie L. Long-term outcome of black diaphragm intraocular lens implantation in traumatic aniridia. *Br J Ophthalmol.* 2010;94(4):456-459.
23. Rosenthal KJ, Osher RH. Video journal of viscosurgery. *Pharmacia.* 2002-2003;10.
24. Burk SE, Da Mata AP, Snyder ME, et al. Prosthetic iris implantation for congenital, traumatic, or junctional iris deficiencies. *J Cataract Refract Surg.* 2001;27:1732-1740.
25. Hermeking H. Iris Prosthetic System (IPS). Germany. VHS Pal-'10, English-1998, Ref. 8v1h021-OPHTEC.
26. Karatza EC, Burk SE, Snyder ME, Osher RH. Outcomes of prosthetic iris implantation in patients with albinism. *J Cataract Refract Surg.* 2007;33(10):1763-1769.
27. Mavrikakis I, Mavrikakis E, Syam PP, et al. Surgical management of iris defects with prosthetic iris devices. *Eye.* 2005;19(2):205-209.
28. Ozturk F, Osher RH, Osher JM. Secondary prosthetic iris implantation following traumatic total aniridia and pseudophakia. *J Cataract Refract Surg.* 2006;32(11):1968-1970.
29. Ziegler SL. Multicolor tattooing of the cornea. *Trans Am Ophthalmol Soc.* 1922;20:71-87.
30. Panda A, Pangtey MS, Sony P. Corneal tattooing. *Br J Ophthalmol.* 2002;86(12):1461.
31. Pitz S, Jahn R, Frisch L, Duis A, Pfeiffer N. Corneal tattooing: an alternative treatment for disfiguring corneal scars. *Br J Ophthalmol.* 2002;86:397-399.
32. Burris TE, Holmes-Higgin DK, Silvestrini TA. Lamellar intrastromal corneal tattoo for treating iris defects (artificial iris). *Cornea.* 1998;17(2):169-173.
33. Islam N, Franks WA. Therapeutic corneal tattoo following peripheral iridotomy complication. *Eye.* 2006;20:389-390.
34. Kim JH, Lee D, Hahn TW, Choi SK. New surgical strategy for corneal tattooing using a femtosecond laser. *Cornea.* 2009;28(1):80-84.

17

Cataract and Corneal Pathology

In situations in which the eye has corneal pathology perhaps requiring keratoplasty, the surgeon should always examine the lens. It is also essential to examine the cornea, in case a cataract operation becomes necessary. It should be remembered that cataract formation is more common in patients with Fuchs' dystrophy and signs of inflammation or trauma. The formation of cataracts is less frequent in younger patients undergoing keratoplasty and those with keratoconus. Thus, when the surgeon examines patients with significant corneal disease, associated with a potentially significant cataract, he or she must determine the relative contribution of each of the conditions[1] and decide whether to just remove the cataract, to remove it during or following keratoplasty, or to perform only the keratoplasty procedure.

Preoperative Evaluation

Preoperative examination of patients having corneal pathology and cataracts must be precise in selecting ideal candidates for surgery.[1-8]

In terms of the cataract, a totally or slightly abnormal cornea may prevent good visualization of the cataract. Mild to moderate epithelial and stromal edema can be temporarily improved during the diagnostic testing with repeated instillation of 10% glycerine. Its application must follow instillation of a topical anesthesia to reduce patient discomfort.

Some of the traditional methods used to determine the significance of a cataract are of little benefit and may be totally useless. For example, direct ophthalmoscopy or determination of the transparency of the lens based on red reflex cannot isolate the lens from the corneal effect on vision.

The condition of the lens in the fellow eye, if visible, can provide useful information as long as the patient does not have pathologies that can accelerate the development of a unilateral cataract (eg, inflammation or trauma).

The pupil must be dilated to visualize the entire lens.

The corneal opacity can be determined based on how cloudy the iris and lens are. Surface irregularities also often interfere with evaluation of concomitant opacities. Biomicroscopy frequently does not reveal surface distortions that are optically significant.

Corneal topography using a Placido disc, with photokeratoscopy or, better yet, computerized tomography, will reveal irregularities; however, this does not determine the relative contribution to visual limitation. Contact lens over-refraction is the best way to quantify surface irregularity and determine its contribution to the overall decrease in vision.

Evaluation of the endothelial cell reserve in patients with guttata is traditionally not precise.

In the patient's clinical history, the surgeon should pay attention to symptoms such as glare, fluctuating drop in contrast sensitivity, and particularly blurred vision in the morning. Edema developing at night, when the eyes are closed, is frequently a first sign of decompensation. Under slit-lamp examination, observation of endothelial striae or microcystic edema indicates incipient decompensation.

Minimal microcystic edema may be very difficult to visualize in the presence of dense guttata; fluorescein may prove useful in this examination.

Two tests can also be used: specular microscopy or confocal microscopy. Specular microscopy is used for functional evaluation of the endothelium, but can produce mixed results, particularly because the corneal endothelial decompensation is in proximity to a variety of cell densities and also because endothelial pump function depends not only on the cell count but also on the integrity of intercellular links, and neither of these is evaluated by specular microscopy. Second, with guttata, the interpretation of specular microscopy is clouded by the dark guttata shadowing of endothelial cells, preventing visualization of the endothelium.

Buratto L, Brint SF, Caretti L.
Cataract Surgery in Complicated Cases (pp 177-201).

It is also not clear whether endothelial cell density, measured in the most transparent peripheral area of the cornea, provides an adequate evaluation of the central cornea.

Optical or ultrasound pachymetry provides only objective measurements that may indicate decreased function of the cell pump. Normal corneal thickness has a Gaussian distribution; it occasionally exceeds 600 microns, and in the majority of patients, this indicates adequate endothelial function. Asymmetry exceeding 20 microns between corresponding areas of both corneas suggests edema in the thicker cornea, even when the thicknesses of both corneas are within normal limits.

Preoperative examination of a patient scheduled for combined cataract and corneal transplant includes measurement of the intraocular pressure (IOP) and fundus examination.

Uncontrolled IOP in patients scheduled for keratoplasty can greatly complicate the postoperative course. Consequently, it is essential to obtain good control of IOP prior to proceeding with keratoplasty[9,10]; topical or systemic hypotensive drugs, surgery, or antiglaucoma perisurgical procedures are indicated.

The surgeon should also determine macular function, so that a potential functional recovery outcome can be determined; this is assisted by tests, such as the potential acuity meter or laser interferometry.

Given that the majority of combined procedures are performed on elderly patients, they should be questioned about their general state of health, including blood pressure and any coagulation abnormalities. These patients are particularly at risk of developing choroidal hemorrhage.

Therapeutic Planning

For therapeutic planning, the ophthalmologist may have patients with varying densities of cataracts and corneal pathology, such as guttata, keratoconus, or corneal scars. The surgeon formulates a therapeutic plan: just cataract surgery, keratoplasty (with successive cataract surgery if required), or the combined operation of cataract, IOL implantation, and keratoplasty (triple procedure). Keratoplasty, alone or combined with cataract surgery, may be full thickness or penetrating (PKP), anterior lamellar (ALK), or posterior lamellar (PLK).

Cataract surgery alone is indicated in patients with the following:

- Guttata, if slit-lamp examination does not reveal stromal edema and/or pachymetry of 600 microns or less
- Early keratoconus with very slow evolution
- Minimal corneal opacities

Combined surgery is indicated in patients with the following:

- Guttata with stromal edema and/or pachymetry greater than 650 microns (a value clearly suggesting endothelial decompensation)
- Keratoconus at a stage that is equal to or greater than Amsler's third stage
- Corneal opacity causing severe visual deficiency

Keratoplasty is also indicated when the lens opacity is mild.

One of the most frequent and controversial questions is when the patient has marked guttata, with no microcystic epithelial edema, how does the surgeon decide when to just operate the cataract or perform a combined procedure of cataract, IOL implantation, and keratoplasty (triple procedure)?

Many patients with significant guttata of the central cornea can have cataract surgery alone, without corneal decompensation. Removal of the cataract alone (without keratoplasty) is determined by the visual significance of the lens opacity, often difficult to quantify in the presence of corneal opacity. The significance of the cataract can generally be obtained with a careful evaluation of the eye prior to keratoplasty. Generally, the surgeon should remove any cataract reducing visual acuity to 20/40 or less. Nevertheless, each case should be individually considered, as regards the visual requirements of the patient, the patient's general state of health, and that of the eye.

Even though dense guttata can sometimes cause a slight drop in vision, the surgeon can perform cataract surgery only with full corneal precautions, when there are no visible signs or symptoms of corneal decomposition. Recovery from cataract surgery is rapid, and the patient may be able to avoid the life-long problems associated with corneal transplants.

If stromal edema is not present and/or pachymetry is 600 microns or less, cataract surgery alone is generally indicated, as typically this will not induce postsurgical corneal decompensation.

The surgeon must take basic precautions. It is known that endothelial damage during cataract surgery is associated with both mechanical and nonmechanical events. Mechanical events include corneal folds, contact between instruments and endothelium, turbulence associated with intraocular fluid flow, and cavitation and bubbles. Nonmechanical events include osmosis, chemicals, toxins, and pressure.

The surgeon should use a viscoelastic substance (VES) providing maximum endothelial protection such as Viscoat (sodium chondroitin hyaluronate) or Healon Endocoat (Abbott Laboratories, Abbott Park, IL).[11,12]

The surgeon should perform cautious and gentle surgery to prevent endothelial damage, including avoiding collapse of the anterior chamber ([AC] pay attention to the height of the infusion bottle and surge). This is facilitated by microincisional phacoemulsification systems (MICS), which reduce turbulence induced by fluid flow and bubbles produced, optimizing balance between ultrasound power and fluid flow. In addition to reducing ultrasound power, the surgeon should use ultrasound only when the phaco tip is occluded.

To prevent endothelial damage, it is important that all surgical preparations and solutions have an appropriate formulation: irrigation solutions (balanced salt solution [BSS], BSS Plus, lactated Ringer's[13]), intraoperative drugs used (lidocaine, epinepherine antibiotics, and miotics), intraoperative dyes (trypan blue), and substances that may be toxic (preservatives, disinfectants, and impurities).

In the majority of cases, modern coaxial MICS and bimanual MICS allow the surgeon to operate confidently and safely with regard to the corneal endothelium in eyes with low endothelial cell counts and with Fuchs' dystrophy.[11-19]

A recent review of the literature[20] has shown that viscoadaptive VES are better than dispersive in protecting the endothelium during cataract surgery. In turn, dispersive VES provides better protection than cohesive VES. Moreover, Arshinoff's soft-shell technique provides better protection than the use of a cohesive VES alone. Comparing all available options for endothelial protection, the difference in the amount of damage seen in this study was less than 100 cells/mm^2 (4% to 5%).

The results from studies comparing changes to the endothelium following phacoemulsification or extracapsular cataract extraction (ECCE) showed no statistically significant difference between the 2 techniques.[21-23]

It was also shown that the surgeon could place the incision according to clinical needs and personal preference, with no negative repercussions on the endothelial cell count.[24] However, prior to surgery one should clearly inform the patient that there is an increased risk of corneal decompensation following surgery due to the preexisting corneal dystrophy. This will avoid subsequent misunderstandings.

Alternatively, if the surgeon feels that a routine cataract procedure will cause corneal decompensation, he or she should opt for a combined operation. If a patient has evident stromal edema and/or the pachymetry is greater than 650 microns, he or she should consider the triple procedure.

If there is a stromal scar associated with a dense nucleus, the surgeon should remember that the anterior corneal surface will have a greater contribution to the overall refractive power of the eye.

Significant scarring of the corneal stroma can sometimes have a minimal effect on visual acuity, as is the case with interstitial keratitis. The surgeon should look for uniformity of the anterior corneal surface with keratometry or better still, with corneal topography, to decide whether to just go ahead with a triple procedure.

When keratoplasty and cataract surgery are clearly indicated, the surgeon should decide whether a single operation (triple procedure) is preferable to 2 separate procedures.

The combined procedure has the following advantages:

- A single procedure is an easier and less expensive option for the patient.
- There is less risk for the endothelium of the transplanted cornea than with a secondary cataract surgery.[25-31]
- Opacification of the posterior capsule (PCO) is less frequent with a combined procedure than with cataract surgery alone.[32]

The following are disadvantages of the triple procedure:

- Lower accuracy determining the power of the IOL, as postoperative keratometry can only be estimated. Following the combined technique, it is difficult to manage patients with significant refractive errors. The problem with accurate calculation of desired IOL power is having to use estimated keratometry readings.
- Higher complication rate, particularly when the surgeon performs an "open-sky" cataract removal. Theoretically, choroidal hemorrhage is more frequent as opposed to a sequential approach in elderly patients; rupture of the blood-aqueous barrier is greater as compared to PKP alone.[33-38]

The IOL power is a problem.[5,6,27,39] Axial length and keratometry values are essential for calculation of the IOL power. The axial length is measured prior to surgery; however, PKP or ALK obviously change the keratometry values. The axial length should be measured and compared in both eyes to increase accuracy and will be less precise in patients with keratoconus.

A number of methods exist for estimating the keratometry values for calculating the power of the IOL.[5,6,27,39,40]

One is based on mean keratometric values obtained on a series of patients undergoing keratoplasty. Others modify this value based on the keratometry measurements of the eye to be operated or the fellow eye. However, this method is not very reliable. For other surgeons, if the patient has a relatively steep cornea, postoperatively, the keratometry readings will be steeper than normal. Similarly, if the cornea is flatter than normal, the keratometry will be flatter postoperatively. Some surgeons use a mean keratometry value. Preoperative values of the eye to be operated are used (or the fellow eye, if accurate keratometry values cannot be obtained). A mean value is added or subtracted (calculated from the mean change in keratometry readings obtained from a large group of patients).

Our personal preference is the first method suggested—the use of a typical corneal curvature following transplantation. This is approximately 45 diopters (D) in all patients. Each surgeon should calculate the keratometry of his or her PKP or ALK patients following surgery. If the technique used is reproducible, the transplant surgeon should have repeatable keratometry readings.

Occasionally following surgery, the residual refractive error may result in symptomatic anisometropia. If the anisometropia is unacceptable, the surgeon can use a contact lens, insert a second lens (piggyback), replace the lens, or use laser refractive surgery such as laser-assisted in situ keratomileusis (LASIK) or photorefractive keratectomy.

The advantage of a consecutive procedure (keratoplasty followed by cataract surgery) is basically greater accuracy in the power of the IOL.[5,6,33,34]

The surgeon should pay attention when removing a slightly brunescent yet optically transparent cataract as the prognosis and visual recovery following keratoplasty is often better in the phakic eye because of the stability of the anterior segment afforded by the lens. The surgeon should also remember that a moderate opacity of the lens tends to increase rapidly following PKP, even when the surgery is uncomplicated[41-44] (using post transplant steroids will accelerate cataract formation), and to a lesser degree following PLK.[45] With gradual cataract formation, both the patient and the surgeon will be disappointed with the visual recovery following keratoplasty, particularly as the optical characteristics of the cornea improve. The patient's visual recovery will be slow, and this is a drawback of the sequential procedure.

Another advantage is that sequential surgery is probably a safer approach, particularly when cataract removal during the triple procedure is open-sky. Debate continues whether sequential surgery or a combined procedure is preferable. Another advantage is that choroidal hemorrhage is less frequent in consecutive treatment than in a combined approach. With a combined procedure, any rupture of the blood-aqueous barrier will be greater as compared to PKP alone.[36-38,41-44]

During a sequential procedure, when a patient previously grafted for keratoconus has cataract surgery, the endothelium of the transplanted cornea is exposed to surgical trauma.[25-31,46] In these cases, the surgeon should use a VES providing maximum endothelial protection. The literature suggests that cataract surgery, following any type of keratoplasty, is a relatively safe and effective procedure associated with a low but real risk that the transplant may fail; following phacoemulsification, eyes having PKP have endothelial cell loss greater than eyes undergoing ALK or those who have not had previous surgery. This is an advantage for the ALK procedure (see the Combined Procedure for Cataract Removal and Anterior Lamellar Keratoplasty section in this chapter). When the cataract is extremely dense and amber in color and there is evidence of previous PKP, recent literature suggests that ECCE appears to have less cell loss than phacoemulsification.[28]

However, there are few comparative findings on endothelial damage caused by cataract surgery after keratoplasty surgery as opposed to simultaneous combined procedure. In a study dating to 2006,[47] no statistically significant difference was reported between the 2 procedures (combined and sequential).

If the surgeon opts for sequential surgery, the cataract should wait at least 1 to 3 months after removal of the keratoplasty suture to allow stabilization of keratometry readings[48]; the corneal curvature completely stabilizes just 2 to 3 months following removal of the suture. Nevertheless, according to some surgeons, keratometry is reliable even with the suture in place 2 or 3 months after surgery, if the corneal sutures are not too tight. Rarely, the surgeon may consider cataract surgery with the corneal suture in place; however, the surgeon should be aware that when the suture is removed, the refraction may change significantly.

As demonstrated by a review of recent literature,[35-39,47,49-55] there is little agreement on whether sequential surgery or a combined procedure is preferable. Some studies suggest that as there is no statistically significant difference in terms of visual acuity, refractive error, risk of rejection, and decompensation of the graft between the 2 procedures, a triple procedure is preferred as this will provide more rapid visual recovery and reduce costs. Others recommend the sequential procedure because of better refractive outcomes with this approach, and cataract surgery can be performed in relative safety.

Combined Penetrating Keratoplasty and Cataract Removal

Preoperative Preparation

The surgery may be performed under general or local/regional anesthesia. General anesthesia is still widely used with this type of surgery, even though intraoperative vitreous pressure may develop from extraocular muscles not having been anesthetized. Retrobulbar anesthesia requires a long acting agent (eg, bupivacaine or ropivacaine); these allow prolonged anesthesia and reduce postoperative discomfort.[56] The amount of anesthetic agent must be appropriate (ie, relative to the size of the patient's orbit). The anesthetic agent can be combined with a small quantity (0.5 to 0.7 cc) of hyaluronidase to facilitate diffusion of the agent inside the orbit.

Some surgeons prefer to use peribulbar anesthesia,[57,58] even though the degree of anesthesia varies.

A facial nerve block is advisable as it is important to ensure that the orbicularis muscle is anesthetized during keratoplasty.

Normal mydriatic drops are used; they should not induce cycloplegia because one may want to use miotic agents after the surgery.

The eye must be "soft" during surgery, which is essential for the success of any open-sky procedure. The globe is softened with gentle pressure following peribulbar or retrobulbar block.

A device, such as a Honan balloon (30 mm Hg; Lebanon Corporation, Lebanon, IN), should be applied at least 20 minutes prior to surgery. Intravenous mannitol can be injected for 1 to 2 minutes while the patient is being prepped. The dose should be calculated based on the patient's weight and general health, avoiding potential congestive heart failure. The most used dose for the majority of adults is 50 mL of 18% mannitol. With this, the maximum hyperosmotic effect is created just as the eye is opened (ie, after 10 to 15 minutes); if too early, the reduction of IOP will peak too soon.

The surgeon should use a speculum resting on the orbital rim, such as the Schott lid speculum ([Katena Products, Denville, NJ] Figure 17-1) or a Smirmaul eye speculum (Katena Products; see the Positive Pressure and Vitreous Loss section in this chapter).

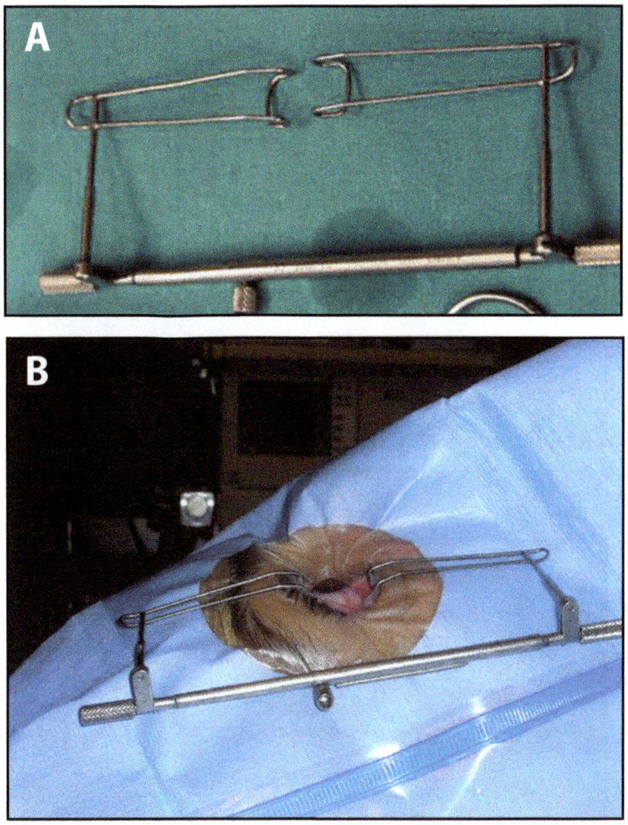

Figure 17-1. (A) Schott speculum. (B) Schott speculum in the surgical field.

Cataract Removal Techniques

In a combined procedure, the cataract can be removed by phacoemulsification or with ECCE technique. However, regardless of whether the surgeon opts for phacoemulsification or for ECCE, it is advisable to prepare the cornea for transplant before the patient is moved to the operating room.

Prior to marking the central cornea (Figure 17-2), the surgeon places the donor sclerocorneal tissue on a Teflon block (Barron Precision Instruments, Grand Blanc, MI) with the endothelium facing upward and proceeds with the punch technique (Figure 17-3). The sclerocorneal ring is then removed, and the corneal button is soaked in its preserving liquid (Figure 17-4).

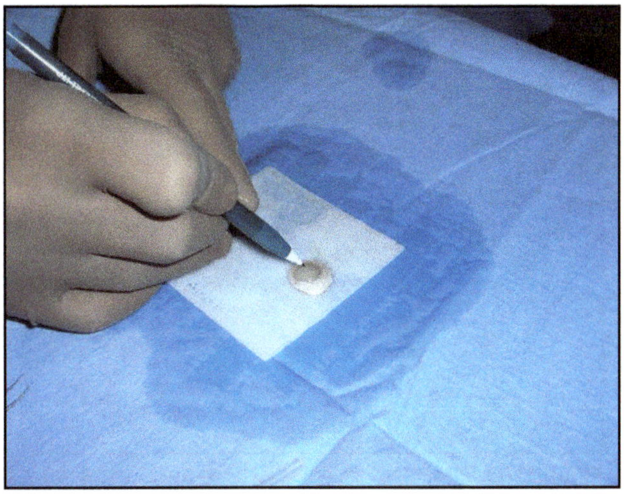

Figure 17-2. Central epithelial marking of donor sclerocorneal tissue using a skin marker.

Some surgeons believe that cutting the button using an artificial AC is more precise with a disposable Hessburg-Barron trephine (Barron Precision Instruments), and this will also be used on the host bed, because in this way the same trephine maneuvers will be replicated on the host.

In both cases, when a transplant is required, the diameter of the trephine varies between 7.50 and 8.50 mm. According to some authors, the diameter of the donor button should be 0.25 mm larger to allow more appropriate positioning of the donor button in the host bed, even though there is not total consensus on this and it should not always be used (eg, keratoconus).

The buttons can be produced using both a classic trephine or using a more modern technique with a femtosecond laser; this creates donor and host flap profiles of complementary shape that in theory will fit together more precisely.

We will now analyze 2 surgical options for cataract surgery.

Phacoemulsification With Penetrating Keratoplasty

Phacoemulsification should be performed prior to the transplant.[59] This technique, now performed using MICS, has the advantage of a closed-chamber procedure with more surgeon confidence.[59,60] There is a less risk of capsular rupture, vitreous pressure, choroidal hemorrhage, and other complications (see the Complications section in the chapter).[61-65] The only cost associated with this technique is the expense of the disposable instruments used in phacoemulsification.

In many cases in which a combined procedure is required, the corneal pathology may prevent good visualization of

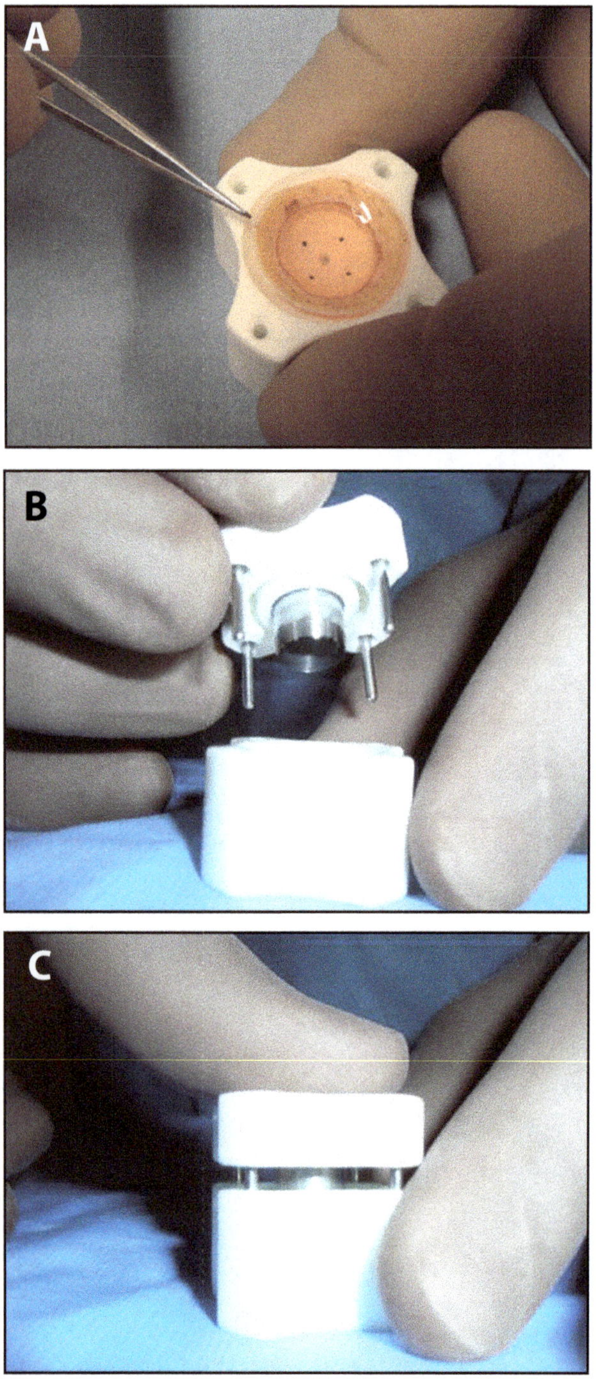

Figure 17-3. Placement of donor sclerocorneal tissue on a Teflon block with the endothelium facing up and then the punch.

the cataract—something considered necessary for many surgeons. Visualization of the posterior chamber (PC) may prove to be particularly difficult. Surprisingly, phacoemulsification is possible under these conditions; adequate visualization of the cataract and the posterior capsule can be achieved by focusing through the opacities and corneal scars.

If corneal edema is present, the surgeon may opt to remove the epithelium to improve visibility. When

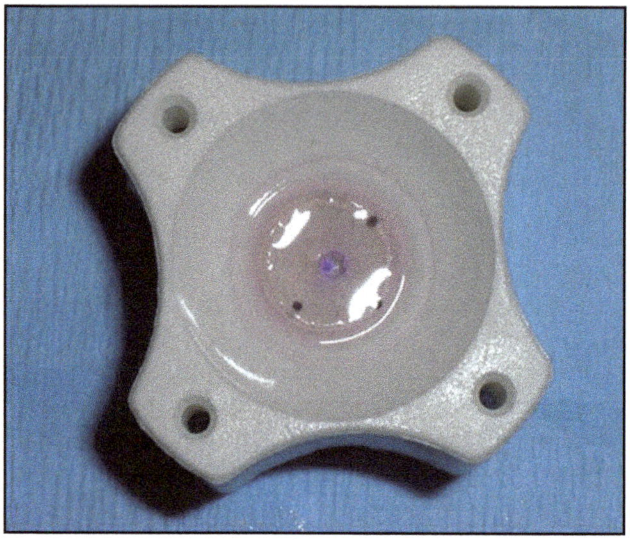

Figure 17-4. The corneal graft that was just created and placed on a Teflon block, after the sclerocorneal ring has been removed.

phacoemulsification is not possible (eg, because of the corneal opacity), the surgeon can remove the anterior corneal opacity,[59,66] apply a temporary donor button,[67] or use a keratoprosthesis.[68,69]

Inexperienced surgeons should not attempt this surgery as it is much more difficult than phacoemulsification with a clear cornea.

Specifically, several points should be explained for phacoemulsification. Phacoemulsification requires a small separate incision. A larger incision for phacoemulsification separate from the keratoplasty incision will require a suture, particularly if the incision is in clear cornea. The suture after keratoplasty may create tension in the peripheral cornea, stretching the tunnel and leading to aqueous leak.

A clear or near clear incision may be created. The corneal incision is more popular; some do not recommend an incision in clear cornea with a combined procedure and prefer the creation of a scleral tunnel. Prior to creating the incision, the surgeon should make a small incision in the conjunctiva at the superior limbus and reflect the conjunctiva away from the limbus. Any bleeding from scleral vessels can be cauterized. Cauterization should not be excessive as the sclera may retract, with potential difficulties with wound healing or scarring. A scleral tunnel is then created. A scleral incision of 1.5 to 2 mm posterior to the limbus is created with steel or diamond knives to half scleral depth, followed by dissection into the peripheral cornea, and then penetration into the AC with 2- to 2.2-mm knives.

Regardless of whether the incision is clear corneal or is scleral, the tunnel into clear cornea should not be excessively long as this may interfere with the keratoplasty. For good scarring, the dissection should be performed in peripheral cornea just beyond the limbal vascular arcade. Microcoaxial phacoemulsification through a 2- to 2.2-mm incision has the advantage of a smaller incision allowing a shorter tunnel; these close well and are ideal for this type of surgery.

Then a limbal paracentesis is created for the introduction of a second instrument and injections into the AC, generally at the 2 o'clock position for right-handed surgeons.

Traditional phacoemulsification follows, with injection of VES, continuous curvilinear capsulorrhexis (CCC), hydrodissection, emulsification of the nucleus, cortical removal, and implantation of a foldable IOL into the bag (with no complications).

Usually, sutures are not required; however, if the surgeon detects any leakage from the incision, a single 10-0 nylon suture should be placed.

After bag implantation of the IOL, the surgeon removes the VES and injects acetylcholine into the AC to induce miosis. He or she then injects additional high viscosity VES into the AC for the transplant part of the surgery.

Four cardinal points of the central and radial corneal epithelium are marked (Figure 17-5).

The circular corneal trephination is full depth using a trephine of desired diameter (usually a disposable Hessburg-Barron trephine [Barron Precision Instruments]); the diameter of the trephine varies depending on the pathology (Figure 17-6). Generally speaking, when the transplant is for optical purposes, the diameter of the trephination varies between 7.50 and 8.50 mm.

Full-depth trephination is frequently performed, but is often not completely 360 degrees and must be completed with corneal scissors. At this point, once the host corneal tissue has been removed (Figure 17-7) under open-sky conditions, dispersive VES should be placed onto the iris (Figure 17-8). The surgeon places the graft once it has been irrigated to remove the residual preserving liquid (Figure 17-9). It is useful to place the first corneal suture at the 12 o'clock position using Pollack forceps (Asico, Westmont, IL), allowing the needle pass without torqueing the button. We then place 4 9-0 silk sutures at the 4 cardinal points. These are removed at the end of surgery. These sutures stabilize the flap.

After the sutures are placed, the surgeon verifies that they have been placed correctly by seeing the formation of a square on the corneal surface.

At this point, the most critical phase is completed, and the surgeon can then place the remaining corneal sutures. Four individual 10-0 nylon sutures are positioned at 2, 4, 8, and 10 o'clock. A Siepser slip knot with a 1-1-1 throw is an elegant technique allowing the creation of a small knot that can be easily buried (Figure 17-10). The surgeon then marks the corneal surface with a skin marker, using the rule of half of the half (Figure 17-11). A continuous suture is then used, normally with 16 passes. The needle must pass through the corneal tissue of the donor and host tissue at the same depth, approximately 90% deep (Figure 17-12). The suture is tightened using an IOL hook, to avoid the need for forceps that may break the suture, and tied with a

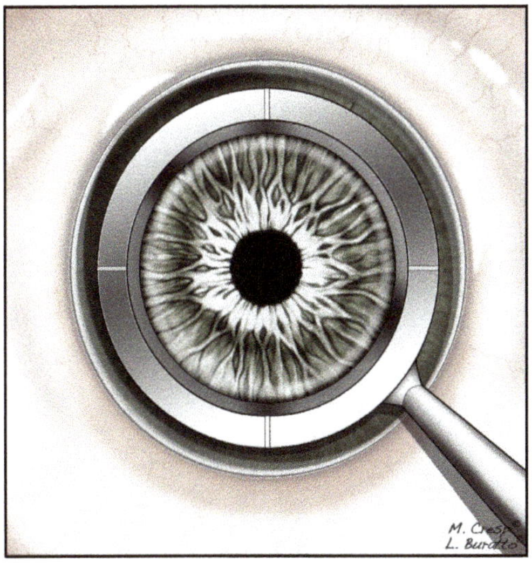

Figure 17-5. Marking of the central and radial corneal epithelium of the host bed at 4 cardinal points.

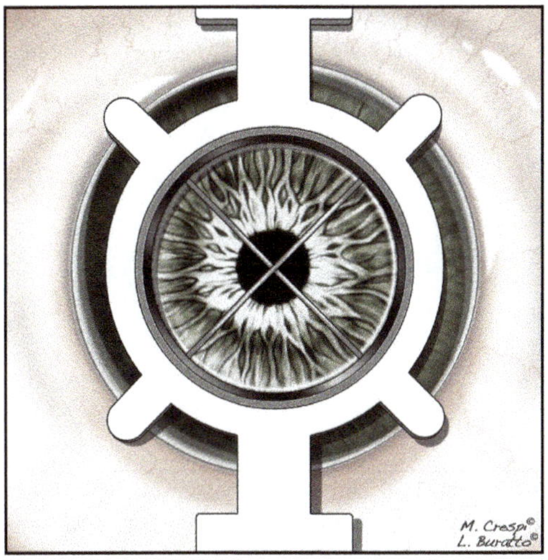

Figure 17-6. Full-thickness corneal trephination of the host bed with a disposable trephine.

2-1-1 knot. The hook slides over the knot and buries it in the tissue. The 9-0 silk sutures are then removed, and subconjunctival cortisone is injected (4 mg betamethasone; Figure 17-13).

Penetrating Keratoplasty With Extracapsular Cataract Extraction

Open-sky ECCE can be performed if phacoemulsification is not possible. There are risks associated with any open-sky procedure and protection against expulsive suprachoroidal hemorrhage is lacking. (The management of these problems will be examined in the Complications section in this chapter.) For this reason, it is essential that the globe has been softened preoperatively.

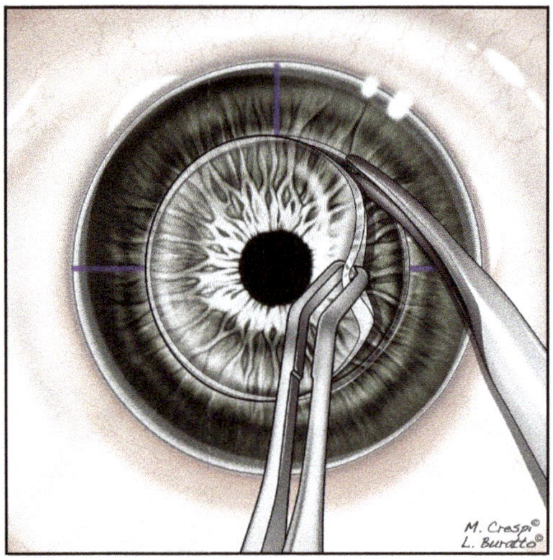

Figure 17-7. Removal of the host bed.

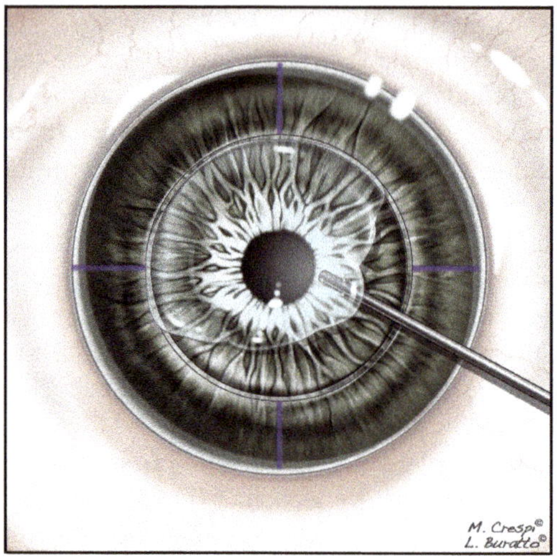

Figure 17-8. Open-sky placement of dispersive VES.

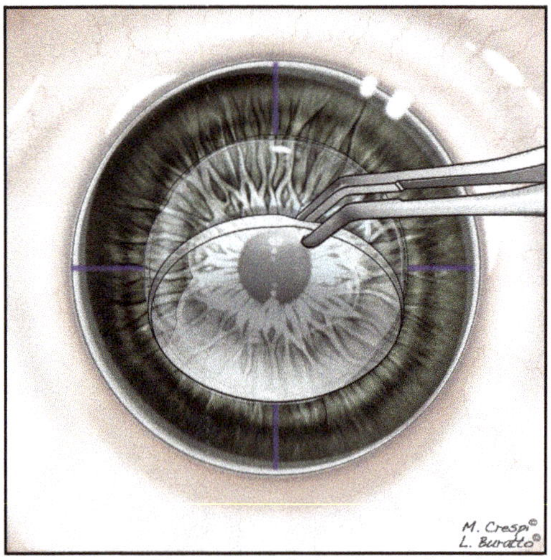

Figure 17-9. Placement of the donor flap following washing. The pupil is in pharmacological miosis and the IOL is in the capsular bag.

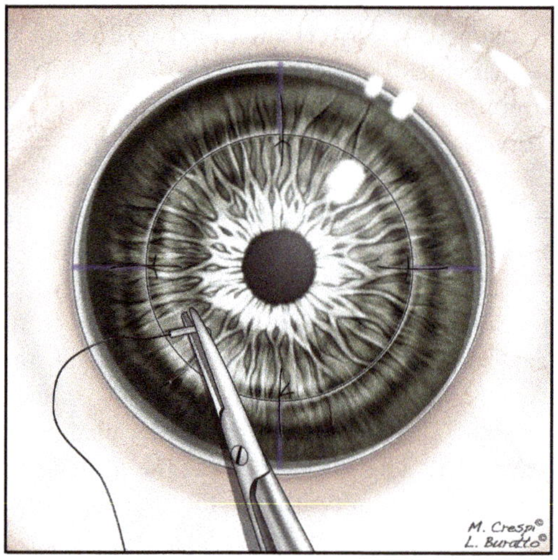

Figure 17-10. Placing 4 individual sutures of 10-0 nylon.

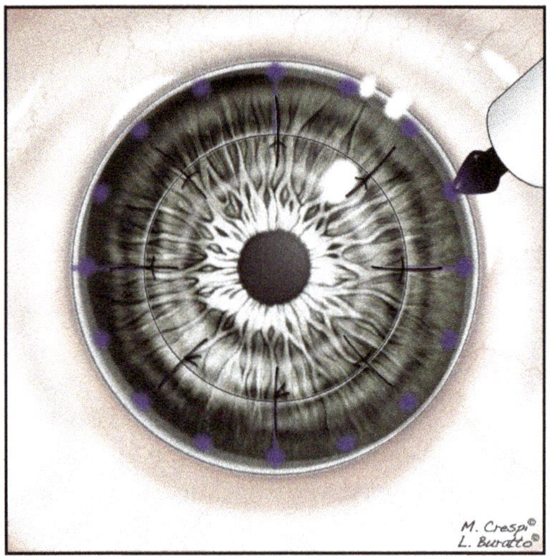

Figure 17-11. Sixteen points are marked.

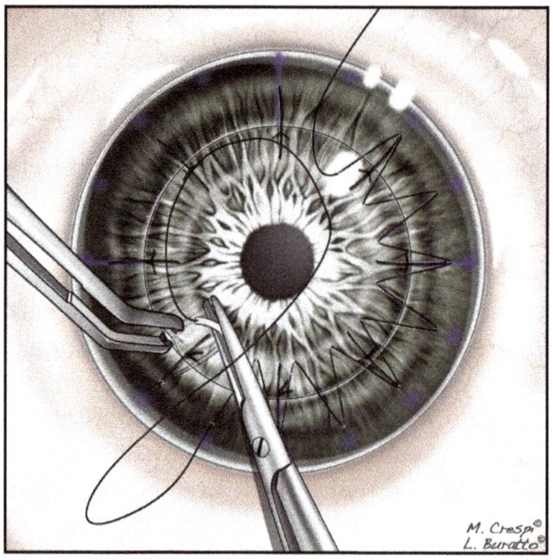

Figure 17-12. Continuous running suture with 16 passes.

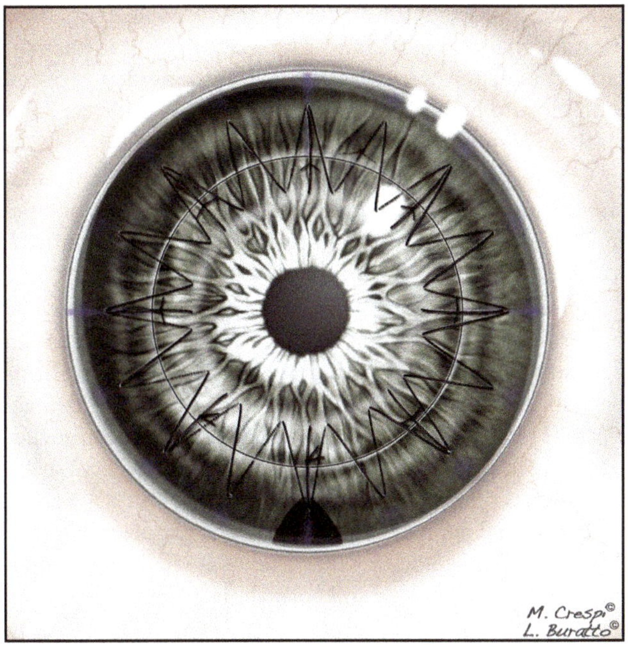

Figure 17-13. Eye with a classical triple procedure.

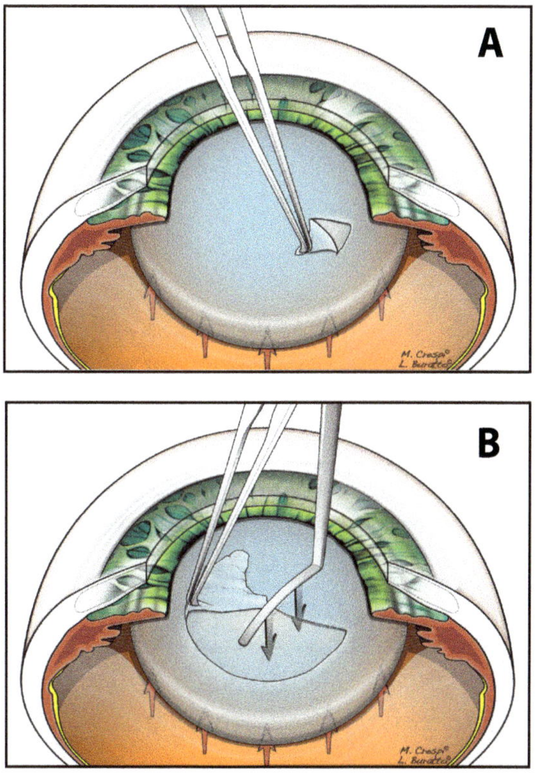

Figure 17-14. (A) Vitreous pressure during PK tends to extend the tear of the rhexis toward the equator and beyond. (B) Positive vitreous pressure can be countered by pushing the nucleus posteriorly with a spatula during capsulorrhexis.

Once the host button has been removed, open-sky ECCE begins with the anterior capsulotomy. Frequently, the surgeon may need to manually retract the iris with an iris hook because of intraoperative miosis. Generally, a can-opener capsulotomy provides satisfactory results, as does a capsulotomy made with scissors; however, CCC is the best technique, ideal for maintaining an intact margin, facilitating cortical aspiration and IOL implantation in the capsular bag. A large diameter rhexis must be created (at least 7 mm) to prolapse the intact nucleus; however, creating a rhexis of this size may be difficult because with the open-sky procedure, a certain degree of positive pressure is inevitable. The posterior pressure on the nucleus tends to encourage escape of the rhexis.

In addition to the preoperative steps mentioned previously, positive pressure can be managed with a spatula, held in the nondominant hand compressing the center of the nucleus during the rhexis (Figure 17-14).

If the tear extends out to 8 mm and cannot be recovered, the surgeon should convert to a scissors capsulotomy before the rhexis extends to the equator.

The experienced surgeon is aware that the critical moment is the open-sky removal of the nucleus and IOL implantation, because of possible vitreous pressure and rupture of the capsule.

The nucleus can be removed in a variety of ways. If the anterior rhexis is continuous, the surgeon can safely proceed with hydrodissection to free the nucleus. If the flow is directed just underneath the anterior capsule, cortical cleavage is straightforward, greatly facilitating cortical removal (Figure 17-15).

When it is not possible to perform hydrodissection, the nucleus should be freed by engaging it and rotating it with a sharp instrument such as a 23-gauge needle or a thin cyclodialysis spatula (Figure 17-16A).

As soon as the surgeon sees the lens equator (the superior portion of the lens itself [Figure 17-16B]), a lens loop is passed underneath the nucleus facilitating its removal through the capsulotomy (Figure 17-16C). If the nucleus falls back into the bag, it can be elevated by injecting a small quantity of VES, avoiding excessive posterior pressure that could extend an existing capsule tear.

Alternatively, a cryoprobe may be used centrally on the nucleus once most of the cortex over it has been removed. If good adhesion is achieved, the nucleus can be removed by "lollipopping," then aspirating the epinucleus and cortex.

A normal irrigation/aspiration technique can be used; however, with open-sky, air will also be aspirated creating aspiration fluctuations. There are also problems with infusion making it difficult to aspirate cortex and clean the anterior capsule, particularly with posterior pressure. Thus, the surgeon should also be familiar with older manual techniques of irrigation/aspiration, such as Simcoe (Eye4Vision Ophthalmics Int'l, the Netherlands) or McIntyre (Millenium Surgical Corp, Narberth, PA).

The inverted Simcoe technique utilizes the advantages of each of the 2 techniques. A 3-mL aspiration syringe is

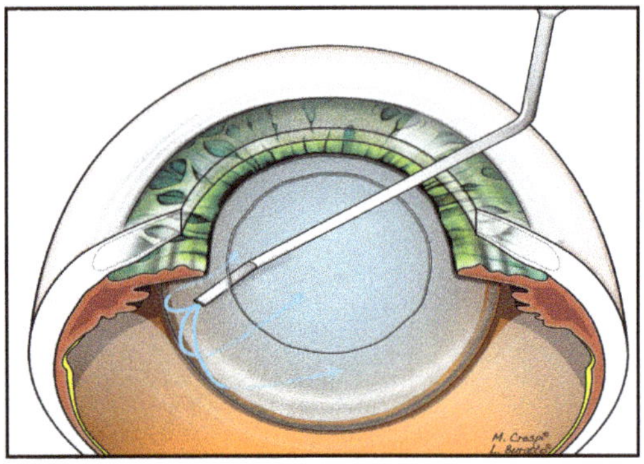

Figure 17-15. Open-sky hydrodissection.

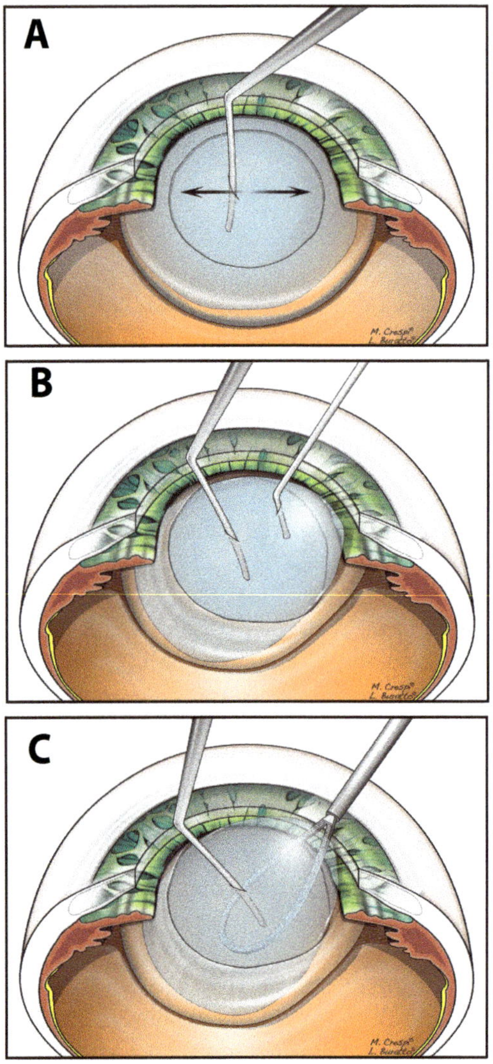

Figure 17-16. (A) Prolapse of the nucleus using the tip of a thin cyclodialysis spatula. Positive vitreous pressure helpful here (if the eye is soft, vitreous pressure can be simulated by gently compressing the sclera). (B) Tilting of the nucleus once the equatorial edge has been exposed. (C) A microsurgical loop is passed underneath the nucleus to extract it intact.

attached directly to the device. As the tip of the irrigation/aspiration device is flat and slightly curved, it is particularly suitable for cortical aspiration with positive pressure with closure between the anterior and posterior capsular leaflets (Figure 17-17).

The surgeon should be careful not to aspirate the anterior capsule and tear the zonules. All of the cortical material must be removed gently to minimize postoperative inflammation that could compromise the corneal transplant.

Once the cortex has been completely removed and the posterior capsule has been cleaned of any debris, a lens can be inserted into the PC. If an intact anterior capsulorrhexis permits bag implantation, a one-piece polymethylmethacrylate (PMMA) lens with a length of 12 mm is recommended. If the implantation of a lens in the sulcus is necessary, a lens 13 or 14 mm in length is better for stability. A patient with a normal pupil will tolerate an optic diameter of 6 mm. The surgeon may opt for a diameter of 6.5 to 7 mm without positioning holes for a pupil with abnormalities.

When the ECCE is completed with IOL implantation in the bag, the surgeon injects acetylcholine to induce miosis, places high viscosity VES into the AC, positions the donor cornea, sutures the graft, and finally subconjunctival injection of cortisone (4 mg betamethasone) is completed.

Complications

Positive Pressure and Vitreous Loss

Positive pressure, appearing as bulging of the posterior capsule with the red reflex of the fundus still present, can be due to many reasons; the most common is pressure on the lids and drape from the lid speculum.

We prefer to use the Schott or the Smirmaul speculum, which rests on the orbital rim. Other speculums may compress the globe.

Regardless of the type of speculum used, if there is positive pressure, the surgeon must manage it. The proof is reduction of the positive pressure when the speculum is lifted or repositioned.

If the positive pressure is great and there is risk of posterior capsule or zonular rupture, the surgeon should consider vitreous aspiration. However, in an open-sky procedure, any attempt to penetrate the globe by introducing a needle through pars plana will increase the pressure and almost certainly lead to vitreous loss.

A delicate scleral incision using a sharp blade such as a diamond knife can reduce this risk; however, usually a rapid increase in positive pressure leaves the surgeon no time to perform this maneuver. Alternately, intravenous mannitol can be used to reduce vitreous pressure. The surgeon should always anticipate suprachoroidal effusion, a complication that will be discussed in the following section.

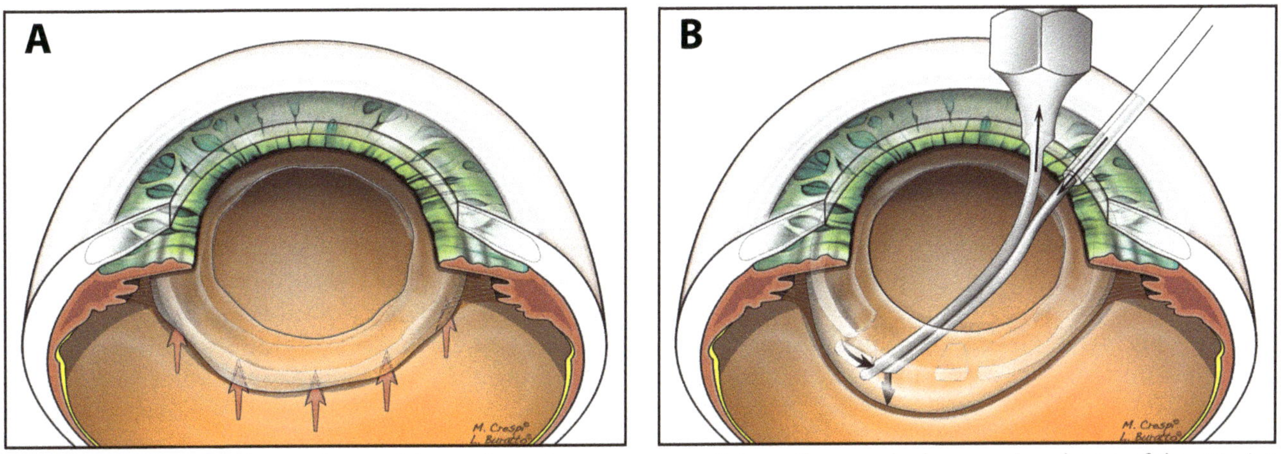

Figure 17-17. (A) Following prolapse of the nucleus, vitreous pressure flattens the capsular bag, causing closure of the anterior and posterior capsular layers. (B) The inverted Simcoe irrigation/aspiration device has both a flat tip and a slightly curved tip. This instrument is ideal for aspiration of the cortex with positive pressure. The tip can slide delicately between the 2 capsular layers, separated by exerting delicate downward pressure, allowing safe aspiration of the equatorial cortex.

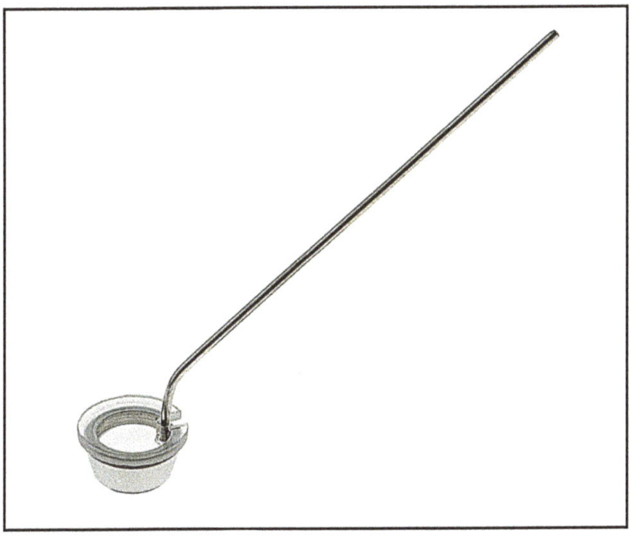

Figure 17-18. Cobo's temporary keratoprothesis.

In the absence of signs of effusion and hemorrhage, vitreous loss requires a vitrectomy.[70] Automated vitrectomy with a guillotine-type probe is preferable as it will minimize traction on the vitreous base.

If automated vitrectomy is not possible, the surgeon can perform open-sky vitrectomy with a cellulose sponge tip and scissors, avoiding excessive traction on the vitreous. At the end of the vitrectomy, the AC must be examined carefully. A sponge tip should be passed over the pupil and the iris to ensure that all of the vitreous strands have been removed. Any strands will tend to become trapped in the keratoplasty wound, at the very least leading to distortion of the pupil and possibly cystoid macular edema.

Hemorrhage and Suprachoroidal Effusion

Once the host button has been removed, the eye invites the devastating complication of effusion and suprachoroidal hemorrhage. The surgeon must always suspect this complication and be ready to manage it immediately if required. The signs of hemorrhage and suprachoroidal effusion in an open-sky procedure include posterior vitreous pressure on the intact posterior capsule, a tear in the posterior capsule and zonules with vitreous loss, loss of the red reflex, or even a combination of these.

If the patient is aphakic, before inserting the IOL, the surgeon can visualize the retina simply by focusing the microscope downward. A smooth retinal elevation, with a normal color, suggests choroidal effusion; however, if the retinal elevation is dark, this probably is a hemorrhage. If the elevation progresses slowly, it can be contained; a more rapid hemorrhage expels the intraocular contents without immediate surgical intervention.

As soon as the surgeon sees a suprachoroidal mass, he or she must immediately place a gloved finger over the corneal opening. It is also a good idea to have a clear lens available, which can be used to keep the eye closed with a suprachoroidal complication; an example is the temporary corneal prosthesis Cobo (Ocular Instruments, Bellevue, WA]; Figure 17-18). This calibrated lens can adapt to a large range of corneal openings, and its placement stabilizes the globe, allowing the surgeon to evacuate the suprachoroidal space.

One reason for suprachoroidal hemorrhage during open-sky maneuvers is that a patient under light general anesthesia begins to resist the endotracheal tube. Given that PKP is relatively painless, only light general anesthesia is required and many anesthetists use even less to prevent lowering the blood pressure. To avoid expulsive hemorrhage, the surgeon should instruct the anesthetist to use an anesthetic agent that will paralyze the patient.

Intraocular Implantation Following Vitreous Loss

If vitreous loss occurs and the surgeon is concerned about the ability of the posterior capsule remnants to support a PC-IOL, there are 3 options for IOL implantation: AC-IOL, PC-IOL with iris fixation, or PC-IOL with scleral fixation.

The literature suggests that all of them can be used with relative efficacy and safety.[61,62,70] If the surgeon opts for scleral fixation, he or she should remember that dissection of the scleral grooves required for scleral fixation is difficult once the cornea has been removed.

The surgeon may secure the PC-IOL to the iris with mid-peripheral sutures or using a technique initially described by Lane, using a scleral suture not requiring a scleral groove (see Chapter 19). This is possible if the PC-IOL has a hole in the haptic. The surgeon uses a permanent suture of 10-0 or 9-0 Prolene; the suture is passed through the positioning hole, and then each end of the suture is passed through the sclera approximately 1 mm behind the ciliary sulcus. The suture is tied, cut, and the knot is buried in the sclera. The conjunctiva is then closed above the smooth Prolene loop that should not erode the conjunctiva.

Combined Cataract Removal and Posterior Lamellar Keratoplasty

PLK or endothelial keratoplasty (EK) is a revolutionary development in the treatment of patients with endothelial pathology, allowing rapid visual recovery.[71]

The advantages of EK are largely due to the fact that the keratometry does not change with time; thus the postoperative corneal power is more predictable than PKP. Visual recovery in these patents is therefore more rapid.

A number of studies indicate that 50% of PKP patients have postoperative astigmatism less than 3 D[5,6,72,73]; they report a mean astigmatism of 5.0 D. Thus, postoperative refractive errors are frequent. The keratometry of a transplanted cornea stabilizes between 1 to 3 months after suture removal compared to the usual postoperative stabilization of 12 to 18 months. During this period, visual acuity fluctuates with suture removal; it may also decrease because of cataract development, with a delay in the patient's visual recovery.

Moreover, PKP is invasive surgery involving a full-thickness vertical corneal scar; a need for sutures; frequent, high irregular postoperative astigmatism; long-term visual recovery; and risk of rejection.

Patients with both a cataract and Fuchs' endothelial dystrophy, having a traditional triple or sequential procedure, may be faced with these complex problems.

In addition to stability of keratometry, the advantages of EK are that only pathological tissue is replaced (selective transplant) and the surgery is performed with a closed eye. Thus, the eye is at a lower risk of intraoperative and postoperative complications. It is more resistant to trauma and less exposed to infections.

Rejection with this technique is a possibility (endothelial rejection is the most frequent and dangerous). However, a small group of researchers suggest that this complication is less frequent as opposed to PKP due to the lack of communication with superficial vessels and tear film.[74]

The disadvantages of this technique include the delicate expensive instruments required (see the following sections).

Since it was introduced, the EK technique has been greatly simplified and improved. The stability and predictability of the keratometry make this procedure even more useful when associated with contemporary cataract surgery. Moreover, in patients with only mild endothelial dystrophy, the surgeon is more confident in doing cataract surgery alone; if there is post surgery endothelial cell loss, the surgeon has the option of offering the patient surgery that is easier than traditional PKP.

Indications

When the endothelium decompensates or the cell count is too low for allowing even the most careful phacoemulsification, the surgeon may offer cataract surgery combined with EK. Essential requisites for EK are below:

- An edematous cornea that is relatively clear and therefore has good optical potential (with no permanent scars or irregularity)
- Corneal edema that allows visibility of the cataract surgery: capsulorrhexis, phacoemulsification, cortical aspiration, and IOL implantation in the bag

EK can be performed with different techniques, including the popular Descemet's stripping EK (DSEK) and Descemet's stripping automated EK (DSAEK). Other, less commonly used techniques include deep lamellar endothelial keratoplasty (DLEK) and Descemet's membrane EK (DMEK). Cataract surgery can be combined with each of these types of posterior keratoplasty, giving rise to the so-called new triple procedure: phacoemulsification, IOL implantation, and EK.

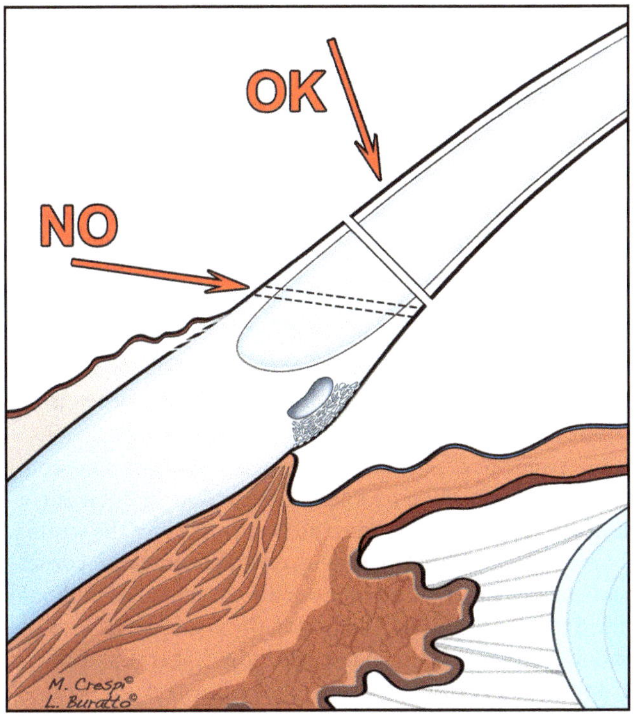

Figure 17-19. The paracentesis must be as small and as short as possible, therefore more vertical. It should be vertical to allow air to be easily injected under the lenticle.

Preoperative Preparation

The patient undergoing the new triple procedure is examined exactly the same way as patients having EK alone. The patient should be informed that postoperatively, he or she must remain supine to allow the air-assisted attachment of the endothelial graft. For patients who cannot comply, the surgeon may use different postoperative management, such as prolonged sedation with the patient in a dedicated area in the hospital or clinic. Alternately, the surgeon may suggest a PKP procedure.

Regarding anesthesia, as mentioned previously, retrobulbar anesthesia is useful with long-acting anesthetic agents[56]; some surgeons prefer topical/intracameral anesthesia.[75,76] Another advantage of retrobulbar anesthesia is the paralysis of the retrobulbar muscles, which reduce the rapid and saccadic eye movements immediately postoperative, which encourages adhesion of the endothelial graft to the host cornea.

EK has a minimal effect on postoperative keratometry—it maintains postoperative corneal power. The surgeon should develop new nomograms for IOL selection in patients having the new triple procedure. Many surgeons report a hyperopic shift following EK; some cases of myopic shift have also been reported.[77-82]

The amount of shift varies with the surgeon and technique used resulting from a number of factors, such as the thickness and shape of the donor tissue, the size of the incision, and other variables.

Surgeons using this new type of keratoplasty should monitor their results to create an algorithm for IOL selection in combined procedures. Given that there are many reports of hyperopic shift of between +0.75 and +1.5 D, the surgeon should target between -0.75 and -1.5 D to achieve emmetropia.

Phaco/Descemet's Stripping Automated Endothelial Keratoplasty Technique

Phacoemulsification is generally microcoaxial through a 2- to 2.2-mm incision, usually performed prior to EK to avoid exposing the new endothelium to ultrasound and other trauma associated with phacoemulsification.

During phacoemulsification, the following technical aspects should be observed as they differentiate the technique from standard phacoemulsification.

The paracentesis is extremely important in this surgery. The final injection and maintenance of air in the AC (essential for the attachment of the donor endothelium) is facilitated by a small, self-sealing vertical paracentesis (as small as possible) (Figure 17-19). Small paracenteses allow insertion of a Sinskey hook or curved 30-gauge cannula for the manipulation of the corneal graft. Nevertheless, the paracenteses should not be excessively small; they must be large enough to accommodate the instruments needed to manipulate the nucleus. Moreover, the paracentesis may be distorted and enlarged during cataract surgery with the introduction, use of, and removal of the instruments. Thus, it may leak and not maintain air inside the AC in the final steps of the procedure. To minimize the risk of air leakage, the paracentesis should be as small as possible. The surgeon should use maximum care and attention when introducing, using, and removing instruments to minimize trauma.

The size and placement of the incisions must be compatible with the phacoemulsification technique and the EK technique preferred by the surgeon. For example, the surgeon normally creates a corneal tunnel for phacoemulsification at 10 o'clock. At the end of the procedure, the incision is enlarged so the surgeon can comfortably use a bimanual technique for lenticle insertion. Ideally, one should place the 2 instruments for insertion of the lenticle almost horizontally, avoiding any interference from the nose or forehead. If the surgeon places the incisions vertically, the forehead or cheekbones may interfere with the maneuvers.

If the surgeon creates a 5-mm scleral incision for EK, typically superior, but prefers to use a temporal approach for phacoemulsification using a clear corneal incision, the best choice may be a temporal scleral tunnel for combined surgery. Moreover, the tunnel should be a compromise between a sealed tunnel, good for easy phacoemulsification, and a direct, almost vertical incision, better for

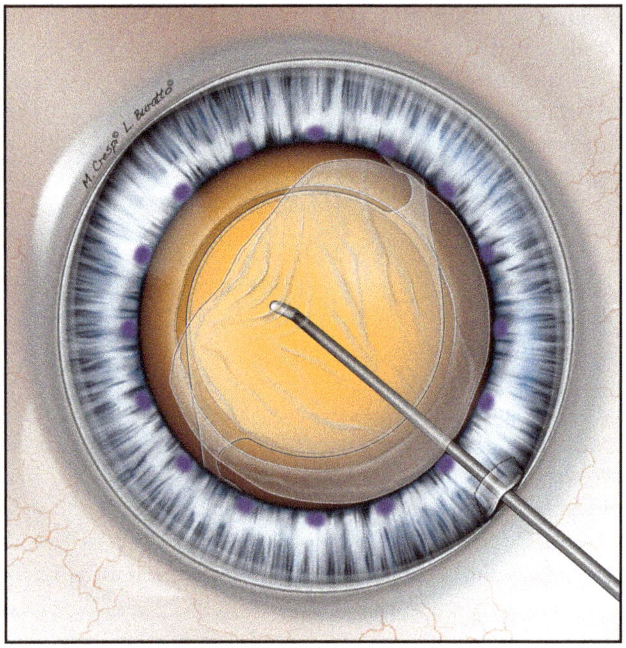

Figure 17-20. Complete removal of the Descemet's-endothelium complex.

introduction of the lenticle into the AC; thus, the tunnel should not be too long.

The use of a capsule dye, such as trypan blue, facilitates visualization of the capsule with an opaque cornea. The dye is injected with aqueous in the AC, left in position for a few seconds, then passively removed by injecting BSS into the AC. Another technique involves injecting the dye beneath the VES; as the dye is also absorbed by the pathological endothelium, the surgeon should use a bubble of highly cohesive VES (eg, Healon 5 AMO) to fill the AC. When the dye is injected underneath the VES spreading over the anterior capsule, one should not inject too much to avoid it staining the corneal endothelium. The capsulorrhexis should not be too large (measuring 5 to 5.5 mm) and should overlap the edge of the optic. If visualization is poor, the surgeon should consider performing the early steps of the EK procedure prior to cataract surgery. If extremely dense guttata are present and obstruct visualization, stripping Descemet's endothelial complex prior to phacoemulsification can improve corneal transparency. If epithelial edema is present, de-epithelialization may prove useful.

The correct VES must be used. Highly dispersive VES should not be used as it can be extremely difficult to remove it later. Retained VES can negatively impact adhesion of the transplanted posterior lenticle. One should use cohesive VES for all steps of the combined surgery. According to some surgeons, small amounts of cohesive VES can be used to coat and protect the donor endothelium. The surgeon must be sure that VES does not remain in the interface between the donor and host tissue, as this compromises adhesion of the tissues.

Following IOL implantation, the eye is prepared for removal of the Descemet's-endothelial complex. Without removing the VES, the surgeon marks the corneal surface with a circular marker the desired size for stripping (generally between 8 to 8.5 mm) on a dry surface. The surgeon then removes the Descemet's-endothelial complex under VES protection. The procedure is generally with mydriasis utilizing the red reflex. A Price hook (Moria Inc, Doylestown, PA) is used for the removal; this instrument is shaped like an inverted IOL hook, with an angled tip facing upward (Figure 17-20). The diameter for the stripping is usually 8.5 mm, with a donor lenticle having a diameter of 8.75 mm, to be fairly sure that a peripheral ring of host cornea is not covered with endothelium.

The Descemet's incision must be very delicate. One commonly made mistake by a less experienced surgeon is cutting too deep, including into the deeper layers of the stroma. This can have a negative impact on adhesion of the corneal lenticle. During removal of the complex, the surgeon should avoid touching the endothelium in the visual axis. He or she should only touch the endothelium peripherally, to avoid risking damage to the tissue in the visual axis.

The removal of the complex can be completed with a Busin spatula (Moria Inc), which is broad, blunt, and angled.

If the cornea has had prolonged stromal edema, the use of a dye such as trypan blue highlights the endothelium for removal.

At this point the surgeon enlarges the paracentesis to 2 clock hours to allow introduction of vitreoretinal 20-gauge crocodile forceps and a new paracentesis is made, usually at 5 o'clock; for the AC maintainer, orient inferiorally, not toward the main incision to prevent the BSS flow from complicating the insertion of the posterior lenticle. The flow from the AC maintainer should create approximately 40 mm Hg of pressure.

At this point the VES is carefully and completely removed from the AC and from behind the IOL. The irrigation/aspiration handpiece is used with repeated gentle depression to the IOL. Because of the cohesive nature of the VES, the compression ensures its complete removal. To remove cohesive VES, it is not necessary to go behind the IOL using maneuvers that are risky to the posterior capsule.

The surgeon then injects acetylcholine into the AC to induce miosis, although not all surgeons agree on this.

The eye is now ready to receive the posterior donor lenticle. Most surgeons believe that a relatively large primary incision is important to minimize endothelial trauma during insertion. As described for combined surgery, after cataract removal, one should enlarge the main incision for insertion of the lenticle (Figure 17-21). The size of the incision depends on the thickness and diameter of the lenticle and also on surgeon preference; many surgeons prefer an incision of around 4 mm, some 4.5 to 5 mm, and others larger than 5 mm. If the lenticle is inserted through an

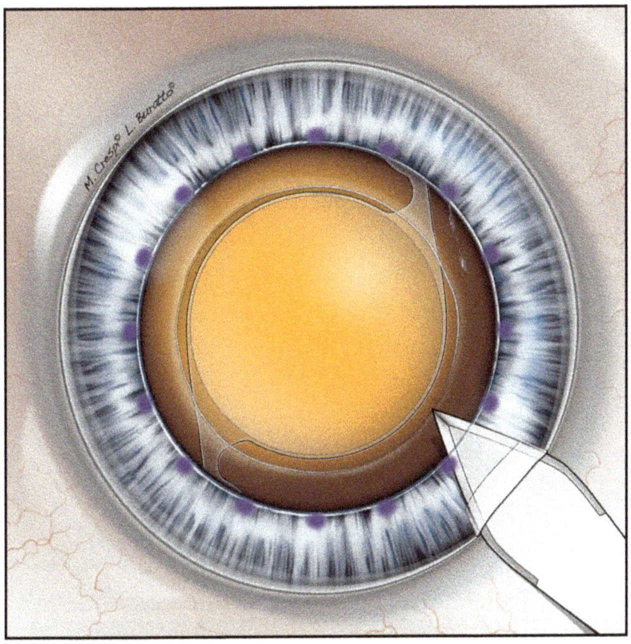

Figure 17-21. Enlargement of the main corneal incision to allow insertion of the lenticle.

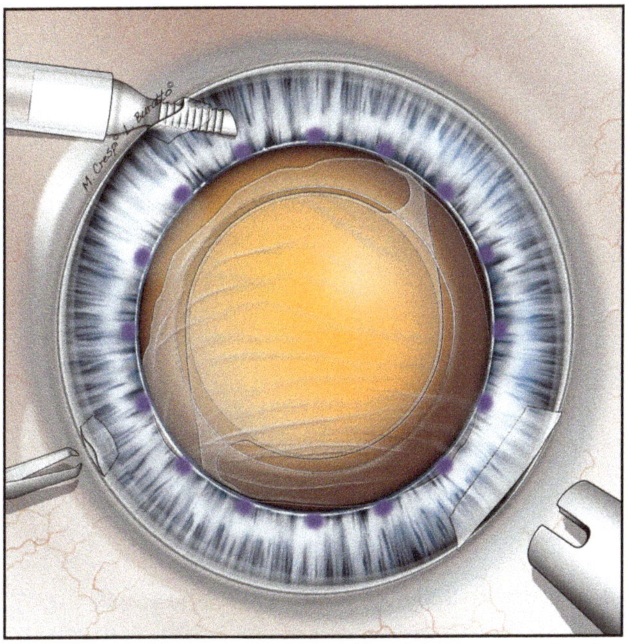

Figure 17-22. The posterior corneal lenticle immediately after insertion into the AC using a glide.

incision that is too small, the compression may cause significant endothelial cell death.[83] With thin lenticles of standard diameter (8.75 mm), the ideal incision is approximately 4.5 mm; if the corneal lenticle is thicker and the diameter is larger, an incision of 5 mm is preferable. New devices allow less traumatic insertion of lenticles through relatively small incisions with less induced astigmatism.[84-86]

The surgeon now uses Colibrì forceps (Katena Eye Instruments) to place the lenticle at the end of a glide. The nondominant hand inserts crocodile forceps through a side-port incision at 2 o'clock; this crosses the AC, and the arms come through the main incision and are ready to grasp the lenticle positioned on the glide, endothelium facing downward. The surgeon places the glide close to the main incision; the crocodile forceps grasp the lenticle, pulling it inside the AC, maintaining the glide in position to reduce BSS leakage.

The assistant stops the BSS flow from the AC maintainer. The surgeon removes the glide and delicately releases the lenticle. It will be almost perfectly centered in the majority of cases (Figure 17-22).

During the insertion of the donor lenticle, AC depth may decrease and the IOL tends to move anteriorly. This may complicate the insertion, damaging the donor lenticle or other structures of the anterior segment. To reduce the tendency to prolapse, it is important that the capsulorrhexis overlaps the edge of the IOL optic and is not too large.

Once the graft has been inserted in the AC, it is released. The surgeon must check that it is correctly positioned: the markings on the stromal edge of the lenticle are excellent reference points. The letter "F" is normally used as it is clearly identifiable when back to front. Repeated movements with the cannula at the edge of the lenticle or in the interface correctly position the lens.

The surgeon now injects air into the AC to attach the corneal lenticle; the air cannula in the AC should be directed to avoid air going behind the pupil. The AC must be filled.

Inflating the AC with air can prove to be difficult if the side-port incision for cataract surgery is used. In some cases, the air will escape from the AC through the paracentesis. Occasionally, fluid escapes because the air flows posteriorly with anterior prolapse of the iris. In these cases, the air should be removed, the AC is reformed with BSS, the paracentesis is sutured with 10-0 nylon, and finally, a new air bubble is injected. Some surgeons recommend the creation of a 20-gauge paracentesis with the nondominant hand to allow introduction of air into the AC. Others prefer to use a 30-gauge needle placed directly under the lenticle.

It is essential that all incisions be well sealed at the end of surgery to ensure stability of the lenticle. Three individual 10-0 nylon sutures close the main incision. Some surgeons believe the sutures are not really necessary to seal the incision; however, they prevent a sudden and dramatic expulsion of the lenticle when it unfolds in the AC using BSS or air. Some surgeons suture the main incision and the side port; other surgeons also suture the incision for the AC maintainer.

There has been debate relative to the length of time the air bubble should remain in the AC.[71,76,78,80] Some surgeons prefer to reduce the size of the air bubble in the operating room after just 10 minutes. However, the majority

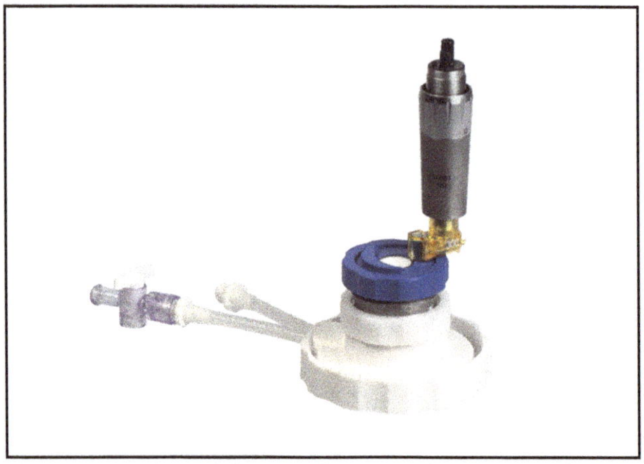

Figure 17-23. Use of the microkeratome for creation of precut corneal tissue ideal for EK.

of surgeons examine the patient a few hours after surgery; they can then reduce the size of the bubble by depressing the paracentesis with a hook.

Some surgeons remove the sutures after just 1 week post surgery[71,76,78,80]; we prefer to leave them in place for 2 to 3 months. They have little or no effect on the postoperative refraction.

Since 2008,[87] this innovative technique has used precut lenticles from the eye bank. A cornea suitable for PKP is cut using a microkeratome with a head that removes a cap 9 mm in diameter and 350 microns thickness; the remaining posterior lamella has a thickness of approximately 150 microns (Figure 17-23).

In the operating room, the surgeon receives a cornea with a free cap that can be temporarily removed. He or she checks the diameter of the cap and the markings on the stromal surface of the lenticle and then repositions the cap on its bed. The cornea is placed on a Teflon block, endothelium facing up; a "punch" maneuver of the desired diameter is done. Finally, the scleral ring is removed and the cap (not to be used) and the posterior corneal lenticle are placed into BSS Plus (Alcon Laboratories, Fort Worth, TX) to expand its thickness (prior to introduction into the eye). Some surgeons believe that by swelling the graft, they can manipulate the corneal tissue more easily, with less chance of causing damage to the corneal endothelium and reducing the incidence of postoperative dislocation of the lenticle.[88] Not all surgeons agree.

The use of precut lenticles has made a contribution in increasing the popularity of this surgical technique. Their use is not associated with any specific complications associated with tissue preparation, with results comparable to those of surgeon-prepared lenticles (Figure 17-24).[87-89]

An added advantage is that the surgeon or clinic does not have the expense of purchasing the instruments for the preparation of the lenticles (artificial AC, microkeratomes, or femtosecond laser).

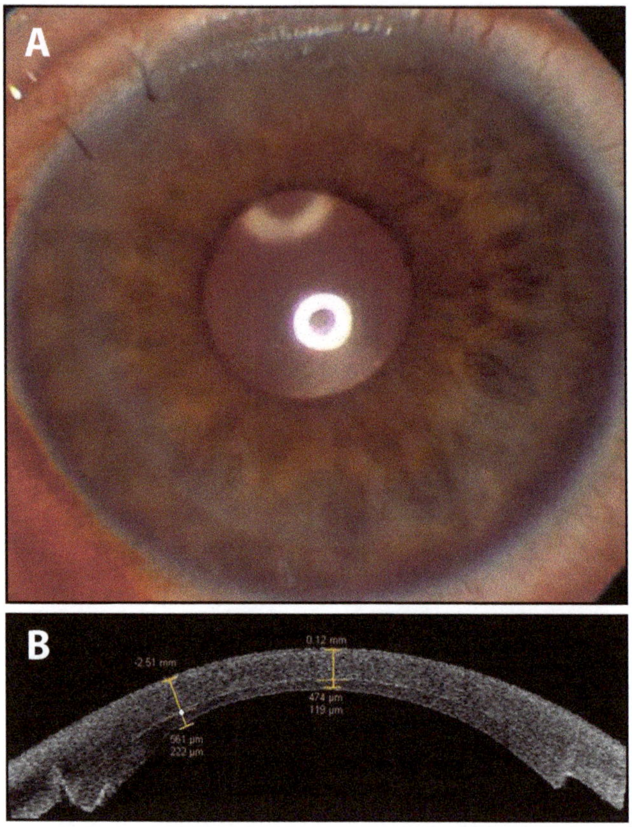

Figure 17-24. (A) Image of the anterior segment of an eye 7 days postoperatively with the new triple procedure. (B) Biomicroscopy.

Results

EK combined with phacoemulsification and IOL implantation is predictable, safe, and efficacious. Terry et al published results on 225 eyes having the triple procedure.[90] Six months postoperative, 93% of the eyes (122 eyes) with no other problems had a best-corrected visual acuity of 20/40 or better. The spherical equivalent was within 1 D of emmetropia in 73% of cases. The study did not report the incidence of dislocation or transplant failure with the triple procedure compared with 90 eyes having only EK during the same period. Similarly, Yoo et al reported increased visual acuity of 92% in 12 eyes following the triple procedure.[81] Postoperative refractive results showed a mean shift of 1.46 D from desired, and all patients were within 3 D of target. In another study,[82] 21 eyes had a triple procedure; there was no statistical difference in the amount of astigmatism, and all patients had a significant increase in visual acuity. In 62%, the refraction was within 1 D of emmetropia, and all were within 2 D.

This demonstrates the big difference from the classical triple procedure of PKP combined with cataract surgery. The outcome with this older type of surgery is much less predictable. An analysis of 10 studies describing postoperative refractive results of the classical triple procedure showed that

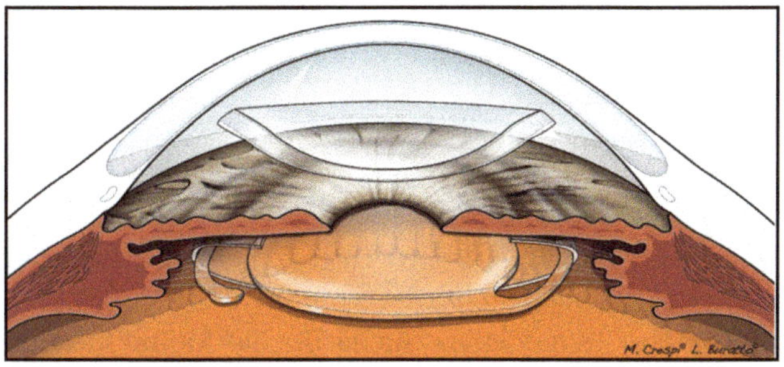

Figure 17-25. Drawing of corneal lenticle dislocation in the AC in a patient undergoing a new triple procedure (phaco/IOL/EK).

refractive results within 2 D of target varied between 26% and 76% with the classical triple procedure.[5,6,47,50,72,73,91-95] A recent study by Hayashi and Hayashi reported only 39% of 39 eyes were within 2 D of the refractive target 1 year following the combined technique.[47] Similarly, the percentage of patients with best-corrected visual acuity of 20/40 or better varied between 37% and 78%.

Consequently, the new triple procedure is much more predictable and effective when compared to the classical technique, with more rapid visual rehabilitation.[71,95]

Complications

The EK surgical technique has a low complication rate even when combined with phacoemulsification.[90-97] The most common complication is detachment or dislocation of the lenticle immediately postoperative; Suh et al[97] reported this in 23% (Figure 17-25) of cases. Terry et al reported a much lower incidence (1.8%).[90]

The patient should be examined the day following surgery and also 3 days later as dislocation several days after surgery has been reported. Dislocation of the lens can be fixed in the majority of cases by repositioning it and/or injecting air into the AC. Rarely with aphakia, the surgeon may have to use short acting gas, such as SF6. In Suh et al's study,[97] there was a 6% rejection rate.

Rarer complications include cystoid macular edema (5%), retinal detachment (4%), pupil block (2%) resolved by removing the air, blood in the interface (1%), epithelial cell growth in the interface (1%), peripheral synechiae between the iris and the lenticle, and limited suprachoroidal hemorrhage (1%). Recently, cases of glaucoma have been reported for patients following EK.[98]

No cases of primary graft failure were reported. In the recent 2009 report from the American Academy of Ophthalmology on EK not combined with cataract surgery,[71] this procedure was judged safe and effective.

The new EK procedure is a better way of treating isolated endothelial dysfunction in cataract surgery. Healing is more rapid compared to the classical triple procedure; the eye is more resistant to trauma, and the refractive result is both excellent and predictable.

Future Trends

The management of patients with both cataract and Fuchs' dystrophy will certainly improve in the future.

The visual results of EK depend on the thickness of the donor tissue. Some have analyzed visual results regarding thickness of donor tissue in 33 eyes (with no comorbidity) having EK because of corneal edema.[99] In 17 eyes with a lenticle thickness less than 133 microns (mean value of 109), 100% achieved 20/25 or better. However, in 16 eyes receiving corneal tissue greater than 133 microns thick (mean 165 microns), only 50% achieved 20/25 or better.

In light of this, many eye banks and a number of surgeons are working to produce thinner corneal lenticles for EK. Moreover, the DMEK procedure has already become popular. The development of ultrathin DSEK and the DMEK technique contribute to better vision in patients with corneal failure.

A future improvement is development of new instrumentation allowing atraumatic (to the endothelium) insertion of donor tissue through increasingly smaller incisions resulting in less induced astigmatism.

Combined Procedure for Cataract Removal and Anterior Lamellar Keratoplasty

ALK is an elegant surgical procedure for treating pathology of the corneal stroma and keratoconus. The corneal criteria for ALK include the following:

- Healthy host ocular surface
- Adequate endothelial cell function
- Corneal opacities not affecting Descemet's membrane or obvious surface abnormalities preventing the use of contact lenses

In addition to improving vision, this type of keratoplasty is also indicated for restoration of normal peripheral corneal thickness in corneas thinned from keratoconus or pellucid marginal degeneration.

Due to its technical difficulty, ALK is less popular than PKP, though it does have advantages.[100-108] Most importantly, it is a closed procedure, with better intraoperative and postoperative safety. Regarding postoperative safety, these corneas have greater resistance to trauma, allowing an earlier return to normal activity including sports and exercise.

The PKP graft has a higher failure rate than that of ALK because of such postoperative complications as glaucoma.[108] As ALK does not include the host endothelium, there is no risk of endothelial rejection.

As the incision is not full thickness, no sutures are close to the AC with consequently less suture-related issues.

Finally, donor tissue is readily available as good endothelium is not required.

Regarding published results,[100-108] final visual acuity is usually one Snellen line worse than that for PKP. Possible reasons include the following:

- Irregular dissection of donor tissue
- Debris in the interface
- Irregular dissection of host tissue
- Folds in the posterior layer involving the visual axis (frequently seen in advanced keratoconus)

A recent report by the American Academy of Ophthalmology[108] reviewed the clinical results of 55 studies comparing deep anterior lamerallar keratoplasty (DALK) and PKP:

- DALK is equal to PKP in terms of best-corrected visual acuity, especially with minimal host corneal thickness
- No difference in terms of postoperative refractive error
- Even though improved graft survival has not been demonstrated, endothelial maintenance is better with DALK
- DALK is safer because it is extraocular

In conclusion, DALK is a good surgical option for visual rehabilitation of patients having corneal pathologies not involving the endothelium.

When a cataract is present and is associated with keratoconus (Amsler third stage or greater), or with stromal opacities not affecting Descemet's creating severe visual loss, the surgeon may consider a triple procedure of phacoemulsification, IOL implantation, and ALK, with good results.[29,109-111] The removal of host corneal tissue in ALK should be deep, resulting in DALK.

Preoperative Preparation

This is similar to that of the classical triple procedure.

Surgical Technique

Surgeons vary in their sequence of the steps in DALK surgery. Some remove the host corneal tissue first, then proceed with cataract surgery, and finally implant the anterior donor corneal tissue.[109,110] Two studies indicate that Descemet's membrane can withstand the intraoperative pressure during phacoemulsification.

Others believe that the complete ALK surgery should be done prior to cataract surgery. The presently recommended sequence is cataract surgery followed by ALK.

The surgeon should remember that the patient's endothelium is subjected to ultrasound and other potential trauma during phacoemulsification. The surgeon should use modern microcoaxial phacoemulsification with a 2- to 2.2-mm incision and a high-viscosity VES providing maximum endothelial protection.

Once phaco is completed, the IOL is implanted in the bag, the VES is removed, acetylcholine is injected to induce miosis, and then the ALK is completed.

The surgeon performs a circular corneal trephination on the host not full thickness. As with PKP, the diameter varies depending on the pathology. Generally, in transplants for visual improvement, the diameter varies between 7.50 and 8.50 mm.

The host trephination should be 300 to 400 microns deep. If a disposable Hessburg-Barron cutter (Barron Precision Instruments) is used, the surgeon should rotate the blade 5 to 6 quarter turns.

Pachymetry should be done at a 6- and 8-mm diameter, with trephination going 100 microns short of the measured thickness. One should position the trephine, contact the epithelium, mark the trephine with a skin marker, and initiate trephination, calculating that a full revolution equals 250 microns.

The surgeon now dissects the deep corneal stroma at a uniform plane, using bevel up blades, with subsequent removal of the tissue (keratectomy).

Given that the deep stromal layers are parallel and this continues as far as Descemet's,[112,113] dissection in a single plane is fairly straightforward, between deep stroma and Descemet's membrane.

In DALK, deep anterior lamellar dissection in one plane (in deep stroma adjacent to Descemet's membrane) can be done with blades or with newer techniques—injection of BSS (hydrodelamination), VES (viscodissection), or air (Big Bubble).[114-118]

Some have also suggested that the keratectomy, possibly because of the thinner corneal stroma, increases the probability of success of the Big Bubble technique.

Air-modulated intrastromal dissection is performed as follows: following the trephination, a dissector with a blunt tip is introduced into the corneal stroma (Fogla dissector [Storz Ophthalmics Inc, Clearwater, FL]). The surgeon then introduces a curved cannula or a 27-gauge needle following the corneal curvature of the eye, attached to a 5-mL syringe filled with filtered air. The insertion of this instrument begins at the trephination extending into the stroma as far as the pupil—a relatively long distance—to reduce air outflow through the passage just created (Figure 17-26). With keratoconus, the surgeon should avoid the peak of the cone; this point is thinnest, with a greater risk of perforation. The syringe should be 5 mL and not less because the amount of air necessary to create the dissection is more than 2 to 2.5 mL. Slow gradual injection of air allows detachment of deep stroma from Descemet's membrane (Big Bubble) even if perforations of Descemet's occur.[104,119-122] Small perforations do not jeopardize successful completion.

Sometimes the introduction of air leads to widespread diffusion at different stromal planes, causing stromal opacification, with no single dissection plane. The surgeon can attempt to correct the situation with additional air injections into the stroma, though usually the results are poor.

Once the surgeon successfully achieves the bubble, he or she should immediately perform a paracentesis to allow dissipation of the increased ocular pressure.

The steepest point of the stroma is dissected using a blade, with a single rapid oblique movement avoiding penetration of Descemet's membrane (Figure 17-27). The surgeon can inject a small amount of dispersive VES through the small opening, maintaining the patency of the space and dividing the stroma into 4 quadrants with long blunt scissors, using an upward movement (Figure 17-28). Following the creation of 4 quadrants, scissors are used to cut peripheral corneal tissue, following the curvature of the trephination to obtain a smoother surface for good attachment of the host cornea (Figure 17-29).

Once the surgeon has removed the corneal tissue, which had been cut into 4 pieces, the residual remnants of cornea are removed. This can be assisted by applying moderate pressure on Descemet's with a damp sponge tip.

The surgeon now prepares the donor graft. The donor button should only be prepared after the Big Bubble is successful. Normally, corneas for PKP are ordered from the eye bank. One should only strip the endothelium off the button, when there are no significant perforations; otherwise, the surgeon may convert to a PKP procedure.

A less popular alternative is to order 2 corneas, one for DALK and one for PKP. The surgeon then uses the cornea he or she needs, returning the unused cornea to the eye bank.

Some surgeons recommend oversizing the donor graft 0.25 mm larger than the bed, resulting in better apposition of the edges and a return to normal corneal curvature (even in eyes with advanced keratoconus); however, others believe they should have the same diameter.

The creation of the donor button involves placing the cornea on a Teflon block and punching or puncturing it. As with PKP, in DALK some surgeons feel creation of the donor button is more precise when performed using an artificial AC, because the trephination on the host is duplicated on the donor tissue. The donor cornea is positioned on a Teflon block, endothelium up; 2 dry, stiff Merocel sponge tips (Beaver Visitec International Inc, Waltham, MA) are used to completely strip the endothelium (Figure 17-30).

The bed is irrigated copiously and tangentially with BSS (taking care not to damage the fragile Descemet's membrane); this removes the VES and any debris.

The surgeon sutures the graft with 16 passes of 10-0 nylon. The level of donor and host corneas should be the same for perfect alignment.

Another exciting development is the use of the femtosecond laser, which creates a perfect round trephination and can be used with the Big Bubble technique.[123]

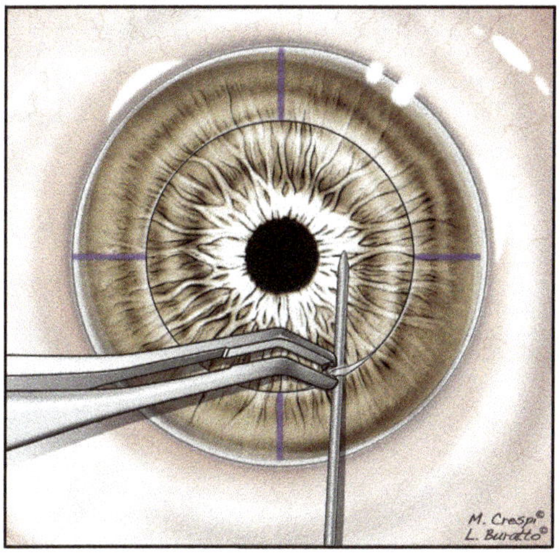

Figure 17-26. During DALK, the surgeon inserts a cannula or a 27-gauge needle on a 5-mL syringe filled with filtered air, into the stromal layer as far as the pupillary edge, for a relatively long distance.

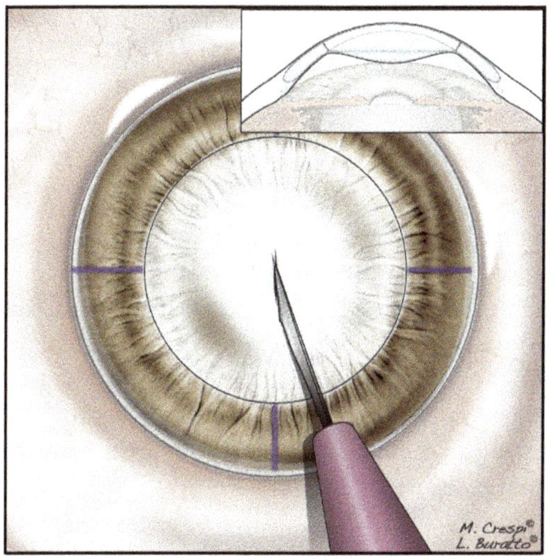

Figure 17-27. Incision of the stroma at its steepest point.

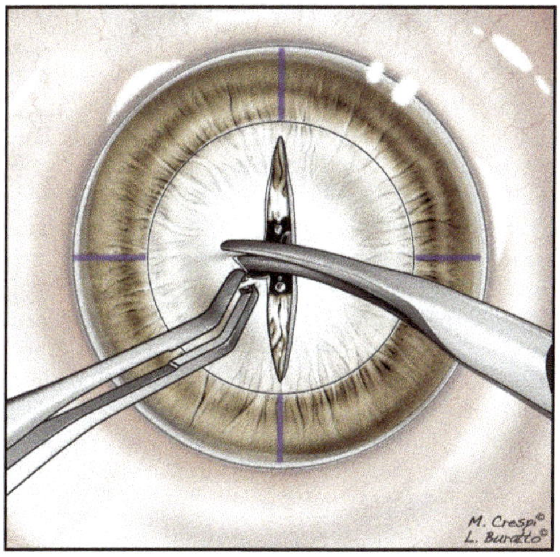

Figure 17-28. The stroma is cut into 4 quadrants with long blunt scissors, using an upward movement.

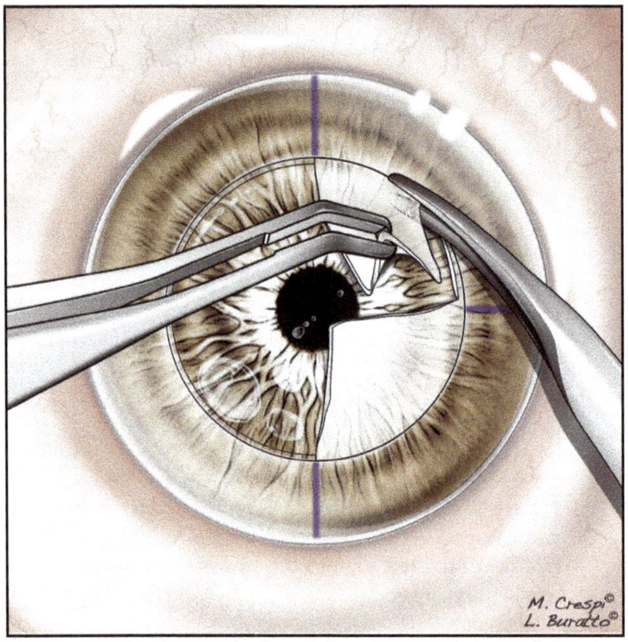

Figure 17-29. Removal of peripheral corneal tissue following the curve that has been created.

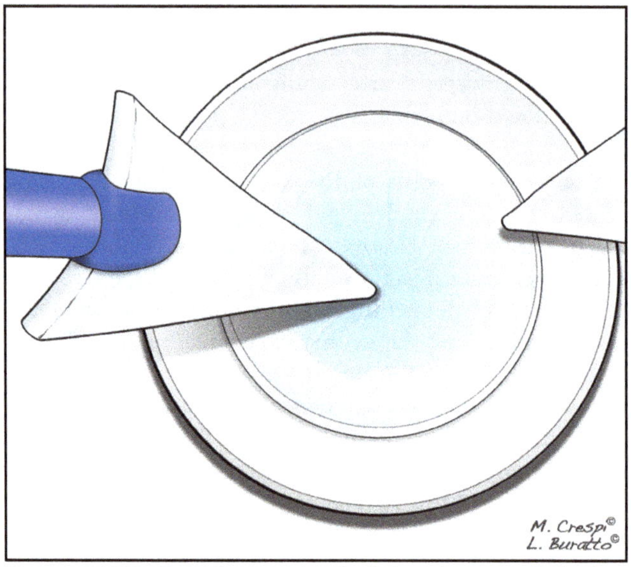

Figure 17-30. Complete removal of the donor endothelium using 2 dry, stiff sponge tips (Merocel).

Conclusion

We recently have seen an increasing trend to perform one or more procedures in the same operating session. This trend continues with combination treatments for cataracts and corneal pathologies. Currently, it is possible to successfully combine cataract surgery with different types of keratoplasty: penetrating, anterior lamellar, or posterior lamellar with improved visual results and a more rapid functional recovery.

References

1. Fine M. Therapeutic keratoplasty and Fuchs' dystrophy. *Am J Ophthalmol.* 1964;57: 371-378.
2. Lindstrom RL, Harris WS, Doughman DJ. Combined penetrating keratoplasty, extracapsular cataract extraction, and posterior chamber intraocular lens implantation. *J Am Intraocular Implant Soc.* 1981;7:130-132.
3. Hunkeler JD, Hyde LL. The triple procedure: combined penetrating Keratoplasty, extracapsular cataract extraction, and posterior chamber intraocular lens implantation: an expanded experience. *J Am Intraocular Implant Soc.* 1983;9:20-24.
4. Kramer SG. Penetrating keratoplasty combined with extracapsular cataract extraction. *Am J Ophthalmol.* 1985;100:129-133.
5. Binder PS. The triple procedure: refractive result. 1985 update. *Ophthalmology.* 1986; 93:1482-1488.
6. Crawford GJ, Stulting RD, Waring GO, et al. The triple procedure: analysis of outcome Refraction, and intraocular lens calculation. *Ophthalmology.* 1986;93:817-824.
7. Busin M, Arffa RC, McDonald MB, et al. Combined penetrating keratoplasty, extracapsular cataract extraction, and posterior chamber intraocular lens implantation. *Ophthalmology Surg.* 1987;18:272-275.
8. Meyer RF, Musch DC. Assessment of success and complication of triple procedure. *Surgery. Am J Ophthalmol.* 1987;104:233-240.
9. Yamagami S, Suzuki Y, Ohya T, Murao M, Miyata K, Tsuru T. Statistic evaluation of prognostic risk factor in penetrating keratoplasty using Cox multiple regression model. *Nihon Ganka Gakkai Zasshi.* 1994;98:777-781.
10. The Australian Corneal Graft Registry: 1990 to 1992 report. *Aust NZ Ophthalmol.* 1993;21:1-48.
11. Craing MT, Olson RJ, Mamalis N. Air bubble endothelial damage during phacoemulsification in human eye bank eyes: the protective effects of Healon and Viscoat. *J Cataract Refract Surg.* 1990;16:597-602.
12. Koch DD, Liu JF, Glasser DB, Merin LM, Haft E. A comparison of corneal endothelial changes after use of Healon or Viscoat during phacoemulsification. *Am J Ophthalmol.* 1993;115:188-201.
13. Lucena DR, Ribeiro MS, Messias A, Bicas HE, Scott IU, Jorge R. Comparison of corneal changes after phacoemulsification using BSS Plus versus Lactated Ringer's irrigating solution: a prospective randomised trial. *Br J Ophthalmol.* 2011;95(4):485-489.
14. Yamazoe K, Yamaguchi T, Hotta K, et al. Outcomes of cataract surgery in eyes with a low corneal endothelial cell density. *J Cataract Refract Surg.* 2011;37(12):2130-2136.
15. Hayashi K, Yoshida M, Manabe S, Hirata A. Cataract surgery in eyes with low corneal endothelial cell density. *J Cataract Refract Surg.* 2011;37(8):1419-1425.
16. Wilczynski M, Supady E, Loba P, Synder A, Palenga-Pydyn D, Omulecki W. Comparison of early corneal endothelial cell loss after coaxial phacoemulsification through 1.8 mm microincision and bimanual phacoemulsification through 1.7 mm microincision. *J Cataract Refract Surg.* 2009;35(9):1570-1574.
17. Seitzman GD, Gottsch JD, Stark WJ. Cataract surgery in patients with Fuchs' corneal dystrophy: expanding recommendations for cataract surgery without simultaneous keratoplasty. *Ophthalmology.* 2005;112(3):441-446.

18. Seitzman GD. Cataract surgery in Fuchs' dystrophy. *Curr Opin Ophthalmol.* 2005;16(4):241-245.
19. Traish AS, Colby KA. Approaching cataract surgery in patients with fuchs' endothelial dystrophy. *Int Ophthalmol Clin.* 2010;50(1):1-11.
20. Van den Bruel A, Gailly J, Devriese S, Welton NJ, Shortt AJ, Vrijens F. The protective effect of ophthalmic viscoelastic devices on endothelial cell loss during cataract surgery: a meta-analysis using mixed treatment comparisons. *Br J Ophthalmol.* 2011;95(1):5-10.
21. Bourne RR, Minassian DC, Dart JK, Rosen P, Kaushal S, Wingate N. Effect of cataract surgery on the corneal endothelium: modern phacoemulsification compared with extracapsular cataract surgery. *Ophthalmology.* 2004;111(4):679-685.
22. Gogate P, Ambardekar P, Kulkarni S, Deshpande R, Joshi S, Deshpande M. Comparison of endothelial cell loss after cataract surgery: phacoemulsification versus manual small-incision cataract surgery: six-week results of a randomized control trial. *J Cataract Refract Surg.* 2010;36(2):247-253.
23. Díaz-Valle D, Benítez del Castillo Sánchez JM, Castillo A, Sayagués O, Moriche M. Endothelial damage with cataract surgery techniques. *J Cataract Refract Surg.* 1998;24(7):951-955.
24. Walkow T, Anders N, Klebe S. Endothelial cell loss after phacoemulsification: relation to preoperative and intraoperative parameters. *J Cataract Refract Surg.* 2000;26(5):727-732.
25. Bourne WM, Nelson LR, Hodge DO. Continued endothelial cell loss ten years after lens implantation. *Ophthalmology.* 1994;101:1014-1022.
26. Zacks CM, Abbott RI, Fine M. Long-term changes in corneal endothelium after keratoplasty. *Cornea.* 1990;9:92-97.
27. Binder PS. Intraocular lens implantation after penetrating keratoplasty. *Refract Corneal Surg.* 1989;5:224-230.
28. Acar BT, Buttanri IB, Sevim MS, Acar S. Corneal endothelial cell loss in post-penetrating keratoplasty patients after cataract surgery: phacoemulsification versus planned extracapsular cataract extraction. *J Cataract Refract Surg.* 2011;37(8):1512-1516.
29. Leccisotti A, Islam T, McGilligan VE, Moore TC. Phacoemulsification after deep anterior lamellar keratoplasty. *Eur J Ophthalmol.* 2010;20(4):680-683.
30. Nagra PK, Rapuano CJ, Laibson PL, Kunimoto DY, Kay M, Cohen EJ. Cataract extraction following penetrating keratoplasty. *Cornea.* 2004;23(4):377-379.
31. Parmar P, Salman A, Kalavathy CM, Thomas PA, Jesudasan CA. Outcome analysis of cataract surgery following therapeutic keratoplasty. *Cornea.* 2005;24(2):123-129.
32. Dangel ME, Kirkham SM, Phipps MJ. Posterior capsule opacification in extracapsular cataract extraction and the triple procedure. *Ophthalmic Surg.* 1994;25:82-87.
33. Hsiao CH, Chen JJ, Chen PY, Chen HS. Intraocular lens implantation after penetrating keratoplasty. *Cornea.* 2001;20:580-585.
34. Geggel HS. Intraocular lens implantation after penetrating keratoplasty improved unaided visual acuity, astigmatism, and safety in patients with combined corneal disease and cataract. *Ophthalmology.* 1990;97:1460-1467.
35. Davis EA, Stark WJ. The triple procedure: is it the best approach for the patient? The triple procedure may be superior to sequential surgery. *Arch Ophthalmol.* 2000;118(3):414-415.
36. Hammil MB. Sequential surgery may be the best approach for the patient. *Arch Ophthalmol.* 2000;118:415-417.
37. Malbran ES, Malbran E Jr, Malbran J. In favour of the triple procedure. *Arch Ophthalmol.* 2001;119(8):1223-1224.
38. Nguyen NX, Langenbucher A, Seitz B, et al. Blood aqueous barrier breakdown after penetrating keratoplasty with simultaneous extracapsular cataract extraction and posterior chamber lens implantation. *Graefes Arch Clin Exp Ophthalmol.* 2001;239(2):114-117.
39. Flowers CW, McLeod SD, McDonnell PJ, et al. Evaluation of intraocular lens power calculation formulas in the triple procedure. *J Cataract Refract Surg.* 1996;22:116-122.
40. Vajpayee RB, Angra SK, Honavar SG. Combined keratoplasty cataract extraction and intraocular lens implantation after corneolenticular laceration in children. *Am J Ophthalmol.* 1994;17:507-511.
41. Martin TP, Reed JW, Legault C, et al. Cataract formation and cataract extraction after penetrating keratoplasty. *Ophthalmology.* 1994;101:101-103.
42. de Chaenace B, Guidi M, Valiere-Vialeiz JP. Short, medium and long-term post-operative complications in 150 patients undergoing penetrating keratoplasty after one year. *Ophthalmology.* 1989;3:11-12.
43. Payant JA, Gordon LW, VanderZwaag R, et al. Cataract formation following corneal transplantation in eyes with Fuchs' endothelial dystrophy. *Cornea.* 1990;9:286-289.
44. Muraine M, Gueudry J, Retout A, Genevois O. Keratoplasty combined with cataract surgery [in French]. *J Fr Ophthalmol.* 2012;35(7):546-554.
45. Price MO, Price FW Jr. Cataract progression and treatment following posterior lamellar keratoplasty. *J Cataract Refract Surg.* 2004;30(6):1310-1315.
46. Acar BT, Utine CA, Acar S, Ciftci F. Endothelial cell loss after phacoemulsification in eyes with previous penetrating keratoplasty, previous deep anterior lamellar keratoplasty, or no previous surgery. *J Cataract Refract Surg.* 2011;37(11):2013-2017.
47. Hayashi K, Hayashi H. Simultaneous versus sequential penetrating keratoplasty and cataract surgery. *Cornea.* 2006;25(9):1020-1025.
48. Isager P, Hjortdal JO, Ehlers N. Stability of graft refractive power after penetrating keratoplasty. *Acta Ophthalmol Scand.* 2000;78:623.
49. Nguyen DQ, Mumford LL, Jones MN, et al. The visual and refractive outcomes of combined and sequential penetrating keratoplasty, cataract extraction, and intraocular lens insertion. *Eye (Lond).* 2009;23(6):1295-1301.
50. Das S, Langenbucher A, Jacobi C, et al. Long-term refractive and visual outcome after penetrating keratoplasty only versus the triple procedure in Fuchs' dystrophy. *Graefes Arch Clin Exp Ophthalmol.* 2006;244(9):1089-1095.
51. Bersudsky V, Rehany U, Rumelt S. Risk factors for failure of simultaneous penetrating keratoplasty and cataract extraction. *J Cataract Refract Surg.* 2004;30(9):1940-1947.
52. Green M, Chow A, Apel A. Outcomes of combined penetrating keratoplasty and cataract extraction compared with penetrating keratoplasty alone. *Clin Exp Ophthalmol.* 2007;35(4):324-329.
53. Pineros OE, Cohen EJ, Rapuano CJ, Laibson PR. Triple vs nonsimultaneous procedures in Fuchs' dystrophy and cataract. *Arch Ophthalmol.* 1996;114(5):525-528.
54. Shimmura S, Ohashi Y, Shiroma H, Shimazaki J, Tsubota K. Corneal opacity and cataract: triple procedure versus secondary approach. *Cornea.* 2003;22(3):234-238.
55. Cazabon S, Quah SA, Jones MN, Batterbury M, Kaye SB. Sequential versus combined penetrating keratoplasty and cataract surgery. *Optom Vis Sci.* 2010;87(7):482-486.
56. Alhassan MB, Kyari F, Ejere HO. Peribulbar versus retrobulbar anaesthesia for cataract surgery. *Cochrane Database Syst Rev.* 2008;Jul 16(3):CD004083.
57. Muraine M, Calenda E, Watt L, et al. Peribulbar anaesthesia during keratoplasty: a prospective study of 100 cases. *Br J Ophthalmol.* 1999;83(1):104-1049.
58. Davis DB, Mandel MR. Posterior peribulbar anesthesia: an alternative to retrobulbar anesthesia. *J Cataract Refract Surg.* 1986;12:182-184.
59. Malbran ES, Malbran E, Buonsanti J, et al. Closed-system phacoemulsification and posterior chamber implant combined with penetrating keratoplasty. *Ophthalmic Surg.* 1993;24:403-406.

60. Keates RH, Rothchild EJ, Bloom R. Endocapsular triple procedure: a new triple procedure technique. *J Cataract Refract Surg.* 1984;15:332-335.
61. Gloor B, Kalman A. Choroidal effusion and expulsive hemorrhage in penetrating interventions: lesson from 26 patients. *Klin Monbl Augenheilkd.* 1993;202(3):224-237.
62. Kalman A. Choroidal effusion and expulsive hemorrhage in penetrating inverventions-lessonsbfrom 26 patients. *Klin Monbl Augenheilkd.* 1992;11:509-513.
63. Egger SF, Huber-Spitzy V, Scholda C, Schneider B, Grabner G. Bacterial contamination during extracapsular cataract extraction: prospective study on 200 consecutive patients. *Ophthalmologica.* 1994;208:767-781.
64. Boke W. Phacoemulsification. Why? Klin Monbl Augenheilkd 1990;197:100-105.
65. Ohrloff C. Comparison of phacoemulsification and planned extracapsular cataract extraction. *Klin Monbl Augenheilkd.* 1993;203:93-98.
66. Baca LS, Epstein RJ. Closed-chamber capsulorhexis for cataract extraction combined with penetrating keratoplasty. *J Cataract Refract Surg.* 1998;24(5):581-584.
67. Nardi M, Giudice V, Marabotti A, Alfieri E, Rizzo S. Temporary graft for closed-system cataract surgery during corneal triple procedures. *J Cataract Refract Surg.* 2001;27(8):1172-1175.
68. Menapace R, Skorpik C, Grasl M. Modified triple procedure using a temporary keratoprosthesis for closed-system, small-incision cataract surgery. *J Cataract Refract Surg.* 1990;16(2):230-234.
69. Duncker G, Eckardt C. Modified temporary keratoprosthesis in the triple procedure: a new surgical technique. *J Cataract Refract Surg.* 1988;14(4):434-436.
70. Wang HS. Management of a posterior capsule rupture in planned extracapsular cataract extraction and posterior chamber lens implantation. *J Cataract Refract Surg.* 2001;27(8):1172-1175.
71. Lee WB, Jacobs DS, Musch DC, Kaufman SC, Reinhart WJ, Shtein RM. Descemet's stripping endothelial keratoplasty: safety and outcomes: a report by the American Academy of Ophthalmology. *Ophthalmology.* 2009;116(9):1818-1830.
72. Katz HR, Forster RK. Intraocular lens calculation in combined penetrating keratoplasty, cataract extraction and intraocular lens implantation. *Ophthalmology.* 1985;92(9):1203-1207.
73. Davis EA, Azar DT, Jakobs FM, Stark WJ. Refractive and keratometric results after the triple procedure: experience with early and late suture removal. *Ophthalmology.* 1998;105(4):624-630.
74. Terry MA, Ousley PJ. Small-incision deep lamellar endothelial keratoplasty (DLEK): six-month results in the first prospective clinical study. *Cornea.* 2005;24(1):59-65.
75. Fang JP, Hamill MB. Descemet's stripping endothelial keratoplasty under topical anesthesia. *J Cataract Refract Surg.* 2007;33(2):187-188.
76. Oberg TJ, Sikder S, Jorgensen AJ, Mifflin MD. Topical-intracameral anesthesia without preoperative mydriatic agents for Descemet-stripping automated endothelial keratoplasty and phacoemulsification cataract surgery with intraocular lens implantation. *J Cataract Refract Surg.* 2012;38(3):384-386.
77. Jun B, Kuo AN, Afshari NA, Carlson AN, Kim T. Refractive change after descemet stripping automated endothelial keratoplasty surgery and its correlation with graft thickness and diameter. *Cornea.* 2009;28(1):19-23.
78. Koenig SB, Covert DJ. Early results of small-incision Descemet's stripping and automated endothelial keratoplasty. *Ophthalmology.* 2007;114(2):221-226.
79. Price MO, Price FW Jr. Descemet's stripping with endothelial keratoplasty: comparative outcomes with microkeratome-dissected and manually dissected donor tissue. *Ophthalmology.* 2006;113(11):1936-1942.
80. Rao SK, Leung CK, Cheung CY, et al. Descemet stripping endothelial keratoplasty: effect of the surgical procedure on corneal optics. *Am J Ophthalmol.* 2008;145(6):991-996.
81. Yoo SH, Kymionis GD, Deobhakta AA, et al. One-year results and anterior segment optical coherence tomography findings of descemet stripping automated endothelial keratoplasty combined with phacoemulsification. *Arch Ophthalmol.* 2008;126(8):1052-1055.
82. Covert DJ, Koenig SB. New triple procedure: Descemet's stripping and automated endothelial keratoplasty combined with phacoemulsification and intraocular lens implantation. *Ophthalmology.* 2007;114(7):1272-1277.
83. Terry MA, Saad HA, Shamie N, et al. Endothelial keratoplasty: the influence of insertion techniques and incision size on donor endothelial survival. *Cornea.* 2009;28(1):24-31.
84. Chen ES, Shamie N, Terry MA, Phillips PM. Busin glide vs forceps in Descemet stripping automated endothelial keratoplasty: not all forceps insertions are created equal. *Am J Ophthalmol.* 2009;148(1):175; author reply 175-176.
85. Gangwani V, Obi A, Hollick EJ. A prospective study comparing EndoGlide and Busin glide insertion techniques in descemet stripping endothelial keratoplasty. *Am J Ophthalmol.* 2012;153(1):38-43.
86. Busin M, Bhatt PR, Scorcia V. A modified technique for descemet membrane stripping automated endothelial keratoplasty to minimize endothelial cell loss. *Arch Ophthalmol.* 2008;126(8):1133-1137.
87. Chen ES, Terry MA, Shamie N, Hoar KL, Friend DJ. Precut tissue in Descemet's stripping automated endothelial keratoplasty donor characteristics and early postoperative complications. *Ophthalmology.* 2008;115(3):497-502.
88. Lee JK, Eghrari AO, Desai NR, Stark WJ, Gottsch JD. Presoaking donor corneas reduces graft detachment rates in descemet stripping endothelial keratoplasty. *Am J Ophthalmol.* 2009;147(3):439-441.
89. Terry MA. Endothelial keratoplasty: a comparison of complication rates and endothelial survival between precut tissue and surgeon-cut tissue by a single DSAEK surgeon. *Trans Am Ophthalmol Soc.* 2009;107:184-191.
90. Terry MA, Shamie N, Chen ES, et al. Endothelial keratoplasty for Fuchs' dystrophy with cataract: complications and clinical results with the new triple procedure. *Ophthalmology.* 2009;116(4):631-639.
91. Taylor DM, Stern AL, McDonald P. The triple procedure: 2 to 10 year follow-up. *Trans Am Ophthalmol Soc.* 1986;84:221-249.
92. Sanford DK, Klesges LM, Wood TO. Simultaneous penetrating keratoplasty, extracapsular cataract extraction, and intraocular lens implantation. *J Cataract Refract Surg.* 1991;17(6):824-829.
93. Mattax JB, McCulley JP. The effect of standardized keratoplasty technique on IOL power calculation for the triple procedure. *Acta Ophthalmol.* 1989;192(suppl):24-29.
94. Djalilian AR, George JE, Doughman DJ, Holland EJ. Comparison between the refractive results of combined penetrating keratoplasty/transsclerally sutured posterior chamber lens implantation and the triple procedure. *Cornea.* 1997;16(3):319-321.
95. Geerards AJ, Hassmann E, Beekhuis WH, Remeyer L, van Rij G, Rijneveld WJ. Triple procedure; analysis of outcome, refraction, and intraocular lens power calculation. *Br J Ophthalmol.* 1997;81(9):774-777.
96. Padmanabhan P, Warade SK, Sejpal K. New endothelial keratoplasty, phacoemulsification, and intraocular lens implantation triple procedure: comparison with conventional triple procedure. *J Cataract Refract Surg.* 2010;36(7):1142-1148.
97. Suh LH, Yoo SH, Deobhakta A, et al. Complications of Descemet's stripping with automated endothelial keratoplasty: survey of 118 eyes at One Institute. *Ophthalmology.* 2008;115(9):1517-1524.

98. Naveiras M, Dirisamer M, Parker J, et al. Causes of glaucoma after Descemet membrane endothelial keratoplasty. *Am J Ophthalmol.* 2012;153(5):958-966.
99. Neff KD, Biber JM, Holland EJ. Comparison of central corneal graft thickness to visual acuity outcomes in endothelial keratoplasty. *Cornea.* 2011;30(4):388-391.
100. Wood TO. Lamellar transplants in keratoconus. *Am J Ophthalmol.* 1977;83(4):543-545.
101. Richard JM, Paton D, Gasset AR. A comparison of penetrating keratoplasty and lamellar keratoplasty in the surgical management of keratoconus. *Am J Ophthalmol.* 1978;86(6): 807-811.
102. Gasset AR. Lamellar keratoplasty in the treatment of keratoconus: conectomy. *Ophthalmic Surg.* 1979;10(2):26-33.
103. Benson WH, Goosey CB, Prager TC, Goosey JD. Visual improvement as a function of time after lamellar keratoplasty for keratoconus. *Am J Ophthalmol.* 1993;116(2):207-211.
104. Shimazaki J, Shimmura S, Ishioka M, Tsubota K. Randomized clinical trial of deep lamellar keratoplasty vs penetrating keratoplasty. *Am J Ophthalmol.* 2002;134(2):159-165.
105. Aggarwal RK. Deep lamellar keratoplasty: an alternative to penetrating keratoplasty. *Br J Ophthalmol.* 1997;81(3):178-179.
106. Ilango B. Comparative cohort study of the outcomes of deep lamellar keratoplasty and penetrating keratoplasty for keratoconus. *Eye (Lond).* 2007;21(3):447; author reply, 447.
107. Jhanji V, Sharma N, Vajpayee RB. Management of keratoconus: current scenario. *Br J Ophthalmol.* 2011;95(8):1044-1050.
108. Reinhart WJ, Musch DC, Jacobs DS, Lee WB, Kaufman SC, Shtein RM. Deep anterior lamellar keratoplasty as an alternative to penetrating keratoplasty a report by the American Academy of Ophthalmology. *Ophthalmology.* 2011;118(1): 209-218.
109. Panda A, Sethi HS, Jain M, Nindra Krishna S, Gupta AK. Deep anterior lamellar keratoplasty with phacoemulsification. *J Cataract Refract Surg.* 2011;37(1):122-126.
110. Muraine MC, Collet A, Brasseur G. Deep lamellar keratoplasty combined with cataract surgery. *Arch Ophthalmol.* 2002;120(6):812-815.
111. Senoo T. Combined surgery with deep lamellar keratoplasty. *Semin Ophthalmol.* 2001;16(3):126-136.
112. Hirano K, Sugita J, Kobayashi M. Separation of corneal stroma and Descemet's membrane during deep lamellar keratoplasty. *Cornea.* 2002;21(2):196-199.
113. The cornea and the sclera. In: Fine BS, Yanoff M, eds. *Ocular Histology.* Hagerstown, MD: Harper and Row; 1979:163-192.
114. Price FW Jr. Air lamellar keratoplasty. Refract *Corneal Surg.* 1989;5(4):240-243.
115. Anwar M, Teichmann KD. Deep lamellar keratoplasty: surgical techniques for anterior lamellar keratoplasty with and without baring of Descemet's membrane. *Cornea.* 2002;21(4):374-383.
116. Alio JL, Shah S, Barraquer C, Bilgihan K, Anwar M, Melles GR. New techniques in lamellar keratoplasty. *Curr Opin Ophthalmol.* 2002;13(4):224-229.
117. Manche EE, Holland GN, Maloney RK. Deep lamellar keratoplasty using viscoelastic dissection. *Arch Ophthalmol.* 1999;117(11):1561-1565.
118. Amayem AF, Anwar M. Fluid lamellar keratoplasty in keratoconus. *Ophthalmology.* 2000;107(1):76-79.
119. Terry MA. The evolution of lamellar grafting techniques over twenty-five years. *Cornea.* 2000;19(5):611-616.
120. Hanna KD, David T, Besson J, Pouliquen Y. Lamellar keratoplasty with the Barraquer microkeratome. *Refract Corneal Surg.* 1991;7(2):177-181.
121. Haimovici R, Culbertson WW. Optical lamellar keratoplasty using the barraquer microkeratome. *Refract Corneal Surg.* 1991;7(1):42-45.
122. Barraquer JI. Lamellar keratoplasty. (Special techniques). *Ann Ophthalmol.* 1972;4(6):437-469.
123. Lee D, Kim JH, Oh SH, Choi SK, Kim JK. Femtosecond laser lamellar keratoplasty to aid visualization for cataract surgery. *J Refract Surg.* 2009;25(10):902-904.

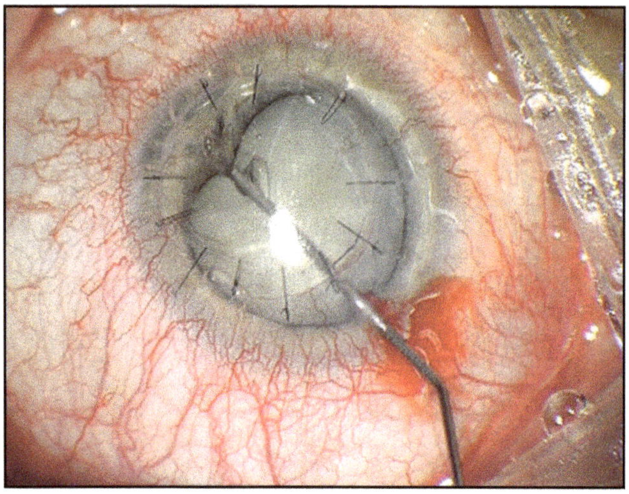

H-1. Hard/mature cataract in penetrating keratoplasty. (Reprinted with permission of Boris Malyugin.)

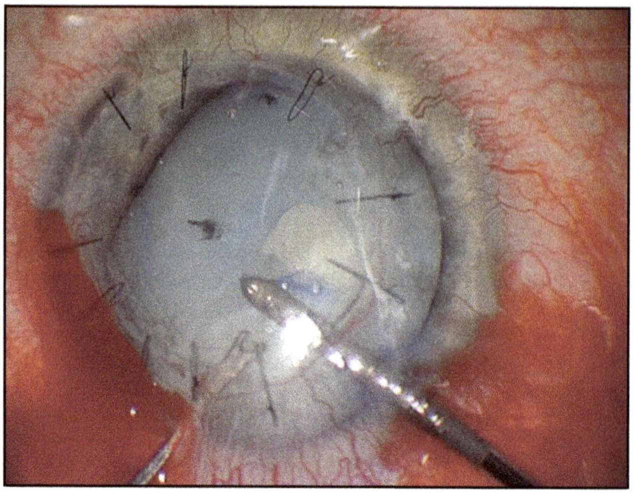

H-2. When the synecchiae have been detached, the capsule is colored with trypan blue and the capsulotomy is performed; the capsulotomy procedure is well controlled by the surgeon. (Reprinted with permission of Boris Malyugin.)

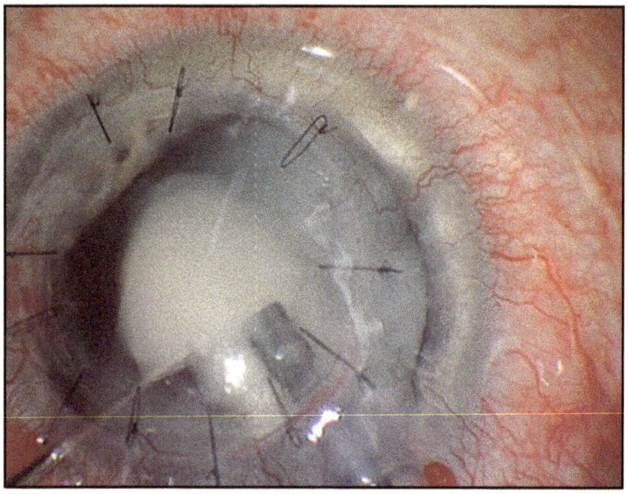

H-3. Phacoemulsification follows. (Reprinted with permission of Boris Malyugin.)

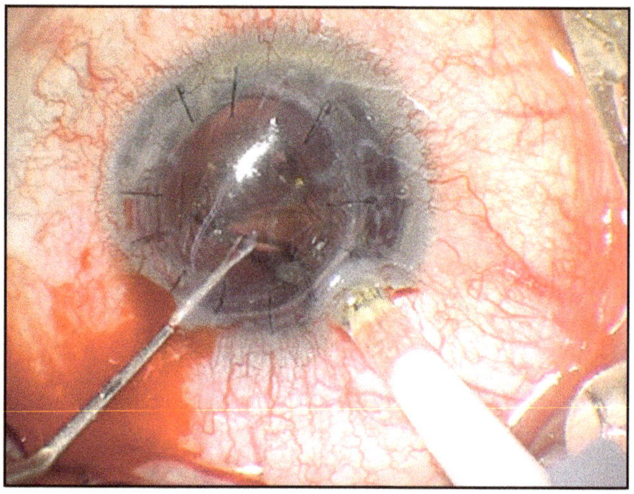

H-4. Implantation of the IOL. (Reprinted with permission of Boris Malyugin.)

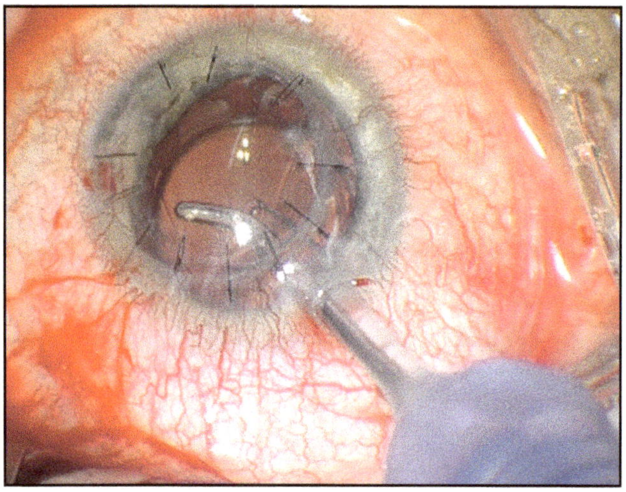

H-5. Removal of the VES. (Reprinted with permission of Boris Malyugin.)

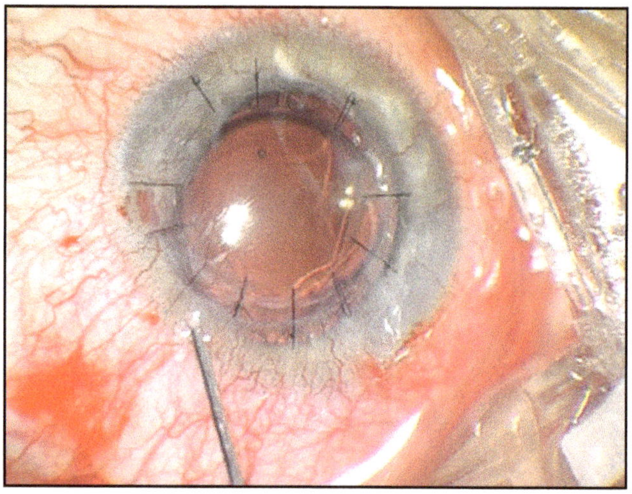

H-6. Final appearance of the surgery. (Reprinted with permission of Boris Malyugin.)

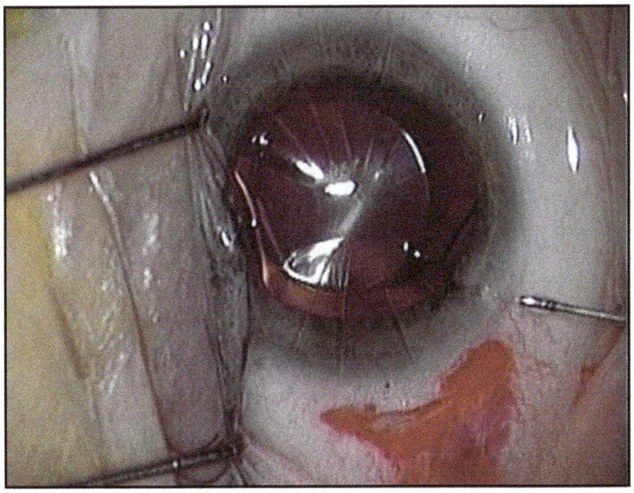

I-1. Cataract surgery in RK eye with 16 incisions: there were no complications with the phaco procedure and the implantation of the IOL in the PC.

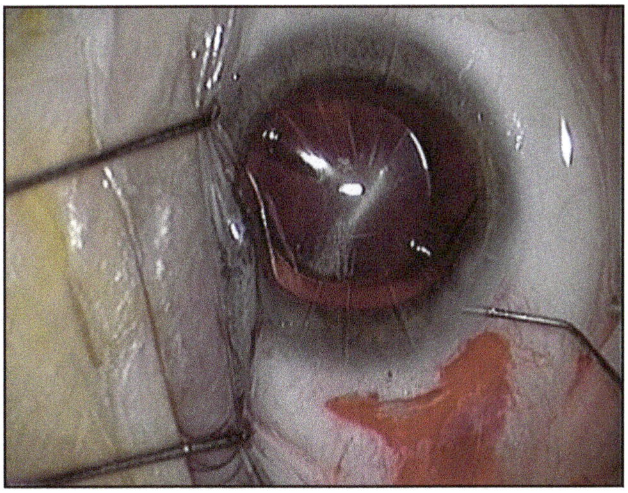

I-2. Hydroclosure of a secondary incision.

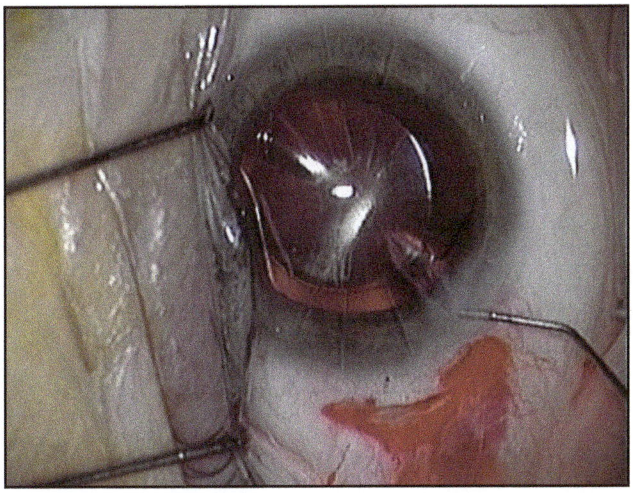

I-3. One of the incisions of the RK procedure, performed 18 years before, opens.

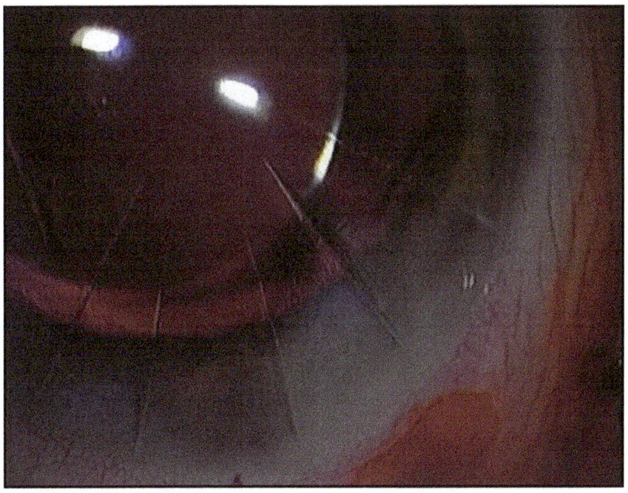

I-4. A suture may be positioned; in this case, must not create traction, otherwise the nearby incisions may open.

18

Cataract Surgery Following Implantation of a Phakic Intraocular Lens

For a number of years, implantation of a phakic intraocular lens (IOL) has been a valid option for the correction of myopic and hyperopic refractive errors in phakic eyes, in addition to correcting residual refractive error associated with cataract surgery.

The refractive IOL for phakic eyes (P-IOL) has been designed for implantation in eyes with a clear lens to correct refractive errors while maintaining accommodation. The IOLs used to correct myopia have negative power, those for the correction of hyperopia have positive power, and toric lenses are used for astigmatism. Refractive correction with P-IOLs is associated with numerous advantages even in eyes with significant refractive error: they are straightforward, potentially the error can be corrected, they are associated with visual rehabilitation, the refractive correction achieved is stable, and the pre-existing curvature and integrity of the cornea and accommodation are preserved. This is more evident in the correction of high myopia and hyperopia, in which surgery with excimer laser has been associated with problems of night vision, regression, and poor optical quality of the remodeled cornea.[1-5]

P-IOLs are used mostly in the treatment of myopia in excess of a −8.00 diopters (D) and hyperopia in excess of +4.00 D.

Some authors continue to question the long-term safety and efficacy of the P-IOLs. This is despite the fact that there are several publications that confirm efficacy, predictability, and stability of the P-IOL in the correction of high myopia and more recently high hyperopia.[1,3-18] These publications include a report by the American Academy of Ophthalmology published in 2009 on the correction of high myopia with a P-IOL[3] and an important paper by Cochrane published in 2010[4] reporting results of treatment with an excimer laser and with a P-IOL in the correction of moderate and high myopia. In particular, this study reported that P-IOLs are safer than using an excimer laser for the correction of myopia ranging from −6.00 to −20.00 D; they are associated with a lower risk of retinal detachment than refractive removal of the clear lens, and patients prefer them. This paper also reports that the P-IOL for high myopia (> 7.00 D) can also be safely implanted in the eyes of patients with moderate myopia (< 7.00 D).

Further evidence supporting safety of P-IOLs was published recently in a report[11] in which the authors described the case of a patient implanted 18 years previously with a first-generation posterior phakic chamber IOL (PC-P-IOL; Fyodorov's IOL) who had a low endothelial cell count; however, there were no signs of cataract or other complications.

Nevertheless, implantation of an anterior or posterior refractive IOL in phakic eyes still raises many questions about potential long-term risks for the normal crystalline lens, the corneal endothelium, the anterior uvea, and other ocular structures.[3,16-21] Complications are rare and associated predominantly with the position and the type of P-IOL. The main complications of the initial (Baikoff) IOL for the anterior chamber (AC) with angle support are glare, haloes, pupillary ovalization, and loss of endothelium cells.[7,11,15,16] The complications associated with the AC P-IOL with iris fixation are mainly chronic subclinical inflammation, endothelial cell loss, dislocation, and glaucoma from pupillary block (without an iridectomy). Finally, complications associated with the PC-P-IOL are in particular anterior subcapsular cataract, pigment dispersion and dislocation, and glaucoma from pupil block.

Numerous articles have been written regarding potential damage to the corneal endothelium by the AC phakic lenses, especially with the first models of these lenses.[3,16-26]

Buratto L, Brint SF, Caretti L.
Cataract Surgery in Complicated Cases (pp 203-211).

As mentioned before, cataracts can develop with these lenses, though this is a rare occurrence.[3,16-20,27-33] In a recent meta-analysis,[27] new-onset or progression of existing cataract was seen in 4.35% of cases (6338 eyes). The incidence of cataract depended on the type of IOL: 1.29% with AC-IOL, 1.11% with an iris-fixated IOL, and 9.6% with a PC-IOL. For the PC-IOLs, the early formation of cataract is frequently associated with surgical trauma, while late-onset cataracts are caused by contact between the IOL and the crystalline lens.

Two types of cataract are associated with the P-IOL: anterior subcapsular and nuclear. In a study from 2003 that examined the development of cataract associated with implantation of a P-IOL in the posterior chamber,[34] the anterior subcapsular is the most frequent and does not tend to progress rapidly, while the nuclear cataract has greater impact in visual terms and is frequently progressive.

It should be remembered that high myopia alone can be a predisposing factor for cataract formation,[35] and the cataract can develop independent of implantation of a P-IOL. Actually, cataract is 4 times more frequent in patients with high myopia compared to the incidence in the general population.

Nevertheless, despite the various reports in the literature that describe complications associated with the P-IOL, the currently available models are considerably safer than the previous models.

Coexistence of a P-IOL and a cataract is a new challenge for surgeons. Factors involved in formation of the cataract following implantation of a P-IOL are still not clear. In order to understand the clinical factors associated with development of the cataract, the surgical result from cataract surgery and the appropriate way of preserving best-corrected visual acuity, we have to clarify the differences of the models of P-IOL, the technical modifications, including explantation of the IOL and phacoemulsification, a topic on which just a few articles have been published, dealing with a small number of cases.

Types of Phakic Intraocular Lenses

As mentioned earlier, a P-IOL can usually be implanted in 3 different fixation sites:

1. In the angle of the AC
2. On the iris surface
3. In the posterior chamber (PC)

Each of the these has its supporters, its specific insertion methods, and its complications.

Cataract Development Following the Implant of the Phakic Intraocular Lens

The cataract can develop as a complication of other procedures of the anterior segment. There are several possible reasons why the lens becomes opaque following the implantation of a P-IOL, and these may differ depending on the model implanted.

Cataracts may also form for reasons not related directly to the implantation of the P-IOL.

Myopic eyes may prematurely develop a cataract following implantation of a P-IOL; some studies[28,31,36] and an unpublished report by Buratto report on the presence of nuclear cataracts in eyes implanted with a P-IOL for the AC (angle support or iris fixation) to correct high myopia. Various authors reported that predisposing factors were patients 40 years of age and older when implanted with a P-IOL and an axial length greater than 30 mm.

It is well-known that nuclear cataracts are more common in highly myopic eyes (see Chapter 8), and one of the early signs may be an increase in the optic power of the myopic eye (induced myopia). Nuclear sclerosis is difficult to recognize early; in some cases, it may actually be the first step in the development of a nuclear cataract. Thus, the surgeon should look for this prior to suggesting implantation of the P-IOL.[36]

Moreover, accidental damage to the lens during the insertion of a P-IOL can lead to the formation of a focal cataract.

Laser iridotomy or surgical iridectomy, mandatory surgeries to avoid glaucoma from pupillary block, can cause opacification of the lens. Normally, the opaque areas are small, localized, and not progressive.

Other ocular pathologies such as uveitis and postoperative inflammation can induce cataract formation. It is possible that higher subclinical values of flare, reported in the AC in myopic eyes with implantation of the AC P-IOL, could also be a factor in the early development of cataract in these eyes.

Other factors include therapies (with cortisone), metabolic dysfunctions (diabetes, hypocalcemia), trauma, familial predisposition, and other systemic disorders.[37,38]

Specific Causes Correlated to the Implantable Contact Lens for the Posterior Chamber

Accidental damage to the lens during the insertion of the IOL can produce an early anterior subcapsular focal cataract that is often of little clinical importance. Moreover, contact between the implantable contact lens (ICL) and the capsule surrounding the lens can chronically alter the metabolic state of the lens and with time produce a nonmechanical cataract.

The anterior subcapsular cataract that may develop with implantation of an ICL is caused by poor vaulting (spacing) of the lens,[39,40] as confirmed by examination with optical coherence tomography (OCT) of the anterior segment and consequent fibroblastic metaplasia of the lens epithelial cells, as shown by histopathological studies.[30] For this reason, the recent designs of the phakic ICL for the PC have a significant vault with 200 to 300 microns of space between the anterior capsule of the lens and the ICL.[29,39-41] Currently, 230 microns is the minimum central vaulting necessary to give the ICL a safe overall space that will avoid contact between the ICL and the lens.[29] This is slightly greater than the minimal measurement of 150 microns considered in the past by Gonvers et al.[39]

In a study reported some time ago, Trindade et al[42] reported contact demonstrated in 6 eyes with ICL examined with ultrasound biomicroscopy. For some cases, they described the contact in the middle periphery between the ICL and the capsule of the lens; however, there was no opacification in that area. During accommodation, the vault is reduced; however, there is still noncontact with the capsule of the lens. At any rate, surgeons can not presume that these relationships stay unchanged during accommodation, rapid eye movement, blinking, and changes of position. In more recent studies, it has been shown with the Visante (Carl Zeiss Meditec, Dublin, CA) OCT that the vaulting does not change between one state of accommodation and another.

In our opinion, it is probable that when the ICL is below the iris, it touches the surfaces of the lens and that the degree of contact may accentuate during accommodation when the iris root moves backward and the lens moves forward. In any case, there will be physiological contact between the posterior pigmented iris epithelium and the capsule of the lens without formation of focal cataracts; this can be seen as the syndrome of pigment dispersion. The constant scraping of the mobile pupil produces pseudoexfoliative material on the lens surface and a focal cataract will not develop.

If the P-IOL is too small, the lens may rotate and cause opacification of the lens. It was recently demonstrated that altered circulation of the aqueous is a factor that can potentially opacify the lens. In a recent study on pig eyes,[43] it was shown that presence of an ICL will cause changes in intraocular dynamics of the aqueous humor, reducing its flow toward the anterior capsule; this is considered to be the cause of a metabolic disorder of the crystalline lens that leads to onset of anterior subcapsular opacities. The same group published another study on changes of the lens in pig eyes following the implantation of an ICL with a hole created at the center of the optic.[44] Using a special software package, the authors calculated the diameter of the central hole (1 mm) as the size that would not alter the optical characteristics of the IOL, and they observed that the size of the opening influenced the dynamics of the aqueous humor and increased the volume of perfusion of the humor itself over the entire anterior surface of the crystalline, suggesting possible clinical applications to prevent cataract development in patients implanted with a P-IOL.

Technical and Surgical Considerations

Planning of Surgery and Preoperative Examinations

The calculation of the IOL power to be implanted during cataract surgery must be accurate. These patients desire a solution for their refractive error (previously corrected with a P-IOL). The surgeon must explain to patients that they will lose their accommodation.

Using a matrix formula, we can calculate the power of the aphakic IOL[45]; it can also be calculated using the Binkhorst II formula adding 1 mm to the preoperative depth of the AC.[46] The refractive target should be approximately -0.5 D.

Another option is to use the SRK-T formula alone to calculate the power of the IOL[46]; this system supplies good predictability of the postoperative refraction.

It has been shown that the presence of an IOL in the AC (with angle support) does not greatly affect the measurement of the axial length[20,36] calculated either with the IOL Master (Carl Zeiss Meditec, Oberkochen, Germany) or with the A-scan ultrasound machine.

Given that the speed of sound passing through the various materials of the P-IOL differs from the speed observed in the media used to measure the various parameters of the eye, a variable but definitive error results. Hoffer[47] stated that in biphakic eyes, the axial length can be measured with greater accuracy by using a simple mathematical formula that differs depending on the material of the specific P-IOL. He found that the greatest effect (the greatest difference) occurs with the silicone P-IOL in eyes with high hyperopia, while a lesser effect is found with the ICLs (IOL Collamer [STAAR Surgical, Monrovia, CA]) in highly myopic eyes.

An alternative proposal was presented by Leccisotti[48] who implanted an IOL of power calculated using an algebraic formula and the results of the intraoperative refraction achieved following phacoemulsification and the reformation of the AC.

In any case, we recommend that axial biometry should be performed by an expert technician and confirmed by B-scan ultrasound. In cases affected by posterior staphyloma, special attention should be paid to the measurement of the axial length along the visual axis. All of the calculations must be performed using the same biometry software. Theoretical and empirical formulas for the power of the lens and the calculation of the dimensions must be prepared for every model of lens.

Essential tests are long-term serial pre- and postoperative specular microscopy to document that endothelial cell loss does not exceed the normal physiological loss for the patient's age. (The surgeon should fill the AC with viscoelastic substance [VES] during surgery to protect the endothelium.)

Intraoperative (or better still, preoperative) use of a goniolens can be used to check the position of the feet. They should be positioned on the scleral spike below the iris insertion without displacing the iris.

The surgeon should examine every portion of the eye carefully, with special attention paid to cases of AC-IOLs or iris fixed IOLs, recording the pupil diameter and the pupillary shape, its ability to be dilated, and the presence or absence of synechiae.

Day of Surgery

As mentioned previously, only a few papers have been published on the subject of the P-IOL and the successive phacoemulsification procedure, and these included a very limited number of cases.[20,33,36,46,48-50] In a recent review,[33] all of the combined procedures (P-IOL extraction and cataract surgery) terminate successfully with implantation of an IOL in the capsular bag. Nevertheless, some pre-, intra-, and postoperative aspects need to be examined more in depth.

Pupil Size and Preoperative Medication

When removing an AC-IOL with angle support or iris fixation, we prefer to dilate the pupil prior to surgery. Other surgeons prefer to constrict the pupil with topical pilocarpine, to protect the anterior capsule of the lens during lens extraction and facilitate the freeing of the foot from its fixation point.

In our experience, there were no problems liberating the foot with the dilated pupil, and there was no damage to the anterior capsule because of the protection provided by the VES.

For PC-IOLs, all surgeons agree that the pupil should be well dilated (with 1% cyclopentolate, 10% phenylephrine, 0.03% flurbiprofen, every 5 to 10 minutes for a total of 3 times immediately prior to surgery).

Anesthesia

Topical Anesthesia

Theoretically, extraction of the P-IOL, phacoemulsification, and implantation of the IOL could be performed using topical anesthesia (1% tetracaine or 4% lidocaine, 3 to 4 times with intracameral supplements of 1% xylocaine). However, for young and anxious patients, other options of anesthesia are available. Which anesthesia is used is a decision made during the preoperative examination.

Peribulbar Anesthesia

It is our opinion that peribulbar anesthesia is ideal for this type of surgery. A peribulbar injection of 0.75% bupivacaine and 2% lidocaine will reduce the eye's movements; however, this type of anesthesia should be used cautiously in severely myopic eyes with posterior staphyloma. Intravenous sedation can be used if required.

Retrobulbar Anestheosa

This is not normally used.

Sub-Tenon's Anesthesia

This type of anesthesia can be instilled using a blunt cannula and provides another alternative. The eye is compressed gently for 5 minutes with Honan's balloon 15 minutes prior to surgery.

General Anesthesia

This is usually not necessary but may be required under special circumstances.

Incision for the Explantation

It is possible to reopen the previous wound (used to implant the lens) or the surgeon can create a new corneal or sclerocorneal incision.

The globe is grasped with forceps or a fixation ring; the surgeon performs a superior conjunctival peritomy followed by light coagulation of the sclera.

The surgeon performs a sclerocorneal or internal limbal corneal valve or hinge incision. Using a calibrated diamond blade or a 45-degree stainless steel superblade, he or she creates an incision with a depth of 200 to 300 microns.

The dissection is extended approximately 1.5 mm in clear cornea using a diamond blade or a blunt steel blade.

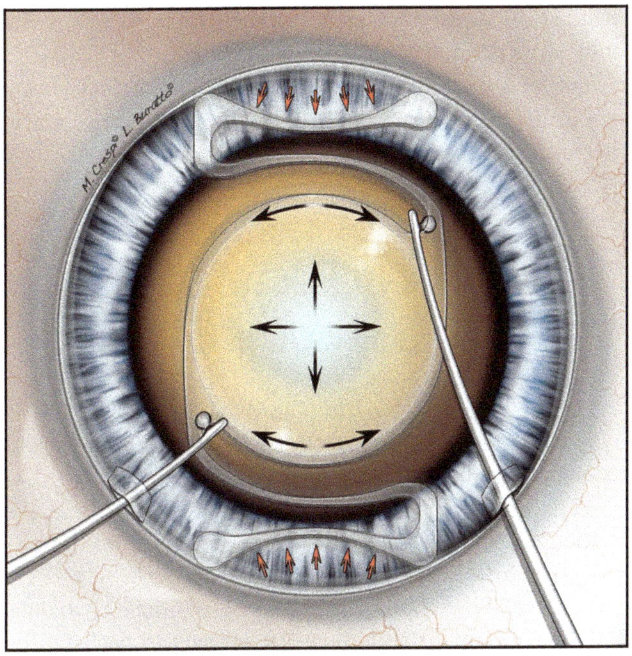

Figure 18-1. Mobilization of the angle-supported IOL to exclude the presence of any angle synechiae.

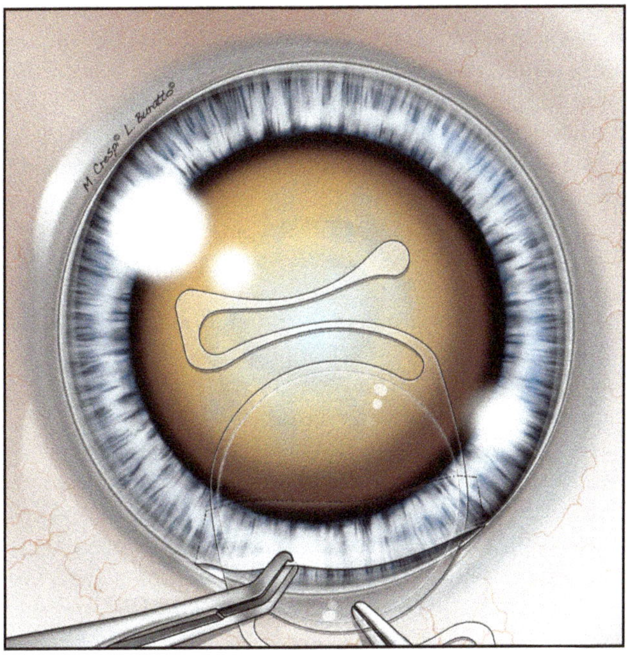

Figure 18-2. Explantation of the IOL from the AC.

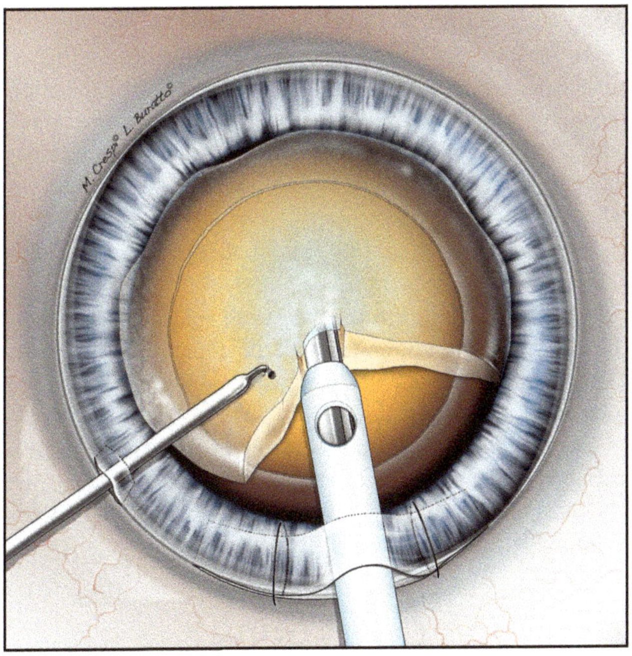

Figure 18-3. Emulsification of the nucleus in the AC of a severely myopic patient.

The surgeon enters the AC by means of a wide keratome (2.2 or 2.75 mm), and VES is injected into the chamber.

For successive intraocular manipulation, the surgeon creates 2 side-port incisions of approximately 1 mm positioned at 60 and 90 degrees with respect to the main incision. The internal incision is then extended to 6.0 mm with a knife.

Filling the AC with VES during the surgery will protect the endothelium and provide the surgeon with a deep chamber for the procedures. It is advisable not to inject VES underneath the iris as the substance can be trapped behind the IOL causing potential problems with the IOL. If the depth of the AC is less than 2.8, VES can be added if necessary to maintain depth. It is our opinion that the use of 2 different and complementary (dispersive-cohesive) products will maximize the benefits, minimize the disadvantages of both types.[51,52]

Explantation Technique

Anterior Chamber Intraocular Lens With Angle Support

The lens is moved slightly using a Lester hook (Katena, Denville, NJ) introduced into the AC through a small paracentesis to exclude the presence of synechiae in the AC angle. When these are present, they must be delicately removed to avoid bleeding or iris dialysis (Figure 18-1). Once VES is introduced, the lens is rotated as much as required, and the proximal loop is extracted from the angle of the corneal tunnel and explanted using Clayman forceps (Asico, Westmont, IL) with no further problems once the cornea has been opened (Figures 18-2 and 18-3).

Intraocular Lens With Iris Enclavation

The most important step is releasing the IOL from its enclavation points. The AC is filled with VES. A bimanual technique is used to extract the lens. The optic is grasped with an instrument held in one hand (preferably special implantation iris-claw forceps). A blunt needle held in the other hand is inserted through a side-port incision to push the iris out of the claw. VES is injected once again, the IOL is rotated slightly using a cannula, and the lens is extracted using iris claw forceps through a 6-mm corneal opening.

Posterior Chamber Intraocular Lens

The most delicate step of the procedure involves sliding the proximal loop of the ICL into the AC; this step can be assisted with Bechert's IOL manipulator inserted through a paracentesis, with or without the help of VES. VES is then injected at the edges of the ICL. One of the loops in maneuvered into the incision (that can measure up to 3.2 mm). The entire loop is then grasped with McPherson forceps inserted through the incision. By rotating the forceps, the lens is gently pulled externally until the surgeon manages to achieve a firm grip on the thickest part of the lens, and this will facilitate the lens extraction.

Phacoemulsification

Following the extraction of the P-IOL, the corneal incision is partially closed with single sutures. An opening of 2 to 2.2 mm should be left to allow insertion of the rhexis forceps and the phaco microtip through the same opening. According to Alio et al,[20] and we agree with them, the use of the MICS technique in surgical bilensectomy will improve the control of the intraocular fluid circulation. Actually, the AC will be more stable with a lower likelihood of iris prolapse. The corneal sutures are positioned radially and must leave enough space for the introduction of the phaco tip. An 8-0 silk suture is used (these will produce tighter closure compared to nylon suture) and will be replaced at the end of surgery.

Another option is the creation of a second incision for the phaco procedure (different from the one used to extract the P-IOL).

After having placed the sutures, the AC is filled once again with VES and the surgeon performs a continuous curved capsulorrhexis with forceps. Hydrodissection is then performed; the nucleus is luxated in the AC with light hydro-expression.

The nucleus is then emulsified using a microaxial pulsed phacoemulsification. The surgeon should always remember that he or she is dealing with a globe that is highly myopic (see Figure 18-3) or highly hyperopic (see Chapters 8 and 9, respectively).

Once the PC-IOL has been implanted, the silk sutures are removed and the large main incision is closed with a continuous 10-0 nylon suture (Ethicon, Edinburgh, Great Britain); this will induce a certain degree of surgically induced astigmatism.

The VES is removed through the 2 side-port incisions.

Finally, the corneal incision is hydrated and if necessary, the surgeon can add a 8-0 silk or 7-0 Vicryl conjunctival suture.

Intra- and Postoperative Difficulties

During surgery, the main objective is to preserve physiological distances between the AC structures and avoid intraoperative collapse or flattening of the chamber.

The most common postoperative complications are residual refractive error and the potential effect on the corneal endothelium.

The use of the appropriate VES can significantly reduce endothelial damage and allow the surgeon to perform the surgical maneuvers in a deep chamber. In our opinion, long-term pre- and postoperative specular microscopy is essential to ensure that the degree of endothelial cell loss does not exceed normal physiological levels.

At the start of surgery, in order to achieve intraoperative dilatation of the pupil, we recommend the injection through a side incision of 1 mL of 1:1000 adrenaline mixed with 9 mL of BSS in a 10-mL syringe; alternately, adrenaline can be added to the infusion bottle (4 IU of 1:1000 in 500 cc BSS).

Intraocular acetylcholine (Miochol) is recommended to achieve intraoperative miosis.

Adding antibiotics to the irrigation solution will reduce the risk of endophthalmitis. Our postoperative therapy is 1% prednisolone acetate 4 times per day for 2 weeks and tobramycin eyedrops.

Despite all of these possible intra- and postoperative variables, bilensectomy is safe and effective in the vast majority of cases and will preserve the refractive benefits obtained with the previous P-IOL implant.

Conclusion

Ophthalmology has witnessed the evolution in implantation of P-IOLs. This direction would appear to be a solution for the correction of many refractive errors, even those of mild to moderate severity. One of the major advantages of the P-IOL is the ease with which the lenses can be removed or replaced. Consequently, this is an adjustable and reversible surgical technique.

The most recent models of these lenses are associated with a low incidence of postoperative complications, though longer follow-up will be necessary to confirm this.

There are numerous causes of cataract and these must be identified before we can clearly under stand the etiology of the postoperative opacification of the crystalline lens.

The outcome of bilensectomy procedure is linked to endothelial cell loss (from the manipulation of the IOL and the successive phacoemulsification procedure), to the intra- and postoperative complications, poor predictability of the final refraction due to the high degree of surgically induced astigmatism secondary to the large limbal incision and the difficulty the surgeon faces in choosing the IOL power of the lens to be implanted.

Consequently, the combination of the P-IOLs and cataract presents a new challenge for the surgeon, and at the time of writing, appears to be heading toward a successful conclusion.

References

1. Alió JL, de la Hoz F, Pérez-Santonja JJ, Ruiz-Moreno JM, Quesada JA. Phakic anterior chamber lenses for the correction of myopia: a 7-year cumulative analysis of complications in 263 cases. *Ophthalmology.* 1999;106(3):458-466.
2. Waring GO 3rd. Comparison of refractive corneal surgery and phakic IOLs. *J Refract Surg.* 1998;14(3):277-279.
3. Huang D, Schallhorn SC, Sugar A, et al. Phakic intraocular lens implantation for the correction of myopia: a report by the American Academy of Ophthalmology. *Ophthalmology.* 2009;116(11):2244-2258.
4. Barsam A, Allan BD. Excimer laser refractive surgery versus phakic intraocular lenses for the correction of moderate to high myopia. *Cochrane Database Syst Rev.* 2010 May 12;(5):CD007679.
5. Rosman M, Alió JL, Ortiz D, Pérez-Santonja JJ. Refractive stability of LASIK with the Visx 20/20 excimer laser vs ZB5m phakic iol implantation in patients with high myopia (>-10.00 d): a 10-year retrospective study. *J Refract Surg.* 2011;27(4):279-286.
6. Pérez-Santonja JJ, Bueno JL, Zato MA. Surgical correction of high myopia in phakic eyes with Worst-Fechner myopia intraocular lenses. *J Refract Surg.* 1997;13(3):268-281; discussion 281-284.
7. Baikoff G, Arne JL, Bokobza Y, et al. Angle-fixated anterior chamber phakic intraocular lens for myopia of -7 to -19 diopters. *Refract Surg.* 1998;14(3):282-293.
8. Menezo JL, Aviño JA, Cisneros A, Rodriguez-Salvador V, Martinez-Costa R. Iris claw phakic intraocular lens for high myopia. *J Refract Surg.* 1997;13(6):545-555.
9. Kaufman HE, Kaufman SC, Beuerman RW. In defense of phakic anterior chamber lenses. *J Cataract Refract Surg.* 1997;23(6):815-817.
10. Davidorf JM, Zaldivar R, Oscherow S. Posterior chamber phakic intraocular lens for hyperopia of +4 to +11 diopters. *J Refract Surg.* 1998;14(3):306-311.
11. Bozkurt E, Yazici AT, Yildirim Y, Alagöz C, Göker H, Yilmaz OF. Long-term follow-up of first-generation posterior chamber phakic intraocular lens. *J Cataract Refract Surg.* 2010;36(9):1602-1604.
12. Qasem Q, Kirwan C, O'Keefe M. 5-year prospective follow-up of Artisan phakic intraocular lenses for the correction of myopia, hyperopia and astigmatism. *Ophthalmologica.* 2010;224(5):283-290.
13. Dick HB, Budo C, Malecaze F, et al. Foldable Artiflex phakic intraocular lens for the correction of myopia: two-year follow-up results of a prospective European multicenter study. *Ophthalmology.* 2009;116(4):671-677.
14. Alfonso JF, Baamonde B, Fernández-Vega L, Fernandes P, González-Méijome JM, Montés-Micó R. Posterior chamber collagen copolymer phakic intraocular lenses to correct myopia: five-year follow-up. *J Cataract Refract Surg.* 2011;37(5):873-880.
15. Knorz MC, Lane SS, Holland SP Angle-supported phakic intraocular lens for correction of moderate to high myopia: three-year interim results in international multicenter studies. *J Cataract Refract Surg.* 2011;37(3):469-480.
16. Kohnen T, Kook D, Morral M, Güell JL. Phakic intraocular lenses: part 2: results and complications. *J Cataract Refract Surg.* 2010;36(12):2168-2194.
17. Güell JL, Morral M, Gris O, Gaytan J, Sisquella M, Manero F. Five-year follow-up of 399 phakic Artisan-Verisyse implantation for myopia, hyperopia, and/or astigmatism. *Ophthalmology.* 2008;115(6):1002-1012.
18. Tahzib NG, Nuijts RM, Wu WY, Budo CJ. Long-term study of Artisan phakic intraocular lens implantation for the correction of moderate to high myopia: ten-year follow-up results. *Ophthalmology.* 2007;114(6):1133-1142.
19. Utine CA, Bayraktar S, Kaya V, Eren H, et al. ZB5M anterior chamber and Fyodorov's posterior chamber phakic intraocular lenses: long-term follow-up. *J Refract Surg.* 2006;22(9):906-910.
20. Alió JL, Abdelrahman AM, Javaloy J, Iradier MT, Ortuño V. Angle-supported anterior chamber phakic intraocular lens explantation causes and outcome. *Ophthalmology.* 2006;113(12):2213-2220.
21. Plainer S, Wenzl E, Saalabian AA, et al. Long-term follow-up with I-CARE phakic IOLs. *Br J Ophthalmol.* 2011;95(5):710-714.
22. van Eijden R, de Vries NE, Cruysberg LP, Webers CA, Berenschot T, Nuijts RM. Case of late-onset corneal decompensation after iris-fixated phakic intraocular lens implantation. J *Cataract Refract Surg.* 2009;35(4):774-777.
23. Patel V, Muhtaseb M. Endothelial cell loss after pIOL implantation for high myopia. *J Cataract Refract Surg.* 2008;34(9):1424-1425.
24. Coullet J, Mahieu L, Malecaze F, et al. Severe endothelial cell loss following uneventful angle-supported phakic intraocular lens implantation for high myopia. *J Cataract Refract Surg.* 2007;33(8):1477-1481.
25. Benedetti S, Casamenti V, Benedetti M. Long-term endothelial changes in phakic eyes after Artisan intraocular lens implantation to correct myopia: five-year study. *J Cataract Refract Surg.* 2007;33(5):784-790.
26. Pérez-Santonja JJ, Iradier MT, Sanz-Iglesias L, Serrano JM, Zato MA. Endothelial changes in phakic eyes with anterior chamber intraocular lenses to correct high myopia. *J Cataract Refract Surg.* 1996;22(8):1017-1022.
27. Chen LJ, Chang YJ, Kuo JC, Rajagopal R, Azar DT. Metaanalysis of cataract development after phakic intraocular lens surgery. *J Cataract Refract Surg.* 2008;34(7):1181-1200.
28. Menezo JL, Peris-Martínez C, Cisneros-Lanuza AL, Martínez-Costa R. Rate of cataract formation in 343 highly myopic eyes after implantation of three types of phakic intraocular lenses. *J Refract Surg.* 2004;20(4):317-324.
29. Schmidinger G, Lackner B, Pieh S, Skorpik C. Long-term changes in posterior chamber phakic intraocular collamer lens vaulting in myopic patients. *Ophthalmology.* 2010;117(8):1506-1511.
30. Khalifa YM, Moshirfar M, Mifflin MD, Kamae K, Mamalis N, Werner L. Cataract development associated with collagen copolymer posterior chamber phakic intraocular lenses: clinicopathological correlation. *J Cataract Refract Surg.* 2010;36(10):1768-1774.
31. Lackner B, Pieh S, Schmidinger G, et al. Long-term results of implantation of phakic posterior chamber intraocular lenses. *J Cataract Refract Surg.* 2004;30(11):2269-2276.
32. Sanders DR. Anterior subcapsular opacities and cataracts 5 years after surgery in the visian implantable collamer lens FDA trial. *J Refract Surg.* 2008;24(6):566-570.

33. Moshirfar M, Mifflin M, Wong G, Chang JC. Cataract surgery following phakic intraocular lens implantation. *Curr Opin Ophthalmol.* 2010;21(1):39-44.
34. Sánchez-Galeana CA, Smith RJ, Sanders DR, et al. Lens opacities after posterior chamber phakic intraocular lens implantation. *Ophthalmology.* 2003;110(4):781-785.
35. Metge P, Pichot De Champfleyrt A. La cataracte du myope fort. In: Hondon H, Metge P, eds. *La Myopie Forte.* Paris, Masson; 1994 :448.
36. Alio JL, de la Hoz F, Ruiz-Moreno JM, Salem TF. Cataract surgery in highly myopic eyes corrected by phakic anterior chamber angle-supported lenses. *J Cataract Refract Surg.* 2000;26:1303-1311.
37. Alio JL, de la Hoz F, Ismail M. Subclinical inflammatory reactions induced by phakic anterior chamber lens for the correction of high myopia. *Ocul Immunol Inflamm.* 1993;1:219-223.
38. Pérez-Santonja JJ, Iradier M, Benítez del Castillo JM, et al. Chronic subclinical inflammation in phakic eyes with intraocular lenses to correct myopia. *J Cataract Refract Surg.* 1996;22:183-187.
39. Gonvers M, Bornet C, Othenin-Girard P. Implantable contact lens for moderate to high myopia: relationship of vaulting to cataract formation. *J Cataract Refract Surg.* 2003;29(5):918-924.
40. Zaldivar R, Oscherow S, Ricur G. The STAAR posterior chamber phakic intraocular lens. *Int Ophthalmol Clin.* 2000;40(3): 237-244.
41. Fernandes P, González-Méijome JM, Madrid-Costa D, Ferrer-Blasco T, Jorge J, Montés-Micó R. Implantable collamer posterior chamber intraocular lenses: a review of potential complications. *J Refract Surg.* 2011;27(10):765-776.
42. Trindade F, Pereira F, Cronemberger S. Ultrasound biomicroscopic imaging of posterior chamber phakic intraocular lens. *J Refract Surg.* 1998;14(5):497-503.
43. Fujisawa K, Shimizu K, Uga S, et al. Changes in the crystalline lens resulting from insertion of a phakic IOL (ICL) into the porcine eye. *Graefes Arch Clin Exp Ophthalmol.* 2007;245(1):114-122.
44. Shiratani T, Shimizu K, Fujisawa K, Uga S, Nagano K, Murakami Y. Crystalline lens changes in porcine eyes with implanted phakic IOL (ICL) with a central hole. *Graefes Arch Clin Exp Ophthalmol.* 2008;246(5):719-728.
45. Fimia A, Alió J, Pascual I, Beléndez A. New theoretical matrix formula for intraocular lens calculation using the optimal bending factor. *J Cataract Refract Surg.* 1993;19(2):293-297.
46. de Vries NE, Tahzib NG, Budo CJ, Webers CA, de Boer R, Hendrikse F, Nuijts RM. Results of cataract surgery after implantation of an iris-fixated phakic intraocular lens. *J Cataract Refract Surg.* 2009;35(1):121-126.
47. Hoffer KJ. Ultrasound axial length measurement in biphakic eyes. *J Cataract Refract Surg.* 2003;29(5):961-965.
48. Leccisotti A. Intraoperative autorefraction for combined phakic intraocular lens explantation and cataract surgery. *J Refract Surg.* 2007;23(9):931-934.
49. Bleckmann H, Keuch RJ. Results of cataract extraction after implantable contact lens removal. *J Cataract Refract Surg.* 2005;31(12):2329-2333.
50. Morales AJ, Zadok D, Tardio E, et al. Outcome of simultaneous phakic implantable contact lens removal with cataract extraction and pseudophakic intraocular lens implantation. *J Cataract Refract Surg.* 2006;32(4):595-598.
51. Arshinoff SA. Dispersive-cohesive viscoelastic soft shell technique. *J Cataract Refract Surg.* 1999;25(2):167-173.
52. Buratto L. Viscoelastic substances and cataract surgery. In: Buratto L, ed. *Phacoemulsification: Principles and Techniques.* Thorofare, NJ: SLACK Incorporated; 1998:263-271.

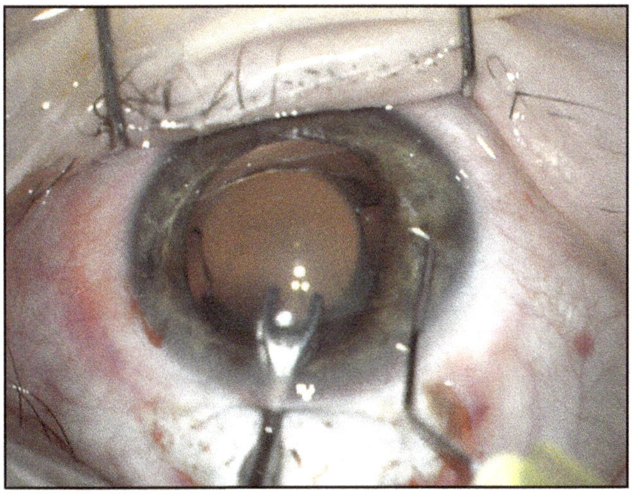

J-1. Cataract after Artisan phakic IOL implantation; after VES injection both claws are disenclaveted.

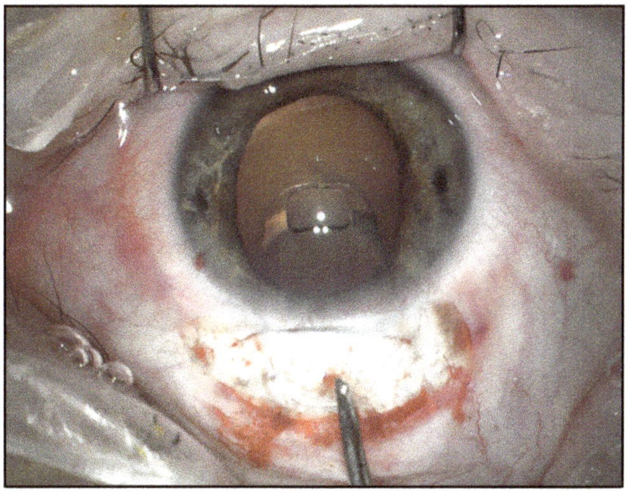

J-2. The phakic IOL is extracted.

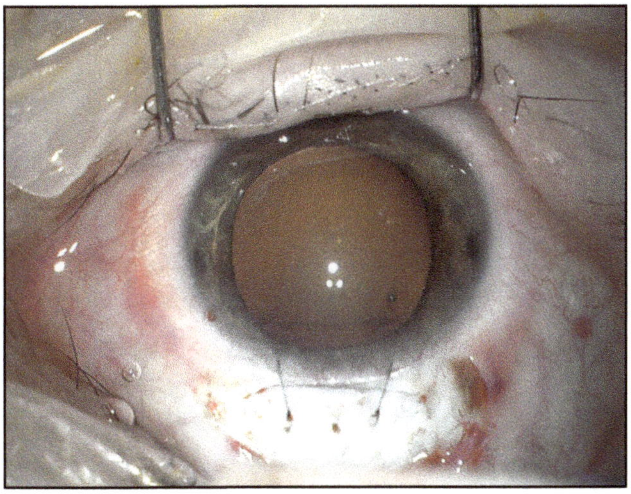

J-3. Two to three sutures are applied.

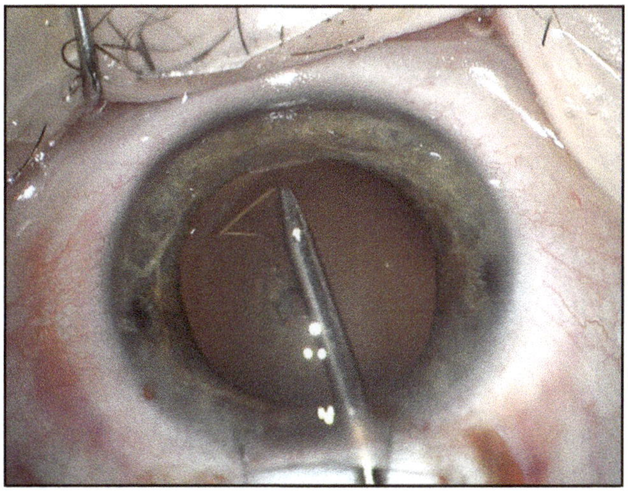

J-4. The capsulotomy follows.

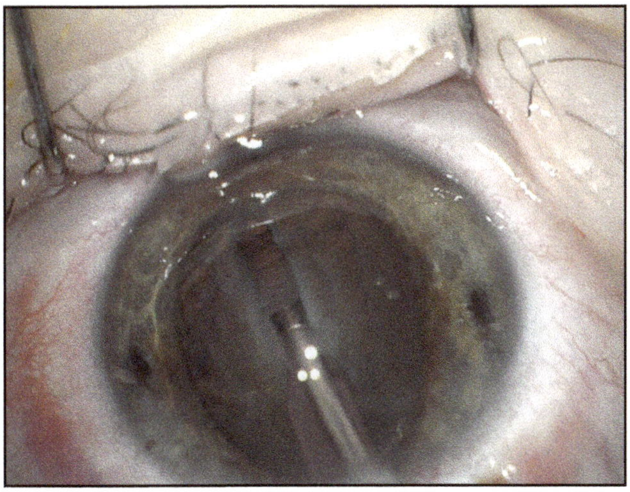

J-5. The phaco.

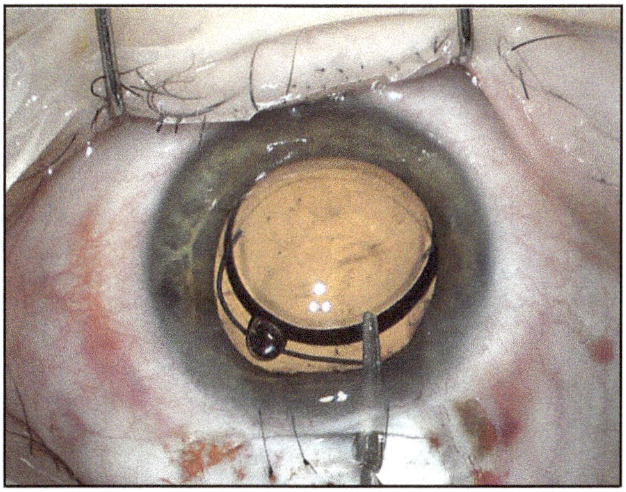

J-6. Finally, IOL implantation in the capsular bag.

19

Secondary Intraocular Lens Implants in Eyes With or Without Capsular Support

There are a number of different strategies in the intraocular approach to correction of postoperative aphakia. The strategy depends on the anatomy and functional conditions of the eye.

A secondary implant can be placed in the bag or in the ciliary sulcus, options available only when there is adequate capsular support. The lens can also be implanted in the anterior chamber (AC) or in the posterior chamber (PC), with IOL fixation to the iris or sclera with sutures. Techniques of intrascleral fixation have been developed recently that do not require sutures, securing the haptics of the IOL in specifically constructed intrascleral tunnels or in the bed of a scleral flap using fibrin glue. The objective is to reduce surgical time, suturing time, and associated complications, while at the same time ensuring ideal positioning of the lens with good centration of the IOL.

A number of studies compared the results of vision and complications associated with secondary implantation of AC-IOLs with those of PC-IOLs. The preferred site for the implant remains a topic of discussion. Even though many believe that secondary implantation of a PC-IOL may be preferable to that of an AC-IOL, some studies suggest that the efficacy and complication rates are similar.

Due to the ease of surgery, the insertion of an AC-IOL is still the choice for many surgeons. Nevertheless, there are many situations where there is poor angle support, which suggest the implantation of a PC-IOL.

Compared to an AC-IOL, potential advantages of a PC-IOL include reduced risk of a number of different complications: endothelial cell loss, corneal edema, secondary glaucoma, cystoid macular edema (CME), inflammation with formation of a fibrin membrane, pupillary capture, and uveitis-glaucoma-hyphema (UGH) syndrome. Other theoretical advantages of a PC-IOL compared to an AC-IOL include reduced incidence of anterior peripheral synechiae, fibrosis of the angle, and iris chafing.

For these reasons, implantation of a PC-IOL is our elective procedure for aphakic secondary lens implantation.

Preoperative Evaluation of the Aphakic Patient

Uncorrected aphakia leads to significant functional disability. The aphakic patient will benefit greatly from a secondary lens implant, particularly if there is intolerance of spectacles and contact lenses.

The surgeon should always make an attempt at visual rehabilitation with aphakic spectacles or contact lenses to avoid the potential risks associated with secondary lens implantation. In binocular aphakia, the patient may tolerate spectacles well. However, with unilateral aphakia, spectacles are not an option because of anisometropia and resulting aniseiconia; the surgeon should attempt to use a soft or hard gas-permeable lens.

Relative or absolute contraindications to contact lenses include giant papillary conjunctivitis, dry eye syndrome, blepharitis, lagophthamos, a large filtering bleb, difficulty inserting and removing the lens, and a history of complications associated with contact lenses such as infective keratitis, corneal edema, or corneal neovascularization. A secondary PC-IOL implant would be the best option in these situations. Intolerance to contact lenses should be adequately recorded. Secondary PC-IOLs should be cautiously recommended in patients with a history of retinal

Buratto L, Brint SF, Caretti L.
Cataract Surgery in Complicated Cases (pp 213-230).

detachment, chronic uveitis, glaucoma, or a borderline endothelial cell count. Inserting the lens may be associated with retinal detachment and CME, and may be a relative contraindication in patients with chronic uveitis. Pre-existing glaucoma may be aggravated by secondary postoperative glaucoma. A low endothelial cell count (<1000 cells/mm^2) may be a relative contraindication to secondary lens implantation, given that any intraocular procedure may lead to endothelial cell loss. Endothelial cell loss can reach up to 26% in patients undergoing cataract extraction or lens implantation.

More than 60% of patients with a secondary PC-IOL lose more than 10% endothelial cells, risking postoperative corneal decompensation.

For every patient considering secondary lens implantation, the surgeon must perform a detailed clinical history and a complete eye examination.

Clinically, it is essential to note all previous ocular surgeries (intracapsular cataract extraction [ICCE], extracapsular cataract extraction [ECCE], complicated phacoemulsification with capsular rupture, anterior vitrectomy, posterior vitrectomy.

As part of the complete eye examination, the surgeon must perform an accurate refraction and determine best-corrected visual acuity for the eye to be operated as well as the contralateral eye. Accurate biomicroscopy of the anterior segment should be performed with special attention to corneal transparency, corneal endothelium, iris anatomy, integrity of the hyaloid face and the posterior capsule, the position of the vitreous, and in particular the presence or absence of capsular support. The surgeon should examine the anterior sclera to exclude scleral ectasia, particularly in patients with severe myopia or patients with rheumatoid arthritis. Gonioscopy and measurement of intraocular pressure (IOP) are also important.

The preoperative exam should also include careful examination of the posterior segment to exclude CME or any other fundus pathology. If the surgeon suspects CME or any other retinal pathology, he or she should perform retinal angiography or/and optical coherence tomography. If the preoperative examination of the peripheral retina shows risk factors for retinal detachment, such as lattice degeneration or retinal tears, the surgeon should consider prophylactic treatment.

Examinations prior to secondary PC-IOLs include endothelial cell count, analysis of cell morphology, corneal pachymetry, calculation of the IOL power, and high resolution ultrasound biomicroscopy. This is useful for examining the anatomy of the angle, the presence of synechiae between the iris and the residual capsule that could impede the insertion of the PC-IOL, and with poor mydriasis, evidence of capsular support.

The general state of health is important, and when necessary, the patient has a full medical examination, in particular, connective tissue diseases to exclude the option of scleral fixation.

Preoperatively one should ascertain the need for a capsular tension ring or a PC-IOL (sutured to the sclera or the iris) or an AC-IOL in phakic patients with weak zonules (Marfan's syndrome, trauma, or pseudoexfoliation).

In these patients, the preoperative examination must be the same as for the aphakic patient. Knowledge of the eye's anatomy will greatly assist the surgeon in the operative plan. In many cases, the surgeon can make the decision to implant the type of lens, if the capsule has ruptured or if the support for sulcus fixation of the IOL is inadequate.

Anesthesia and Preparation of the Patient

In general, when the surgeon opts for a secondary IOL without capsular support, local or general anesthesia can be used, depending on the patient's general health and the surgeon's personal preference. If the surgeon opts for a retrobulbar or peribulbar block, he or she can compress the eye after the block to improve anesthetic distribution. Topical anesthesia may be sufficient for implanting an IOL in the bag or sulcus.

With the exception of AC-IOL implantation, the eye is dilated either with Mydriasert inserts (Thea Farma SpA, Milan, Italy) or with a drop of 2.5% phenylephrine hydrochloride and a drop of 1% cyclopentolate instilled every 5 minutes for 3 applications during the hour prior to surgery.

For the implantation of an AC-IOL, 2% pilocarpine drops are instilled 30 minutes prior to surgery to induce miosis.

All patients should also have a drop of an antibiotic/steroid combination and a drop of nonsteroid anti-inflammatory drug (0.1% diclofenac sodium, 0.3% flurbiprofen sodium, or 0.5% ketorolac tromethamine) for 3 applications preoperatively. These drops act as prophylaxis against bacterial infections, minimize postoperative inflammation, and increase pupil dilation.

The patient is prepped for surgery and draped as usual. The speculum is positioned and surgery proceeds as planned.

Surgery

Careful preoperative planning is crucial for the success of surgery. Fundamental is the evaluation of whether the capsular support is adequate for the procedure.

A candidate for a secondary IOL implant may have had an ICCE, ECCE, or phacoemulsification with capsular rupture.

If there is adequate post-phaco or post-ECCE capsular support, the most appropriate choice is the implantation of an IOL in the bag or in the ciliary sulcus.

However, if the capsular support is not adequate or if the patient has had ICCE, the surgeon must decide whether he or she should implant an AC-IOL or PC-IOL with scleral fixation or iris sutured.

Intraocular Lens in the Bag or Sulcus

In the patient having undergone phaco or ECCE with an intact anterior and posterior capsule, a secondary PC-IOL can be positioned directly in the capsular bag or in the sulcus with no fixation sutures (the technique preferred with minimal complications).[1,2] The first option is rarely feasible; it is seldom possible to insert a secondary PC-IOL in the capsular bag in a patient with an intact posterior capsule. With this situation, opening the bag is the most important surgical problem. In cases without extensive fibrosis, the anterior and posterior capsules can be separated fairly easily; the key element is to identify an area of the anterior capsule that is not firmly adhered to the posterior capsule. At this point, viscoelastic substance (VES) can be injected to separate the 2 layers. If the layers are tightly adhered, the surgeon can attempt mechanical dissection using a cannula or similar blunt instrument. Sometimes a focal adhesion can be left, creating a peripheral extension of the anterior capsulotomy with scissors or rhexis forceps. Another alternative is a dissection with a blade inserted between the anterior and posterior capsules, though this option is risky as it may penetrate the posterior capsule.

A secondary implant in the sulcus can be inserted much easier, following phaco or ECCE with complications, such as posterior capsular rupture (with an intact anterior capsule), radial tears of the anterior capsule, zonule rupture, and/or loss of vitreous or unsuccessful reopening of an intact capsular bag. In these situations, determination of whether or not capsular support is adequate is absolutely critical.

Capsular support adequate for an IOL requires at least 6 hours of residual peripheral capsule, with at least half of this in the inferior quadrant, and relatively intact zonules. The most favorable situation is when the anterior capsulorrhexis is intact in this case, the haptics of the IOL are placed in the ciliary sulcus, with the optic captured in front of the anterior capsulorrhexis, providing optimal centration and stability of the IOL.[3-5]

The technique includes 2 important steps: choice of IOL and positioning of the haptics in the sulcus.[6]

The ideal IOL for secondary sulcus implantation with adequate capsular support should be a standard PC-IOL, a 3-piece acrylic lens with an optic diameter of 6 to 6.5 mm and overall length of 13 to 13.5 mm. It should have long, thin, flexible haptics, rounded edges, and a 5-degree posterior angle. The large size of the optic offers an additional margin of safety to minimize edge glare if the lens decenters postoperatively. Even one-piece polymethylmethacrylate (PMMA) IOLs with a diameter of 6.5 mm provide an extremely satisfactory solution. The rigidity of the one-piece PMMA lens has the advantage of providing stability in the sulcus.

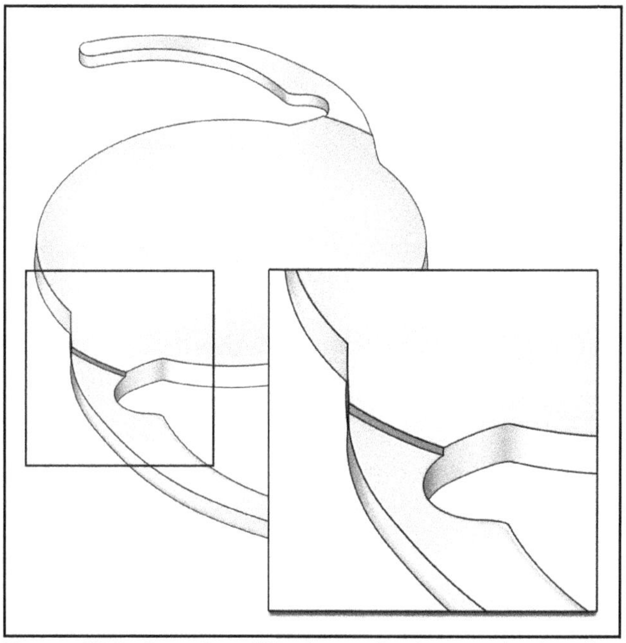

Figure 19-1. One-piece IOL. Squared edges at the junction between the optic and the haptics.

The one-piece acrylic IOL with thick, stiff haptics and square edges can damage delicate uveal structures and thus is not ideal for implantation in the sulcus (Figure 19-1).

The second important aspect is correct positioning of the haptics in the sulcus and this is the most difficult part. One study estimated that in 42% of eyes, the sulcus IOL was not in the correct position; malpositioned haptics have important clinical implications.[7] If one of the 2 haptics is positioned anterior to the ciliary sulcus, the peripheral iris will have an anterior vault with angle-closure for about 2 hours and contact between the edge of the optic and the posterior surface of the iris, resulting in iritis and pigment dispersion. If the haptic is posterior to the sulcus, the haptic may become trapped in the ciliary body giving rise to chronic inflammation and possible hemorrhage.

Refractively, malpositioned haptics will lead to[8] chromatic aberration (asymmetrical decentration or tilting of the optic), myopic shift (symmetrical anterior positioning of the optic), or hyperopic shift (symmetrical posterior positioning of the optic).

Aphakic patients with residual capsule often have synechia formation between the anterior capsule and the posterior surface of the iris (or between the anterior and posterior capsules). These synechiae must be severed to reconstruct the ciliary sulcus prior to IOL implantation.

During insertion, it is important to ensure that the haptics of the IOL do not go under the anterior capsule as this will compromise adequate support of the IOL and risk vitreous rupture. If the surgeon is not confident about the capsular support, the haptics of the IOL may be sutured to the iris or to the sclera.

Anterior Chamber Intraocular Lens

If capsular support post-phaco, post-ECCE is absent or ICCE, the surgeon must decide whether to proceed with a secondary AC-IOL, PC-IOL with scleral fixation or sutured to the iris.

Secondary implantation of an AC-IOL is widely used, even though its correct indication should be based on the following parameters:

- Corneal endothelial function
- AC depth ≥3 mm
- Horizontal corneal diameter >10.5 mm
- Integrity of iris tissue for at least 270 degrees
- Pupil diameter <6 mm

AC-IOLs have angle support or iris enclavation. The implantation of an angle-supported AC-IOL is technically more straightforward; however, constant contact between the haptics and the iris root and the trabecular meshwork can lead to a series of complications that will be discussed later in this chapter.

Open loop AC-IOLs and those with iris enclavation can be implanted without capsular support, except in eyes with extensive congenital or traumatic abnormalities of the angle that will not allow sufficient support for the lens.[9,10]

The correct surgical procedure for implanting an open loop AC-IOL includes the following steps:

- Correct sizing of the IOL
- Miosis of the pupil preoperatively (2% pilocarpine instilled 30 minutes prior to surgery)
- Ensuring that the haptics of the IOL are far from the peripheral iridectomies; the incisions should be created at the axis of steeper curvature to reduce postoperative astigmatism: the size of the incision depends on the type of IOL implanted
- Insertion of high viscosity VES to maintain AC depth and protect the endothelium
- The surgeon may opt for an anterior vitrectomy to remove vitreous from the AC and incisions
- Special IOL implantation techniques will avoid iris tuck and iridodialysis; some surgeons use Sheets' glides (BD Medical, Franklin Lakes, NJ)
  - Careful check of support: the Bounce test will evaluate the fixation stability and the absence of iris tuck
  - Peripheral iridectomy, if not already present
  - Removal of viscoelastic from the AC
  - 10-0 nylon corneal suture (interrupted or running sutures).

Despite the relative ease of primary and secondary implantation techniques used for these open-loop AC-IOLs, many surgeons do not use them because of the well-known side effects associated with closed-loop AC-IOLs.[11] These were associated with a high incidence of complications such as progressive loss of corneal endothelium, chronic ocular inflammation, secondary glaucoma, UGH syndrome, and CME. These complications are caused by excessive vaulting of the IOL with resulting chronic endothelial damage and chafing; moreover, the fibrosis of the loops in the angle can lead to erosions of uveal tissue leading to rupture of the blood-eye barrier and intraocular release of inflammatory mediators.[11-14]

Fortunately, the implantation site is the only similarity between modern open loop AC-IOLs and the older closed-loop AC-IOLs.[9] The new AC-IOLs result in minimal vaulting with less damage to the corneal endothelium.[9] Moreover, the minimal contact area because of the design of the loops greatly reduces the tendency of fibrosis of the haptics and erosion of the angle structures.[9] Open loop IOLs are associated with a lower incidence of complications and a lower rate of explantation.[10] Several studies showed an increase in IOP following secondary implantation of an AC-IOL with angle support.[15,16]

In studies of open loop AC-IOLs alone[17-35] or in comparison to scleral sutured PC-IOLs[16,36-39] or iris sutured,[37-39] there is no scientific evidence to suggest that the visual results with open loop AC-IOLs are worse. These studies looked at both primary and secondary implants and when combined with penetrating keratoplasty (PKP).[15]

The second type of AC-IOL, with iris enclavation, requires greater surgical skill but is associated with a lower incidence of complications. The surgical technique of iris enclavation is as follows:

1. Constriction of the pupil preoperatively (2% pilocarpine instilled 30 minutes prior to surgery)
2. Creation of a paracentesis incision for insertion of high viscosity VES to maintain AC depth and protect the endothelium
3. Creation of corneal incisions: the main incision measuring 5.2 mm is created at 12 o'clock; 2 paracentesis incisions are created at 2 and 10 o'clock

4. Vitrectomy if required to remove vitreous from the AC and incisions
    - Insertion of the iris claw AC-IOL. It is centered on the pupil with the loops oriented at 3 and 9 o'clock. The optic of the lens is held firmly with special forceps. An enclavation needle is inserted first through one side incision and then through the other. The surgeon completes the enclavation of the haptics of the IOL into the anterior surface of the mid-peripheral iris through a down-up movement of the hook (Figure 19-2). Fixation of the "crab claw" haptics occurs in the mid-peripheral iris distant from the delicate angle structures. Another advantage is that in the mid-peripheral iris, the blood vessels are small and encapsulated, arranged radially resulting in a lower risk of bleeding. Enclavation is the most critical phase of the entire operation and is associated with the fact that the aphakic iris is thicker and less fragile than the iris in phakic patients.
    - Peripheral iridectomy if not already present.
    - 10-0 nylon corneal suture (individual or running).
    - Removal of the VES from the AC.

The literature published since 1970[40] to today[41-44] has shown that IOLs with iris enclavation are a safe and secure method for correcting aphakia (Figure 19-3). In a recent study,[45] the results of eyes with iris enclavation of the IOL were compared to the results of eyes in which the IOL was sutured to the iris; the results of the 2 procedures are similar in terms of efficacy and safety.

The potential complications are similar to those of iris sutured PC-IOLs; they include increased IOP (also because of pupillary block), iris atrophy at the enclavation site, dislocation of the IOL, pigment deposits on the IOL, retinal detachment, and pupil deformation (resulting from an inappropriate enclavation site).

A multicenter trial with the Artisan (Ophtec, Boca Raton, FL) phakic IOLs[46] showed that endothelial cell loss stabilized at a physiological level after 3 years. As an alternative to enclavation on the anterior surface of the iris, the AC-IOL with iris claw may also be implanted behind the pupil.[47] The most frequent complication of these retropupillary implants is secondary glaucoma. Nevertheless, this implantation technique is valid even in association with PKP.

Posterior Chamber Intraocular Lens Sutured to the Iris

In 1976, Malcom McCannel[48] described a technique of iris fixation for a subluxated PC-IOL. He had the idea of suturing the loops of the IOL to the peripheral portion of the iris using a 10-0 Prolene suture when the globe was

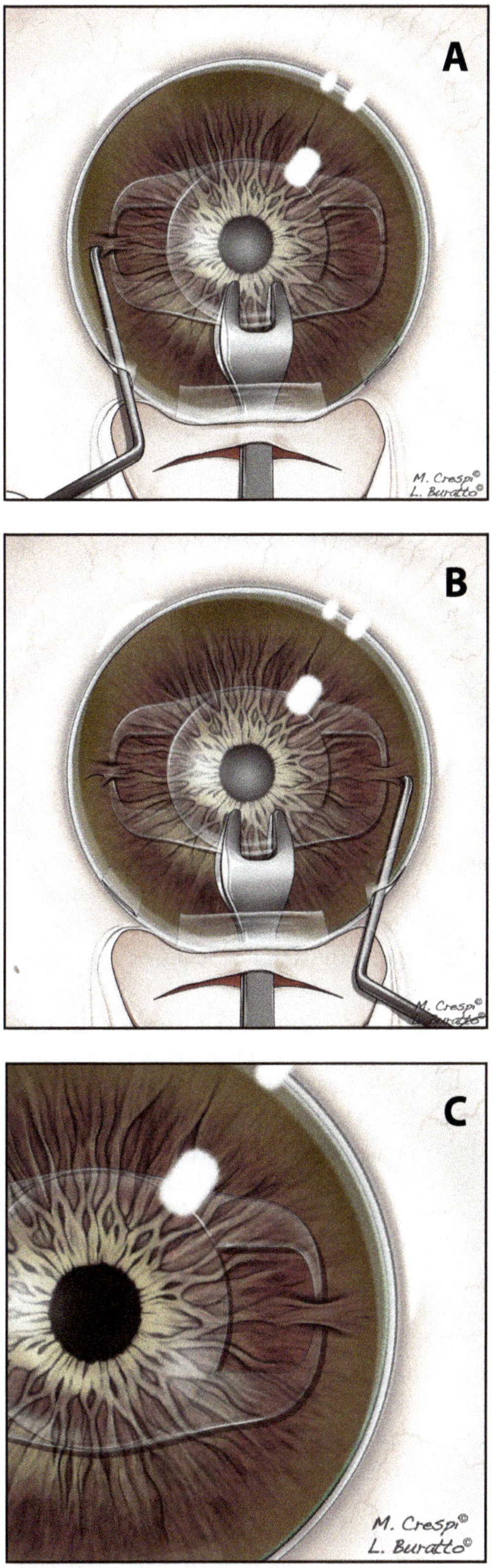

Figure 19-2. (A) Enclavation of the nasal mid-peripheral iris in the claws of the Artisan IOL. (B) Enclavation of the temporal mid-peripheral iris in the claws of the Artisan IOL. (C) Enclavation viewed under high magnification.

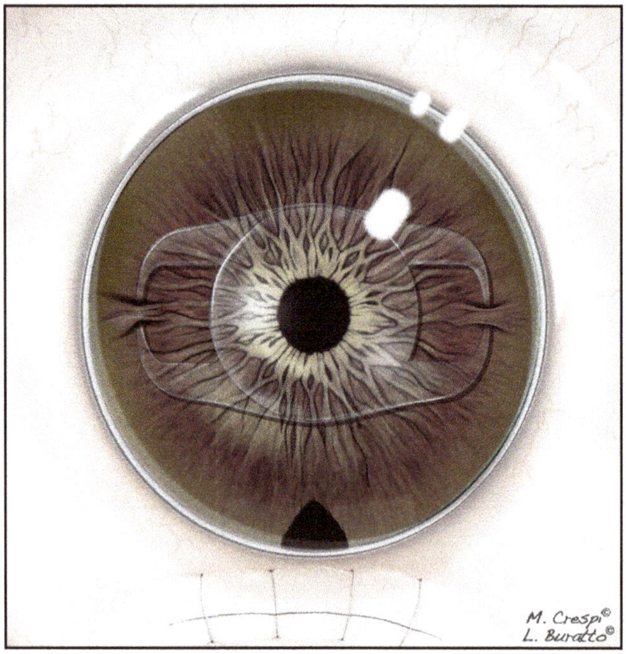

Figure 19-3. Postoperative outcome of a secondary iris-fixed IOL implant.

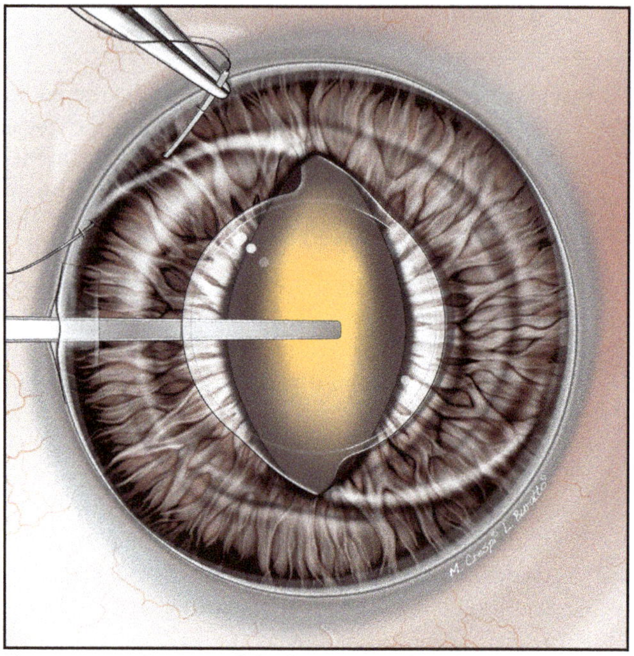

Figure 19-4. Capture of the loop sutured with 10-0 propylene to the iris.

open during PKP. Some years later, Stark et al[49] followed by Stutzman and Stark[50] and Condon[51] described this suture technique with a closed eye, for repositioning a subluxated IOL or as a secondary implant. The PC-IOLs sutured to the iris can be implanted in eyes without capsular support; however, they cannot be sutured to the iris in eyes with significant damage to the anterior segment due to congenital abnormalities or trauma.[52]

The essential requisites for this are good rigidity of the iris and normal pupil movement. This type of implant is also suitable for patients with glaucoma, in which implantation of an AC-IOL is neither advisable nor possible, or when the conjunctiva should be preserved for successive glaucoma surgery or if a filtering bleb is present and needs to be protected. It is also indicated during phacoemulsification under topical anesthesia in which the capsular support is considered to be inadequate. The technique can be used in the majority of cases under intracameral 1% lidocaine, not an option with the scleral fixation technique.

The insertion of these IOLs, particularly when the limbal approach is used, is a more difficult procedure as compared to open loop AC-IOLs.

The surgical steps of this technique are summarized here. The corneal incisions are created (2 paracentesis incisions and a main incision measuring 2.5 mm). High viscosity VES is injected into the AC, and some may also be injected behind the iris to move it away from the vitreous and the capsule. An injector introduces a hydrophobic 3-piece acrylic IOL into the AC. A Hirschman hook (Katena Products Inc, Denville, NJ) or Kuglen hook (Katena Products Inc) is inserted through the 2 side incisions, using the nondominant hand; an Osher probe (Katena Products Inc) is introduced using the dominant hand. In this way, the surgeon can temporarily "capture" the optic of the PC-IOL in the moderately dilated pupil anterior to the iris plane, with the haptics remaining in the PC. A nonabsorbable 10-0 Prolene suture with a long narrow needle (STC6 [Ethicon, Cornelia, GA]) is passed through a side incision. It penetrates the peripheral iris close to the haptic entering into the iris stroma, exiting from the iris immediately after engaging the haptic, and finally exits through the peripheral area of the clear cornea (Figure 19-4). An elegant system uses the tip of a 25-, 27- (insulin), or 28-gauge needle that acts as a guide to assist the needle exiting from the eye.

At this point the suture can be tightened and secured with a "slip knot" (created outside of the eye); an alternative elegant technique is as follows. The needle is removed, and a hook is introduced into the AC through the side incision used for the passage of the needle to grasp the suture and pull it outside of the eye through the same incision. The knot is tied outside the eye and brought close to the corneal incision. The ends of the suture are grasped with forceps to tighten the knot. Using the other hand, the knot is slipped inside the AC using the Osher instrument (Katena Products Inc) and pushed as far as the iris plane (Siepser's slip knot). This procedure is repeated another 2 times to secure the haptic stably to the iris.

The same sequence of maneuvers is repeated for the other haptic. Normally, the haptics of the IOL are sutured to the iris at 3 and 9 o'clock.

Then the optic of the IOL is pushed into the PC. The VES is removed from the AC using a system of infusion aspiration and then the incisions are hydrated.

Soong et al[53] described fixation of the PC-IOL to the iris in 2 and 4 points during PKP.

The technique used to suture the IOL to the iris requires good surgical skills, particularly in the following steps:

1. Positioning of the haptics behind the iris with pupillary capture of the optic of the PC-IOL
2. Capture of the haptic with McCannel sutures
3. Creation of the Siepser's slip knot[54]

A round, centered pupil can be achieved with short needle passes in the peripheral iris. The length of the suture creases the iris tissue, while passes too close to the pupil inhibit pupil movements. Both of these errors result in a distorted nonreactive pupil.

The iris fixation technique allows PC centration of a PC-IOL; this allows correct positioning from an anatomical, functional point of view. The final position is close to the original planned one (bag fixation) with all of the advantages of implantation in the PC.

The fixation of the flexible loops to the iris creates a posterior vault of the haptic-optic junction, separating the optic from the posterior surface of the iris, reducing chafing and pigment dispersion. From a refractive point of view, this procedure creates an optical effect similar to that as planned in original position, avoiding a reduction in the optic power as required by anterior displacement of the IOL.[55]

Another advantage of this technique is stability of the sutures; compared to scleral fixation, where blinking can create mechanical stress with the possibility of erosion, here, the technique is not associated with stress or damage. The lens position is stable over time[15] with a minimal risk of dislocation[56] and endophthalmitis, sometimes seen with scleral sutures.[57] On the other hand, the peripheral iris is the ideal site for suspension of the lens, because of its lack of tone, its elasticity, and the type of vascularisation.

A recent study using ultrasound biomicroscopy by Mura et al,[58] demonstrated that the site of the suture is the point in which the haptic and the posterior iris are in contact, thus a minimal risk of pigmentary dispersion.

PC-IOLs sutured to the iris have potential advantages of good anatomical position of the implant (in the PC) and the disadvantage of increased surgical time, similar to a PC-IOL with scleral fixation.

Iris fixation of the IOL is technically more difficult than scleral fixation. This may explain the fewer reports on this type of lens implantation.[55,56,59-61] On the other hand, many eye surgeons consider iris fixation techniques during PKP to be simpler than scleral fixation techniques.[37-39,62-65]

Theoretically, iris fixation and scleral fixation should have fewer serious complications, as opposed to open loop AC-IOLs. Doubts persist on potential problems associated with chronic irritation of the iris perhaps leading to chronic inflammation and CME.

The other complications are similar to those associated with iris claw AC-IOLs; they include high IOP (due to pupillary block), IOL dislocation, iris atrophy at the enclavation site, pigment deposits on the IOL, retinal detachment, capture of the IOL, and endothelial cell loss (of no great importance over time).

A study by Guttman in 2009[55] had a postoperative complication rate varying between 1% and 8% (with a mean follow-up of 8 months). In 144 eyes, 8% showed a transient increase in IOP, 7% of the lenses were redislocated, 1% developed bullous keratopathy, and 1% iris hemorrhage.

Chronic inflammation of the iris is another possible complication that appears in 2 situations: incorrect positioning of the sutures in the mobile portion of the iris or excessive tension in the suture.[56] Iridodialysis is a rare event that can result from incorrect manipulation of the iris base.[59]

Price et al[66] reported cases of spontaneous late onset rupture of the Prolene suture fixing the IOL to the iris with subsequent dislocation of the IOL, breakage of the suture that appears to be associated with constant chafing over time and occurs on average 9 years after surgery.

Pathology has shown that sutures are the only and main fixation method for IOLs sutured to the iris[67]; there is no postoperative fibrosis and no inflammatory reaction around the Prolene suture.

Rupture of the Prolene suture is sometimes followed by dislocation of the IOL into the vitreous chamber, a displacement often occurring a long time after the suture has ruptured, suggesting that the haptics can be engaged in the tissue for a certain amount of time but not indefinitely.

Some authors[45] suggest that fixation of the haptics of the IOL at 12 and 6 o'clock will reduce the probability of decentration because of rotation (slippage; eg, following blunt trauma).

Overall, the visual results with this technique are excellent both as a primary and a secondary implant and in combination with PKP, and as mentioned the percentage of complications does not differ greatly from that of other types of implants discussed in this chapter.[15]

Posterior Chamber Intraocular Lens Sutured to the Sclera

When capsular support is inadequate, we prefer a technique with transscleral fixation suturing because of secondary positioning of the PC-IOL, when there is significant congenital or traumatic damage to the anterior segment.[68]

The scleral fixation technique was introduced by Girard in 1981[69] and was successively revived by Malbran et al in 1986 for secondary implantion in previous ICCE patients.[70] The implant requires fixation of the IOL haptic to the sclera, behind the iris, below 2 basic limbal incisions at 3 and 9 o'clock, using 10-0 Prolene sutures (single or dual; Ethicon, Cornelia, GA) with a long straight or curved needle. The incisions allow the knots of the fixation sutures to be embedded.

Prolene is not reactive, rarely reabsorbed, and it is relatively nondegradable, so it is relatively stable over time, and rigid.[15,71] It is a single strand polymer of crystalline isotactic propene.

Over the years, many authors have described variations of the technique; however, the basic technique remains the same.

This type of implantation has enjoyed greater use among surgeons than was expected; because of the position of the implant in the PC, there are less complications (endothelial cell loss, glaucoma, and CME) compared to implantation of open loop AC-IOLs (see later in the chapter). However, this technique is more difficult and requires longer surgical times compared to open loop AC-IOLs: 35 to 60 minutes compared to 8 to 16 minutes[16] and is associated with additional surgical risks.

In our opinion, the elective lens for a PC-IOL sutured secondary implantation without adequate capsular support is a large-diameter one-piece PMMA lens with buttonholes of 180 degrees on the internal surface of each haptic. The diameter of the optic should be 6.5 mm (eg, P366UV [Storz Ophthalmics Inc, Clearwater, FL]) or 7 mm (eg CZ70BD [Alcon Surgical Inc, Fort Worth, TX]). A lens with an optic diameter of 7 mm should be considered if the IOL is either secondary or a replacement associated with PKP, as a lens with a large optic diameter can be easily introduced through a large opening.

With transscleral fixation sutures, the rigidity of the one-piece model decreases the possibility of displacement as compared to a 3-piece model in which the haptics are less stable. The larger optic minimizes the risk of glare if the lens is not centered perfectly during surgery, is decentered postoperatively, or if an iridoplasty does not completely cover the lens edges. The buttonholes prevent the migration of the suture along the haptic and ensure that the sutures are secured to the haptics at 180 degrees.

There are a number of different types of IOLs available for scleral fixation; the unusual feature here are the buttonholes.

A number of foldable IOLs for scleral fixation are available; these allow the surgeon to perform the ab interno technique with a smaller incision than the larger incision needed to insert a PMMA IOL, extremely important if capsular support has been lost during small-incision phacoemulsification.

The power of the IOL should be calculated using one of the approved formulas taking into account the patient's visual requirements. The incision site is an extremely important factor in PC-IOLs with scleral fixation, depending on preoperative astigmatism and the anatomy.

The incision should be centered on the axis of steeper preoperative cylinder, as determined by keratometry or corneal topography. Thus, the incision in patients having with-the-rule astigmatism should be centered at 12 o'clock; conversely, the incision in patients having against-the-rule astigmatism should be placed at 180 degrees. With time, the astigmatic power of the meridian of the incision will tend to decrease. In patients with significant preoperative cylinder (in excess of 2 diopters), an astigmatic keratotomy can be performed intraoperatively, or as a separate procedure postoperatively, when refraction and keratometry readings have stabilized.

Anatomical factors that may influence the orientation of transscleral sutures include the location of filtering blebs, scleral thickness, nerves, and ciliary vessels.

If the sclera is thin, suture erosion may lead to dislocation of the PC-IOL. Ideally, transscleral sutures should be positioned at an oblique axis to avoid nerves and the long ciliary arteries. Fixation at 3 and 9 o'clock should be avoided because of the risk of damaging the nerves and the long ciliary arteries present here. If the astigmatism is with the rule, the incision is normally at 12 o'clock and the transscleral sutures at 2 and 8 o'clock.

In summary, preoperative planning for secondary implantation of a PC-IOL requires the surgeon to carefully determine whether capsular support is adequate and the optimal position for the incision and transscleral suture.

Using this technique, IOLs can be sutured from the inside to the outside of the globe (ab interno technique) or vice versa, by passing the needle from the outside to the inside of the eye (ab externo technique). The main advantage of the ab interno approach is that it is more straightforward (even during PKP) and it is also less time consuming than the ab externo. The disadvantages are the needle passing below the iris without a clear view and the necessity to be based on an indentation of the iris (from below) with the needle to achieve correct positioning in the sulcus.

Regarding the ab interno surgical technique, it may be useful to position a traction suture superiorly or inferiorly. A 12-incision radial keratotomy marker dipped in methylene blue is used to mark the cornea and ensure the position of the transscleral sutures at the appropriate axis 180 degrees from the first.

If there are no contraindications such as a filtering bleb or scleral ectasia, the surgeon performs a conjunctival peritomy with a fornix base of 4 clock hours, centered on the axis of steeper astigmatism. This initial peritomy should be large enough to expose bare sclera above the site for the fixation of the transscleral suture. A second peritomy is made at 2 o'clock, 180 degrees away from the first site of the transscleral suture. For example, in a patient having with-the-rule astigmatism at 90 degrees, the surgeon should make a peritomy of 4 hours at 12 o'clock. This peritomy should be large enough to expose bare sclera at 2 o'clock to place the transscleral suture. A second peritomy should be centered at 8 o'clock for the second transscleral suture. The haptics of the PC-IOL should therefore be fixed at

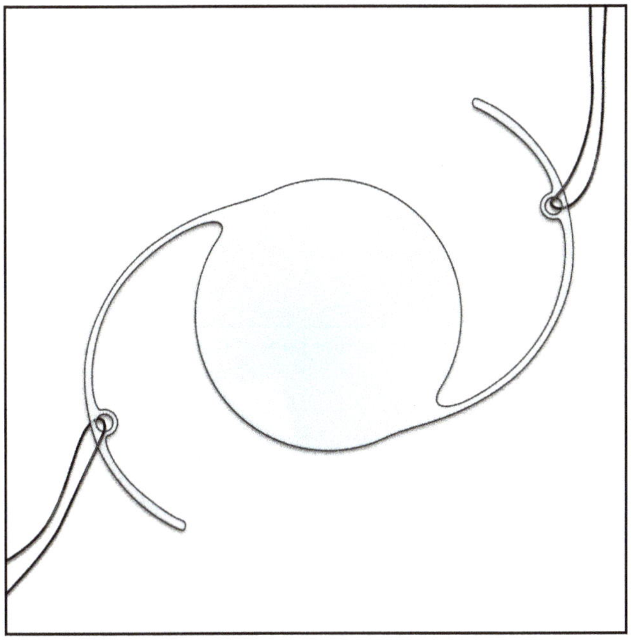

Figure 19-5. Preparation of a PC-IOL for transscleral fixation with a double strand of 10-0 polypropylene passed through the holes in the loops.

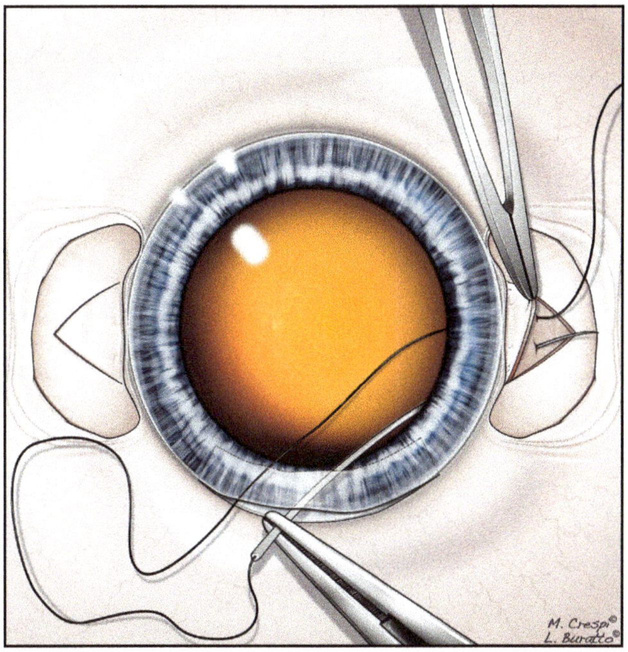

Figure 19-6. Technique for the ab externo approach: the long needles pass first underneath the iris, then through the sulcus to exit through the sclera underneath the flap.

2 and 8 o'clock, to avoid impenging on the nerves, long ciliary arteries as mentioned before.

Wet cauterization is performed to stop bleeding. When conjunctival dissection occurs in the area of previous cataract surgery, dissection of tissue and hemostasis may prove to be more difficult. A no. 67 blade can be used to clean the sclera.

A vertical scleral groove is created approximately 6.5 to 7 mm in length, 1 to 1.5 mm posterior to the surgical limbus. It is approximately 50% of tissue depth. The sclera is then dissected in a plane perpendicular to the groove and extends forward into clear cornea. A supersharp or crescent blade enters the AC just behind Schwalbe's line parallel to the scleral groove to create a 3-planed incision. This type of incision minimizes postoperative astigmatism and creates a watertight closure. The initial opening into the eye should not be more than 3.5 mm in width allowing maintenance of the chamber death for a possible subtotal anterior vitrectomy.

A vitrectomy is necessary in the majority of cases as it will allow correct positioning of the lens without engaging the vitreous. An anterior bimanual vitrectomy is performed through the primary incision with automated irrigation through a second paracentesis. Attention must be paid to removing all of the vitreous from the AC. A light pipe is useful for identifying the vitreous during vitrectomy. In order to decrease the incidence of CME, vitreous should be removed from the wound, the iris, and anything coming into contact with the lens.

Following the vitrectomy, VES is used to push any remaining vitreous away from the insertion site, reform the AC, and protect the endothelium during implantation. The maximum width of the incision is 6.5 to 7.0 mm.

In the ab interno technique, the secondary PC-IOL is prepared for transscleral fixation by passing the end of a double strand 3-inch 10-0 Prolene suture with a long needle (Sharpoint SSL-15, JA2559 [Sharpoint, Surgical Specialties Corp, Reading, PA]) through the eyelet of the lower haptic (Figure 19-5). Long needles such as the STC-6 and the CIF-4 by Ethicon are commonly used; the latter is thicker and provides the surgeon with greater control.

The needle attached to this suture is grasped firmly by a small needle-holder. This needle is passed under the base of the iris and through the ciliary sulcus 0.5 mm above the 8 o'clock axis. The needle should exit the sclera 0.5 to 1 mm behind the surgical limbus.

The second needle of the same suture is then passed under the base of the iris through the ciliary sulcus with the needle exiting 0.5 to 1 mm behind the surgical limbus. This second needle must also pass about 0.5 mm below at 8 o'clock so that the 2 ends of the same suture exit from the sclera approximately 1 mm apart.

A short needle with a 2-inch 10-0 Prolene suture (Sharpoint SSL-5, JA-2560) should be passed through the opposite eyelet.

The needles should therefore be passed through the ciliary sulcus about 0.5 mm above and below the axis at 2 o'clock, 0.5 and 1 mm behind the surgical limbus (Figure 19-6).

It should be remembered that the ciliary sulcus is located just 0.83 mm behind the limbus at the vertical meridian and only 0.46 mm from the limbus at the horizontal meridian.[72]

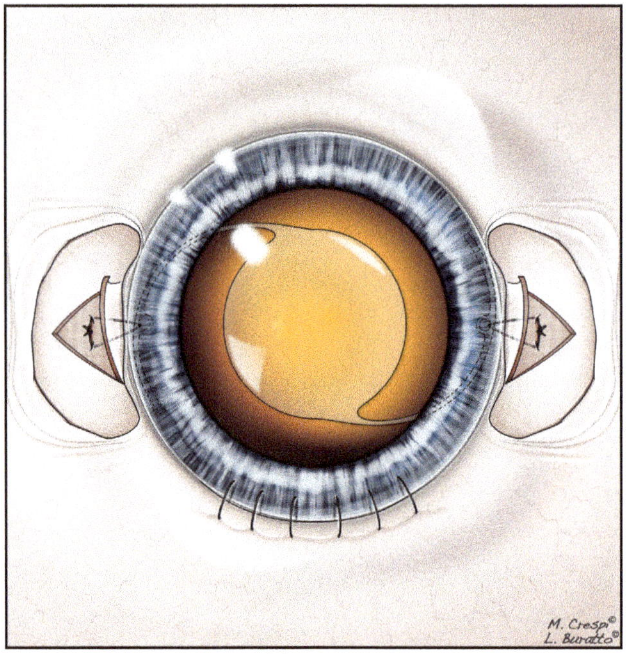

Figure 19-7. The sutures of the PC-IOL are suitably tightened to guarantee perfect centration of the IOL.

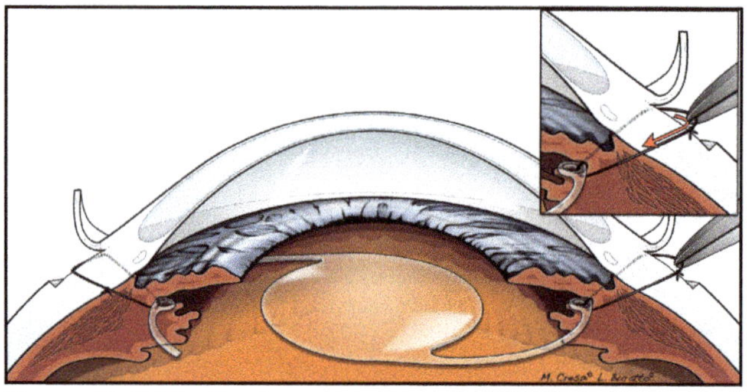

Figure 19-8. The fixation suture knot of the PC-IOL is buried.

One frequent mistake made by inexperienced surgeons is positioning the haptics excessively posterior. This will be obvious as the needle passes in an excessively anterior position noting movements of the iris when this penetrates the peripheral iris stroma close to the angle.

When determining the correct position, the surgeon must make a perfectly perpendicular pass of the needle with respect to the sclera. If the passage of the needle through the sclera is oblique, the successive scleral exit will be more posterior position with respect to the internal sclera, because this will be at the ciliary sulcus.

The superior and inferior transscleral fixation sutures must pass through the sclera 180 degrees opposite to ensure optic centration.

The AC is filled with additional VES. The one-piece PMMA PC-IOL is grasped with lens forceps, through the scleral incision, in the ciliary sulcus (see Figure 19-5). The suture must be held firmly as the lens in inserted to avoid a loop of suture wrapping around the implant. The superior haptic of the lens is then positioned in the ciliary sulcus with the suture pulled tightly. The sutures are then gently pushed forward and backward across the pass for a few millimeters to ensure easy rotation of the knot (Figure 19-7). Each suture is then tied, cut, and the knot buried in the sclera. The suture is rotated with forceps (Figure 19-8). The needles exit from the sclera about 1 mm from the edge and must be strong enough to rotate easily.

Burying the knot in the sclera eliminates the need for scleral flaps and largely decreases suture erosions through the scleral flap and the conjunctiva. An eroded suture can increase the risk endophthalmitis.

If necessary, the surgeon may elect a pupilloplasty or an iridoplasty. A superior peripheral iridectomy can be performed if required and not already present. Positioning of symmetrical sutures between the 2 haptics in the ciliary sulcus and with equal tension will ensure good centration.

Once the PC-IOL has been positioned, VES is removed with irrigation/aspiration to prevent increase in postoperative IOP. The corneoscleral wound is then closed with the surgeon's standard technique. Our method consists of a continuous 10-0 nylon suture. The conjunctiva is sealed with bipolar cauterization or with a suture.

Alternative to the ab interno technique, the ab externo technique suggested by Lewis can be used. [73] This involves passage of the needle through the sclera from outside to in. The sutures are 10-0 Prolene with a long strong needle (such as STC-6). Alcon produces a Pair Pack Fixation Suture (Alcon Laboratories, Fort Worth, TX), which is a hybrid that combines a long needle, SC-5, on one end and a corneal needle, AUM-5, on the other, specific for the ab externo fixation. The long strong needle passes perpendicularly through the sclera (generally below a partial thickness sclera flap), approximately 0.75 mm behind the limbus. The needle should penetrate the ciliary sulcus. The tip of a 25-, 27-, or 28-gauge needle then guides the needle that has penetrated the sulcus from the opposite side. Again with the ab externo technique, the Prolene is pulled through the eye (Figure 19-9). A hook is used to extract the suture through the superior corneal incision. The suture is cut and tied to the IOL haptic (Figure 19-10). At this point the IOL is positioned and the suture fixed to the sclera (Figure 19-11).

This procedure can also be performed with 2 sutures at each haptic, if the surgeon prefers 4 scleral fixation points. Finally, the sutures are tightened on the haptics and the knots buried under the scleral flap.

The advantage of the ab externo technique is greater accuracy in identifying the internal penetration point of the sclera at the ciliary sulcus. Avoiding the highly vascularized pars plicata can minimize bleeding. Moreover, the AC remains closed during the needle passes, reducing the duration of hypotony. The disadvantages are longer procedure times and that it cannot be performed during open-sky

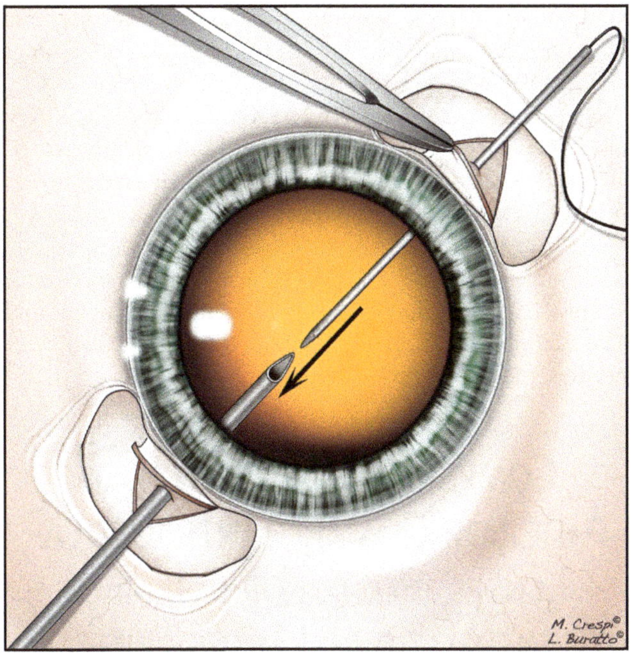

Figure 19-9. Technique for the ab interno approach: the polypropylene suture passes through the eye.

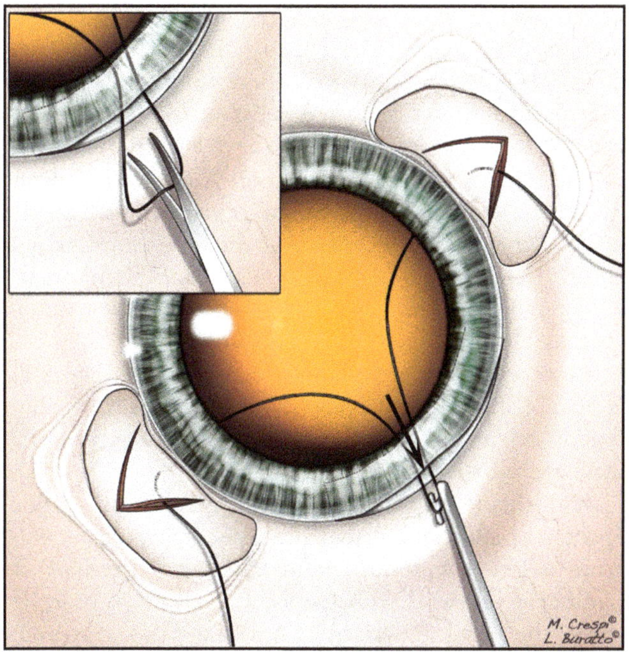

Figure 19-10. A hook is used to draw the suture through the superior corneal incision. The suture is cut and each end is then tied to the haptic of the IOL.

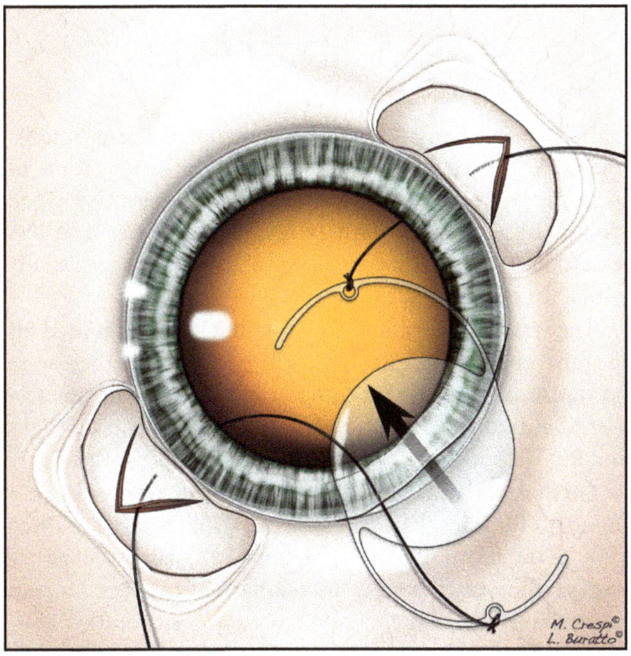

Figure 19-11. After each end has been tied to the haptic of the IOL, the IOL is maneuvered into position, and the suture is fixed to the sclera.

PKP. Also, if several sutures are passed, it is difficult to maintain the same trajectory for each suture.

PC-IOLs with scleral fixation produce excellent visual results and have an acceptable safety profile when implanted as a primary procedure during complicated cataract surgery. In these eyes, however, there are complications associated with capsule rupture, such as retinal detachment and CME, and these may affect recovery. They can also be used in secondary procedures, even with PKP.

The advantages of implanting a scleral fixated PC-IOL come from its position reducing the risk of implantation in AC (progressive endothelial cell loss, synechiae with pupil deformation, chronic inflammation).

In the recent review by Wagoner et al[15] on IOL implants with no capsular support between 1980 and 2001, sponsored by the American Academy of Ophthalmology (AAO), it was concluded that PC-IOLs with scleral fixation are safe and effective in adults. This study included 5 groups of primary implants following complicated cataract surgery, 4 with secondary implants, and 9 implanted during PKP.

Subluxation of the IOL due to suture rupture was not reported in any of the patients. The mean follow-up was 17 months (range, 5.8 to 29 months). Overall, secondary PC-IOL implantation is an effective way to rehabilitate an aphakic patient.

Complications with this type of implant are rare and tend not to induce significant visual disturbances. In relation to the visual results, many of the complications occurred in patients associated with PKP. Careful attention must be paid to the choice of appropriate surgical techniques, as this will avoid some of these complications.

A number of complications have been reported following this type of implantation, some of which are specific to this technique[15,56,67,74-82]: inaccurate placement of the scleral sutures, suprachoroidal hemorrhage, AC or vitreous hemorrhage, retinal detachment, while erosion of the suture may be associated with endophthalmitis. Finally, rupture of the suture can lead to IOL displacement. For these reasons, some surgeons believe that this technique is associated with a greater number of complications as opposed to iris sutured or foldable open loop AC-IOLs.[37]

The transscleral pass of the needle close to the ciliary sulcus carries with it a risk of intraocular hemorrhage (in the AC or vitreous), even though these are rare occurrences. Hemorrhages in the vitreous chamber are usually self-limiting and reabsorb spontaneously; massive suprachoroidal hemorrhages are extremely rare.

As we will see later, numerous studies demonstrate risks of PC-IOL dislocation because of suture rupture or deterioration[77] or endophthalmitis caused by infected sutures and these are statistically significant.[78]

With this technique, suture erosion and/or dislocation of the lens are rare but they are a possibility. Many surgeons believe that erosion and the exposure of the knot are significant problems with the technique.[71,79] In order to reduce this problem, seen in up to 17% of cases, numerous techniques have been developed to bury the knots partially or completely, with a procedure similar to the nylon sutures used in corneal incisions.[80]

A number of studies[56,81,82] have shown that 10-0 Prolene can degrade over time, leading to the spontaneous subluxation of the IOL. A tilted or decentered IOL has been reported in 3% to 10% of cases. This may occur years after implantation of the IOL, typically 4 to 5 years or more and is the result of trauma or biodegradation. We believe that in the older findings (that suggested good results in both adults and children), the observation period was too short, particularly in children.

AAO *Focal Points*, published September 2006 (based on a previously published report[15]) focused on sutured PC-IOLs and recommended using 9-0 and 10-0 Prolene sutures; however, it did not mention the real potential long-term deterioration of 10-0 Prolene.[71,79]

If the surgery suggestions are followed, the vast majority of eyes will have the sutures positioned in the ciliary sulcus with a development of a fibrous membrane around the haptics. However, up to 23% of the lenses are actually located posterior to the ciliary sulcus.[83]

The use of a lens that is too large or too small for the sulcus, with a suture that is too tight, may induce astigmatism, especially in PKP eyes.[84]

Other complications possible following a secondary IOL implant (such as corneal edema, glaucoma, and CME) occur in percentages comparable to the open loop AC-IOLs.[15]

Macular edema (ME) is probably the most frequent complication after this type of implant; 2% to 36% of cases are reported for various groups.[11,15,16,36-39] Some feel ME is less frequent with PC-IOLs sutured to the iris, compared to foldable open loop AC-IOLs or PC-IOLs with scleral fixation.

CME and retinal detachment appear more frequently after vitreous loss or vitrectomy. For this reason, manipulation of the vitreous should be avoided unless vitreous presents on the iris or in the implantation. Retinal detachment occurs in 2.6% to 5.4% of cases.[16,36-39]

Secondary glaucoma may be the result of pupillary block, hyphema, or inflammation, and is frequently associated with PKP. Aqueous inhibitors should be used if necessary. Untreatable cases may require a filtering procedure.

Progressive corneal edema or secondary failure of corneal transplants are rare and can be minimized by careful use of VES to coat the endothelium during lens implantion. The surgeon should avoid touching the endothelium with needles, the lens, or instruments.

Comparison of Open Loop Anterior Chamber Intraocular Lenses, Posterior Chamber Intraocular Lenses With Scleral Fixation, and Iris-Sutured Posterior Chamber Intraocular Lenses

In the few clinical trials that compare these 3 techniques[16,36-39] or in studies specific for each type of implant,[17,65] there is no evidence of clear superiority. Open loop AC-IOL implantation is technically easier and less time consuming than the other 2 techniques, especially with a limbal approach.[16]

The visual results are similar for all 3 IOLs when used for the same clinical indication.[16-39,60-68,74-78] In fact, there were no statistically significant differences in visual outcomes in 2 randomized trials[16,36] that compared open loop AC-IOLs and PC-IOLs with scleral fixation after cataract surgery.

Furthermore, no significant differences were seen in a number of studies that evaluated the visual results obtained with different IOLs.[21,22,25,26,60,61] Following secondary implantation in eyes with uncomplicated cataract surgery, more than 90% of the eyes achieved a postoperative best-corrected visual acuity equal to or greater than 1 Snellen line compared to the preoperative best-corrected visual acuity, regardless of the technique used.[21,22,25,26,60,61]

Regarding complications, the percentage of endothelial cell loss, glaucoma, and CME is relatively low for open loop AC-IOLs[16-39] and perhaps slightly lower for lenses with scleral fixation[16,24,30,34,36,37,39] or iris suture[16,36-39,60-65] (Table 19-1).

For eyes undergoing simultaneous PKP, there was no statistically significant difference in terms of visual acuity among the 3 types of IOLs and in terms of postoperative complications (particularly endothelial cell loss) between

Table 19-1.

Complications

COMPLICATION	IOL IN THE SULCUS	AC-IOL	PC-IOL	
			With Scleral Fixation	*With Iris Fixation*
Acute cystoid macular edema	+	++	++	++
Chronic cystoid macular edema	-	+	+	+
Glaucoma	-	++	+	+
IOL tilt/decentrataion	-	+	++	++
Suture eosion	No	No	++	No
Endophthalmitis associated with the suture	No	No	+	No
Endophthalmitis not associated with the suture	+	+	+	+
Corneal edema	+	++	+	+
Intraoperative bleeding	+	+	++	++
Synechiae	-	++	-	+
Retinal detachment	-	+	++	+
Choriodal detachment	-	+	++	+
Uveitis	-	++	-	+
Long-term corneal decompensation	-	+	-	-
Risk of failure of Prolene	No	No	+	+

the open loop AC-IOLs and iris sutured PC-IOLs in the first 2 years after surgery.[38]

In studies on the individual IOLs, the incidence of postoperative corneal edema or endothelial cell loss of a transplanted cornea was not a significant problem, regardless of the type of IOL implanted.[16-39,60-65] Only one study reported nonstatically significant corneal edema after secondary implantation of an open loop AC-IOL with cataract surgery compared to the implantation of PC-IOL with scleral fixation.[36]

There were no statistically significant differences in the incidence of postsurgery glaucoma in 2 studies that compared the 3 techniques during PKP.[37,39]

The interpretation of CME is more complex, as it is difficult to make an accurate assessment of its impact (probably high) in many eyes. The incidence of this complication is relatively high in several patient groups for all 3 types of IOLs.[11,15] In 2 clinical studies that compared secondary implantation of open loop AC-IOLs and PC-IOLs with scleral fixation during PKP, it appeared that the incidence of CME is not different.[37-39] In another study on PKP, there was a statistically lower incidence of CME with a PC-IOL sutured to the iris as opposed to open loop AC-IOLs and PC-IOLs with scleral fixation.[37]

Secondary Intraocular Lens Implants in Children

Good results of secondary implants have been reported in children with or without adequate capsular support. Pediatric patients implanted with an AC-IOL face significant long-term complications, such as endothelial cell loss, iris sphincter erosion, pupillary ectopia, and glaucoma; consequently, this procedure is not recommended.[85,86]

On the other hand, the iris claw IOLs (always located in AC) are not angle supported, but remain enclavated to the iris using small PMMA clips that are part of the IOL lens. These are frequently used in Europe (not in the United States) and have produced satisfactory results for more than 20 years. Good results have been published with these implants in children.[87]

The implant of a PC-IOL with scleral fixation is the choice for many surgeons for pediatric patients; the benefit is the anatomical site of the implant.[86,88-90] After a PC-IOL with scleral fixation, most cases showed a significant improvement in vision, as reported in several studies. However, all (except one) had a relatively short follow-up.

The longest had a mean period of just 3 years.[86,91-93] The procedure is therefore considered safe and effective, and the material of the fixation suture seems to be strong enough to resist deterioration over the years.

The most important factor that limits functional results in children is amblyopia, regardless of the type of implant used.

A review of the literature[56,71,79,81,82] shows that breakage of 10-0 Prolene suture is not an issue. However, it should be pointed out that follow-up in most of these studies was probably too short to demonstrate the true incidence of this late onset complication.[56,71,79,81,82] A study based on IOLs sutured in the PC in pediatric cases with a longer follow up was published by Buckley.[71] The mean observation period was 5 years with one-third of patients followed for over 7 years. Spontaneous rupture of the 10-0 Prolene suture (spontaneous biodegradation of the suture thread) was seen frequently (ie, in 9% of cases, no trauma had been reported). Spontaneous deterioration of the suture had been documented by Drews several years ago in a study using scanning electron microscopy.[94]

Moreover, as children are more physically active than adults, they run a greater risk of chafing by suture; so as suggested earlier, a different type of suture may be indicated.

Another interesting work was published by Jongebloed and Worst[95] who studied a 10-0 Prolene suture to fix an IOL for a period of 6.5 years. The degradation phenomena, presumably related to the activation of enzymatic tissue fluid, were as follows: cracks appeared in the fixation suture perpendicular to its longitudinal axis, a portion of the surface layer was partially or completely detached, the overall diameter of both ends of the suture was reduced by 50% of the initial diameter, and the substrata layer exposed had a fibrillar structure.

Subsequent reports suggest that these degradation phenomena affecting the suture are related to the molecular orientation of the Prolene used in the sutures, since they are also observed in the Prolene used in the haptics of the IOLs.[96]

Clearly, integrity of the sutures is important for long-term scleral fixation of the IOL because the formation of fibrous membranes, formed around the haptic when they are positioned accurately in the sulcus, contributes little to the stability of this type of implant.

To secure the IOL to the sclera, 10-0 Prolene should be used with caution in children; other materials should be considered as alternatives or slightly larger dimensions.[71]

As previously mentioned, the AAO *Focal Points* article on sutured PC-IOLs recommended sutures of 9-0 to 10-0 Prolene for this type of surgery. Also, Price et al[56] and Stewart and Landers[96] recommend the use of 9-0 Prolene as opposed to 10-0 Prolene. The physical characteristics of 9-0 Prolene are the same as 10-0 Prolene, yet the tensile strength of 9-0 Prolene is 60% greater and the diameter 50% greater, with a surface area 125% greater, resulting in greater resistance to degradation over time than 10-0 Prolene.

Moreover, the 9-0 Prolene suture is available with the CIF-4 needle, but not with the STC-6. Alternatively, some surgeons proposed a simple needle hook combination to obtain the same effect as the STC-6 needle using a 9-0 Prolene suture.[63]

In the literature,[56,63,71,79,81,82,86-90,94] there are no cases of IOL dislocation secondary to rupture of a 9-0 Prolene suture. The only difficulty associated with the use of these sutures is the size of the knot being larger, requiring deeper burying to avoid conjunctival erosion.

Assia et al,[97] in cases of suture rupture, implant AC-IOL or iris fixation instead of a resuturing the IOL to the sclera.

Surprisingly, none of the authors who suggested resuturing suggested a different size or type of suture.[98]

Sutureless Scleral Fixation Techniques

Sutureless implantation with scleral fixation is performed with 2 strategies:

- Scleral tunnel
- Fibrin glue

The creation of "intrascleral tunnels" to fix the haptic of a PC-IOL is a technique that combines the control of a closed eye system with the axial stability of the PC-IOL.[99-101]

The steps of the procedure are as follows:

1. Using a standard 25-gauge blade, 2 sclerotomies are performed 1.5 to 2.0 mm from the limbus, placed 180 degrees apart.
2. Two scleral tunnels are created with a 24-gauge cannula starting from the sclerotomy and extending clockwise for 4 mm to about 50% of scleral thickness.
3. A PC-IOL injector for a standard 3-piece acrylic lens is introduced through an incision in clear cornea (2.5 mm).
4. Stabilization of the haptics: At first the proximal haptic is left outside the globe, while the distal tip of the haptic is grasped with a 25-gauge microforceps toward the sclerotomy and pulled into the tunnel. After positioning of the distal haptic, the proximal haptic is placed into the AC, and the tip is grasped with 25-gauge forceps and positioned into the second tunnel.

After securing the haptics, the IOL is positioned behind the pupil and correct centration of the PC-IOL is achieved through small adjustments of the intrascleral position of the haptic.

The intrascleral tissue is a good anatomical site because it is avascular and has a low tendency to inflammation.

The haptic can also be attached to the sclera with fibrin glue. This is a biological glue containing human fibrinogen

(20 mg/0.5 mL), thrombin (250 UI/0.5 mL), a solution of aprotinin (1500 KIU in 0.5mL), and has a triple action—it is adhesive, hemostatic, and stimulates tissue regeneration.

Fibrin glue in ophthalmology has several applications: conjunctival closure after pterygium surgery, strabismus, closure of corneal perforations, descemetoceles, and closure of a conjunctival bleb following trabeculectomy.[102] Recently, Agarwal et al[103] used fibrin glue to attach the haptic of a PC-IOLs to the sclera.

The steps of surgery follow:

1. Creation of limbal-based scleral flaps in the inferior temporal and superior nasal areas 180 degrees apart
2. Creation of 2 sclerotomies with a 23-gauge blade—the inferior one is positioned near the lower edge of the inferior temporal scleral flap, the upper one near the top edge of the superior nasal flap
3. Introduction of standard PC-IOLs following the creation of a 2.5-mm tunnel in clear cornea
4. Externalization of the haptics: The distal end of the haptic is grasped with 25-gauge forceps and externalized through the sclerotomy below the superior nasal flap, following its curvature, and finally positioned on the bed of the scleral flap
5. Insertion of the tips of the haptic in the scleral tissue (a useful tip)
6. Externalization of the proximal haptic through the sclerotomy of the inferior temporal flap and positioning in the bed of the flap
7. Application of fibrin glue under the flaps using a special delivery system
8. Compression of the scleral flap for 20 seconds
9. Perfect adhesion of the scleral flap was obtained from the first postoperative day and was finally complete 6 weeks after surgery

Postoperative Treatment

Immediately after implantation of a secondary IOL, the patient should have an injection of antibiotics and steroids in the lower conjunctival fornix, followed by a moderate compression patch and a protective shell on the operated eye.

The patient is examined on the first postoperative day. The eye is examined for any degree of inflammation, hyphema, any increase in IOP, or wound leak.

The patient uses antibiotic/steroid eye drops for the first 4 to 6 weeks postoperatively. Any excessive inflammation is treated by increasing the topical steroids. Postoperative hyphema is frequent, but does not normally require surgical intervention. Increase in IOP is treated with aqueous inhibitors.

After the initial check, the patient is examined at regular intervals based on the clinical situation. We usually see the patient at the end of the first postoperative week, and after the third and eighth weeks. The fundus is examined regularly 12 to 18 months after surgery to avoid the risk of retinal detachment and postoperative CME.

Conclusion

The secondary implantation of a lens with or without capsular support is a relatively safe and effective option for visual rehabilitation of the aphakic eye, even for children, when the patient cannot tolerate spectacles or contact lenses. However, presently, none of the techniques are felt to be superior to the other techniques presented. Through careful surgical planning and adequate discussion with the patient regarding potential surgical benefits and risks, secondary IOL implantation will often produce great satisfaction for both the patient and the surgeon.

References

1. Collins JF, Gaster RN, Krol WF, Colling CL, Kirk GF, Smith TJ; Department of Veterans Affairs Cooperative Cataract Study. A comparison of anterior chamber and posterior chamber intraocular lenses after vitreous presentation during cataract surgery: the Department of Veterans Affairs Cooperative Cataract Study. *Am J Ophthalmol.* 2003;136(1):1-9.
2. Yilmaz A, Başer Z, Yurdakul NS, Maden A. Posterior chamber lens implantation techniques in posterior capsular rupture. *Eur J Ophthalmol.* 2004;14(1):7-13.
3. Chang DF, Masket S, Miller KM, Braga-Mele R, Little BC, Mamalis N, Oetting TA, Packer M; ASCRS Cataract Clinical Committee. Complications of sulcus placement of single-piece acrylic intraocular lenses: recommendations for backup IOL implantation following posterior capsule rupture. *J Cataract Refract Surg.* 2009;35(8):1445-1458.
4. Amino K, Yamakawa R. Long-term results of out-of-the-bag intraocular lens implantation. *J Cataract Refract Surg.* 2000;26(2):266-270.
5. Pavlin CJ, Harasiewicz K, Foster FS. Ultrasound biomicroscopic analysis of haptic position in late-onset, recurrent hyphema after posterior chamber lens implantation. *J Cataract Refract Surg.* 1994;20(2):182-185.
6. Vasavada AR, Raj SM, Karve S, Vasavada V, Vasavada V, Theoulakis P. Retrospective ultrasound biomicroscopic analysis of single-piece sulcus-fixated acrylic intraocular lenses. *J Cataract Refract Surg.* 2010;36(5):771-777.
7. Loya N, Lichter H, Barash D, Goldenberg-Cohen N, Strassmann E, Weinberger D. Posterior chamber intraocular lens implantation after capsular tear: ultrasound biomicroscopy evaluation. *J Cataract Refract Surg.* 2001;27(9):1423-1427.
8. Mimura T, Amano S, Sugiura T, et al. Refractive change after transscleral fixation of posterior chamber intraocular lenses in the absence of capsular support. *Acta Ophthalmol Scand.* 2004;82(5):544-546.
9. Dick HB, Augustin AJ. Lens implant selection with absence of capsular support. *Curr Opin Ophthalmol.* 2001;12:47-57.

10. Auffarth GU, Wesendahl TA, Brown SJ, Apple DJ. Are there acceptable anterior chamber intraocular lenses for clinical use in the 1990s? An analysis of 4104 explanted anterior chamber intraocular lenses. *Ophthalmology.* 1994;101:1913-1922.
11. Smith PW, Wong SK, Stark WJ, et al. Complications of semi-flexible, closed-loop anterior chamber intraocular lenses. *Arch Ophthalmol.* 1987;105:52-57.
12. Apple DJ, Brems RN, Park RB, et al. Anterior chamber lenses. Part I (Complications and pathology and review of designs). *J Cataract Refract Surg.* 1987;13:157-174.
13. Apple DJ, Hansen SO, Richards SC, et al. Anterior chamber lenses. Part II (A laboratory study). *J Cataract Refract Surg.* 1987;13:175-189.
14. Miyake K, Asakura M, Kobayashi H. Effect of intraocular lens fixation on the blood-aqueous barrier. *Am J Ophthalmol.* 1984;98:451-455.
15. Wagoner MD, Cox TA, Ariyasu RG, Jacobs DS, Karp CL; American Academy of Ophthalmology. Intraocular lens implantation in the absence of capsular support: a report by the American Academy of Ophthalmology. *Ophthalmology.* 2003;110(4):840-859.
16. Bellucci R, Pucci S, Morselli S, Bonomi L. Secondary implantation of angle-supported anterior chamber and scleral-fixated posterior chamber intraocular lenses. *J Cataract Refract Surg.* 1996;22:247-252.
17. Hennig A, Evans JR, Pradhan D, et al. Randomised controlled trial of anterior-chamber intraocular lenses. *Lancet.* 1997;349:1129-1133.
18. Rattigan SM, Ellerton CR, Chitkara DK, Smerdon DL. Flexible open loop anterior chamber intraocular lens implantation after posterior capsule complications in extracapsular cataract extraction. *J Cataract Refract Surg.* 1996;22:243-246.
19. Bergman M, Laatikainen L. Long-term evaluation of primary anterior chamber intraocular lens implantation in complicated cataract surgery. *Int Ophthalmol.* 1996;97;20:295-299.
20. Hykin PG, Gardner ID, Corbett MC, Cheng H. Primary or secondary anterior chamber lens implantation after extracapsular cataract surgery and vitreous loss. *Eye.* 1991;5:694-698.
21. Bayramlar HS, Hepsen IF, Cekic O, Gunduz A. Comparison of the results of primary and secondary implantation of flexible open loop anterior chamber intraocular lens. *Eye.* 1998;12:826-828.
22. Weene LE. Flexible open loop anterior chamber intraocular lens implants. *Ophthalmology.* 1993;100:1636-1639.
23. Kazemi S, Wirostko WJ, Sinha S, et al. Combined pars plana lensectomy-vitrectomy with open loop flexible anterior chamber intraocular lens (AC-IOL) implantation for subluxated lenses. *Trans Am Ophthalmol Soc.* 2000;98:247-251.
24. Omulecki W, Nawrocki J, Sempinska-Szewczyk J, Synder A. Transscleral suture fixation and anterior chamber intraocular lenses implanted after removal of posteriorly dislocated crystalline lenses. *Eur J Ophthalmol.* 1997;7:370-374.
25. Ellerton CR, Rattigan SM, Chapman FM, et al. Secondary implantation of open loop, flexible, anterior chamber intraocular lenses. *J Cataract Refract Surg.* 1996;22:951-954.
26. Drolsum L, Haaskjold E. Secondary implantation of flexible open loop anterior chamber IOLs. *Acta Ophthalmol (Copenh).* 1993;7:482-486.
27. Malinowski SM, Mieler WF, Koenig SB, et al. Combined pars plana vitrectomy-lensectomy and open loop anterior chamber lens implantation. *Ophthalmology.* 1995;102:211-216.
28. Mittra RA, Connor TB, Han DP, et al. Removal of dislocated intraocular lenses using pars plana vitrectomy with placement of an open loop, flexible anterior chamber lens. *Ophthalmology.* 1998;105:1011-1014.
29. Lois N, Cohen EJ, Rapuano CJ, Laibson PR. Long-term graft survival in patients with flexible open loop anterior-chamber intraocular lenses. *Cornea.* 1997;16:387-392.
30. Brunette I, Stulting RD, Rinne JR, et al. Penetrating keratoplasty with anterior or posterior chamber intraocular lens implantation. *Arch Ophthalmol.* 1994;112:1311-1319.
31. Hassan TS, Soong HK, Sugar A, Meyer RF. Implantation of Kelman-style, open loop anterior chamber lenses during keratoplasty for aphakic and pseudophakic bullous keratopathy. A comparison with iris-sutured posterior chamber lenses. *Ophthalmology.* 1991;98:875-880.
32. Kornmehl EW, Steinert RF, Odrich MG, Stevens JB. Penetrating keratoplasty for pseudophakic bullous keratopathy associated with closed-loop anterior chamber intraocular lenses. *Ophthalmology.* 1990;97:407-412.
33. Zaidman GW, Goldman S. A prospective study on the implantation of anterior chamber intraocular lenses during keratoplasty for pseudophakic and aphakic bullous keratopathy. *Ophthalmology.* 1990;97:757-762.
34. Lass JH, DeSantis DM, Reinhart WJ, et al. Clinical and morphometric results of penetrating keratoplasty with one-piece anterior-chamber or suture-fixated posterior-chamber lenses in the absence of lens capsule. *Arch Ophthalmol.* 1990;108:1427-1431.
35. Koenig SB, Apple DJ, Hyndiuk RA. Penetrating keratoplasty and intraocular lens exchange (open loop anterior chamber lenses versus sutured posterior chamber lenses). *Cornea.* 1994;13:418-421.
36. Lyle WA, Jin JC. Secondary intraocular lens implantation (anterior chamber vs posterior chamber lenses). *Ophthalmic Surg.* 1993;24:375-381.
37. Schein OD, Kenyon KR, Steinert RF, et al. A randomized trial of intraocular lens fixation techniques with penetrating keratoplasty. *Ophthalmology.* 1993;100:1437-1443.
38. Sugar A. An analysis of corneal endothelial and graft survival in pseudophakic bullous keratopathy. *Trans Am Ophthalmol Soc.* 1989;87:762-801.
39. Davis RM, Best D, Gilbert GE. Comparison of intraocular lens fixation techniques performed during penetrating keratoplasty. *Am J Ophthalmol.* 1991;11:743-749.
40. Worst JG, Massaro RG, Ludwig HH. The introduction of an artificial lens into the eye using Binkhorst's technique. *Ophthalmologica.* 1972;164(5):387-391.
41. Evereklioglu C, Er H, Bekir NA, Borazan M, Zorlu F. Comparison of secondary implantation of flexible open loop anterior chamber and scleral-fixated posterior chamber intraocular lenses. *J Cataract Refract Surg.* 2003;29(2):301-308.
42. Güell JL, Velasco F, Malecaze F, Vázquez M, Gris O, Manero F. Secondary Artisan-Verysise aphakic lens implantation. *J Cataract Refract Surg.* 2005;31(12):2266-2271.
43. Koss MJ, Kohnen T. Intraocular architecture of secondary implanted anterior chamber iris-claw lenses in aphakic eyes evaluated with anterior segment optical coherence tomography. *Br J Ophthalmol.* 2009;93(10):1301-1306.
44. Acar N, Kapran Z, Altan T, Kucuksumer Y, Unver YB, Polat E. Secondary iris claw intraocular lens implantation for the correction of aphakia after pars plana vitrectomy. *Retina.* 2010;30(1):131-139.
45. Hirashima DE, Soriano ES, Meirelles RL, Alberti GN, Nosé W. Outcomes of iris-claw anterior chamber versus iris-fixated foldable intraocular lens in subluxated lens secondary to Marfan syndrome. *Ophthalmology.* 2010;117(8):1479-1485.
46. Budo C, Hessloehl JC, Izak M, et al. Multicenter study of the Artisan phakic intraocular lens. *J Cataract Refract Surg.* 2000;26(8):1163-1171.
47. Rüfer F, Saeger M, Nölle B, Roider J. Implantation of retropupillar iris claw lenses with and without combined penetrating keratoplasty. *Graefes Arch Clin Exp Ophthalmol.* 2009;247(4): 457-462.
48. McCannel MA. A retrievable suture idea for anterior uveal problems. *Ophthalmic Surg.* 1976;7(2):98-103.

49. Stark WJ, Goodman G, Goodman D, Gottish J. Posterior chamber intraocular lens implantation in the absence of posterior capsula support. *Opthalmic Surg.* 1988;19:240-243.
50. Stutzman RD, Stark WJ. Surgical technique for suture fixation of an acrylic intraocular lens in the absence of capsule support. *J Cataract Refract Surg.* 2003;29(9):1658-1662.
51. Condon GP. Simplified small-incision peripheral iris fixation of an AcrySof intraocular lens in the absence of capsule support. *J Cataract Refract Surg.* 2003;29(9):1663-1667.
52. Hall JR, Muenzler WS. Intraocular lens replacement in pseudophakic bullous keratopathy. *Trans Ophthalmol Soc UK.* 1985;104:541-545.
53. Soong HK, Musch DC, Kowal V, Sugar A, Meyer RF. Implantation of posterior chamber intraocular lenses in the absence of lens capsule during penetrating keratoplasty. *Arch Ophthalmol.* 1989;107(5):660-665.
54. Siepser SB. The closed chamber slipping suture technique for iris repair. *Ann Ophthalmol.* 1994;26(3):71-72.
55. Guttman C. IOL dislocation management differentiated by complication profiles. *Ophthalmology Times.* 2009
56. Price MO, Price FW Jr, Werner L, Berlie C, Mamalis N. Late dislocation of scleral-sutured posterior chamber intraocular lenses. *J Cataract Refract Surg.* 2005;31(7):1320-1326.
57. Schechter RJ. Suture-wick endophthalmitis with sutured posterior chamber intraocular lenses. *J Cataract Refract Surg.* 1990;16(6):755-756.
58. Mura JJ, Pavlin CJ, Condon GP, et al. Ultrasound biomicroscopic analysis of iris-sutured foldable posterior chamber intraocular lenses. *Am J Ophthalmol.* 2010;149(2):245-252.
59. Hoffman RS, Packer M, Fine IH. Decentered and subluxed IOLs need not be intimidating. *Ophthalmology Times.* 2005.
60. Hoh H, Ruprecht K, Nikoloudakis N, Palmowski A. Preliminary results following implantation of iris-suture-fixated posterior-chamber lenses. *Ger J Ophthalmol.* 1993;2:70-75.
61. Navia-Aray EA. Suturing a posterior chamber intraocular lens to the iris through limbal incisions (results in 30 eyes). *J Refract Corneal Surg.* 1994;10:565-570.
62. Zeh WG, Price FW. Iris fixation of posterior chamber intraocular lenses. *J Cataract Refract Surg.* 2000;26:1028-1034.
63. Gaster RN, Ong HV. Results of penetrating keratoplasty with posterior chamber intraocular lens implantation in the absence of a lens capsule. *Cornea.* 1991;10:498-506.
64. Busin M, Brauweiler P, Boker T, Spitznas M. Complications of sulcus-supported intraocular lenses with iris sutures, implanted during penetrating keratoplasty after intracapsular cataract extraction. *Ophthalmology.* 1990;97:401-405.
65. Chu MW, Font RL, Koch DD. Visual results and complications following posterior iris-fixated posterior chamber lenses at penetrating keratoplasty. *Ophthalmic Surg.* 1992;23:608-613.
66. Price FW Jr, Whitson WE, Collins K, Johns S. Explantation of posterior chamber lenses. *J Cataract Refract Surg.* 1992;18(5):475-479.
67. Lubniewski AJ, Holland EJ, Van Meter WS, Gussler D, Parelman J, Smith ME. Histologic study of eyes with transsclerally sutured posterior chamber intraocular lenses. *Am J Ophthalmol.* 1990;110(3):237-243.
68. Stark WJ, Gottsch JD, Goodman DF, et al. Posterior chamber intraocular lens implantation in the absence of capsular support. *Arch Ophthalmol.* 1989;107:1078-1083.
69. Girard LJ. Pars plana phacoprosthesis (aphakic intraocular implant): a preliminary report. *Ophthalmic Surg.* 1981;12(1):19-22.
70. Malbran ES, Malbran E Jr, Negri I. Lens guide suture for transport and fixation in secondary IOL implantation after intracapsular extraction. *Int Ophthalmol.* 1986;9(2-3):151-160.
71. Buckley EG. Hanging by a thread: the long-term efficacy and safety of transscleral sutured intraocular lenses in children (an American Ophthalmological Society thesis). *Trans Am Ophthalmol Soc.* 2007;105:294-311.
72. Duffey RJ, Holland EJ, Agapitos PJ, Lindstrom RL. Anatomic study of transsclerally sutured intraocular lens implantation. *Am J Ophthalmol.* 1989;108(3):300-309.
73. Lewis JS. Ab externo sulcus fixation. *Ophthalmic Surg.* 1991;22(11):692-695.
74. LeeJG, Lee JH, Chung H. Factors contributing to retinal detachment after transscleral fixation of posterior chamber intraocular lenses. *J Cataract Refract Surg.* 1998;24:697-702.
75. Pavlin CJ, Rootman D, Arshinoff S, et al. Determination of haptic position of transsclerally fixated posterior chamber intraocular lenses by ultrasound biomicroscopy. *J Cataract Refract Surg.* 1993;19:573-577.
76. Durak A, Oner HF, Kocak N, Kaynak S. Tilt and decentration after primary and secondary transsclerally sutured posterior chamber intraocular lens implantation. *J Cataract Refract Surg.* 2001;27:227-232.
77. Cahane M, Chen V, Avni I. Dislocation of a scleral-fixated, posterior chamber intraocular lens after fixation suture removal. *J Cataract Refract Surg.* 1994;20:186-187.
78. Heilskov T, Joondeph BC, Olsen KR, Blankenship GW. Late endophthalmitis after transscleral fixation of a posterior chamber intraocular lens. *Arch Ophthalmol.* 1989;107:1427.
79. Solomon K, Gussler JR, Gussler C, Van Meter WS. Incidence and management of complications of transsclerally sutured posterior chamber lenses. *J Cataract Refract Surg.* 1993;19(4):488-493.
80. Lewis JS. Sulcus fixation without flaps. *Ophthalmology.* 1993;100(9):1346-1350.
81. Kim J, Kinyoun JL, Saperstein DA, Porter SL. Subluxation of transscleral sutured posterior chamber intraocular lens (TSIOL). *Am J Ophthalmol.* 2003;136(2):382-384.
82. Vote BJ, Tranos P, Bunce C, Charteris DG, Da Cruz L. Long-term outcome of combined pars plana vitrectomy and scleral fixated sutured posterior chamber intraocular lens implantation. *Am J Ophthalmol.* 2006;141(2):308-312.
83. Holland EJ, Djalilian AR, Pederson J. Gonioscopic evaluation of haptic position in transsclerally sutured posterior chamber lenses. *Am J Ophthalmol.* 1997;123(3):411-413.
84. Hardten DR, Holland EJ, Doughman DJ, Nelson JD. Early post-keratoplasty astigmatism following placement of anterior chamber lenses and transsclerally sutured posterior chamber lenses. *CLAO J.* 1992;18(2):108-111.
85. Sharpe MR, Biglan AW, Gerontis CC. Scleral fixation of posterior chamber intraocular lenses in children. *Ophthalmic Surg Lasers.* 1996;27(5):337-341.
86. Epley KD, Shainberg MJ, Lueder GT, Tychsen L. Pediatric secondary lens implantation in the absence of capsular support. *J AAPOS.* 2001;5(5):301-306.
87. Van der Pol BA, Worst JG. Iris-claw intraocular lenses in children. *Doc Ophthalmol.* 1996-1997;92(1):29-35.
88. Trivedi RH, Wilson ME Jr, Facciani J. Secondary intraocular lens implantation for pediatric aphakia. *J AAPOS.* 2005;9(4):346-352.
89. Biglan AW, Cheng KP, Davis JS, Gerontis CC. Secondary intraocular lens implantation after cataract surgery in children. *Am J Ophthalmol.* 1997;123(2):224-234.
90. Lambert SR, Lynn M, Drews-Botsch C, et al. Intraocular lens implantation during infancy: perceptions of parents and the American Association for Pediatric Ophthalmology and Strabismus members. *J AAPOS.* 2003;7(6):400-405.
91. Buckley EG. Scleral fixated (sutured) posterior chamber intraocular lens implantation in children. *J AAPOS.* 1999;3(5):289-294.
92. Bardorf CM, Epley KD, Lueder GT, Tychsen L. Pediatric transscleral sutured intraocular lenses: efficacy and safety in 43 eyes followed an average of 3 years. *J AAPOS.* 2004;8(4):318-324.
93. Jacobi PC, Dietlein TS, Konen W. Multifocal intraocular lens implantation in pediatric cataract surgery. *Ophthalmology.* 2001;108(8):1375-1380.

94. Drews RC. Polypropylene in the human eye. *J Am Intraocul Implant Soc.* 1983;9(2):137-142.
95. Jongebloed WL, Worst JF. Degradation of polypropylene in the human eye: a SEM-study. *Doc Ophthalmol.* 1986;64(1): 143-152.
96. Stewart MW, Landers MB 3rd. Transscleral intraocular lens fixation with a "homemade" needle and hook. *J Cataract Refract Surg.* 2006;32(2):200-202.
97. Assia EI, Nemet A, Sachs D. Bilateral spontaneous subluxation of scleral-fixated intraocular lenses. *J Cataract Refract Surg.* 2002;28(12):2214-2216.
98. Balta FN. Surgical technique for repositioning subluxated previously scleral-fixated intraocular lenses. *Am J Ophthalmol.* 2004;138(4):676-677.
99. Gabor SG, Pavlidis mm. Sutureless intrascleral posterior chamber intraocular lens fixation. *J Cataract Refract Surg.* 2007;33(11):1851-1854.
100. Sharioth GB, Prasad S, Georgalas I, Tataru C, Pavlidis M. Intermediate results of sutureless intrascleral posterior chamber intraocular lens fixation. *J Cataract Refract Surg.* 2010;36(2): 254-259.
101. Kheirkhah A. Long-term results of scleral fixation of posterior chamber intraocular lenses in children. *Ophthalmology.* 2008;115(1):67-72.
102. Scharioth GB, Prasad S, Georgalas I, Tataru C, Pavlidis M. Intermediate results of sutureless intrascleral posterior chamber intraocular lens fixation. *J Cataract Refract Surg.* 2010;36(2): 254-259.
103. Agarwal A, Kumar DA, Jacob S, Baid C, Agarwal A, Srinivasan S. Fibrin glue-assisted sutureless posterior chamber intraocular lens implantation in eyes with deficient posterior capsules. *J Cataract Refract Surg.* 2008;34(9):1433-1438.

20

Intraocular Lens Explantation and Replacement

Even though most eyes undergoing cataract surgery with intraocular lens (IOL) implantation have rapid and long-lasting anatomical and visual recovery, a small percentage develop complications that require repositioning, removal, or replacement of the IOL.

A number of factors may require exchange of an IOL. In the past, dislocation of the lens and chronic intraocular inflammation were much more frequent indications for IOL exchange.[1] Currently, one of the more frequent causes is incorrect IOL power with possible anisometropia or asthenopia associated with the refractive error.

On rare occasions, a manufacturing defect of the IOL may be the cause; this can lead to chronic inflammation or opacification of the optic with a reduction in vision. In other cases, the reason may be the interaction of the IOL material with other substances, such as the absorption of trypan blue by the optic of a hydrophilic IOL with consequent blue dyschromatopsia.[2]

A lens that is too small may lead to excessive movement of the IOL and possible onset of uveitis-glaucoma-hyphema (UGH) syndrome, which may necessitate the explant of the anterior chamber (AC) IOL.

If an AC-IOL is positioned incorrectly, it may induce iris tuck, uveal irritation, and UGH syndrome. Other complications of a badly positioned AC-IOL that has moved in the AC include uveitis, glaucoma, hyphema, cystoid macular edema (CME), and corneal decompensation.

A posterior chamber (PC)-IOL may be decentered for a number of reasons: inadequate capsular or zonular support, asymmetric positioning of the haptics, inappropriate IOL-capsular bag sizing, posterior synechia formation with pupillary block, endocapsular fibrosis, late-onset zonular dehiscence, post-YAG (yttrium-aluminum-garnet) extension of a Nd:YAG laser capsulotomy, or postoperative trauma.[3,4]

Inadequate capsular support is the most common cause of PC-IOL dislocation and occurs most frequently in the early postoperative period. Even if the dislocation of the IOL in the bag (dislocation of the IOL-capsular bag complex) is late onset and typically observed several months or even years following perfect cataract surgery, it is associated with progressive zonular dehiscence, increasingly reported in the literature (see the Posterior Chamber Intraocular Lens section later in this chapter).

The complications associated with a dislocated PC-IOL tend to be less serious and predominantly refractive in nature, even though UGH syndrome, uveitis, vitreous hemorrhage, and retinal holes/detachment may develop. For example, PC-IOLs can induce diplopia for a number of reasons, with development of binocular symptoms caused by anisiconia or the prismatic dislocation of the image. There are numerous monocular symptoms, and these include blurred vision and monocular diplopia caused by an image refracted through the edge of the optic, 2 competing images. Glare may be due to the refractive and diffractive effects that originate on the edges of the IOL or in older model IOLs, from positioning holes.

On some rare occasions, a well-centered IOL of the correct dioptric power can cause a severe positive or negative dysphotopsia for no specific reason; the condition may be so severe as to necessitate the replacement or repositioning of the IOL. Similarly, halos or severe glare may appear following implantation of multifocal (M-IOLs) or accommodative IOLs.

Finally, the IOL may be explanted at the patient's request (eg, if he or she wishes to replace the monofocal IOL with a lens that can correct presbyopia or oppositely, if he or she is extremely disturbed by the rings of a diffractive M-IOL).

Though a surgical procedure may be indicated, it is not the only option available for the management of cases with complications associated with implantation of IOLs; observation and drug therapy must also be taken into consideration.[3,4]

Buratto L, Brint SF, Caretti L.
Cataract Surgery in Complicated Cases (pp 231-246).

The procedure and timing depend on the type and the position of the IOL, the age and state of health of the patient, symptoms, visual acuity, condition of the corneal endothelium, the presence and severity of intraocular inflammation, and the situation of the contralateral eye.

Conservative management and observation may be suitable for an eye with an AC-IOL with a pupil with a notch or is oval shaped, if the symptoms and signs of intraocular inflammation are absent.

Even with dislocation of an IOL into the vitreous, patients often maintain excellent visual acuity under conditions of corrected aphakia with no surgical intervention, while maintaining a stable eye.

Management with drugs often involves the use of topical steroids and may be indicated in cases of moderate flare and cells, in association with subjective symptoms and a reduction in visual acuity. Nonsteroidal anti-inflammatory drugs (NSAIDs) accompanied by steroids is justified as a first step in the treatment of symptomatic CME in pseudophakia. Moreover, the effects induced by the edge of the optic, diplopia, and glare can sometimes be managed successfully using topical pilocarpine or apraclonidine. Topical sodium chloride may be preferable to surgery with peripheral corneal edema in very elderly patients with a low endothelial cell count.[5] A poorly positioned iris support IOL with refractive or inflammatory symptoms can be managed less easily with conservative treatment due to the design of the IOL itself, compared to an AC-IOL and many other PC-IOLs. The posterior dislocation of a single loop of the Copeland IOL, a loop of the Binkhorst IOL, or the Medallion IOL, all older generation IOLs, may be associated with posterior synechiae or a fixed pupil. Sometimes pharmacological manipulation of the pupil can allow the optimal repositioning of these older IOLs.[5-7]

Following decentration of an IOL, the most frequently reported symptom is unwanted optical images caused by the edge of the IOL optic. If these disturbances are mild and are limited to night when the pupil is more dilated, the surgeon may decide to treat the patient conservatively using a topical miotic agent.

Repositioning, explanting, and replacing the IOL can manage more severe debilitating symptoms. In the event of complete dislocation of an IOL, the options available include the following:

- Observation
- Repositioning the IOL
- Removal and/or replacement of the IOL[7-9]

Suturing techniques, indicated for secondary PC-IOL implants and for repositioning of dislocated IOLs, have improved the efficacy of the various surgical options.[10,11] Moreover, intrascleral techniques have recently been suggested that do not require sutures; these ensure the correct positioning of the IOL haptics in specially constructed intrascleral tunnels or in the scleral flap bed using a fibrin glue (see Chapter 19).

Preoperative Evaluation

When considering surgery for a dislocated IOL, initial preoperative evaluation includes determination of bilateral best spectacle-corrected visual acuity (BSCVA), biomicroscopy with the slit lamp, gonioscopy, and the examination of the fundus. The surgeon should also perform keratometry, corneal topography, A-scan ultrasonography, endothelial microscopy, and on some occasions the potential acuity meter. B-scan ultrasonography can provide useful anatomical-physiological-pathological information relative to the condition of the eye.[12,13]

Important information regarding the patient's clinical history can be found in the original operative report, from the type of IOL implanted, its dioptric power, its design, its A-constant, the position of implantation during the primary surgery, and postoperative refraction (following the first surgery)—all of this information may prove useful for providing a postoperative pseudophakic refraction that is as close as possible to emmetropia.

Measurement of the axial length with the IOL Master (Carl Zeiss Meditec, Dublin, CA) has considerably improved calculation accuracy for the dioptric power of the IOL in the event of its exchange in eyes that are already pseudophakic, particularly when previous data are no longer available. When the surgeon decides to replace an IOL implanted in the bag with another fixed in the sulcus, with or without sutures, the power of the IOL should be reduced by 0.5 to 1 diopters (D) compared to the previous power calculated for emmetropia.

Following an examination considering all the clinical history, the surgeon can plan a preliminary surgical strategy for repositioning, removing, and/or replacing the IOL. Things to consider regarding the surgery include the timing of surgery, the approach (anterior or posterior), the composition of the surgical team (surgeons specialized in the anterior or posterior segment or both), and how the management of the IOL should be done (repositioning, explantation, and replacement).

If the surgeon decides to intervene, repositioning of the lens is always preferable to removal/replacement of the IOL because of the benefits associated, namely less trauma to the corneal endothelium, the possibility of using smaller incisions with less postoperative astigmatism, and a lower risk of vitreous prolapse and choroidal hemorrhage associated with removal of the IOL. Even if the surgeon opts for the most suitable technique for the management of the specific clinical case, each patient is an individual and consequently necessitates a personalized approach. Moreover, each surgeon needs to consider his or her own experience and confidence with each of the techniques available.

If the surgeon decides to reposition the IOL, the preoperative plan must always include measurements and calculations for the replacement of the IOL, in the event repositioning is not possible. Consequently, the type of luxated IOL and its precise dioptric power must be known.

Important factors in deciding whether to reposition or replace the IOL include the stability of the IOL and the dimensions and the design of the haptics. For example, foldable silicone IOLs are less suitable for repositioning compared to polymethylmethacrylate (PMMA) lenses due to their greater structural instability. IOLs with small optics and shorter haptics will be more inclined to induce effects associated with the edge of the optic and to have lower stability when sutured to the sclera compared to other types of IOLs. Similarly, very thin or short IOLs, in particular the J loops, and acrylic one-piece IOLs are poorer choices for scleral fixation.

During the preoperative exam, if mydriasis is not optimal, the surgical plan may need to be revised during surgery when there is maximum pupil mydriasis, allowing direct visualization of the anatomy. For a full understanding of the malpositioned PC-IOL, there must be optimal visualization of the anatomy. During surgery, poor visualization of the anatomy can be improved using Fry's stretch technique,[14] using iris retractors or pupil expansion rings (see Chapter 5).

The surgeon can also reduce any residual refractive error during surgery; moderate or severe astigmatism can be reduced by carefully positioned corneal incisions, astigmatic keratotomy, limbal relaxing incisions, or the replacement of the dislocated IOL with a toric IOL (though this is not always possible and is not always a simple procedure). Moreover, during the operation, the surgeon may resolve other associated problems including synechiolysis, reopening of the bag, removal of Soemmering's rings, cleaning of the capsule, repair of the iris defects (with sutures or with a prosthetic iris device), expansion, contraction or displacement of the pupil, and finally, the implantation of a capsular tension ring (CTR) to reinforce weakened zonules (a procedure that can be performed only if it is possible to reopen the capsular bag and if the second surgery is performed shortly after the first one).

Surgical Techniques

Anterior Chamber Intraocular Lens

Repositioning an AC-IOL should be considered when one of the loops engages iris tissue, when the iris prolapses, when marked ovalization of the pupil is induced, when the haptic of the IOL migrates through the iridectomy, decentering the IOL, or when it vaults forward and comes into contact with the corneal endothelium.

If diagnosed early, the trapped iris and the malpositioned haptics can be corrected by bending, shaping, and repositioning the responsible haptic(s). The optical images created by the decentered optic can occasionally be corrected by repositioning the iris and the AC-IOL; nevertheless, explanting the lens may be necessary if the symptoms are not acceptable to the patient.

Even though repositioning may be sufficient in selected cases, removal of the IOL will be necessary if its dimensions are inappropriate (the lens is too large or too small). Rotation of the IOL or a change in its position between one postoperative visit and the next indicates that the lens is too small; ovalization of the pupil or indentation of ciliary body suggests that the IOL is too large and rigid. In both of these cases, gonioscopy provides useful information. Explantation of an AC-IOL will be necessary if chronic UGH syndrome develops and proves resistant to medical therapy.[7,10]

Management of the AC-IOL replacement depends on the type of IOL and any trapping of the loops. The loops of older AC-IOL (closed loops) may be trapped in peripheral anterior synechiae; this situation requires the surgeon to perform a delicate procedure of separation by cutting the loop to allow removal of the IOL. He or she must avoid bleeding, iridodialysis, and serious damage to the angle. This can be achieved using intraocular scissors during surgery or the YAG laser before surgery.[15] The optic of the IOL must be handled very carefully because the cut loops have sharp edges and can be dangerous. Once viscoelastic substance (VES) has been injected into the AC, a spatula is positioned underneath the optic of the IOL to prevent contact with the edges of the corneal incision during the removal procedures. Given that almost all AC-IOLs are PMMA, the incision must approximate the size of the rigid optic that will be removed intact. Following the removal of the optic, if possible, the remaining loops of the IOL are "unthreaded" in the AC from the synechiae that trap them and then grasped with forceps and removed (Figures 20-1 and 20-2).

If there is residual posterior capsule that will offer adequate peripheral support, the AC-IOL can be replaced with a PC-IOL. If the posterior capsule is intact and the capsular membranes are fused together, fixation in the sulcus will be sufficient. Sutures that fix the PC-IOLs to the iris or the ciliary sulcus are an excellent alternative, particularly in patients with glaucoma or with an abnormal anterior segment (eg, extensive synechiae or angle recession).[16-21] Alternately, the surgeon can remove as much of the loop material as possible, leaving the parts that are firmly adhered in position. Alternately, the posterior capture of the optic is an elegant alternative through the creation of a primary posterior capsulorrhexis with capture of the PC-IOL optic[22] (see Chapter 19).

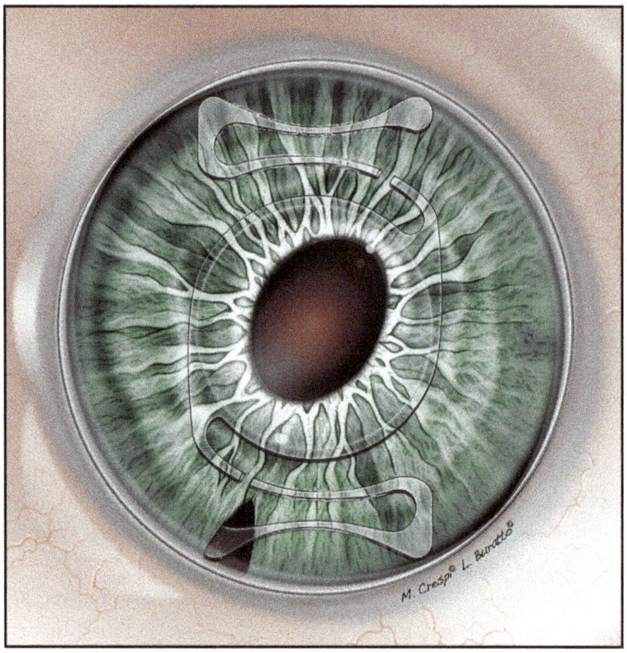

Figure 20-1. AC-IOL with the haptics trapped in peripheral anterior synechiae. Scissors are used to cut the haptic from the optic.

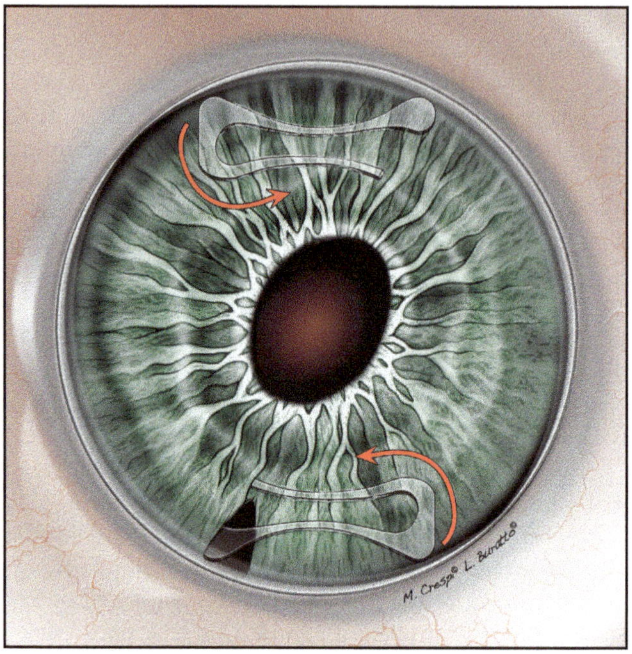

Figure 20-2. Following the removal of the optic, the remaining haptics are teased into the AC and then removed.

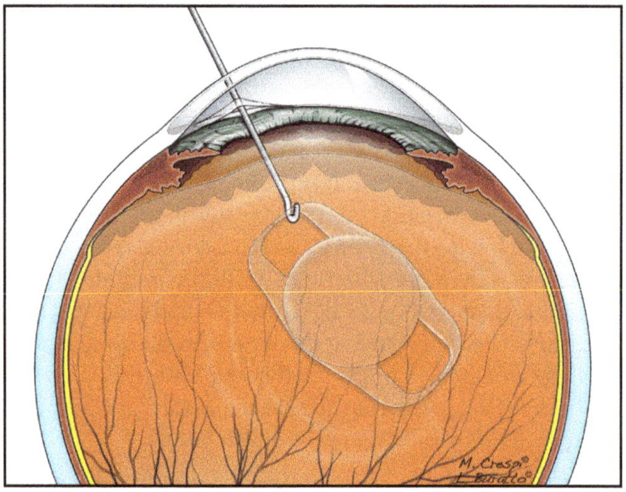

Figure 20-3. A dislocated IOL with iris fixation is removed from the anterior portion of the vitreous chamber using a C-hook and a limbal approach.

Intraocular Lens With Iris Claw Fixation

As a general rule, repositioning of these lenses should be considered in situations in which the more extensive procedure of exchange may be risky, for example, in elderly patients with a low endothelial cell count, and when the endothelium still has good vitality.

Prior to repositioning the IOL (which will be free floating in the AC in the majority of cases), the surgeon may inject an air bubble into the AC through a paracentesis incision. This will assist the identification of the exposed vitreous face and avoid its rupture. Alternately, and preferentially, the surgeon should inject a dispersive VES; this can be used relative safely as the probability of a postoperative increase in the IOP is lower as opposed to the other cohesive agents. If vitreous is present and has prolapsed around the IOL, the surgeon must perform a vitrectomy to prevent traction on the vitreous base and a possible retinal detachment and/or CME.

The surgeon introduces an enclavation hook through a strategically constructed limbal incision; this will re-enclavate the free loop. It is advisable that the incision is created just in front of the corneoscleral junction to avoid intraocular bleeding. The optic is grasped with iris-fixation IOL forceps while the hook engages the iris and draws it between the loops of the lens.

Preoperatively, the pupil is constricted with miotics and intraoperatively with acetylcholine to improve the stability of the IOL and facilitate the repositioning procedure.

When an IOL with iris fixation is associated with chronic irritation or progressive loss of endothelial cells, explantation of the IOL is necessary. Separation of posterior synechiae, frequently associated with the anterior vitrectomy, facilitates less traumatic explant procedures.

If the dislocation is in the anterior part of the vitreous chamber, recovery can be achieved using 2 anterior incisions to engage the visible loop with a C-shaped hook and luxating the IOL anteriorly toward the pupil in the AC (Figure 20-3). A second hook is then positioned under the IOL to reduce the possibility of losing the IOL. At this point,

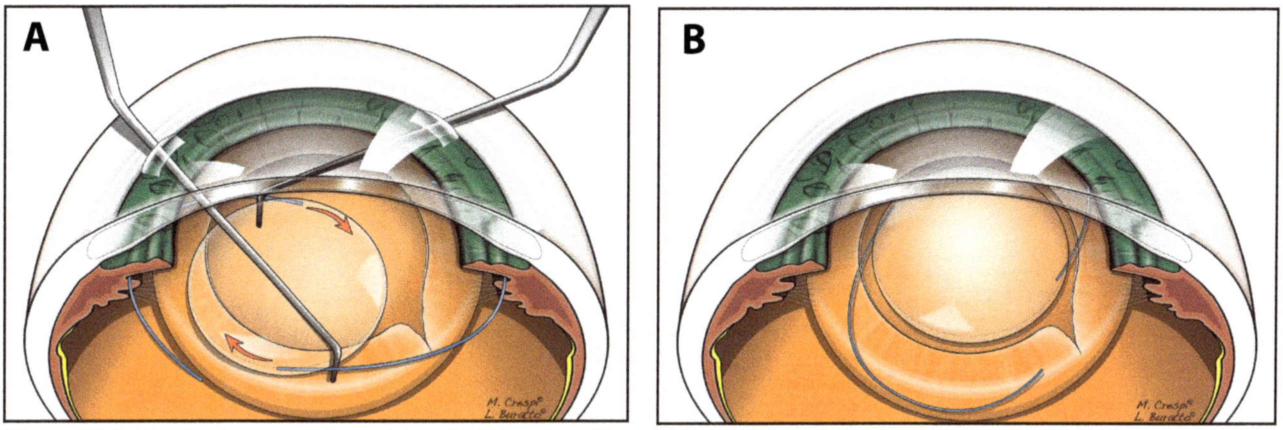

Figure 20-4. Two hooks are used to rotate a PC-IOL malpositioned in the ciliary sulcus.

the pupil is constricted with a miotic injected into the AC, and this will trap the IOL in the AC.

Now the corneal incision can be safely opened and the IOL can be explanted using a second instrument as a glide and eliminating vitreous traction with a vitrectomy.

In the event there is significant vitreous involvement, that is, tight adhesion between the vitreous and the IOL, or an IOL that has dislocated more posteriorly in the vitreous chamber, the most appropriate procedure is the primary vitrectomy technique (see the Management of Posteriorly Luxated Posterior Chamber Intraocular Lens section in this chapter).

Following removal of a dislocated IOL with iris support, the surgeon can choose to implant an AC-IOL or a PC-IOL with iris or scleral sutures.

Posterior Chamber Intraocular Lens

The surgical options for dislocated PC-IOLs include repositioning with or without scleral fixation sutures (dependent on the presence or absence of residual capsular support) and the removal of the IOL with or without the reimplantation of the same IOL or the implantation of another IOL.

Repositioning of a Posterior Chamber Intraocular Lens

In these situations, the surgeon must carefully examine the eye and determine whether or not there is adequate capsular support.

1. With adequate capsular support, several procedures can be used to reposition a decentered PC-IOL.

- If the capsular bag is intact, it is generally possible to reposition the PC-IOL in the capsular bag. In these situations, cohesive VES can be injected just below the anterior capsule, and the capsular bag can usually be reopened with appropriate maneuvers. The IOL can be rotated in the bag and in the sulcus if it is not possible to reopen the sac. This will allow symmetrical positioning of the haptics to center the IOL.
- A useful suggestion for the surgeon is to engage the dislocated loop with an Osher manipulator (Asico LLC, Westmont, IL) in one hand; the instrument in the other hand rotates the lens in a clockwise direction. The surgeon uses the Osher hook to push the lens downward, repositioning it in the bag. Alternately, the haptics of the IOL can be rotated into the sulcus with the optic captured in the anterior capsulorrhexis (Figure 20-4).
- A one-piece acrylic IOL that has been unexpectedly implanted in the sulcus can be repositioned in the bag reopened with VES and a successful delicate manipulation of the soft and extremely flexible loops, as described.
- All of the IOLs trapped in the pupil can be correctly repositioned, with the release of any synechiae and the optic repositioned in the PC.
- If an IOL is mistakenly implanted upside down, it can be rotated into the correct position inside the eye; cohesive VES is injected to protect the structures and to expand the AC and the bag, cautiously avoiding damage to the endothelium.
- A small IOL, decentered in a bag of unusually large dimensions, can be repositioned with anterior and posterior capture of the optic.
- It should be remembered that there will be a slight change in the IOL effective power when the optic prolapses far back in the bag or when it is positioned anteriorly in the event the IOL is captured anteriorly through the capsulorrhexis (0.5 to 1 D, as mentioned earlier).
- In the situation of a dislocated one-piece acrylic IOL with sufficient residual capsular support, some

surgeons suggest the repositioning of the IOL by fixing the haptic that was outside of the bag to the sclera with a single suture.

2. If the posterior capsule is open (therefore capsular support is inadequate), the dislocated PC-IOL can be repositioned (or replaced) in a number of different ways. In these situations, the bag cannot be reopened by injecting VES as this would flow into the vitreous chamber. Nevertheless the surgeon can still reposition the IOL.

- For example, if a one-piece IOL is decentered inside a damaged sac, the optic can be brought forward and captured anterior to an intact capsulorrhexis.
- An acute central rupture of the posterior capsule can sometimes be converted into a primary posterior capsulorrhexis and the optic can be captured posteriorly. Even when the rupture extends peripherally, it is possible to capture the optic between 2 flaps of the capsule. With a 3-piece IOL, the 2 haptics can be positioned in the ciliary sulcus.
- A long-standing posterior capsular rupture can allow the creation of a new capsulotomy in the single tissue formed from the fusion of the anterior and posterior capsule, providing another possibility to capture the optic.
- The technique with scleral fixation sutures requires the presence of undamaged open loops. It is important to remember that when the ciliary sulcus is used in the presence of capsular rupture, the surgeon must be very cautious. Presently, many commonly used PC-IOLs have a smaller overall diameter than the IOLs of previous generations, often measuring 13.5 to 14 mm and therefore suitable for fixation in the sulcus.
    - A decentered PC-IOL can be repositioned using a suture, described for the first time by Osher during a Video Symposium on dislocated IOLs at the AAO Meeting in 1997.[23] A double-needle 10-0 Prolene suture (Ethicon, Cornelia, GA) is introduced through a paracentesis incision. The first needle is passed below the haptic of the IOL and successively through the sclera at the ciliary sulcus. The second needle is introduced through the same incision, but this time the needle is oriented above the haptic prior to its exit through the sclera in the ciliary sulcus, in a position close to the first pass. The sutures are tightened on the outside of the globe; the haptic is engaged and secured to the scleral wall. The knot is then cut and buried in the scleral tissue. Alternately, the sutures can be passed under a scleral flap or Hoffman tunnel.
    - Later, Steinert modified the loose suture to apply it specifically to stabilize the dislocated IOL totally contained within the bag. In Steinert's technique, a 10-0 Prolene suture with a long slightly curved needle is inserted ab externo through the ciliary sulcus and directed behind the haptic, and then through the capsule between the haptic and the optic, finally exiting from the eye through a paracentesis incision. The suture is secured with 4 single passes and rotated beneath the sclera, so that only a conjunctival flap will be needed to cover it safely. The same maneuver is then repeated for the second haptic of the IOL. A number of different techniques are available for suturing the haptics of a decentered PC-IOL to the sclera through the ciliary sulcus.[24-32]
    - A loop can be externalized through a paracentesis incision where a knot can secure it to the sclera prior to repositioning the IOL.
    - A clever technique that avoids conjunctival dissection was proposed by Hoffman.[33]
    - Agarwal et al published a technique to fix the PC-IOL under the scleral flap using fibrin glue.[34]
    - Osher described the use of a CTR to stabilize the IOL by creating artificial zonules.[35]
    - Fine and Hoffman[36] described repositioning the subluxated IOL-capsular bag-CTR complex by suturing the ring to the scleral wall (see Chapter 19).
    - The PC-IOL repositioning technique with iris fixation proposed by Stark is widely used.[37,38] Through the pupil, the surgeon captures the optic of a PC-IOL and successively injects a viscoadaptive VES (such as Healon 5 [Abbott Laboratories, Abbott Park, IL]) into the AC. The loops become visible underneath the iris as soon as the VES deepens the AC and compresses the iris against the loops. Each loop is secured to the mid-peripheral iris using Siepser's modified suture technique with 10-0 Prolene. If the needle passes in an excessively close position, the pupil will have a cat-eye appearance.[39] Finally, the optic is positioned behind the pupil and centered in the PC while the iris supports the sutures.
    - Finally, Gimbel et al[40] recently proposed a new technique called "capsule membrane suture fixation" to attach an IOL, implanted in the sulcus but subluxated or decentered, to the residual capsule or the fibrotic elements of a capsular membrane. This technique can also be used in secondary fixation surgeries, repositioning, or replacement of IOLs.

In order to check that the IOL is centered and well supported, Osher's Bounce test can be performed (Figure 20-5). This involves delicately decentering the optic toward each of the haptics, with successive spontaneous recentration of the IOL. Vice versa, the absence of spontaneous IOL recentration may indicate serious problems with capsular support, permanent deformation of the loops, or inadequate sizing of the IOL, all events that may require sutures for

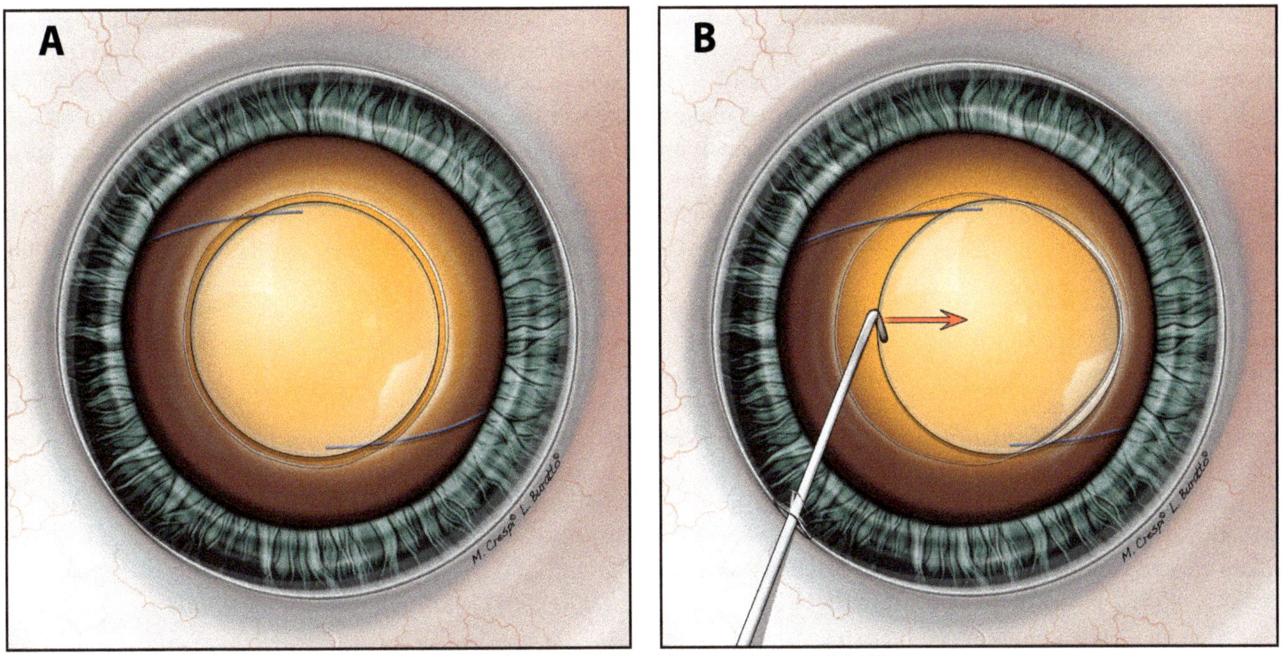

Figure 20-5. The Bounce test to check the successful recentering of a repositioned PC-IOL.

fixation, explantation, or replacement of the IOL, depending on the nature of the problem. Alternately, the surgeon may consider capturing the optic.

Exchange of the Posterior Chamber Intraocular Lens

A PC-IOL can be replaced with a sutured PC-IOL or an AC-IOL. In many cases, repositioning of a dislocated IOL may not be possible or desirable because of structural abnormalities of the implant or concomitant ocular conditions that require the IOL to be removed or replaced.

The haptic of a dislocated IOL may have existing structural damage (distortion or tear) that will preclude adequate repositioning. When repositioning is not possible, our first choice would be to replace the PC-IOL with another PC-IOL, if there is adequate capsular support. It may be easier to determine when the pupil is well dilated and when all of the posterior synechiae between the iris and the capsule have been severed, with complete reconstruction of the PC. Direct inspection of the peripheral anatomy will guide the surgeon toward the best orientation for implantation and the best IOL fixation site. Once the presence of adequate residual capsular support has been determined, foldable 3-piece acrylic or rigid one-piece PMMA IOLs with a large optic (6 to 6.5 mm) and large overall diameter (12.5 to 13.5 mm) are preferable to AC-IOLs or sutured PC-IOLs; however, recent scientific evidence supports the safety of AC-IOLs in these complex cases.[41]

Currently, the surgeon will rarely explant an IOL without simultaneously replacing it with another.

Replacement of the Posterior Chamber Intraocular Lens With an Intact Bag

As mentioned previously, the most common indication for replacing the IOL is incorrect power of the IOL with consequent anisometropia or patient dissatisfaction. In this situation, surgeons who have access to an excimer laser will tend to use laser-assisted in situ keratomileusis (LASIK) to correct the refractive error. Other surgeons prefer a piggyback implant to correct the refractive error. However, this technique can lead to opacification of the interface and undesirable optic phenomena, particularly with M-IOLs (see Chapter 9).

The surgeon may replace a monofocal IOL implanted in the bag with an M-IOL or accommodative IOL because the patient requests correction of presbyopia.

The integrity of the bag is essential. The bag can be reopened by injecting VES into the AC and successively dissecting the partially open capsular bag. A number of VESs are useful with the choice left to the surgeon. Sometimes it may be difficult to elevate the anterior capsulorrhexis from the anterior surface of an acrylic PC-IOL. The surgeon can create a cleavage plane by sliding a thin spatula underneath the edge of the rhexis. If this maneuver is not successful because the adhesion is too strong, the edge of the capsulorrhexis can be delicately raised from the optic using a 25- or 30-gauge needle in the bevel-down position.

At this point, the VES cannula can be inserted underneath the elevated capsular edge and the bag can be expanded by the progressive injection of VES; this viscodissection is frequently necessary for all quadrants and can be performed through a number of paracentesis incisions or by using a variety of cannulas.

Once the bag has been opened, the method used to remove the optic will depend on its material (whether it is foldable or not foldable). PMMA optics require an incision similar to the diameter of the optic. However, there are a number of different possibilities available for removal of foldable optics through small incisions.

Following the injection of VES to protect intraocular structures, the optic can be cut in half with scissors or with lassos created with a suture of 10-0 Prolene with successive removal of the 2 pieces of the optic from the AC.

Batlan and Dodick[42] promoted the Hinge technique; in this procedure, the optic is partially sectioned, leaving the distal portion intact. When half of the optic is grasped and pulled out of the smaller incision, the hinge opens and the other half of the optic follows.

Ernest[43] developed an interesting system of IOL folding. Under the protection of VES, the IOL is manipulated into the AC by prolapsing the presenting haptic through the incision. Successively, a spatula slides under the optic; it is introduced through a paracentesis incision positioned diametrically opposite the main incision. A forceps designed for implantation of the IOL is inserted in the AC through the main incision above the optic. The simultaneous upward pressure with the spatula and the downward pressure with the forceps will fold the optic inside the eye. The IOL can then be rotated 90 degrees and explanted.

Another innovative technique has been developed by Eguchi.[44] After having prolapsed the proximal haptic in the AC, scissors are used to create a radial cut in the optic. The lens is then rotated and a second radial cut is created 90 degrees from the first. At this point, one-quarter of the IOL is explanted and the remaining three-quarters are rotated and removed through a small incision.

The criss-cross technique was developed to explant the plates of silicone IOLs through a small incision. Osher developed it according to Eguchi's principles.[45] The surgeon creates a radial incision along the longitudinal axis of the IOL; the lens is rotated 90 degrees and the surgeon creates a second radial incision that intersects with the first. This produces a rectangular piece of IOL small enough to be removed. The IOL is rotated a further 90 degrees, and a third radial cut is created along the longitudinal axis. Following a final rotation of 90 degrees, the surgeon creates the last radial incision that intersects and creates a second rectangle that is then explanted. The remaining segment of the IOL can be removed through a small incision. The toothed scissors designed by Osher (P1870B, Duckworth & Kent, Hertfordshire, England) to cut the IOL are extremely good in cutting both acrylic and silicone; the toothed blade reduces the tendency of the IOL to rotate during the cut.

During the operation, if the surgeon sees, for example, that the haptics of an IOL are stuck, the haptic must be amputated and the IOL removed in segments. When the cut haptic is stuck in the intact bag, the surgeon should attempt to inject VES under the edge as this may distend the bag, allowing the fragments to be removed. The delicate repetition of this maneuver under VES protection may lead to successful removal, even though it is better to leave a cut loop in situ rather than try to remove it and risk damaging the capsular bag.[46]

Once the IOL has been removed with one of the above-mentioned techniques, the surgeon implants a new IOL in the capsular bag.

Replacement of the Posterior Chamber Intraocular Lens When the Bag Is Torn

The intraoperative situation and type of IOL are factors that determine the possibility of repositioning or replacing an IOL.

If an IOL with a C- or a J-loop cannot be easily rotated, it is likely that a loop has hooked to the zonules or that it has prolapsed through a rupture in the zonules or in the capsular bag.

The trapped loop may be released if the surgeon rotates clockwise, followed by decentration toward the trapped loop and a successive rotation. The lens can be rotated 90 degrees and a Bounce test can be performed to confirm good centration and fixation of the IOL.

If the haptic has a buttonhole or a button-end, the removal procedure may prove to be much more difficult. Resistance to rotation may require amputating the haptics, and it may be necessary to remove the IOL in fragments to avoid causing further damage to the capsular bag.[46]

Regardless of how the IOL is removed, the surgeon should be ready to manage vitreous prolapse. If even a minimal quantity of vitreous has prolapsed, a dry monomanual vitrectomy should be performed with a limbal approach following introduction of dispersive VES. This technique allows the removal of a limited amount of vitreous with a low tendency for AC collapse. If, on the other hand, a large quantity of vitreous presents, the surgeon may decide to perform a bimanual limbal vitrectomy with a low irrigation flow through a second paracentesis incision.[47] Alternately, the surgeon can perform a pars plana vitrectomy 3.5 mm behind the limbus (see later in this chapter).

Some years ago, Burke et al described the use of triamcinolone acetate to highlight the presence of vitreous in the AC and facilitate its removal.[48] Triamcinolone acetate is the most widely used drug for this purpose and prior to being injected it should be purified of its preservatives (alcohol) as it is supplied in an alcohol-based suspension. The alcohol must be eliminated and replaced with balanced salt solution (BSS). At this point, triamcinolone acetate can be introduced into the AC. It will deposit on the vitreous in the AC, and this greatly facilitates its complete removal.

The surgeon should use the automated vitrectomy, setting a high cut rate and a moderate level of vacuum: the parameters should be 800 cpm and 150 to 180 vacuum. If the posterior capsule is open and the vitreous has been removed, it is crucial to keep the AC inflated to prevent any further prolapse of vitreous at the end of the procedure. The VES can be removed manually in small amounts and replaced with BSS; alternately, it can be removed by a bimanual system of irrigation/aspiration with the cannulas inserted through the side-port incisions once the primary incision has been closed.

Once the IOL has been removed, the surgeon can evaluate the possibility of implanting a new IOL (a sutured PC-IOL or an AC-IOL).

Injection of acetylcholine and instillation of pressure-reducing drugs into the AC will reduce the risk of sharp spikes in intraocular pressure postoperatively.

Management of a Posteriorly Luxated Posterior Chamber Intraocular Lens

Previously, we described many efficient techniques for the management of IOLs dislocated in the anterior segment, in other words, subluxated IOLs (AC, iris plane, ciliary sulcus, in the capsular bag, in the anterior vitreous). In any of these situations, the anterior segment surgeon can independently and safely use any of the techniques described previously.

However, when the IOL is completely dislocated posteriorly, is trapped in the vitreous, and/or is in contact with the retina, the surgery must be performed by a vitreoretinal surgeon on his or her own or as part of a team with the anterior segment surgeon.

Prior to describing these techniques, it is important to consider the management of the IOL's dislocated position, but not completely luxated, considering that currently, the majority of the lenses implanted are PC-IOLs.

A patient with a PC-IOL that is completely luxated in the vitreous chamber and lying on the surface of the macula must be referred immediately to the vitreoretinal surgeon. On the other hand, some anterior segment surgeons may (and should) feel confident in managing PC-IOLs that are severely subluxated with a loop hanging in the central part of the vitreous chamber in patients previously having a complete vitrectomy or where both loops are clearly visible, and not enmeshed by the vitreous.

The strategic plan is not as clear when the surgery requires a vitrectomy; the main problem is the determination of the amount of vitreous to be removed.

The 2 most common vitrectomy techniques for anterior segment surgeons are the anterior limbal vitrectomy and the limited pars plana vitrectomy. In the anterior limbal vitrectomy, the vitrectomy probe is inserted into the anterior segment through a limbal incision, frequently with the infusion, through a separate paracentesis incision.

With the limited pars plana anterior vitrectomy, the probe enters the globe through a single sclerotomy or a single 23- or 25-gauge trocar introduced 3 mm posterior to the surgical limbus. Irrigation is supplied by a cannula inserted into the anterior segment through a paracentesis incision. The purely anterior vitrectomy techniques should be used to perform simple vitrectomies; the limited pars plana anterior vitrectomy is indicated in those cases where manipulation of the anterior vitreous inside the vitreous chamber is required. It is important to remember that neither of the 2 techniques will completely remove the vitreous, the peripheral vitreous, and dissection of the posterior vitreous.

The most important consideration is the position of the IOL and its haptics in relation to the vitreous. The surgeon must carefully evaluate whether the haptics are trapped in the vitreous, through thorough indentation of the periphery during the examination of the fundus. If the haptics are trapped, it is not enough to liberate the optic from the vitreous with a limited anterior vitrectomy; manipulation of the IOL without complete dissection of the peripheral vitreous may have disastrous consequences such as retinal detachment with gigantic tears.

The patient should therefore be referred immediately to a vitreoretinal surgeon, particularly because the percentage of retinal lesions possible under these circumstances is very high.[49-53]

The decision to proceed with one of the anterior vitrectomy techniques or to refer the patient to the vitreoretinal surgeon depends on the precise identification of this and other important pre-, intra-, and postoperative anatomical relationships.

The mini-invasive pars plana vitrectomy techniques (MIVS) 23- and 25-gauge also deserve mention[54-59]; by positioning a transconjunctival trocar, this allows the vitrectomy procedure to be performed sutureless. These have also been suggested for the limited pars plana anterior vitrectomy.[60-62]

If the surgeon decides to manage a luxated IOL with a 3-port pars plana vitrectomy, the first step is a central vitrectomy and meticulous and complete peripheral vitrectomy, which always includes peeling of the posterior hyaloid. A careful peripheral dissection is then followed by cleaning of the vitreous base and liberation of the optic and haptics of the IOL from residual vitreous. The IOL is then

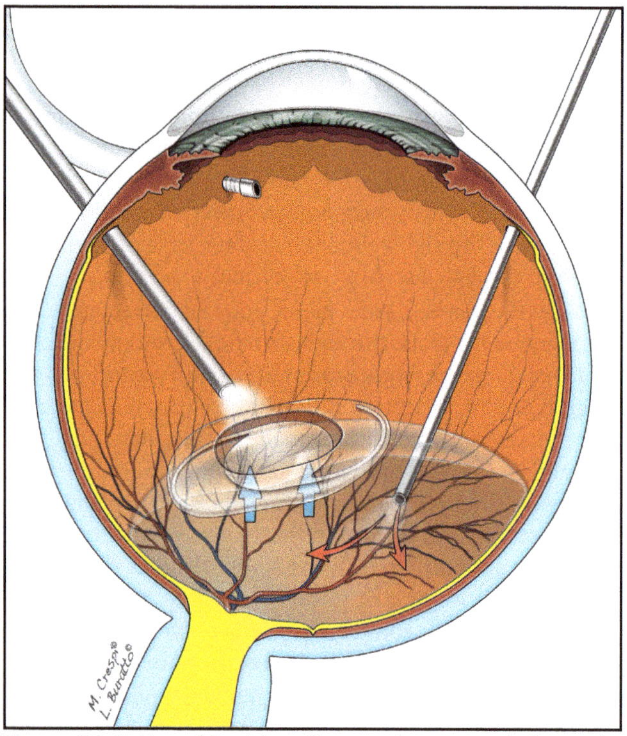

Figure 20-6. Use of liquid perfluorocarbon to push forward a PC-IOL luxated in the vitreous chamber.

mobilized by injecting a bubble of liquid perfluorocarbon, which displaces it anteriorly[63] (Figure 20-6) or with simultaneous aspiration with the vitrectomy probe or an extrusion cannula and forceps.

Once the IOL has been grasped, the surgeon must decide whether to reposition it (with or without fixation sutures) or to explant it and replace it with a sutured PC-IOL or an AC-IOL.

There are a number of different techniques for positioning an IOL that has dislocated in the vitreous chamber.[62-75] The options for fixation include iris, scleral with suture, and residual capsule. They are described in another chapter (see the Chapter 19).

As mentioned previously, with progressive zonular weakness, such as pseudoexfoliation, subluxation of the IOL-capsular complex may occur postoperatively, even with the simultaneous implantation of a CTR. If the subluxation is contained, a suture can pass initially through the peripheral zone of the bag around the haptic apex or around the CTR and then through the sclera. This procedure can be performed with a number of techniques. If the zonules are seriously damaged, it may be easier to remove the entire IOL-capsular sac complex, intact or in several steps, and replace it with a sutured PC-IOL.

There are encouraging results that describe the repositioning or the primary replacement of the IOL luxated in the vitreous chamber with pars plana vitrectomy; in 58% of cases[41-64] the visual acuity is equal to or better than 20/40 (see the following section). In 10% to 20% of cases, depending on different studies, CME developed, although it is generally transitory and responds to medical treatment (see the following section). In 3% to 14% of cases, there may be retinal detachment. Retinal detachment can appear between 10 days and 2 years after surgery; however, most appear after 2 months. There are a number of complications that may result from repositioning the IOL in the sulcus with a scleral fixation suture with a vitrectomy, including IOL tilting, redislocation, erosion of sutures, retinal phototoxicity, persistent hypotony, corneal opacity, iris capture, formation of epiretinal membranes, exposure of the sutures, persistent uveitis, wound leakage with hypotony, choroidal effusion, and vitreous hemorrhage. For these reasons, the surgeon should be aware of other surgical techniques for the optimal management of these complex cases.

Discussion

The surgical treatment of malpositioned and dislocated IOLs should be dealt with by expert surgeons and it can even be difficult for them to manage.

As discussed previously in this chapter, there are a number of situations reported in the literature that necessitate the removal of the IOL.

Solomon et al[74] examined 2500 explants performed between 1982 and 1988. In this study, AC-IOLs accounted for 59% of cases; the lenses were usually explanted because of pseudophakic bullous keratopathy or because of inflammatory complications. IOLs with iris claw fixation account for 21% of cases. PC-IOLs account for 20% and are the IOLs that are most frequently explanted because of decentration, malpositioning, and inflammation.

Apple et al[76] demonstrated that many older style AC-IOLs were explanted because of manufacturing defects, namely roughness of the edge of the optic or loops, and responsible for chromic iris irritation.

Kraff et al[77] reported their results of explant procedures of IOLs performed in 1986, a period in which the AC-IOLs were frequently explanted due to endothelial cell loss and chronic inflammation. The PC-IOLs in this study accounted for 20% of the IOLs explanted and were removed because of dislocation, decentration, and refractive error.

Mamalis et al[78] reviewed the clinical records of 102 IOLs removed between 1982 and 1989. AC-IOLs (66.7% of cases) were removed due to pseudophakic bullous keratopathy, UGH syndrome, and CME. PC-IOLs accounted for 15.7% of cases, and the most commons reasons for explantation were dislocation and decentration of the IOL. In this study, following replacement of the IOL, the visual acuity improved in 39% of patients, was unchanged in 46%, and was worse in 15% of cases after surgery, particularly due to the onset of corneal decompensation, glaucoma, and CME.

In a series of 1400 cases implanted in 1980, Kline and Yang[79] reported an incidence of IOL removal of 1.7%.

Corneal edema, CME, uveitis, and iris erosion were the most frequent causes for the explant.

It has been reported that approximately 90% of patients with replacement of the IOL with the implantation of a PC-IOL have a positive clinical result.[80] Equally good results, similar to those described, have been reported in more recent studies[80-84]; these studies also analyzed cases of IOL replacement with or without penetrating keratoplasty,[84] even though not all of the reports agree with the findings. In their study, Hayashi et al[85] reported that, following replacement of the IOL, the BSCVA did not show a marked increase, and they suggested careful evaluation of the use of alternative surgical techniques to IOL replacement with scleral fixation because this appears to be associated with a high rate of postoperative complications.

The largest retrospective study on the management of dislocated IOLs was performed in 2008.[86] It reported excellent visual results achievable with the various modern surgical techniques and with the latest generation of IOLs; there were low percentages of complications. The new foldable IOLs can now be replaced through very small incisions, and this facilitates rapid visual recovery. This recent study includes a large group of 284 eyes, and consequently the results appear accurate. The eyes included were implanted with different types of lenses: 113 PMMA, 60 one-piece acrylic, 51 with a silicone plate, 38 silicone, and 12 others (AC-IOLs and IOLs with iris claw support). In 51 cases (18%) the dislocation of the IOL was limited to the bag; according to the study, this situation appears to be on the rise and can be managed with scleral fixation sutures or by replacing the IOL. The IOLs that were replaced included AC-IOLs in 24 cases (8%), PMMA PC-IOLs with scleral sutures in 11 (4%), and acrylic PC-IOLs with scleral sutures in 13 cases (3%). The surgical methods examined were repositioning without scleral sutures in 109 eyes (38%), repositioning with scleral sutures 48 eyes (17%), removal and replacement in 6 cases (2%), and other techniques for 11 eyes (4%). Technically, the one-piece acrylic IOLs and those with a silicone plate tend to slip from the instruments; however, they can be fixed to the sclera with sutures or subsequently replaced with sutured foldable PC-IOLs.

The visual results and postoperative refractive results for 184 eyes with a follow-up greater than 3 months are similar for all of the surgical methods used.[86] Intraoperative complications included retinal tears in 5 eyes (2.1%) and one case of massive suprachoroidal hemorrhage during the removal of an AC-IOL. In terms of postoperative complications, the frequency of which is similar to other reports in the literature, the most common was CME (29 eyes, 10%), followed by a repeat dislocation of the IOL (28, 10%), vitreous hemorrhage (26, 9%), secondary glaucoma (14, 5%), retinal detachment (11, 4%), tilted or decentered IOL (11, 4%), persistent corneal edema (10, 4%), exposure of the suture (7, 3%), transitory ocular hypotony (3, 1.1%), error in the calculation of the IOL (2, 1%), severe, uncorrectable astigmatism (2, 0.7%), retinal holes not associated with detachment (1, 0.4%), suprachoroidal hemorrhage (1, 0.4%), and progressive opacification of the IOL (1, 0.3%).

These complications required further surgery in 18% of cases (51 eyes), a percentage that reflected the incidence (3% to 35%) described in other studies.[75-85]

As mentioned, the frequency of complications reported in this important study is similar to published results. For example, the range of incidence of severe complications was 4% to 21% for repeat dislocation, 10% to 20% for CME, and 3% to 14% for retinal detachment. Another fairly frequent complication that is usually benign (due to self-limitation) is intraocular hemorrhage.

As pertains to transscleral sutures, they may be exposed, and they may cause fistulas, intraocular hemorrhage, and endophthalmitis. This type of complication is observed less frequently when a scleral flap or Hoffman tunnel is created. The onset of CME or the formation of epiretinal membranes are other possible complications. However, these events are not very frequent in cases of scleral suture or IOL exchange.

The dislocation of an IOL within the capsular bag is a late onset complication in cataract surgery and is reported to have increased over recent years. Gimbel et al[87] identified a predisposing condition in 90% of cases; in more than 50%, pseudoexfoliation is the cause; however other associated conditions may be uveitis, myopia, previous trauma, retinitis pigmentosa (4% to 10% of cases), previous vitrectomy, and other pathologies associated with progressive zonular weakness and capsular contraction. It is probable that CTRs will reduce but do not completely prevent this complication. In their study, the authors used an AC-IOL in 48% of cases and a PC-IOL in 26% of eyes.

In 2001, Gross et al[88] conducted a multicenter study of 25 eyes in 22 patients with dislocation of the IOL-capsular bag complex, secondary to zonular dehiscence. The authors concluded that this condition was not common, that it was occasionally a bilateral late onset complication of cataract surgery, frequently associated with pseudoexfoliation (44% of cases). In addition, the complication was also associated with uveitis (16%) and trauma (16%). Other causes were not identified in 24% of eyes. The dislocated IOL-capsular bag complex was replaced with an AC-IOL in 60% of cases and repositioned or replaced and sutured to the sclera in 40% of cases.

In 2003, Dick et al[89] reported that the most frequent reasons for replacement of a foldable monofocal IOL included opacification of the IOL (findings for year 2000) and refractive error (findings for year 2001). In addition to error in the power of the IOL and decentration, opacification of hydrophilic IOLs is a major cause of IOL explantation (46%).

The findings from a study by members of the American Society of Cataract and Refractive Surgery and the European Society of Cataract and Refractive Surgeons in 2001 and

2003 were reported.[90,91] The most frequent complications associated with foldable IOLs and leading to explantation or a second surgery include residual ametropia, followed by malpositioning and opacification of IOL.

This increase in incorrect refractive error as the cause for replacement of the IOL has been corroborated by Jin et al[92]; they examined 51 eyes with replacement of the IOL between 1998 and 2004. The overall percentage was 0.77% for all cataract surgeries. The power of the IOL (41.2%), decentration/dislocation (37.3%), and glare (7.8%) were the most common causes of IOL explantation. In the cases in which the IOL was replaced, an AC-IOL was implanted in 14 eyes (27.5%) and a PC-IOL in 37 eyes (72.5%). None of the PC-IOLs were sutured to the sclera or to the iris.

Overall, 90.2% of patients[92] achieved BSCVA that was equal to or greater than 20/40. All of the eyes implanted with an AC-IOL and 94.6% of those implanted with a PC-IOL achieved visual acuity of between −1 and +5 lines compared to preoperatively. These authors also suggested that flexible open-loop AC-IOLs were not associated with greater risks of complication than PC-IOLs in terms of functional results and safety, a claim supported by the published scientific literature.

More recently, Jin et al[93] examined patients undergoing IOL replacement necessary because of postoperative refractive error. Of the 22 cases they examined, the causes were keratometry error in 5 cases (22%) and incorrect determination of the axial length in 3 cases (14%). An additional 3 postoperative refractive errors were associated with the implantation of the wrong IOL. Following the replacement of the IOL, 82% (18/22 eyes) were within ±0.5 D and 86% (19/22 eyes) within ±1 D from emmetropia. Uncorrected visual acuity was 20/40 or better in 82% of eyes, and the BSCVA was 20/40 or better in 95% (21/22) of the eyes.

Regarding the repositioning or exchange of IOLs in children, recent literature has shown that the endothelial cell density was greatly reduced in a study with a mean follow-up of 44 months (for lens repositioning) and 66 months (for explantation).[94] However, no change in the endothelial cell count was reported in another recent publication.[95]

Conclusion

Given that in ophthalmology the clinical management of patients is constantly evolving, we are witnessing a gradual drop in the need for IOL repositioning or exchange. The same applies to the incidence of pseudophakic bullous keratopathy, UGH syndrome, chronic CME, and even the determination of IOL powers. On the other hand, patient expectations are increasing, particularly following the introduction of presbyopia-correcting IOLs (multifocal or accommodating lenses). Currently, the patient now expects excellent uncorrected visual acuity following cataract surgery; for his or her part, in the absence of other ocular problems, the surgeon can now satisfy the enormous expectations of the patient in the majority of cases.

The surgeon must be able to clearly identify the causes that may lead to IOL exchange and must proceed with surgery only when it proves to be strictly necessary.

Thanks to modern surgery techniques, dislocated IOLs (normally foldable lenses contained in the capsular bag) can be successfully repositioned (with or without fixation sutures) or replaced.

The explantation or exchange of an IOL is always a difficult condition that the surgeon has to encounter. However, careful preparation and modern surgery techniques usually produce satisfactory results, even when pre-existing conditions and postoperative complications may limit the visual results.

References

1. Brown DC, Swead JW. Intraocular lens implant exchanges. *J Am Intraocular Implant Soc* 1985;11:376-379.
2. Werner L, Apple DJ, Crema AS, et al. Permanent blue discoloration of a hydrogel intraocular lens by intraoperative trypan blue. *J Cataract Refract Surg.* 2002;28:1279-1286.
3. Flynn HW Jr. Management and repositioning of posteriorly dislocated intraocular lenses. In: Stark WJ, Terry AC, Maumenee AE, eds. *Anterior Segment Surgery: Oils, Lasers, and Refractive Keratoplasty.* Baltimore, MD: William & Wilkins; 1987:321-329.
4. Blumenkranz M, Maguire A. Modern management considerations in dislocation of crystalline and intraocular lenses. In : Stirpe M, editor. *Advances in Vitroretinal Surgery.* Rome, Italy: Fondazione GB Bietti/Ophthalmic Communications Society; 1992:39-46.
5. Insler M, Benefield D, Ross V. Topical hyperosmolar solution in the reduction of corneal edema. *LAO J.* 1987;13:149.
6. Osher RH. Surgical management of the malpositioned posterior chamber lens. *Audiovisual J Cataract Implant Surg.* 1991;VII.
7. Ellington FR. The uveitis-glaucoma-hyphema syndrome associated with the Mark VIII anterior chamber lens implant. *Am Intracellular Implant Soc J.* 1978;4:50-53.
8. Keates RH, Ehrlich DR. "Lenses of chance" complications of anterior chamber implants.. *Ophthalmology.* 1978;85:408-414.
9. Percival SPK, Das SK. UGH syndrome after posterior chamber lens implantation. *J Am Intraocul Implant Soc.* 1983;9:200-201.
10. Koch DD. Scleral fixation of posterior chamber implants. *Audiovisual J Cataract Implant Surg.* 1990;VI.
11. Lubniewski AJ, Holland EJ , Van Meter WS, et al. Histologic study of eyes with transsclerally sutured posterior chamber intraocular lens. *Am J Ophthalmol.* 1990;110:237-243.
12. Ozdal PC, Mansour M, Deschenes J. Ultrasound biomicroscopy of pseudophakic eyes with chronic postoperative inflammation. *J Cataract Refract Surg.* 2003:29:1185-1191.
13. Loya N, Lichter H, Barash D, et al. Posterior chamber intraocular lens implantation after capsular tear: ultrasound biomicroscopy evaluation. *J Cataract Refract Surg.* 2001;27:1423-1427.
14. Fry L. Pupil stretching. *VJCRS* 1995; XI
15. Marques FF, Marquess DM , Smith CM, Osher RH. Intraocular lens exchange assisted by preoperative neodymium: YAG laser haptic fracture. *J Cataract Refract Surg.* 2004;30:247-249.
16. Gimbel HC, DeBroff BM. Intraocular lens optic capture. *J Cataract Refract Surg.* 2004;30:200-206.
17. Chang DF. Use of Malyugin pupil expansion device for intraoparative floppy-iris syndrome: results in 30 consecutive cases. *J Cataract Refract Surg.* 2008;34:835-841.

18. Price FW. Iris fixation of posterior chamber implants. Audiovisual *J Cataract Implant Surg.* 1990;VI.
19. Moretsky SL. Suture fixation technique for subluxated posterior chamber IOL through stab wound incision. *J Am Intraocular Implant Soc.* 1984;10:455-480.
20. Girard LJ , Nino N, Wesson M, et al. Scleral fixation of subluxed posterior chamber intraocular lens. *J Cataract Refract Surg.* 1986;14:326-337.
21. Anand R, Browman RW. Simplified technique for suturing dislocated posterior chamber intraocular lens to the ciliary sulcus. *Arch Ophthalmol.* 1990;108:1205-1206. [letter]
22. Lubniewski AJ, Holland EJ, Van Meter WS, et al. Histologic study of eyes with transsclerally sutured posterior chamber intraocular lens. *Am J Ophthalmol.* 1990;110:237-243.
23. Osher RH. Sewing through the capsular bag: a brief history. *Cataract & Refract Surgery Today.* 2004;4:72-73.
24. Hoffman RS, Fine IH, Packer M, Rozenberg I. Scleral fixation using suture retrieval through a scleral tunnel. *J Cararact Refract Surg.* 2006;32:1259-1263.
25. Hoffman RS, Fine IH, Packer M. Scleral fixation without conjunctival dissection. *J Cataract Refract Surg.* 2006;32:1907-1912.
26. Epley KD, Levine ES, Katz HR. A simplified technique for stable transscleral suture fixation of posterior chamber intraocular lenses. *Ophthalmic Surg Lasers.* 1999;30(5):398-402.
27. Chan CK, Agarwal A, Agarwal S, Argawal A. Management of dislocated intraocular implants. *Ophthalmol Clin North Am.* 2001;14:681-693.
28. Hannush SB. Sutured posterior chamber intraocular lenses: indication and procedure. *Curr Opin Ophthalomol.* 2000;11:233-240.
29. Kulkarni K, Zarbin M, Del Priore LV, Tezel TH. Ab externo technique for accurate haptic placement of transscleral sutured posterior chamber intraocular lenses. *Ophthalmic Surg Lasers Imaging.* 2007;38:72-75.
30. Leon Ja, Leon CS, Aron-Rosa D. Endoscopic technique for suturing posterior chamber intraocular lenses. *J Cataract Refract Surg.* 2000;26:644-649.
31. Arkin MS, Steinert RF. Sutured posterior chamber intraocular lenses. *Int Ophthamol Clin.* 1994;34:67-85.
32. Gimbel HV, Condon GP, Kohnen T. Late in-the-bag intraocular lens dislocation: incidence, prevention, and management. *J Cataract Refract Surg.* 2005;31:2193-2204.
33. Hoffman RS, Fine IH, Packer M. Scleral fixation without conjunctival dissection. *J Cataract Refract Surg.* 2006;32:1907-1912.
34. Agarwal A, Kumar DA, Jocob S, et al. Fibrin glue-assisted sutureless posterior chamber intraocular lens implantation in eyes with deficient posterior capsules. *J Cataract Refract Surg.* 2008;34:1433-1438.
35. Osher RH. Synthetic zonules. *Ophthalmology Times.* 1997;15.
36. Fine IH, Hoffman RS. Phacoemulsification in the presence of pseudoexfoliation: challenges and options. *J Cataract Refract Surg.* 1997;23:160-165.
37. Stark WJ, Goodman G, Goodman D, Gottsch J. Posterior chamber intraocular lens implantation in the absence of posterior capsular support. *Ophthalmic Surg.* 1998;19:240-243.
38. Stark WJ, Gottsch JD, Goodman DF. Posterior chamber intraocular lens implantation in the absence of capsular support. *Arch Ophthalmol.* 1989;107:1078-1083.
39. Osher RH, Snyder ME, Cionni RJ. Modification of the Siepser slip-knot technique. J Cataract Refract Surg. 2005;31:1098-1100.
40. Gimbel HV, Camoriano GD, Shah CR, Dardzhikova AA. Capsule membrane suture fixation of decentered sulcus intraocular lenses. *Arch Ophthalmol.* 2012;130(1):101-105.
41. Kwong YY, Yuen HK, Lam RF, et al. Comparison of outcomes of primary scleral-fixated versus primary anterior chamber intraocular lens implantation in complicated cataract surgeries. *Ophthalmology.* 2007;114:80-85.
42. Batlan SJ, Dodic JM. Explantation of foldable silicone intraocular lens. *Am J Ophthamol.* 1996;122:270-272.
43. Ernest P. Intraocular refolding. *VJCRS.* 1996; XII.
44. Eguchi S. Quadrantotomy. *VJCRS.* 2005; XXI.
45. Osher RH . Criss-cross lensectomy. *VJCRS.* 2005;XXI.
46. Trindade FC. Haptic-induced recurrent vitreous hemorrhage and increased intraocular pressure with a hydrophobic acrylic intraocular lens. *J Cataract Refract Surg.* 2009:35:399-402.
47. Snyder Me, Foster RE. Anterior vitrectomy. *Comp Ophyhalmol Update.* 2001:2:149-158
48. Burke SE, Da Mata AP, Snyder ME. Visualizing vitreous using Kenalog suspension. *J Cataract Refract Surg.* 2003;29:645-651.
49. Winslow RL, Taylor BC. Spontaneous vitreous hemorrhage: etiology and management. *South Med J.* 1980;73:1450-1452.
50. Butner RW, McPerson AR. Spontaneous vitreous hemorrhage. *Ann Ophthamol.* 1982:14:268-270.
51. Dana MR, Werner MS, Viana MA, Shapiro MJ. Spontaneous and traumatic vitreous hemorrhage. *Ophthalmology.* 1993;100:1377-1383.
52. Lindgren G, Sjodell L, Lindblom B. A prospective study of dense spontaneous vitreous hemorrhage. *Am J Ophthalmol.* 1995;119:458-465.
53. Hasenfratz G. Acute vitreous hemorrhage: possibilities for differential diagnostic, echographic assessment. *Fortschr Ophthalmol.* 1990;87:641-645.
54. De Juan E Jr, Hichingbotham D. Refinements in microinstrumentation for vitreous surgery. *Am J Ophthalmol.* 1990;109:218-220.
55. Fujii GY, De Juan E Jr, Humayun MS, et al. A new 25-gauge instrument system for transcon-junctival sutureless vitrectomy surgery. *Ophthalmology.* 2002;109:1807-1812.
56. Lakhanpal RR, Humayun MS, de Juan E Jr, et al. Outcomes of 140 consecutive cases of 25-gauge transconjunctival surgery for posterior segment disease. *Ophthalmology.* 2005;112:817-824.
57. Ibarra MS, Hermel M, Prenner JL, Hassan TS Long-term outcomes of transconjunctival sutureless 25-gauge vitrectomy. *Am J Ophthalmol.* 2005;139:831-836.
58. Eckardt C. Transconjunctival sutureless 23-gauge vitrectomy. *Retina.* 2005;25:208-211.
59. Chalam KV, Shah VA. Successful management of cataract surgery associated vitreous loss with sutureless small-gauge pars plana vitrectomy. *Am J Ophthalmol.* 2004;138:79-84.
60. Shah VA, Gupta SK, Chalam KV. Management of vitreous loss during cataract surgery under topical anesthesia with transconjunctival vitrctomy system. *Eur J Ophthalmol.* 2003;13:693-696.
61. Lewis H, Sanchez G. The use of liquid perfluirocarbon in the repositioning of posteriorly dislocated intraocular lenses. *Ophthalmology.* 1993;100:1055-1059.
62. Sternberg P, Michels RG. Treatment of dislocated posterior chamber intraocular lens. *Arch Ophthalmol.* 1986;104:1391-1393.
63. Flynn HW Jr, Buus D, Culbertson WW. Management of subluxated and dislocated intraocular lenses using pars plana vitrectomy instrumentation. *J Cataract Refract Surg.* 1990;16:51-56.
64. Smiddy WE, Flynn HW Jr. Needle assisted scleral fixation technique for relocating posteriorly dislocated IOLs. *Arch Ophthalmol.* 1993;111:161-162.
65. Smiddy WE, Flynn HW Jr. Management of dislocated posterior chamber intraocular lenses. *Ophthalmology.* 1991;98:889-894.
66. Maguire AM, Blumenkranz MS, Ward TG, et al. Scleral loop fixation for posteriorly dislocated intraocular lenses. *Arch Ophthalmol.* 1991;109:1754-1758.
67. Chan CK. An improved technique for management of dislocated posterior chamber implants. *Ophthalmology.* 1992;99:51-57.
68. Smiddy WE, Ibanez GV, Alfonso E, et al. Surgical management of dislocated intraocular lenses. *J Cataract Refract Surg.* 1995;21:64-69.
69. Mello MO, Scott IU, Smiddy WE, et al. Surgical management and outcomes of dislocated intraocular lenses. *Ophthalmology.* 2000;107:62-67.

70. Trach AB, Dugel PU, Sipperley JO, et al. Outcome of sulcus fixation of dislocated posterior chamber intraocular lenses using temporary externalization of the haptics. *Ophthalmology.* 2000;107:480-484.
71. Sarrafizadeh R, Ruby AJ, Hassan TS, et al. A comparison of visual results and complications in eyes with posterior chamber intraocular lens dislocation treated with pars plana vitrectomy and lens repositioning or lens exchange. *Ophthalmology.* 2001;108:82-89.
72. Wong KL, Grabow HB. Simplified technique to remove posteriorly dislocated lens implants. *Arch Ophthalmol.* 2001;119:273-274.
73. Kokame GT, Atebara NH, Bennett MD. Modified technique of haptic externalization for scleral fixation of dislocated posterior chamber lens implants. *Am J Ophthalmol.* 2001;131:129-131.
74. Johnson MW, Schneiderman TE. Surgical management of posteriorly dislocated silicone plate intraocular lens. *Curr Opin Ophthalmol.* 1998;9:11-15.
75. Solomon K, Apple D, Mamalis N, et al. Complications of intraocular lenses with special reference to an analysis of 2500 explanted intraocular lenses (IOLs). *Eur J Implant Ref Surg.* 1991;3:195-200.
76. Apple DJ, Brems RN, Park RD, et al. Anterior chamber lenses. Part I. Complications and pathology and a review of designs. *J Cataract Refract Surg.* 1987;13:157-173.
77. Kraff M, Sanders DR, Lieberman HL, et al. Secondary intraocular lens implantation. *Ophthalmology.* 1983;90:324-326.
78. Mamalis N, Crandall A, Pulsipher M, et al. Intraocular lens explantation and exchange: a review of lens styles, clinical indication, clinical results, and visual outcome. *J Cataract Refract Surg.* 1991;17:810-818.
79. Kline OR, Yang HK. A review of 1400 intraocular lens implant cases. *Contact Lens.* 1981;7:262-278.
80. Smiddy WE, Flynn HW Jr. Management of dislocated posterior chamber intraocular lenses. *Ophthalmology.* 1991;98:889-894.
81. Doren G, Stern G, Dribe W. Indications for and results of a large series of intraocular lens exchanges. *J Cataract Refract Surg.* 1992;18:79-85.
82. Sinskey RM, Amin P, Stoppel JO. Indication for and results of a large series of intraocular exchanges. *J Cataract Refract Surg.* 1993;19:68-71.
83. Lyle W, Jin JC. An analysis of intraocular lens exchange. *Ophthalmic Surg.* 1992;23:453-458.
84. Marques FF, Marques DM, Osher RH, et al. Longitudinal study of intraocular lens exchange. *J Cataract Refract Surg.* 2007;33:254-257.
85. Hayashi K, Hirata A, Hayashi H. Possible predisposing factors for in-the-bag and out-of-the-bag intraocular lens dislocation and outcomes of intraocular lens exchange surgery. *Ophthalmology.* 2007 May;114(5):969-75.
86. Kim SS, Smiddy WE, Feuer W, Shi W. Management of dislocated intraocular lenses. *Ophthalmology.* 2008;115(10):1699-1704.
87. Gimbel HV, Condon GP, Kohnen T, et al. Late in-the bag intraocular lens dislocation: incidence, prevention, and management. *J Cataract Refract Surg.* 2005;31:2193-2204.
88. Gross JG, Kokame GT, Weinberg DV. In-the-bag intraocular lens dislocation. *Am J Ophthalmol.* 2001;137:630-635.
89. Dick HB, Tehrani M, Brauweiler P, et al. Complications of foldable intraocular lenses requiring explantation. Results of the 2000 and 2001 survey in Germany. *Ophthalmologe.* 2003;100:465-470.
90. Mamalis N. Complication of foldable intraocular lenses requiring explantation or secondary intervention-2001 survey update. *J Cataract Refract Surg.* 2002:28:2193-2201.
91. Mamalis N, David B, Nislin CD, et al. Complication of foldable intraocular lenses requiring explantantion or secondary intervention—2003 survey update. *J Cataract Refract Surg.* 2004;30:2009-2218.
92. Jin GJ, Crandall AS, Jones JJ. Changing indications for and improving outcomes of intraocular lens exchange. *Am J Ophthalmol.* 2005;140:688-694.
93. Jin GJ, Crandall AS, Jones JJ. Intraocular lens exchange due to incorrect lens power. *Ophthalmology.* 2007;114:417-424.
94. Kim MJ, Kim JH, Kim SJ, Yu YS. Long-term follow-up of changes in corneal endothelium after primary and secondary intraocular lens implantations in children. *Graefes Arch Clin Exp Ophthalmol.* 2012;250(6):925-930.
95. Wang Y, Wu M, Zhu L, Liu Y. Long-term corneal endothelial cell changes in pediatric intraocular lens reposition and exchange cases. *Graefes Arch Clin Exp Ophthalmol.* 2012;250(4):547-555.

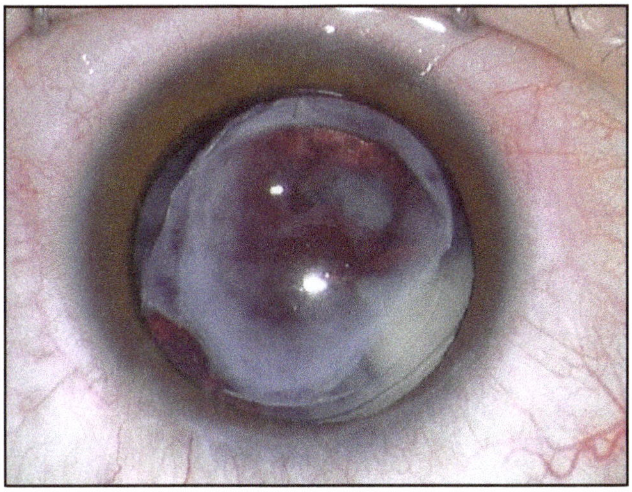

K-1. Explantation of an opaque PMMA IOL.

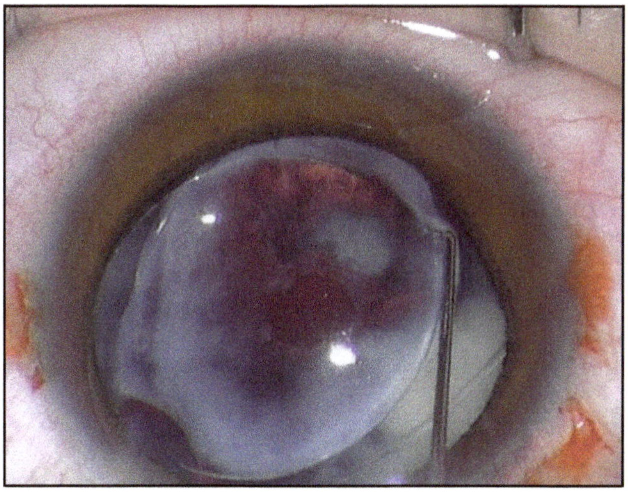

K-2. Removal of some adhesions between the haptics and the capsular bag.

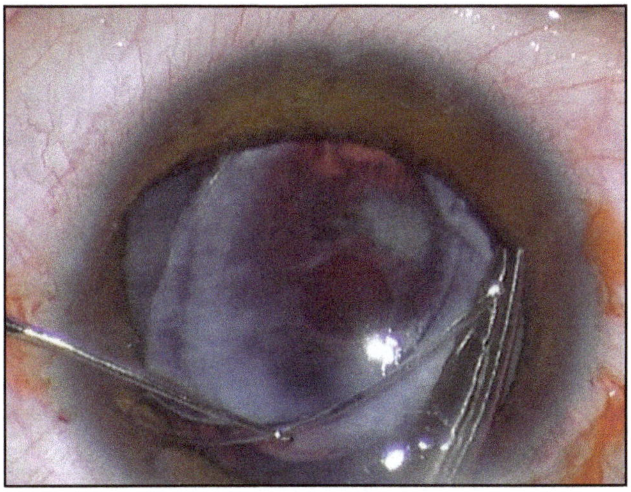

K-3. Cutting of one haptic to adherent at the capsular bag.

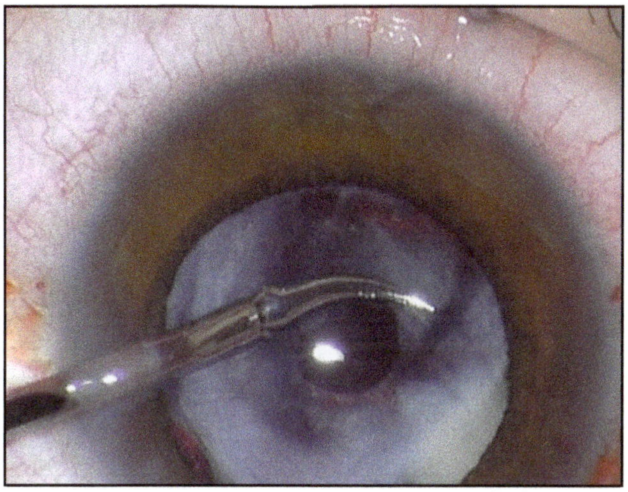

K-4. Enlarging of the opening in the posterior capsule.

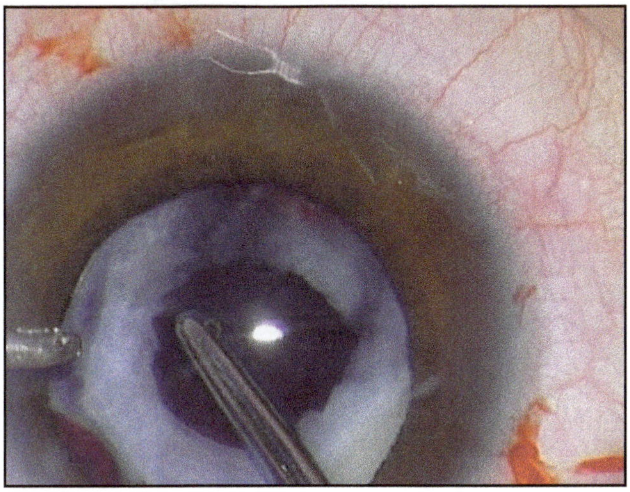

K-5. Anterior vitrectomy.

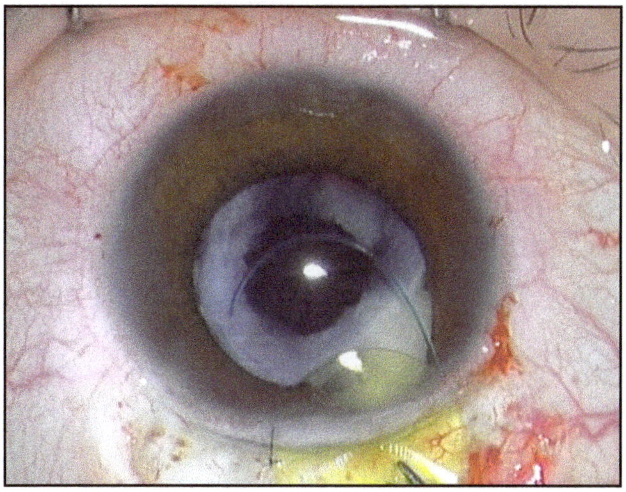

K-6. Implantation of a 3-piece PC-IOL in the sulcus.

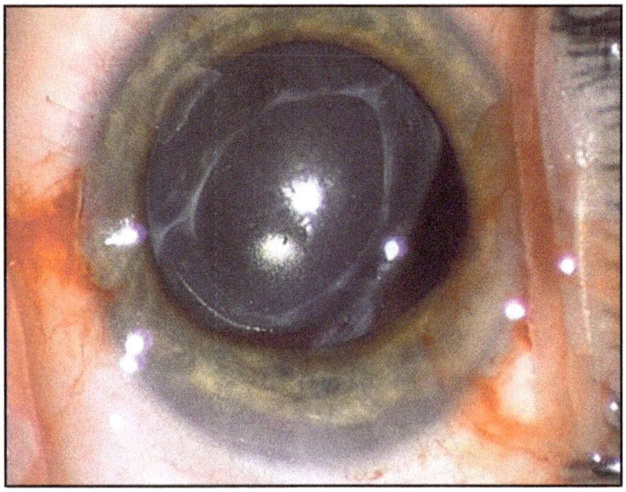

L-1. Opaque IOL: explantation is scheduled.

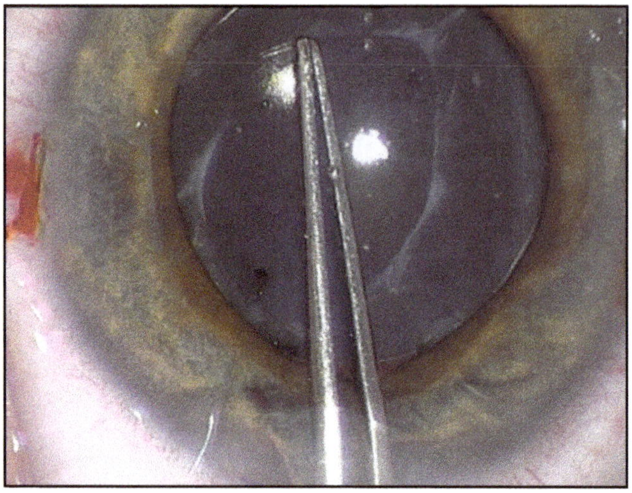

L-2. Following insertion of VES the surgeon attempts to enlarge the anterior rhexis: not possible.

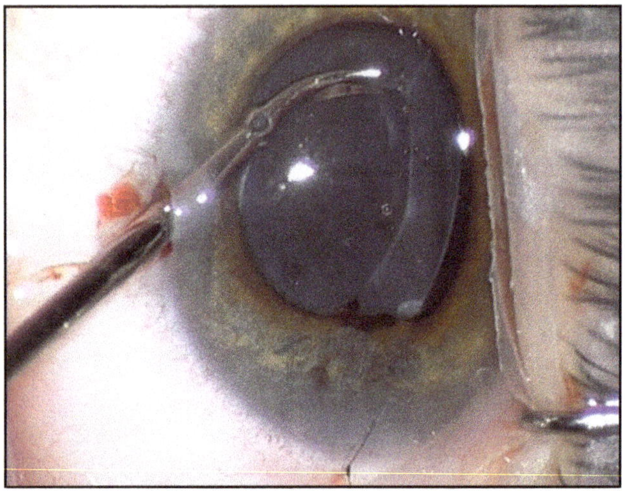

L-3. The anterior capsule is then cut with scissors to enlarge the opening and facilitate the removal of the IOL.

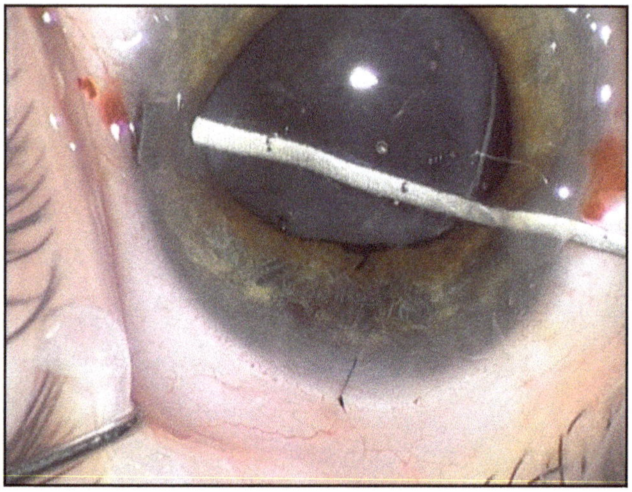

L-4. The lens cannot be released from the adhesions to the anterior capsule using VES and a spatula.

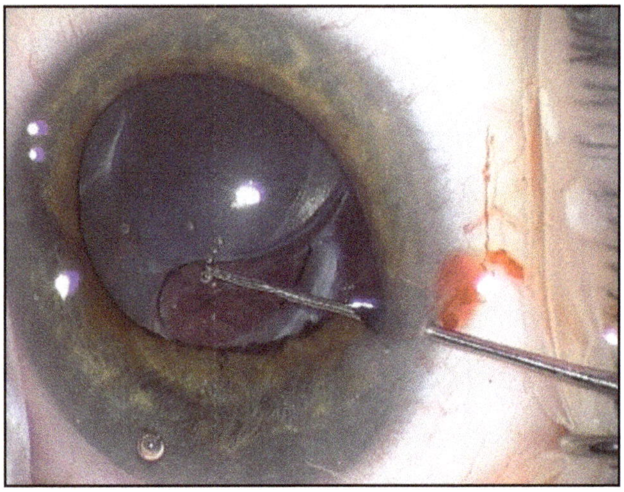

L-5. The IOL with the capsular bag is disinserted.

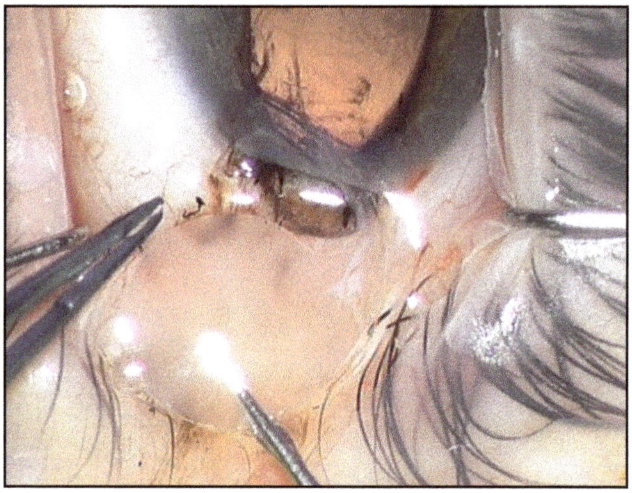

L-6. The IOL is extracted with the capsular bag; anterior vitrectomy follows and then the implantation of an iris-fixed IOL.

Index

acetylcholine (Miochol), intraocular, 208
amblyopia
with pediatric cataract surgery, 7, 10
postoperative prevention of, 8-9
aminoglycoside, in phacotrabeculectomy, 38
AMO Sovereign phaco, 102
amyloid substance, 60-61
anesthesia
for cataract surgery after phakic IOL implantation, 206
for cataract surgery with high myopia, 108
for penetrating keratoplasty with cataract removal, 180
for phacoemulsification and trabeculectomy, 34
for secondary IOL implantation, 214
for traumatic cataract surgery, 157
aniridia, cataracts with, 169-174
anisometropia, after cataract surgery, 107
anterior capsule procedure
age-related macular degeneration and, 96
problems with in pseudoexfoliation syndrome, 65
anterior chamber
collapse of, 109
depth of
in hyperopia, 111-112
in myopic eye, 105
penetration of, 30
anterior lamellar keratoplasty. *See* keratoplasty, anterior lamellar
anterior segment
cleaning, 162
in hyperopic eyes, 112
short, 112
cataract surgery in, 112-114
antibiotic eye drops
postoperative, for secondary IOLs, 227
prophylactic, 208
in phacotrabeculectomy, 38
antifibrotic agents, for glaucoma, 53
anti-inflammatory therapy
for glaucoma and uveitis with cataracts, 124
for uveitis with cataracts, 122
antimetabolites
in deep sclerectomy, 48
for glaucoma and uveitis with cataracts, 124-125
in phacotrabeculectomy, 37-38, 39
aphakia, postoperative
preoperative evaluation of, 213-214
secondary IOL implants for, 213-227
Arpa pupil dilator ring, 84-86
atropine
for floppy iris syndrome, 137
in pupil dilation, 78
axial length, in hyperopia, 111-112

B-scan examination, for traumatic cataracts, 156
basal membrane, in pseudoexfoliation syndrome, 61
Beehler's pupil dilator, 81, 82
betamethasone, postoperative, 8
Big Bubble technique, 194
biomicroscopy, 177
Birmingham Terminology System, 155
blindness, total and partial, definition of, 94
blood-eye barrier stabilization, 157
Bounce test, 236-237

C-shaped PMMA dilating rings, 86
canaloplasty
intraocular pressure in, 30
phacoemulsification and, 51-52
versus trabeculoplasty or trabeculectomy, 52
capsular tension rings
for brunescent cataracts, 101
with coloboma diaphragm, 171-173
implantation technique for, 18
in iris defect repair, 171
modified, 17-19, 21
in myopic eyes, 109-110
in phacoemulsification, 31
for pseudoexfoliation syndrome, 68-69
for subluxated lens, 12, 13, 16-21
capsular tension segments, for subluxated lens, 19-21
capsule
laceration of, 156, 162-163
thin and fragile, 99, 102
capsule retractors, 16-21
capsulorrhexis
age-related macular degeneration and, 96
for brunescent cataracts, 99-100
contraction of, 21
with high myopia, 108
in pediatric cataract surgery, 3-5, 7
in phacoemulsification, 31
phimosis of, 68
for pseudoexfoliation syndrome, 65-66
in subluxated lens removal, 13, 24
capsulotomy
anterior
with small pupil, 88
for traumatic cataracts, 168
retinal detachment with, 106
in subluxated lens removal, 23
for traumatic cataract, 158-159
cataract surgery. *See also* specific procedures
after phakic IOL implantation, 203-211
in age-related macular degeneration, 93-96
combined with vitreoretinal surgery, 151-152, 153, 154
in eyes with small anterior segment, 112-114
following vitreoretinal surgery, 149-151
indications for, 178
risk factors in with pseudoexfoliation syndrome, 64
for traumatic cataracts, 157-168
with uveitis, 121-127
cataracts
in aniridic eyes, 169-174
brunescent, 23, 94, 99
capsulorrhexis for, 99-100
complications of, 104
difficulties and solutions for, 99-103
hydrodissection and hydrodelineation for, 100
phacoemulsification for, 101-103
postoperative care for, 103
removal of, 104
zonular fragility in, 100-101
corneal pathology and, 177-196, 200-201
in diabetic patients, 141-145
extracapsular, intraocular inflammation in, 95
glaucoma associated with, 27, 54
canaloplasty and phacoemulsification for, 51-52
combined surgery for, 33-34
deep sclerectomy and phacoemulsification for, 47-51
determining surgery for, 27-28
implants for, 53
management of, 71-72
new glaucoma surgical techniques for, 53
phacoemulsification for, 28-33
trabeculectomy and phacoemulsification for, 34-40

trabeculotomy and phacoemulsification for, 41-42
viscocanalostomy and phacoemulsification for, 42-47
hereditary transmission of, 1-2
in high myopia, 105
anatomical-surgical considerations in, 105-106
IOLs for, 107-108
postoperative refraction for, 106-107
preoperative evaluation of, 106
surgical procedures for, 108-110
incidence of, 27
luxated, 25
membranous, 165
nigra, 99
pathogenesis of after vitreoretinal surgery, 149-150
pediatric, 1, 9-10
age at surgery for, 2, 3
intraocular lens implantation for, 6-8
outcomes of, 1
postoperative period for, 8
postoperative re-education and amblyopia prevention in, 8-9
preoperative examination for, 1-2
prognostic signs in, 2
surgery for, 2-6
pseudoexfoliation syndrome and, 60
in retinitis pigmentosa, 117-119
in severe hyperopia, 111-116
traumatic, 155
anterior segment cleaning in, 162
capsulotomy and hydrodissection of, 158-159
clinical evaluation of, 155-157
cortical removal for, 160-161
dense nucleus and lacerated posterior capsule in, 162
incision location for, 157-158
intraocular lens implantation for, 163-164
lacerated capsule in, 162-163
lens removal in, 161-162
long-standing changes in, 165
nucleus removal for, 159-160
phacoemulsification with compromised zonules in, 160
repairing iris and restoring pupil opening in, 164-165
surgical planning and technique for, 157
surgical technique for, 168
viscoelastic substance for, 158
cephalosporins, in phacotrabeculectomy, 38
cephtazidime, 38
cephuroxime, 38
children
with cataracts and uveitis, 127
cataracts in, 1-10
IOLs for traumatic cataracts in, 164
secondary IOLs in, 225-226
chop phacoemulsification, 119
for brunescent cataracts, 101-102
choroid
in myopic eye, 105
neovascularization of, 93
active, 94
cataract surgery and, 96
chronic ocular ischemic syndrome, 61
ciliary body
in myopic eye, 105
in pseudoexfoliation syndrome, 62
collagen inserts, in deep sclerectomy, 49
coloboma, iris, 23
suturing of, 169-170
coloboma ring with diaphragm, 170-171
computed tomography, for traumatic cataracts, 156
confocal microscopy, 177
conjunctival bleb, 42
contact lenses
after pediatric cataract removal, 9
after subluxated lens removal, 11
cornea
anatomy of, 28
decompensation of, 179, 214
opacity of, 177, 178
scarring of, 179
topography of, 177
corneal edema
evaluation of, 177
posterior lamellar keratoplasty for, 188
postoperative, 103
stromal, 178
corneal pathology
with cataracts, 196, 200-201
combined anterior lamellar keratoplasty and cataract removal for, 193-194
surgical techniques in, 194-195
combined penetrating keratoplasty and cataract removal for
complications of, 186-188
preoperative preparation for, 180-181
combined posterior lamellar keratoplasty and cataract removal for, 188-193
complications of, 193
future trends for, 193
preoperative preparation for, 189
results of, 192-193
techniques for, 181-186
preoperative evaluation of, 177-178
stromal, keratoplasty for, 193-196
therapeutic planning for, 178-180
corneal scleral laceration, open, 156-157
corneal tattoo, 174
corneal tunnel
in brunescent cataract surgery, 99
with small pupil, 88
corneoscleral component, 33-34
cortical removal, for traumatic cataracts, 160-161
cortisone, after pediatric cataract surgery, 8
cribriform, 34
crystalline lens
as barrier to UV light, 94
congenital subluxation of, 11, 21-22
capsular tension rings, capsule retractors, and capsular tension segments for, 16-21
capsulorrhexis and hydrodissection with, 13
clinical evaluation for, 11-12
IOL implantation for, 15
phacoemulsification and cortex removal for, 13-15
preoperative evaluation of, 12
progressive, 11
removal of, 23-25
surgical treatment of, 12-13
dislocated, surgical management of, 70-71
hydration of, 99, 149
PEX, 61-63
cyclitic membrane, for uveitis with cataracts, 125
cyclodialysis, in trabeculotomy, 42
cyclopentolate
after pediatric cataract surgery, 8
in pupil dilation, 78
cycloplegic drugs, 78

De Juan iris dilator hooks, 83
De Juan iris retractors, 85

deep sclerectomy
  for glaucoma and uveitis with cataracts, 125
  intraocular pressure in, 30
  phacoemulsification and, 47-48
    indications and contraindications to, 50
    results and complications of, 50-51
    technique of, 48-50
Descemet's membrane detachment
  in canaloplasty, 52
  in trabeculotomy, 42
Descemet's window
  creating, 44-46
  in deep sclerectomy, 48-49
  perforation of, 47
dexamethasone eye drops, postoperative, 125
  in pediatric patients, 8
diabetes
  cataract management with, 141-145
  epidemiology of, 141
  types of, 141
diclofenac, postoperative, 126

elastic microfibrils, in pseudoexfoliation syndrome, 61
elderly, subluxated lens in, 12
Ellipse transversal system, 102
Elschnig pearls, proliferation of, 115
emmetropia, refraction formulas for, 108
endocapsular lensectomy with vitrectomy, in diabetic patients, 145
endophthalmitis, postoperative, 208
epikeratophakia, after subluxated lens removal, 11
epinephrine
  for floppy iris syndrome, 134
  in pupil dilation, 78
episcleral surgery, versus vitreoretinal surgery, 149
explantation technique, after phakic IOL implantation, 207-208
extracapsular cataract extraction (ECCE), 27
  after vitreoretinal surgery, 150
  for cataracts with high myopia, 106
  with corneal pathology, 179
  in diabetic patients, 141
  with penetrating keratoplasty, 183-186
  versus phacoemulsification, 29, 34, 40
  secondary IOL implantation after, 214-215
eye, anatomy of, 28

fibrin glue, in scleral fixation of IOLs, 226-227
fibrinoid reactions, after pediatric cataract surgery, 8
fibrinous membranes, postoperative, 126
finasteride, for floppy iris syndrome, 132-133
floppy iris syndrome
  combined strategies for, 137
  etiology and pathogenesis of, 131-133
  grading, 133
  management strategies for, 133-134
  pharmacological strategies for, 134
  pupil expansion devices for, 135-137
  signs of, 131
  surgical risks of, 137-138
  viscoelastics for, 134-135
fluorescein dye, 159
flurbiprofen, in pupil dilation, 78
5-flurouracil, in phacotrabeculectomy, 37-38

gentian violet dye, 159
gentamycin, in phacotrabeculectomy, 38
glare, 15, 77, 118, 119, 122, 163, 170-174, 231-232
glaucoma
  after pediatric cataract surgery, 8
  angle-closure
    cataract removal in, 29
    lens removal in, 27
  with cataracts, 27-54
    in pseudoexfoliation syndrome, 71-72
  combined surgery for uveitis with cataracts and, 124-125
  narrow angle, 46
  neovascular, 46, 52
  new surgical techniques for, 53
  open-angle, 27-28, 29
  piggyback IOLs and, 115
  in pseudoexfoliation syndrome, 60
    pathogenesis of, 71-72
glaucoma drainage devices (GDDs), 28, 53
Graether 2000 pupil expander system, 86
Graether pupillary expansion ring, 135-136
graft failure, with phaco/DSEAK, 193
Grieshaber flexible iris retractors, 3
guttata, 177, 178

Healon 5 VES, 3, 31, 79, 99, 134-135, 137, 143, 158, 190, 236
Healon GV VES, 158
hemorrhage
  after penetrating keratoplasty with cataract removal, 187-188
  subchoroidal, in myopic eye, 105
  suprachoroidal, 156-157
  vitreous, 149
Honan balloon, 181
hyaluronic acid inserts, 49
hydrodelineation, 100
hydrodissection
  after vitreoretinal surgery, 150
  for brunescent cataracts, 100
  in eyes with retinitis pigmentosa, 119
  in eyes with small anterior segment, 113
  for floppy iris syndrome, 133-134
  in high myopia, 108-109
  in pediatric cataract surgery, 3
  in phacoemulsification, 31
  for pseudoexfoliation syndrome, 66
  with small pupil, 88
  for subluxated lens removal, 13
  for traumatic cataract, 158-159
hyperopia
  after cataract surgery, 107
  after pediatric cataract surgery, 8-9
  cataract surgery in, 112-116
  causes of, 111
  determining axial length and IOL power for, 111-112
  refraction formulas for, 108
  surgical anatomy of, 112
hyperpulsated technology, 102
hyphema
  with canaloplasty, 52
  with viscocanalostomy, 47
hypotony
  with canaloplasty, 52
  with viscocanalostomy, 47

immunosuppressive therapy, for uveitis with cataracts, 122
in-the-bag dislocation, 69-70
  in pseudoexfoliation syndrome, 67
infection, in pseudoexfoliation syndrome, 61
inflow surgeries, for glaucoma, 53
INTACS lamellar dissectors, 174
intracameral α-agonists, for floppy iris syndrome, 131-132, 137
intracapsular cataract extraction (ICCE)
  for cataracts with high myopia, 106
  in diabetic patients, 141
  secondary IOL implantation after, 214-215
  for subluxated lens removal, 11-12
intraocular gas, in cataract formation, 149
intraocular inflammation, in macular degeneration, 95
intraocular lens (IOL) capsular bag complex, rupture of, 68-69
intraocular lens (IOL) implantation
  after vitreoretinal surgery, 154
  after vitreous loss, 188
  age-related macular degeneration and, 96
  for cataracts in diabetic patients, 143-144

  combined with vitreoretinal surgery, 152
  for congenital subluxation of lens, 11
  in eye with retinitis pigmentosa, 119
  for hyperopic eyes, 114
  in myopic eyes, 110
  in pediatric cataract patients, 5-8
    with uveitis, 127
  in phaco/DSEAK, 191, 192
  in phacoemulsification, 32
  in phacotrabeculectomy, 35-36
  secondary, 213-227
    anesthesia in, 214
    preoperative evaluation of aphakic patient for, 213-214
  with small pupil, 88
  for subluxated lens, 14, 24
  for uveitis with cataracts, 123-124, 127
intraocular lens (IOL) implants
  anterior chamber, 216-217
    with angle support, 207
    repositioning or replacing, 233-234
  in bag or sulcus, 215-216
  blocking UV rays, 94
  for cataracts and glaucoma, 53
  choice of for pseudoexfoliation syndrome, 67-70
  decentrated, 232
  delayed dislocation of, 20
  diaphragm, 171-172
  dislocated, 231, 232
    management of, 240-242
    in phaco/DSEAK, 193
  explantation and replacement of, 231-232, 240-242, 245-246
    preoperative evaluation for, 232-233
    surgical techniques for, 233-240
  for hyperopia, 8-9
  inadequate capsular support for, 231
  with iris claw fixation, 234-235
  with iris enclavation, 207-208
  for myopic eye, 107-108
  for myopic eyes, 105, 107-108
  in pediatric patients
    positioning of, 6-7
    power of, 7
  phakic, 203
    cataract development with, 204-205
    cataract surgery after implantation of, 205-211
    safety and efficacy of, 203
    types of, 204
  piggyback, 114--116, 180
  posterior chamber, 208
    decentered, 231, 236
    exchange of, 237
    posteriorly luxated, 239-240
    replacement of, 237-239
    repositioning of, 235-237
    sutured to iris, 217-219
    sutured to sclera, 219-224
    with torn bag, 238-239
  for pseudoexfoliation syndrome, 67-70
  refractive formulas for, 107-108
  repositioning of, 232-233
  secondary
    in children, 225-226
    comparison of, 224-225
    complications of, 223-224, 225
    postoperative treatment of, 227
    subluxation of, 223
    sutureless scleral fixation techniques for, 226-227
  for traumatic cataracts
    in pediatric cases, 164
    positioning, 163-164
    selecting, 163
intraocular lens (IOL) power
  calculation of, 2
    formulas for, 205
    for vitreoretinal surgery, 150
  dioptric, 115
  preoperative measurement of, 179
  for severe hyperopia, 111-112
intraocular pressure
  after phacoemulsification, 33
  after viscocanalostomy, 50
  increased
    after trabeculotomy, 42
    with canaloplasty, 52
    YAG laser gonio-puncture for, 51
  before phacoemulsification, 29-30
  phacotrabeculectomy effect on, 39, 40
  preoperative measurement of, 178
iridectomy, 24, 87
  peripheral, in phacotrabeculectomy, 36-37
iris
  atrophy of, 77-78
  coloboma of, 23, 169-170
  defects in
    cataracts with, 169-174
    repair of, 164-165
    repair options for, 169-174
  disinsertion of in traumatic cataracts, 168
  posterior chamber IOL sutured to, 217-219, 224-225
  problems of in pseudoexfoliation syndrome, 64-65
  in pseudoexfoliation syndrome, 62
  surgery on with small pupil, 87-88
  thinning stroma of, 132
iris cerlage, 170
iris claw fixation, 234-235
iris dilator hooks, 83-84, 85
iris implants, 170-171
Iris Prosthetic System (IPS), with PMMA ring, 172-174
iris retractors
  for floppy iris syndrome, 136-137
  irrigating, 84
  in subluxated lens removal, 21, 22
iris rings, in pupil expansion, 82
iris sutures, 87-88
  for iris defect repair, 169-170
  for traumatic cataracts, 168
irrigation/aspiration (I/A) technique
  in pediatric cataract surgery, 3, 5
  in phacoemulsification, 32, 35
  with small pupil, 88

keratectomy, photorefractive, after keratoplasty, 180
keratoconus, 177, 178
  keratoplasty for, 193-196
keratoplasty
  anterior lamellar, 178
    with cataract removal, 193-195
  deep anterior lamellar keratoplasty (DALK), 194
  endothelial
    deep lamellar (DLEK), 188
    Descemet's membrane (DMEK), 188, 193
    Descemet's stripping automated (DSEAK), 188
      with phacoemulsification, 189-193
    Descemet's stripping (DSEK), 188
  indications for, 178
  penetrating (PKP), 178, 200
    versus anterior lamellar keratoplasty, 194-195
  posterior lamellar, 178
    with cataract removal, 188-193
    complications of, 193
    indications for, 188-189
    preoperative preparation for, 189
    results of, 192-193
    techniques in, 189-192
  prognosis for, 180
  types of, 178
keratoprothesis, Cobo's temporary, 187
ketorolac
  postoperative, 126
  in pupil dilation, 78

LASIK
  after keratoplasty, 180
  for hyperopic eyes, 116

latent transforming growth factor, type-1 (LTBP-1), 60
lens. *See* crystalline lens; intraocular lens (IOL) implants
lensectomy, in vitreoretinal surgery, 151
limbal paracentesis, 170
limbus, anatomy of, 28, 33-34
lipofuscin fluorophore A2E, 94
LOXL1 gene, 60, 61

Mackool iris dilator hooks, 83, 85
macula
edema of
cystoid, 32, 118, 142
in diabetic patients, 142-143
with phaco/DSEAK, 193
in uveitis, 121
evaluation of, 178
macular degeneration, age-related
cataract surgery and, 95-96
forms of, 93
physiopathological mechanisms of, 93-95
risk factors for, 93
Malyugin's pupil expander, 86-87
for floppy iris syndrome, 136
mannitol
for preoperative intraocular pressure reduction, 30
in suprachoroidal hemorrhage, 157
methylene blue dye, 159
microincisional cataract surgery (MICS)
bimanual, 133
coaxial (C-MICS), 102, 133
microincisional phacoemulsification systems (MICS), 178-179
microkeratome, 192
mini-sphincterotomies, 82
mitomycin C
for glaucoma and uveitis with cataracts, 124-125
with phacoemulsification, 28
in phacotrabeculectomy, 37-38
Morcher pupil expansion ring, 84, 86
for floppy iris syndrome, 135
Mydriacyl (tropicamide), for floppy iris syndrome, 134
Mydriasert, in pupil dilation, 78
mydriasis
in cataract surgery, 77
correction of, 170
poor, causes of, 77
post-traumatic, 165
in pupil dilation, 78
mydriatics
after pediatric cataract surgery, 8
for small pupil, 78
myopia
anatomy of, 105
cataracts in, 105-110
refraction formulas for, 108

nepafenac, in pupil dilation, 78
nonsteroidal anti-inflammatory drug (NSAID) eye drops
after phacoemulsification, 32
postoperative, 126
in pupil dilation, 78
nuclear sclerosis, progressive, 152
nucleus
hardiness of, 99
removal of in traumatic cataracts, 159-160
nystagmus, in pediatric cataracts, 2

open globe, in traumatic cataracts, 156-157
Ophtec implant, 172
Osher hook, 81
outflow surgeries, for glaucoma, 53
Ozil torsional system, 102

pachymetry, in anterior lamellar keratoplasty, 194
panphotocoagulation, for cataracts in diabetic patients, 142-143
paracentesis, 30, 79, 82-83, 164, 183
pars plana lensectomy, 152
pars plana vitrectomy
mini-invasive, 239-240
for subluxated lens removal, 12
for traumatic cataracts, 156, 162
Perfect Pupil dilator ring, 84
peribulbar anesthesia
for phacoemulsification and trabeculectomy, 34
for phacoemulsification in high myopia, 108
phaco roll technique, 109
phacoemulsification. *See also* chop phacoemulsification
after phakic IOL implantation, 208
after vitreoretinal surgery, 150-151
age-related macular degeneration and, 96
for brunescent cataracts, 101-103
canaloplasty and, 51-52, 51-54
for cataracts
in diabetic patients, 141-145
with glaucoma, 27
with high myopia, 106
deep sclerectomy and, 47-51
with dense nucleus and lacerated posterior capsule, 162
with endothelial keratoplasty, 188-193
versus extracapsular cataract extraction, 29, 34
in eye with retinitis pigmentosa, 119
for floppy iris syndrome, 133-134
in glaucomatous eyes, 28-29
capsular tension ring implantation in, 31
capsulorrhexis in, 31
complications of, 32-33
entrance to anterior chamber in, 30
hydrodissection in, 31
incision in, 30
IOL implantation in, 32
irrigation/aspiration in, 32
paracentesis in, 30
postoperative therapy for, 32
preoperative intraocular pressure reduction in, 29-30
pupils in, 30-31
surgical difficulties with, 29
in high myopia, 108
in hyperopic eyes, 112-116
with penetrating keratoplasty, 181-183
secondary IOL implantation after, 214-215
with small pupil, 77, 89, 91
anterior capsulotomy in, 88
corneal incisions in, 88
hydrodissection in, 88
IOL insertion in, 89
iris surgery in, 87-88
irrigation/aspiration in, 89
pharmacological treatment of, 78
preoperative evaluation for, 77-78
procedures in, 88-89
surgical methods to expand pupil, 79-87
in subluxated lens removal, 12-14, 23
supracapsular, 66
in therapeutic planning for corneal pathology, 178-179
trabeculotomy and, 41-42
for traumatic cataracts, 159-160, 168
for uveitis with cataracts, 122-123
viscocanalostomy and, 42-47
with vitrectomy, 144-145
with vitreoretinal surgery, 152
phacoemulsification machines, hyperpulsated, 102
phacotrabeculectomy, 34
anesthesia in, 34
complications of, 39-40
postoperative period of, 38-39
with single incision superiorly, 35-37
surgical technique in, 35
using separate incisions, 37-40
phenylephrine
for floppy iris syndrome, 134
in pupil dilation, 78
phimosis, of capsulorrhexis, 68
photokeratoscopy, 177
Placido disc, 177
PMMA ring, 173-174
polypseudophakia, 115

posterior capsule opacification (PCO)
after subluxated lens removal, 20
in diabetic patients, 143
in phaco-vitrectomy patients, 145
postoperative, 32, 40, 123-124, 126-127, 143
in retinitis pigmentosa, 118-119
in uveitis, 121
posterior chamber, length of in myopic eye, 105
posterior lamellar keratoplasty. *See* keratoplasty, posterior lamellar
posterior segment disruption, 155
prednisolone eye drops
after pediatric cataract surgery, 8
postoperative, 125
pseudoexfoliation syndrome, 59
cataract and, 60
clinical aspects of, 63-64
dislocated lens in, 70-71
epidemiology of, 59-60
factors associated with, 59-60
glaucoma and, 60, 71-72
histopathological and ultrastructural, 61-63
IOL choice for, 67-70
pathogenesis of, 60-61
preoperative diagnosis of, 64-65
risk factors in cataract surgery in, 64
surgical technique for, 65-67
uni- or bilateral ocular involvement of, 60
pupil
fixed, 31, 77
of glaucomatous eyes, 30-31
hyporeactive, 77
iris surgery for expansion of, 87-88
restoration of in traumatic cataract surgery, 164-165
rim removal, 80
size of with phakic IOL implantation, 206
small, 30-31
in eyes with small anterior segment, 113
mydriatic drugs for, 78
phacoemulsification with, 77-89, 91
stretching, 80-82
with small anterior segment, 113
surgical methods to expand, 79-87
under-reactive, 31
pupil dilators, 81, 82-87
pupillary expansion devices, 84-86, 135-137
for floppy iris syndrome, 137
Purkinje's phenomenon, 156

red reflex, absence of, 99
refraction, postoperative, 106-107
refractive error
after cataract surgery with phakic IOL, 208
postsurgical, 179-180
refractive lensectomy, 114
retina
detachment of
after pediatric cataract surgery, 8
with cataract surgery, 105-106
in myopic eye, 105-106
retinal carotenoids, 93-94
retinitis pigmentosa
age of onset and severity of, 117
cataract associated with, 118-119
cataract surgery in, 119
clinical signs of, 117
diagnosis of, 117
pathologies of, 117
progression of, 118
retinopathy, diabetic, 141, 142
retrobulbar anesthesia, 34, 108

Schlemm's canal, 28, 34
dilation of, 44
failure of, 47
in trabeculotomy, 41
sclera
anatomy of, 28
in myopic eye, 105
posterior chamber IOL sutured to, 219-226
scleral bed
perforation of, 47
preparing for deep sclerectomy, 48
preparing for phacotrabeculectomy, 35
preparing for trabeculotomy, 41
preparing for viscocanalostomy, 43
scleral fixation sutures, 236
scleral flap
deep, 43-44, 46, 48, 49-50
superficial, 48
scleral tunnel, 35
shunts, for cataracts and glaucoma, 53
Siepser pupil expansion ring, 136
slit-lamp biomicroscopy, 156
sodium flurbiprofen, 78
spectacles
after pediatric cataract removal, 9
after removal of subluxated lens, 11
specular microscopy, 177
sphincterectomy, 82
of iris, 169
sphincterotomy, 82
in eyes with small anterior segment, 113
steroids
for dislocated IOLs, 232
postoperative, 227
strabismus, after pediatric cataract surgery, 8
sub-Tenon's anesthesia
for cataract surgery after phakic IOL implantation, 206
for phacoemulsification and trabeculectomy, 34
suprachoroidal effusion, after penetrating keratoplasty, 187-188
suprofene, in pupil dilation, 78
sutures, 236
for iris defect repair, 87-88, 168-170
in deep sclerectomy, 49-50
in phacotrabeculectomy, 37
in secondary IOLs
for traumatic cataracts, 168
to iris, 217-219, 224-225
rupture or erosion of, 223-224
to sclera, 219-226
in trabeculotomy, 41
for viscocanalostomy, 46
synechiolysis, 79-80
for iris defect repair, 169
synechiotomy, 23

tamsulosin, for floppy iris syndrome, 131-132, 134
trabecular meshwork, 33
in pseudoexfoliation syndrome, 62-63
trabeculectomy
versus canaloplasty, 52
for glaucoma and uveitis with cataracts, 124-125
phacoemulsification and, 34
anesthesia in, 34
single incision superiorly, 35-37
surgical technique in, 35
using separate incisions, 37-40
in phacotrabeculectomy procedure, 36
versus viscocanalostomy, 42-43, 50
trabeculoplasty
anti-inflammatory prophylaxis after, 126
versus canaloplasty, 52
trabeculotomy, phacoemulsification and, 41
complications of, 41-42
technique in, 41
trabeculum, 33-34
laceration of, 42
traumatic injury, 155-156. *See* cataracts, traumatic
tropicamide
after pediatric cataract surgery, 8
for floppy iris syndrome, 134
in pupil dilation, 78
trypan blue dye, 159

ultrasound biometry devices, 111
ultraviolet light
in macular degeneration, 94-95
retinotoxic effects of, 96
uveal trabeculum, 33-34
uveitis, 121
cataract surgery with
cyclitic membrane in, 125
follow-up and results of, 126-127
with glaucoma surgery, 124-125
IOL implantation in, 123-124
perioperative treatment of, 122
techniques of, 122-123
timing of, 122
vitrectomy in, 125
physiopathology, signs and symptoms of, 121
postoperative treatment for, 125-126
uveitis-glaucoma-hyphema (UGH) syndrome, 231

vancomycin prophylaxis, 38
viscocanalostomy
contraindications to, 46
intraocular pressure in, 30
phacoemulsification and, 42-43
contraindications to, 46
indications for, 46
results and complications of, 47
technique in, 43-46
versus trabeculectomy, 42-43, 50
viscodissection, for traumatic cataracts, 161
viscoelastic substance (VES) injection
in brunescent cataract treatment, 100, 102-103
in corneal evaluation, 178
to expand pupil, 79
in eyes with small anterior segment, 112-113
for floppy iris syndrome, 134-135, 137
in phaco/DSEAK, 190
preoperative, 78
pseudoadaptive, 112
removal of in hyperopic eyes, 116
in synechiolysis, 79-80
in traumatic cataract surgery, 158, 161
for uveitis with cataracts, 123
viscomydriasis, 79
vision loss
after cataract and vitreoretinal surgery, 152
postoperative, 126
in uveitis, 121
visual acuity loss, 52
visual axis opacification (VAO), 3-6, 8
vitrectomy, 24, 25, 154
for cataracts in diabetic patients, 145
endocapsular lensectomy with, 145
with phacoemulsification, 145
for posterior chamber IOL replacement, 239-240
for uveitis with cataracts, 125
for vitreous loss, 187
vitreoretinal complex
in myopic eye, 105-106
surgery on, 153
cataract development after, 149-150
cataract surgery after, 150-151
clinical situations and indications for, 151-152
functional results of, 152
preoperative evaluation for, 150
surgical options for, 152
vitreous
aspiration of, 186
asteroid degeneration of, 154
hemorrhage in, 149
loss of
after penetrating keratoplasty with cataract removal, 186-187
IOL implantation after, 188
pressure of
in eyes with small anterior segment, 113
positive, 186-187

YAG laser gonio-puncture, 51
YAG laser therapy, after subluxated lens removal, 21

zonular fibers, in myopic eye, 105
zonules
absent, 99
compromised, 160
damaged in traumatic cataract surgery, 161-162
dialysis of in pseudoexfoliation syndrome, 65
fragility of in brunescent cataracts, 100-101
loose, 68
in pseudoexfoliation syndrome, 62

For Product Safety Concerns and Information please contact our EU
representative GPSR@taylorandfrancis.com
Taylor & Francis Verlag GmbH, Kaufingerstraße 24, 80331 München, Germany

www.ingramcontent.com/pod-product-compliance
Ingram Content Group UK Ltd.
Pitfield, Milton Keynes, MK11 3LW, UK
UKHW052223190926
475702UK00006B/1180
9781617116070